MODERN PERSPECTIVES IN PSYCHIATRY
Edited by John G. Howells

8

MODERN PERSPECTIVES IN THE PSYCHIATRY OF INFANCY

MODERN PERSPECTIVES IN PSYCHIATRY

Edited by John G. Howells

Modern Perspectives in the Psychiatry of Infancy

Edited by

JOHN G. HOWELLS
M.D., F.R.C.Psych., D.P.M.
Director, the Institute of Family Psychiatry
The Ipswich Hospital
England

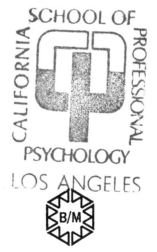

BRUNNER/MAZEL, Publishers ● New York

EDITOR'S PREFACE

Reviewers have been kind to the *Modern Perspectives in Psychiatry* Series. A few, perhaps in a mood of over-optimism, have been inaccurate; they have referred to each volume as a textbook in the field it covers. The volumes do not claim to be textbooks. The aim of the Series, as defined in the first volume, remains the same—to bring the facts from the growing points in the various fields of psychiatry to the attention of the clinician. A complete coverage of each field is not attempted. The emphasis is on the growing points. Each chapter is written by an acknowledged expert in a particular field, who makes his or her expertise available to colleagues in clinical practice who are less acquainted with that field.

This, the eighth volume in the Series, is on *The Psychiatry of Infancy*. Infancy is defined here by its usual meaning of early childhood and, for the purpose of this volume, extends from birth to the age of five. This volume stands, as it were, on the shoulders of its predecessors, and profits thereby, for in almost all the previous volumes there is material relevant to the study of the psychiatry of infancy.

The reader may wish to know that in Volume I, *Modern Perspectives in Child Psychiatry*, there are chapters on The Development of Perception, Piaget's Theory, Disorders of Speech, Adoption, The Aetiology of Mental Subnormality. In Volume III, *Modern Perspectives in International Child Psychiatry*, there are chapters on the Child's Hazards in Utero, The Genesis of Behaviour Disorders, Mother-Infant Relations at Birth, Separation and Deprivation, Culture and Child Rearing, Psychogenic Retardation, Dysfunctions of Parenting. In Volume V, *Modern Perspectives in Psycho-Obstetrics*, there are chapters on Spontaneous Abortion and Miscarriage, Lactation and its Psychological Components, Infanticide, Illegitimacy, and The Psychological Management of Handicapped Children in the First Year of Life. In Volume VII, *Modern Perspectives in the Psychiatric Aspects of Surgery*, there are chapters on Emotional Response to Burns in Children, Psychiatric Aspects of Children Undergoing Surgery, and The Psychological

Care of a Dying Child and his Relatives. The attention of the reader is brought to the cumulative index at the end of Volume V.

The contributors come from Australia, Canada, Czechoslovakia, Denmark, Switzerland, the United Kingdom and the U.S.A. and thus maintain the international outlook of the Series. Indeed, the Series now has an established place as an international reference work—an international encyclopedia of psychiatry.

My work as editor has been made easier by the understanding and eager cooperation of the contributors; rarely has an editor been so well served. The guiding hand of my editorial assistant, Mrs. M. Livia Osborn, has always been at work and she completes this volume also with a major index.

CONTENTS

CLINICAL ISSUES

BASIC THEORY

1

DEVELOPMENT OF THE CHILD'S PERSONALITY IN THE FIRST FIVE YEARS

LEON J. YARROW, Ph.D.

Social and Behavioral Sciences Branch,
National Institute of Child Health and Human Development,
Bethesda, Maryland

Personality is an amorphous concept, one that has been used very loosely. Some years ago Nevitt Sanford (62) observed that even psychologists do not agree about "what the elements of personality are, how they are organized, what the boundaries of personality are, and how personality interacts with other phenomena" (p. 587). The debate still goes on about whether personality is a useful concept and more basically about what it encompasses (52).

Sidestepping the debate, we shall not attempt to define personality, but shall consider the development in young children of a number of characteristics whose varying strengths and patterns contribute to the impression of a unique individual. We shall also note what is known about the origins of individual differences in these characteristics. From the almost endless list of attributes that might be considered components of "personality" we have selected a few that emerge during the first five years of life: the development of a sense of self and feelings and attitudes toward the self, growth in autonomy of functioning and initiative, individualized ways of coping with difficulty and frustration, the development of the child's motivation to have an impact on the environment and to influence other people, the capacity to show concern and empathy for others, the growth in ability to share feelings and material possessions with others. These characteristics are only some of the important attributes of personality that emerge during this earliest period of development.

NORMATIVE DEVELOPMENTAL PATTERNS

We shall first consider the normative patterns of growth during the first five years. Within these normative patterns, there are great individual differences in expression and intensity. These normative stages are important for several reasons. One is that they may index sensitive periods of development, periods in which the particular functions that are emerging may be most sensitive to disruption. It should be clear that these are emerging functions; they do not suddenly appear—their appearance and consolidation extend over a period of many months. These normative patterns emerge as a result of the maturation of the central nervous system and are molded by the experiences of the child. There is a continuous reciprocal interaction. The maturing nervous system allows the child to engage in certain behaviors; in turn, these expressed behaviors influence the behavior of caregivers and other people who interact with the child.

Although the child changes throughout the life cycle, the changes are probably greatest during the first five years. The differences between a neonate and a five-year-old are dramatic. At every stage of development the child elicits a response from others, but the apparent helplessness of the neonate has special influence on the caregiver's behavior. The infant's physical appearance, the shape of the head, the short face, large forehead, protruding cheeks are elicitors of maternal protective behavior. The very young human infant in turn is attuned to the human voice; he attends to and responds to it (19). The sensory and motor systems of parent and infant seem to be sensitively matched from the beginning.

Children differ from the moment of birth. Constitutional or temperamental differences have been distinguished on a variety of dimensions. Differences exist in general sensitivity to stimulation as well as differential sensitivity in particular modalities, i.e., in differing thresholds for visual, auditory or tactile stimuli. Infants also differ in activity level and vigor of responsiveness to stimulation; in how quickly they become habituated to stimuli, in responsiveness and adaptability; in irritability and ease of being soothed, in capacity to direct and maintain focus on an object or person; in the ease or difficulty with which their attention can be distracted. There are also individual differences in regularity of functioning, in the day-to-day predictability of patterns of rest and activity, in orientation and responsiveness to people and to objects.

Individual differences have been noted as early as the newborn period; they have been observed by impartial observers (12, 61), and reported by parents (17, 69). We assume that these early patterns of individuality have a significant influence on personality development, but the relationships are not simple or direct. Although we would like to think of these early temperamental characteristics as precursors of later personality characteristics, the links, if there are any, are extremely complex. Few investigators have found consistencies between early dimensions of infant functioning and later characteristics, nor have any easy rules of dynamic transformation been established. Aside from the question of continuity, one way in which these initial differences in children may influence personality development is through their impact on parents and caregivers. Caregivers may tailor their behavior to their perceptions of infant characteristics. They are likely to initiate different behaviors and respond differently towards an infant they see as predominantly irritable than to one they see as predominantly happy and easygoing; they are likely to interact more with an infant who is socially responsive than with one who gives little response in return. This reciprocal interaction increases the likelihood of these characteristics being reinforced and consolidated.

From birth to the end of the second month, much of the infant's time is spent sleeping, thus limiting the amount of time available for response to stimulation. There are individual differences in patterns of sleep, as well as in the amount of time the infant is awake. Whereas we once thought the neonate was insensitive to most stimuli, recent research has shown that neonates are responsive to a variety of tactile, kinesthetic, auditory and visual stimuli. There are individual differences in intensity and quality of responsiveness to all kinds of stimulation (37).

Between the second and third month there are significant changes in visual accommodation, orienting and habituation (22). The infant attends to objects for increasingly longer periods of time; after sustained attention he adapts to stimuli and gives increasing attention to new stimuli. Towards the end of the second month the infant's longer periods of wakefulness are accompanied by increased social interaction with caregivers. Both a decrease in fussiness and signs of positive social responsiveness occur. The infant engages in mutual regard and eye-to-eye contact with caregivers; his positive affect, expressed through smiling, is also directed towards caregivers, as distinguished from earlier smiles which appear to be undirected. Vigorous smiling to a human face shows a rapid increase during the second and third month of life.

By the end of the second month there is a striking change in the modifiability of the infant's behavior. Although some neonatal behaviors can be conditioned to specific stimuli, Papousek (59), comparing newborns and three-month-olds, found much more rapid conditioning after three months.

After the third month of life, the infant indicates in many ways his receptivity and eagerness for stimulation. The infant not only gives visual attention to the environment, but he also engages in tactile exploration of inanimate objects and attempts to manipulate them. He is also becoming aware of his own body and beginning to differentiate himself from his environment. It is during this developmental period that the infant begins to form a focused relationship with parents and familiar caregivers. This period is also one of increasing autonomy and self-assertion. The infant shows increasingly complex vocalizations which are directed towards people.

During the second half of the first year, infants become aware of being dependent on the mother; they distinguish their mother from other persons and often become anxious in the presence of a stranger. They may become very disturbed if separated from the mother even for a short period of time. For a long time it was assumed that if infants were separated from their mothers permanently or for long intervals during this developmental stage, there would be permanent damage to their capacity to form and establish significant relationships (10). Subsequently, it has been found that children who are separated from their parents but reunited with them within a reasonable period of time are not necessarily irreparably damaged. They do not become affectionless psychopaths who are unable to establish meaningful relationships with anyone. The clinical observations and research on which the conclusions of severe damage were based are derived mainly from studies of children who had persisting or repetitive disruptions in relationships (74).

The Emergence of a Self-Concept and the Development of Focused Relationships

Among the significant developments during the first year are the emergence of a rudimentary self-concept and the development of focused relationships with the parents. As we have pointed out elsewhere (75, 78), the development of focused relationships is part of a chain of social and cognitive developmental changes which extends across a wide age span. It does not appear suddenly, but is a gradual process involving a number of steps.

Early in infancy the child does not differentiate himself from his environment; the boundaries between the inner and outer world are not sharp; a clear sense of self has not emerged. The differentiation of the self from the external environment is a first step in the development of the infant's responsiveness to people. Inasmuch as there are no definitive normative data, we can only speculate about the sequence of this developmental milestone. We can assume that one of the earliest steps is the development of the capacity to distinguish between internal and external sources of stimulation. It is likely that this capacity is influenced by maturation as well as by experiences in being handled by caregivers. Feelings of gratification attendant on tactile and kinesthetic stimulation as well as feelings of hunger, cold and discomfort all undoubtedly contribute to an infant's awareness of her own body and thus to the awareness of boundaries between the self and the external environment. Mahler, Pine and Bergman (49), in discussing the separation-individuation process, see the child's emergence from a symbiotic fusion with the mother as a step in the development of autonomy. Probably the differentiation of self from the external environment is also associated with the developing recognition by the infant that she can have some impact on the environment. When the young child cries or vocalizes, if mother approaches and speaks, picks her up or tries to alleviate distress, the infant begins to associate her own actions with changes in the environment. The differentiation of self from the environment also involves perceptual and cognitive processes; the separation of self from non-self requires a separation of figure from ground. When the infant attains a definite concept of self is not completely clear; it depends on the criteria used as indices. For instance, Lewis and Brooks (44) report that, by nine months, the infant has attained a rudimentary concept of self.

Coincident with the infant's defining the boundaries of the self is the development of awareness of dependence on the external world. The child becomes aware that changes in internal states are associated with the behavior of other people. At this point these changes may not be associated with any specific person; the infant may not yet recognize the mother or have any specific affect associated with her. This differentiation of self from the environment emphasizes the interdependence of cognitive and personality development.

Very early in life the infant begins to respond selectively to familiar and unfamiliar people. We can distinguish two levels of selective responsiveness: passive and active. First, the infant shows differences in visual attention to mother and stranger, orienting to mother and maintaining a longer fixation time on her. When the infant advances to the stage of active responsiveness to the familiar caregiver, he shows more overt preferential behavior, such as making approach movements, smiling and vocalizing towards her (75, 78).

For the infant to be able to respond differentially to the mother, to show selective responsiveness to mother and strangers, he or she must be able to make complex perceptual-sensory discriminations. In recent years, studies have shown that very young infants are capable of making such discriminations much earlier than had been previously assumed (26, 27).

After the infant shows the capacity to discriminate mother from strangers, the next step in the development of focused relationships is the development of specific expectations towards the mother, an event of great psychological significance. When an infant is approached by the mother, he or she may make postural adjustments indicating an expectation of being picked up. When in distress, the infant may stop crying when mother appears. The young child soon acquires a repertoire of responses—cooing, smiling, reaching out to mother accompanied by the expectation that she will respond. This stage is logically followed by the development of trust. The infant is now able to wait for the mother to respond, secure in the expectation that she will meet her needs by providing food, changing diapers or engaging in play. This "confidence relationship" (6) is dependent on a number of cognitive attainments, among which is the acquisition of object and person permanence, i.e., the concept that objects and persons exist outside of the immediate perceptual field. It is also dependent on the development of a differentiated schema of the mother and the development of a rudimentary memory.

Again, we need to recognize that there are great individual variations in the age at which these levels of focused relationships appear, as well as in the behaviors associated with them. There are varying degrees of trust, ranging from the expectation that the mother will respond in ways that are gratifying, to the expectation that she will give an inappropriate, harsh or restrictive response, or to uncertainty about how she will respond. These differing degrees of confidence may be generalized to other people in the immediate environment and may color the child's continuing relationship with parents and other people.

Between seven and 12 months a most important development is the marked increase in wariness to strangers. This wariness is probably a reflection of a number of cognitive attainments. It is a clear indication that the infant is able to discriminate between stranger and familiar caregiver. Wariness may also be a sign that the infant has developed specific expectations towards familiar people, and the appearance of a person who does not fulfill these expectations may be jarring and anxiety-evoking. If the infant has a stable caregiver who is relatively consistent in her behavior, she is more likely to develop confidence and the feeling that the world is predictable. If, on the other hand, she has changing caregivers or the behavior of her mother shows marked inconsistency, she is likely to see the world as unpredictable. This is also a period when the infant spends a good bit of time learning about the environment through exploratory behavior. If she is not securely attached to her mother, it is thought that she may be less free to engage in exploration. This restriction in exploratory behavior may retard not only cognitive development, but also the beginnings of a sense of mastery.

The Development of Autonomy and Mastery

From 12 to 18 months the infant is acquiring increasing control of the environment. She is acquiring the capacity to move on her own through space and her fine motor coordinations are improving, thus enabling her to obtain objects through her own power; these advances in both fine and gross motor coordination allow greater freedom to explore the environment, to find out how objects work and the various consequences of manipulating them. She is also acquiring language and is able to communicate her needs to others, to engage them in reciprocal interactions and to directly affect their behavior. Children's increased responsiveness to others is demonstrated in a variety of ways. At this time they begin to share with others; they show, call attention to or give objects to parents and siblings. By two years, children express in words their awareness of self as distinguished from others; they use the word "mine" to refer to objects that belong to them. The acquisition of language also marks the beginning of the use of symbols; the young children are able to substitute symbols for concrete objects. In play they show signs of beginning to conceptualize and are able to use objects symbolically.

Between 18 months and three years, the motor and perceptual-motor coordinations that were beginning at 12 months are being elaborated and consolidated. The child's feeling of control over the environment is being strengthened as she becomes increasingly adept in activities involving fine motor skills. Her sense of autonomy is also being consolidated as she becomes capable of moving on her own through larger segments of the home environment. Her comprehension of language is growing and her expressive vocabulary is increasing. She is using new language skills to control the behavior of caregivers, to express her wishes and to elicit and maintain social interaction. This is a period of intense socialization training when she is becoming aware of the rules of society. Toilet training is one of many ways by which the infant is taught to conform.

These pressures, coupled with the consolidation of the sense of self, may lead her to resist adult demands. It is a time of ambivalence about conformity; she is both negativistic and conforming. The development of a positive self-concept and feelings of efficacy are associated not only with her growing skills, but with a contingent environment. If caregivers are responsive to her signals and if she is given experiences with objects that are responsive, the infant can make direct associations between her behavior and response from the environment and is likely to develop a sense of competence. We are not yet at all clear about the course of development of the infant's recognition that she can have effects. By two months infants have been observed to work on problems almost to the point of exhaustion, and they seem to develop an intrinsic motivation to do so, that is, their efforts become independent of hunger or nutritional rewards (60). By three years the child's sense of competence has become an extremely significant aspect of her personality. She is also becoming increasingly social, not only sharing treasured possessions with others, but showing sympathy as well. Although her response to other children's distress may often be quite inappropriate, she is showing awareness of feelings other than her own (56). We are just beginning to obtain data on the developmental course of the child's empathic responses (8, 31).

Between three and six years the child's environment broadens considerably. Increasingly she becomes more independent of her mother and engages in much more social interaction with her father, siblings and peers. Young infants form significant relationships with fathers and siblings and they influence the infant's behavior very early, but in our culture the mother is still usually the primary caregiver. Gradually replacing exclusive concern about the parent's attention and approval, the child begins to internalize the norms and values of the larger society and culture and begins to adapt her behavior to these requirements. Children learn to modify, inhibit or delay behaviors rather than demand immediate gratification. Individual children may, of course, interpret these norms and values idiosyncratically. This is a time when the self-concept is becoming differentiated; boys and girls learn their gender identity (53) and show the behaviors considered sex-appropriate. The child identifies with the parent of the same sex and tries to take on his or her standards and emulate the like-sexed parent's behavior. Children are acquiring their own idiosyncratic likes and dislikes and are asserting their own desires and preferences. Boys and girls become sensitive to others' evaluations of them and to approval and disapproval from others. Their play becomes increasingly cooperative and they are willing to take on roles defined by the group, subordinating, to some extent, their own desires for the goals of the group. Competitiveness, as well as cooperation, begins to emerge during this developmental period.

The developmental characteristics we have described from birth to the end of the preschool years parallel the first three stages of personality development—trust, autonomy, and initiative—described by Erikson (24). For most of the early developmental changes described, it is difficult to sharply distinguish cognitive from personality characteristics; they are highly interdependent at least for the first year of life. Within these general patterns of personality development there are great individual differences from the moment of birth. In the next section we shall consider what is known about the determinants of these differences.

THE IMPACT OF THE EARLY ENVIRONMENT

The significance of the early environment for later development has been a recurrent theme throughout the history of mankind and a focus of controversy throughout the history of psychology. In emphasizing the importance of the early years of life, Freud stimulated behavioral scientists and psychiatrists to look at the environment and behavior of the infant in fine detail. The findings of this research have not given clear support to the view that early experiences are decisive for later development; they have, however, led to significant reformulations and reconceptualizations which have advanced our understanding of the impact of the early environment on development. There is increasing recognition that the extent to which early experiences influence development is an exceedingly complex question that belies simple answers.

The research on early experience is diverse in methodology and varied in the categories of experience and the personality dimensions with which it has been concerned. For a long time, early experience was studied solely by retrospective reconstruction of disturbed adults. Later, there was a concentration on prospective studies using parental interview. More recently, we have moved from interview to direct observation in contrived situations in the laboratory and, finally, we have come to direct observations of parent and infant in the natural situation, the home.

The question of whether early experiences have effects has many ramifications. There are many different levels on which we have conceptualized the early environment. At the one extreme, we have analyzed the environment into very simple elements; at the other, we have dealt with experience in terms of very broad and exceedingly complex parameters. Allied to the issue of conceptualization is the question of how to measure experience. Some studies have used simply the frequency of discrete events; others, the intensity of these events; still others have described qualitative variations among events.

An entirely different issue is the question of the relation between immediate and long-term effects. If environmental events influence contemporaneous functioning, do they necessarily have long-term impact? If an infant is sensitive to environmental events and these experiences affect his immediate behavior, what are the conditions under which these behaviors persist and under what conditions are they predictive of later functioning? An allied but not identical question is whether behaviors associated with early experiences are reversible.

In studying the effects of early experience we have not until recently given systematic consideration to the environment. We have not analyzed the kinds and levels of stimulation and human interactions to which the child is sensitive and responsive. Until recently, most studies have used global caregiver behaviors, such as, warmth, hostility, acceptance, rejection; they have not analyzed the environment into its components. These global characteristics have been inferred from a great number of behaviors without precise definition of the bases for these broad inferences. Just as in nutrition we have begun to define specific elements required for physical growth and have discovered relationships between lacks in specific nutritive substances and specific deviations or retardation in growth, so it would seem desirable to define more precisely the elements of early experience, for example, to distinguish the amount and intensity of tactile, kinesthetic, auditory and visual stimulation and the relative balance between parent-initiated stimulation and contingent stimulation (in response to the child). It is questionable whether the frequency of occurrence of these stimuli is a meaningful index of their importance to the child. Obviously, the number of times a parent touches a child or speaks to her or picks her up cannot be a simple index of the relationship (80). Having reduced experience to a level on which independent observers can agree in describing a given setting, then we must reconstruct the patterns of which these elements are a part and try to understand their meaning or psychological significance to the young child. Although we have been dimly aware that stimuli must register to have effects and we recognize that there are individual differences in response to stimuli, we have largely ignored the affective environment. We have not designed studies to take into consideration the fact that the impact of any experience is mediated through individual and developmental differences in sensitivities.

Infant Receptivity to Environmental Events

The belief that the young organism is most sensitive and most vulnerable to environmental events during the early months of life and that the effects of early experience are irreversible needs to be examined critically. Sensitivity has several meanings. One is the capacity to make fine discriminations of quantitative or qualitative variations in stimuli. Another meaning of sensitivity is a lowered threshold of responsiveness to stimuli; still another is a vulnerability to trauma, i. e., an increased susceptibility to damage by noxious stimulation.

Research in recent years has documented the receptivity of neonates to various kinds of sensory stimulation. Neonates respond differentially to sounds of various pitches and loudness (29); they respond to variations in visual (26, 27), olfactory (23), and tactile stimuli (73). As infants develop, they become capable of making increasingly fine discriminations and of processing increasingly complex information (37). Evidence that the young infant is capable of responding to all kinds of sensory stimuli and that his behavior can be modified by these stimuli can be taken as indirect confirmation of the impact of the early environment. There is also considerable clinical evidence that extreme trauma or deprivation can lead to disturbed, withdrawn behavior in infants and is frequently associated with deviant behavior during the preschool years. We cannot, however, extrapolate from these findings to the long-term impact of essentially normal variations in experiences during the early years of life. We do not know how these experiential variations are associated with the nuances in personality that make each individual distinctive. The research is limited and the findings are not consistent.

Interview Studies of the Early Environment

Interview studies of the early environment have concentrated on a small number of broad environmental variables and a limited number of personality attributes. Parents have been interviewed about such global dimensions of child-rearing as restrictiveness-permissiveness and warmth-hostility. The personality variables most often studied have been dependency-autonomy, aggression, achievement and mastery (16).

On the whole, the results of these earlier studies are divergent; they do not add up to clear conclusions. There is some consistency in the findings that parental hostility tends to be associated with problems in the child's adaptation and that parental warmth tends to facilitate good adjustment. There are many methodological problems in these studies (80, 85). One source of contamination is that the data are often based on parental report of their own behavior, and the data on the children are derived from parental evaluation of their offspring. It is likely that the parent who reports feelings of warmth towards the child may evaluate the child's behavior positively, whereas parents who report hostile feelings are more likely to see their children's behavior in an unfavorable light.

The simplistic formulations that tied personality attributes, such as dependency, autonomy, orderliness, obstinacy and optimism, to harshness in weaning or toilet training stimulated much research in the 1930s and early 1940s. On the whole, the findings of these interview studies do not provide much support for these simple formulations; some studies find significant relationships, but many more report no meaningful relationships. It seems clear that the extent to which these parental practices are related to the child's functioning depends on whether they are indices of larger patterns of parental feelings and behavior towards the child, for instance, whether harsh toilet training is a marker of harshness in other areas of relationship between parent and child.

Observational Studies of the Early Environment

Increasingly in recent years parental report has been supplemented or replaced by direct observation in the laboratory and in the home. These observational studies have found significant relations between a number of aspects of the observed environment and the infant's contemporaneous functioning (5, 13, 18, 21, 25, 32, 40, 44, 54, 55, 65, 81). Although the parental and child behaviors in these observational studies have generally been more precisely defined and the environmental characteristics and child characteristics have been evaluated independently, nevertheless, the categories of behaviors examined in many of these studies have been limited, and the psychological meaning of these categories has often been obscure.

The young child's capacity to become involved in exploration of objects, his preference for novel objects, persistence in working on difficult tasks and in eliciting feedback from objects have been studied by investigators with different theoretical orientations. There are some findings linking these attributes in young infants to a number of environmental variables: the amount of kinesthetic stimulation, the responsiveness of the mother to the child's signals, the variety of objects available to the infant and the responsiveness of these objects (14, 28, 39, 42, 70, 76, 81). Intervention attempts with apathetic and withdrawn infants have also found increased responsiveness associated with kinesthetic stimulation and the caregiver's contingent responsiveness (15, 71). It appears that the infant's natural curiosity is strengthened and his motivation and capacity to assimilate new information are influenced by his opportunities to see and handle a wide range of responsive objects. Yarrow, Rubenstein and Pedersen (81) interpret the findings on contingent responsiveness as indicating: "response to an infant's cries does more than reinforce crying. It reinforces active coping with the environment, reaching out to obtain feedback from people and objects. Moreover, in time, an infant whose mother is responsive to his distress may come to feel that through his own actions he can have an effect on other people and his environment" (p. 86). Similar interpretations of the role of contingent responsiveness have been made by Watson (70), Bronson (14), Lewis and Goldberg (44). In a study of mastery motivation these same variables were found to be related to the infant's attempts to master emergent skills, to his persistence in working on difficult problems and persistent attempts to secure feedback from objects (84).

Most observational studies of the early environment have been concerned with cognitive development; few have studied early experience and personality functions. Moreover, the aspects of personality development explored in these studies have been very limited, and the bases for the choice of the functions studied have not often been clear. The diverse characteristics that have been investigated and the little overlap between studies contribute to the difficulty in drawing any general conclusions from this research.

Long-term Effects of Early Experience

In spite of the firmness of the conviction of a relationship between early experience and later functioning, there are relatively few long-term studies that have followed children from early infancy to adolescence or adulthood. Although many studies of children who were subjected to severe deprivation during infancy find severe disturbances at later ages (1, 9, 10, 74), increasingly there are reports of children who were institutionalized in infancy and then moved to more adequate environments who do not show any obvious scars from the earlier trauma and deprivations; they appear to be functioning competently in later life (20, 46, 67). There have also been successful attempts to undo earlier deprivations in animals (68). A recent study documents the severe retardation, depression and withdrawn behavior of infants in Guatemala who during the first year of life are given minimal stimulation. This experiential pattern is changed during the second year when these children are given much more varied stimulation. Although these children continue to show retardation on tests of memory and reasoning until around 11 years of age, by adolescence their cognitive functioning is appropriate for their age (35). It appears that a pattern of continuing deprivation or trauma throughout childhood may be necessary for permanent damage.

Several reports from the Fels longitudinal study on normal children report moderate relations between personality characteristics and the early environment. Baldwin, Kalhorn and Breese (3) found that preschool children from democratic and from authoritarian homes differed in important aspects of personality. The democratic homes were characterized by general permissiveness, avoidance of arbitrary decisions, involvement of children in family decisions and explanations of reasons for family rules. Authoritarian homes, on the other hand, were characterized by arbitrary and rigid rules, authoritarian parental attitudes and many restrictions. The children from democratic homes were outgoing, aggressive, high in curiosity, independent and non-conforming, whereas children from homes rated high in control were quiet, conforming, socially non-aggressive, relatively restricted in curiosity and originality.

Kagan and Moss (36), in a later report from the Fels study, concluded that there were few maternal behaviors that were predictive of later personality. Basically, they analyzed four maternal variables: *maternal protectiveness*, the degree to which the mother rewarded dependent overtures; *maternal restrictiveness*, the extent to which the mother attempted to force the child to adhere to her standards; *maternal hostility*, a variable reflecting the mother's dissatisfaction and active rejection of the child; and *maternal acceleration*, the degree to which the mother pushed the child to achieve beyond his abilities. Protectiveness and maternal acceleration were significantly associated with independence in boys. Although there were a few significant relationships between maternal behavior and the personality variables studied, on the whole, maternal behavior was not highly predictive of either emotional or instrumental dependency or of passivity. There were no consistent relations between ratings of maternal hostility during the first three years and the child's aggressive behavior or anger arousal; nor were there any relations between maternal-overprotection and adult dependency or withdrawal in the face of stress.

In another study (4), nursery school children who were rated by their teachers and trained observers as showing such positive characteristics as maturity, competence, self-reliance, self-control, and self-assertion were found to have parents who were highly consistent, warm, loving, conscientious and secure in their interactions. The nursery school children who were most immature, highly dependent, who lacked self-reliance and self-control, and who withdrew from novel experiences had parents who, although warm and nurturant, made relatively few demands, were overprotective and at the same time lax in discipline, and did not reward their children's attempts at self-reliant, independent behavior.

Some studies find stronger relationships between the early environment and later functioning than between the environment and contemporaneous functioning. Bradley and Caldwell (11), for example, found that the six-month home environment was more highly related to development at 54 months than at either six or 12 months. Three types of environmental stimulation were especially important: emotional and verbal responsivity of the mother, maternal involvement with the child, and provision of appropriate play materials. They conclude that: "Mothers who interact frequently with their children and who are responsive to their emotional needs may develop in their children a sense of trust and enjoyment in the environment. The sense of trust and enjoyment may allow children to behave in accordance with motives for competency and curiosity thus facilitating cognitive growth" (p. 1174).

Yarrow, Goodwin, Manheimer and Milowe (82) found some relationships between maternal care in infancy and personal-social functioning at 10 years of age. The mother's responsiveness to the child's communications, her warmth and expression of positive feelings, her sensitivity to the infant's special characteristics, likes, dislikes and vulnerabilities, and the extent to which she adapted her behavior to this awareness were significantly associated with the child's capacity to relate with closeness and discrimination to parents, siblings and peers. These maternal characteristics were also related to social effectiveness, a measure of the degree to which the child contributes constructively in social interactions with others, and to dominance, the child's capacity to express his own ideas and wishes in attempting to influence others. These relationships, however, were significant only for boys; there were no significant relationships for girls.

In recent years interest in prosocial behavior has stimulated research on young children's sharing, showing concern for and helping others. Although there are almost no definitive findings, there are indications that these behaviors are fostered by a warm relationship with caregivers who provide models for the child to imitate. These behaviors are also significantly affected by the child's level of cognitive development, especially his ability to empathize with the feelings of others and to take the other person's perspective (58).

Analysis of environment-personality relationships by sex has suggested that mothers and fathers handle boys and girls differently and the relations between experiences and later functioning may differ for boys and girls (7, 47). These findings introduce still another complication in interpreting the role of early experiences on development. They indicate that both biological and cultural contexts of experiences must be considered.

On the whole, the findings of the longitudinal studies of normal children do not permit any simple conclusions; they emphasize again the complexity of the determinants of personality. There is increasing recognition that the significance of any environmental event depends on its meaning for the child. Meaning is partly determined by the child's sensitivities and his previous experiences with similar events. The concept of the psychological environment is an old one (43), but few studies of early experience have given adequate attention to the child's perception of events in obtaining, analyzing or interpreting the data.

Continuity in Personality Characteristics

The long-term impact of early experience is intimately tied to questions of continuity in personality characteristics and the reversibility of behavior patterns laid down during infancy. Until recently, personality theory has been dominated by the conception of traits, a view which assumes enduring personality predispositions. As longitudinal studies began to find little consistency over time in personality characteristics, there has been a tendency to discard the concept of traits in favor of the view that behaviors indexing personality are completely controlled by situational events (34, 51).

There have been many studies of consistency of personality and cognitive characteristics. Some are investigations of simple consistency in behavior patterns across situations; others are concerned with continuity across time. On the whole, correlations across situations tend to be higher for cognitive and intellectual characteristics than for dimensions of personality. On a variety of personality characteristics, there seems to be little consistency across situations and over time; there is, however, some continuity in broad personality styles.

Murphy (55, 57) found *some* persistence from infancy to the preschool years in *some* children in *certain* basic coping patterns such as withdrawal, protest, flexibility, contentment, exuberance, smooth growth patterns as contrasted with irregular growth patterns, and in aspects of cognitive style such as tendencies towards delay, differentiated perception and complexity of integrative style. She recognizes that all of these patterns of coping are subject to modification through interaction with the environment, but feels that they are not so likely to change as are affective characteristics such as shyness, affectionateness, anger and destructiveness, or characteristics related closely to interpersonal experience such as dominance, leadership, competitiveness, generosity and nurturance.

MacFarlane (48), in reviewing individual case histories, notes both continuity and dramatic changes. She concludes that what we find with regard to continuity may depend on the level of variables with which we are concerned, the ages at which the measures are taken and the span between the points at which continuity is measured. She suggests that behaviors referring to how one copes with a specific situation are less likely to be consistent across developmental stages than broad inferential concepts reflecting personality style. She also points out that "behavior-personality measures are more subject to variability in times of biological or situational stress and change." Thus, measures made during infancy when the organism is in a relatively unstable equilibrium may show less consistency than measures in middle childhood. Similarly, there is likely to be less continuity between the neonatal period and six months than between four and five years.

Kagan and Moss (36) report very few relationships between behavioral characteristics during the first three years and personality characteristics in adulthood. The only significant association was between passivity in infancy and dependency in adult life for males. Practically no relationships were found with adult behavior before the child was six years old. For many variables there were distinct sex differences in continuity. In a later study, Kagan (34) found even less continuity between four and 27 months. For instance, neither activity level nor irritability showed any stability. On the basis of these findings and the results of other studies he (33) concludes, "The data offer no firm support for the popular belief that certain events during the first year can produce irreversible consequences in either human or infrahuman infants."

We know that adults see themselves in terms of certain predominant dimensions that remain relatively stable over time (50) but we do not know at what age the child begins to see himself in relatively stable terms. Parents and others who follow the course of a child's development from infancy to adulthood also see a core of similarity that stands out within the many developmental changes that occur. It is difficult to know whether these perceived similarities are objectively "true" or whether these impressions of continuity are based primarily on a *need* for constancy. It may be cognitively more satisfying to see continuity than to attempt to reconcile perceptions of change with our deep-rooted conviction of the stability of a person.

Implicit, but not often stated, in predictive statements about personality continuity is that there is a greater likelihood of consistency in personality if there is environmental consistency. Although the data are limited, they indicate that we cannot make any simple assumptions about environmental consistency. For instance, Schaefer and Bayley (63) report maternal behavior on the love-hostility dimension to be quite consistent over time. On the whole, they found some aspects of maternal behavior to be more stable than others; however, they found differing degrees of stability in parental behaviors towards boys and girls. Other research suggests that there may be systematic changes in parental attitudes and behavior at different developmental periods in children's and parents' lives (2, 41). Baldwin found that parents of nine-year-olds were less warm, less indulgent and more restrictive than parents of three-year-olds. He also found significant changes in maternal behavior during pregnancy. Pregnant mothers were more understanding and less directive with their children than they had been before becoming pregnant. After the birth of a child, mothers showed less warmth and became more restrictive and severe in their discipline toward their older children. Studies of other cultures report sharp discontinuities in some cultures between infancy and later childhood (35, 72).

In discussing the problem of personality continuity previously (77), I noted that we recognize that individuals change throughout their life history. Therefore, it is necessary to consider the child's changing capacities, changing relationship to the environment and changing roles at different developmental periods. I suggested, "In attempting to deal with the question of how the same characteristic may be expressed at different developmental periods, it is useful to distinguish between two concepts of consistency—a phenotypic concept and a dynamic concept. The assumption of an isomorphic identity in traits or behavior patterns throughout the developmental cycle—phenotypic continuity—is not meaningful. The concept of dynamic continuity seems to be more tenable. Changes in overt characteristics are seen as developmental transformations, which can be dynamically related to earlier personality patterns" (p.68).

Related to the issue of dynamic and phenotypic continuity is the question of the level at which we conceptualize personality, whether we deal with highly abstract integrative concepts or specific concrete behaviors. Our conclusions about continuity of personality may differ if we are referring to physiological-psychological characteristics, such as activity level, whether we are concerned with characteristics such as dominance, shyness, or empathy which are defined in relation to other people, whether we are concerned with structural aspects of personality and broader aspects of functioning, such as personality style. Some of these characteristics will vary more with situational influences; in fact, they may be largely subject to situational factors. Other aspects of personality may be influenced by repeated or continuous environmental reinforcement; still others may be relatively immune to situational or environmental influences.

We know that the child's response to the same stimulus will vary at different times. It will be influenced by his immediate state, by the situational context, how immediately preceding events influence his perceptions of a specific stimulus event. It is also likely that there are great individual differences in consistency of behavior across situations. The changing behaviors of an individual may be predictable if we are able to take into account all the mediating variables or if we understand the dynamic links.

CONCLUSIONS

In contrast to earlier views of personality development which held that the structures and patterns of functioning were laid down at least by five years of age, we are coming to recognize a much longer period of personality formation. There is a growing acceptance of the view that changes in adaptive modes and defenses continue through the life cycle. The rate of change may be greatest during the first five years, but personality changes probably go on constantly as long as physical, structural and physiological changes occur, and as long as the person is sensitive or vulnerable.

The organism is constantly changing and evolving throughout the life cycle. The changes are probably most dramatic during the first five years of life. Although we now know that the young infant is capable of manipulating and responding to large number of stimuli, he/she is still essentially a helpless being, dependent on parents for both physical and emotional nurturance. The child changes from an essentially dependent being to one who is increasingly capable of initiating behaviors and eliciting response from others, who enjoys exploring objects in the environment and mastering them, one who derives pleasure from solving problems and meeting challenging tasks. She/he changes from an organism in an essentially symbiotic relationship with its caretaker to a being who distinguishes its own needs from others and who has a defined self-concept. The infant also changes from an essentially egocentric being to a person who is sensitive to nuances of feelings of others, from a concern with primarily gratifying its own needs to an interest in sharing with others and to some extent responding to their needs. The child becomes capable of expressing a wide range of feelings, not only joy and sorrow, but also affection, sympathy and hostility. Because the young child is an immature organism, it is probably most vulnerable during this period of life; it can be easily hurt by inadequate nurturance or traumatic events. Whether this damage is reversible, however, depends on many factors.

More than 30 years ago, Hartmann, Kris and Lowenstein (30) pointed out that personality development does not stop at the end of the preschool years: "we feel that the potentialities for its transformation throughout latency and adolescence have for some time been underrated in psychoanalytic writings. But it seems that the basic structure of the personality and the basic functional interactions of the systems have been fixed to some extent. The child does not stop growing and developing, but after that age, both growth and development modify existing structure" (p. 34).

The belief that experiences in early infancy have a significant impact on later development is based largely on reconstructions of the early life histories of disturbed—neurotic and psychotic—individuals. Data were obtained mainly by interview in a treatment setting, a setting in which a basic assumption was that the roots of disturbance resided in early traumatic experiences. We seem to know much more about the origins of disruptive personality patterns and the development of severe disturbances than about the origins of strengths and healthy patterns of adjustment. We know relatively little about the factors associated with the development of capacities to master the environment and cope effectively with stress and frustration.

Until quite recently there were no prospective longitudinal data on normal individuals. The data on personality development are still sparse; there are much more data on cognitive development. The longitudinal studies, on the whole, have failed to establish clear-cut relationships between specific dimensions of early experience and personality characteristics in childhood or adulthood. Some studies do find small positive relationships with some childhood events, but more often the findings are equivocal. If one tallies the conclusive and inconclusive findings, the balance is in favor of the inconclusive. The significance of the negative and equivocal findings has been interpreted in many ways, depending on the interpreter's theoretical biases. Often, the results of this research have been interpreted as disproof of psychodynamic hypotheses regarding the importance of early experiences for personality development. Others have questioned the meaningfulness of the data obtained from this research, pointing out that only surface characteristics have been studied.

The research does not offer strong support for the belief that early experience is decisive and its effects are irreversible. A single event is unlikely to have long-term effects, but it may set in motion a chain of interactions with far-reaching consequences. There is evidence that continuing or recurrent traumatic or depriving experiences have cumulative effects. There is also evidence that children who had experienced trauma or deprivation in infancy, but who were later exposed to more beneficent influences, do not show gross disturbances later in life. As I have noted elsewhere (79):

"It is likely that experiences early in life affect the young, vulnerable organism and these effects may be pervasive and long-term, but not in the simple sense that the organism is unalterably damaged by a single event. Rather there may be a series of interactions, certain experiences predisposing the organism to respond in ways that elicit reinforcing responses. Thus, some events may set in train a cyclical pattern of adverse interactions" (p.901). Other events may mitigate or reverse the distorting influences.

The construct of personality is difficult to defend on an empirical basis, yet it is equally difficult to discard. We perceive ourselves and others as possessing a stable core of characteristics that transcend situations. At the same time, we are aware that dramatic changes take place in the first five years and more gradual changes in adaptive modes and defenses continue throughout the life cycle. The basic dilemma is to conceptualize change within continuity.

REFERENCES

1. AINSWORTH, M. D. 1962. The effects of maternal deprivation: A review of the findings and controversy in the context of research strategy. In *Deprivation of Maternal Care: A Reassessment of its Effects*. Public Health Papers No. 14, Geneva: WHO.
2. BALDWIN, A. L. 1947. Changes in parent behavior during pregnancy: An experiment in longitudinal analysis. *Child Development*, 18, 29.
3. BALDWIN, A. L., KALHORN, J., and BREESE, F. 1945. Patterns of parent behavior. *Psychological Monographs*, 58.
4. BAUMRIND, D. 1971. Current patterns of parental authority. *Developmental Psychology Monographs*, 1, 1.
5. BECKWITH, L. 1972. Relationship between infants' social behavior and their mothers' behaviors. *Child Development*, 43, 397.
6. BENEDEK, T. 1938. Adaptation to reality in early infancy. *Psychoanalytic Quarterly*, 7, 200.
7. BLOCK, J. In Press. Another look at sex differentiation in the socialization behaviors of mothers and fathers. *Psychology of Women: Future Directions of Research*. New York: Psychological Dimensions, Inc.
8. BORKE, H. 1973. The development of empathy in Chinese and American children between three and six years of age. *Developmental Psychology*, 9, 102.
9. BOWLBY, J. 1969. *Attachment*. New York: Basic Books.
10. BOWLBY, J. 1951. *Maternal Care and Mental Health*. Geneva: World Health Organization.
11. BRADLEY, R. M., and CALDWELL, B. M. 1976. Early home environment and changes in mental test performance in children from 6 to 36 months. *Developmental Psychology*, 12, 93.
12. BRAZELTON, T. B. 1973. *Neonatal Behavioral Assessment Scale*. Philadelphia: J. B. Lippincott Co.
13. BRODY, S. 1956. *Patterns of Mothering: Maternal Influences during Infancy*. New York: International Universities Press.
14. BRONSON, W. C. 1971. The growth of competence: Issues of conceptualization and measurement. In: H. R. Schaffer, (Ed.), *The Origins of Human Social Relations*. New York: Academic Press.
15. BROSSARD, L. M., and DÉCARIE, T. G. 1968. Comparative reinforcing effect of eight stim-

ulations on the smiling response of infants. *Journal of Child Psychology and Psychiatry, 9,* 51.

16. CALDWELL, B. M. 1964. The effects of infant care. In: Hoffman, M. L. and Hoffman, L. W. (Eds.), *Review of Child Development Research, 1.* New York: Russell Sage Foundation.

17. CAREY, W. B. 1970. A simplified method of measuring infant temperament. *Journal of Pediatrics, 77,* 188.

18. CLARKE-STEWART, K. 1973. Interactions between mothers and their young children: Characteristics and consequences. *Monographs of the Society for Research in Child Development 38,* (Serial Number 153).

19. CONDON, W. S. and SANDER, L. W. 1974. Neonate movement is synchronized with adult speech: Interactional participation and language acquisition. *Science, 183,* 99.

20. DENNIS, W. 1973. *Children of the Creche.* New York: Appleton-Century-Crofts.

21. ELARDO, R., BRADLEY, R., and CALDWELL, B. M. 1975. The relation of infants' home environments to mental test performance from six to thirty-six months: A longitudinal analysis. *Child Development, 46,* 71.

22. EMDE, R. N., GAENSBAUER, T. J., and HARMON, R. J. 1976. *Emotional Expression in Infancy.* New York: International Universities Press.

23. ENGEN, T., and LIPSITT, L. P. 1965. Decrement and recovery of responses to olfactory stimuli in the human neonate. *Journal of Comparative and Physiological Psychology, 59,* 312.

24. ERIKSON, E. H. 1950. *Childhood and Society.* New York: Norton.

25. ESCALONA, S., and HEIDER, G. M. 1959. *Prediction and Outcome: A Study in Child Development.* New York: Basic Books.

26. FANTZ, R. L. 1958. Pattern vision in young infants. *Psychological Record, 8,* 43.

27. FANTZ, R. L., and NEVIS, S. 1967. Pattern preferences and perceptual cognitive development in early infancy. *Merrill-Palmer Quarterly, 13,* 77.

28. GOLDBERG, S. 1977. Infant development and mother-infant interaction in urban Zambia. In P. H. Leiderman, S. R. Tulkin, and A. Rosenfeld (Eds.), *Culture and infancy.* New York: Academic Press.

29. GRAHAM, F. K., CLIFTON, R. K., and HATTON, H. M. 1968. Habituation of heart rate response to repeated auditory stimulation during the first five days of life. *Child Development, 39,* 35.

30. HARTMANN, H., KRIS, E., and LOWENSTEIN, R. 1946. Comments on the formation of psychic structure. *Psychoanalytic Study of the Child. Vol. 2,* 11, New York: International Universities Press.

31. HOFFMAN, M. L. 1975. Developmental synthesis of affect and cognition and its implications for altruistic motivation. *Developmental Psychology, 11,* 607.

32. JONES, S. J., and MOSS, H. A. 1971. Age, state, and maternal behavior associated with infant vocalizations. *Child Development, 42,* 1039.

33. KAGAN, J. 1976. Emergent themes in human development. *American Scientist, 64,* 186.

34. KAGAN, J. 1971. *Change and Continuity in Infancy.* New York: John Wiley.

35. KAGAN, J., and KLEIN, R. E. 1973. Cross-cultural perspectives on early development. *American Psychologist, 28,* 947.

36. KAGAN, J., and Moss, H. A. 1962. *Birth to Maturity.* New York: John Wiley.

37. KESSEN, W., HAITH, M. M., and SALAPATEK, P. H. 1970. Human infancy: A bibliography and guide. In: P. H. Mussen, (Ed.), *Carmichael's Manual of Child Psychology,* Vol. 1, 3rd Ed. New York: John Wiley.

38. KLAUS, R. A., and GRAY, S. W. 1968. The early training project for disadvantaged children: A report after five years. *Monographs of the Society for Research in Child Development, 33* (Serial Number 120).

39. KONNER, M. E. 1977. Infancy among the Kalahari Desert San. In: P. H. Leiderman, S. R. Tulkin, and A. S. Rosenfeld, (Eds.), *Culture and Infancy: Variations in the Human Experience.* New York: Academic Press.

40. KORNER, A. F., and THOMAN, E. B. 1970. Visual alertness in neonates as evoked by maternal care. *Journal of Experimental Child Psychology, 10,* 67.
41. LASKO, J. K. 1954. Parent behavior towards first and second children. *Genetic Psychology Monographs, 49,* 97.
42. LEIDERMAN, P. H., and LEIDERMAN, G. F. 1977. Familial influences on infant development in an East African agricultural community. In: P. H. Leiderman and S. Tulkin (Eds.), *Cultural and Social Influences in Infancy and Early Childhood.* New York: Academic Press.
43. LEWIN, K. 1946. Behavior and development as a function of the total situation. In: L. Carmichael (Ed.), *Manual of Child Psychology.* New York: Wiley.
44. LEWIS, M., and BROOKS, J. 1976. Infants' social perception: A constructivist view. In: L. Cohen and P. Salapatek (Eds.), *Infant Perception: From Sensation to Cognition.* New York: Academic Press.
45. LEWIS, M., and GOLDBERG, S. 1969. Perceptual-cognitive development in infancy: A generalized expectancy model as a function of the mother-infant interaction. *Merrill-Palmer Quarterly, 15,* 81.
46. MAAS, H. 1963. The young adult adjustment of twenty wartime residential nursery children. *Child Welfare, 42,* 57.
47. MACCOBY, E. and JACKLIN, C. 1974. *The Psychology of Sex Differences.* Stanford, Ca.: Stanford University Press.
48. MACFARLANE, J. W. 1964. Perspectives on personality consistency and change from the Guidance Study. *Vita Humana, 7,* 115.
49. MAHLER, M. S., PINE, F., and BERGMAN, A. 1975. *The Psychological Birth of the Human Infant: Symbiosis and Individuation.* New York: Basic Books.
50. MISCHEL, W. 1969. Continuity and change in personality. *American Psychologist, 24,* 1012.
51. MISCHEL, W. 1968. *Personality and Assessment.* New York: John Wiley.
52. MISCHEL, W. 1973. Towards a cognitive social learning reconceptualization of personality. *Psychological Review, 80,* 252.
53. MONEY, J. and EHRHARDT, A. A. 1972. *Man and Woman, Boy and Girl: Differentiation and Dimorphism of Gender Identity from Conception to Maturity.* Baltimore, Md.: Johns Hopkins University Press.
54. MOSS, H. A. 1967. Sex, age and state as determinants of mother-infant interaction. *Merrill-Palmer Quarterly, 13,* 19.
55. MURPHY, L. B. and ASSOCIATES 1962. *The Widening World of Childhood: Paths toward Mastery.* New York: Basic Books.
56. MURPHY, L. B. 1937. *Social Behavior and Child Personality.* New York: Columbia University Press.
57. MURPHY, L. B. 1964. Factors in continuity and change in the development of educational style in children. *Vita Humana, 7,* 96.
58. MUSSEN, P., and EISENBERG-BERG, N. 1977. *Roots of Caring and Sharing.* San Francisco: Freeman Press.
59. PAPOUSEK, N. 1961. Conditioned head rotation reflexes in the first months of life. *Acta Paediatrica* (Stockholm), *50,* 565.
60. PAPOUSEK, H. and PAPOUSEK, M. In Press. The infant's fundamental adaptive response system in social interaction. In: E. B. Thoman, (Ed.), *Origins of Social Responsiveness.* New York: Erlbaum.
61. PRECHTL, M. F. R., and BEINTEMA, D. J. 1964. The neurological examination of the full-term newborn infant. *Clinics in Developmental Medicine, 12,* 281.
62. SANFORD, N. 1968. Personality: The field. In: D. K. Sills (Ed.), *International Encyclopedia of the Social Sciences,* Vol. 2. New York: Free Press, 587.
63. SCHAEFER, E. S., and BAYLEY, N. 1963. Maternal behavior, child behavior, and their intercorrelations from infancy through adolescence. *Monographs of the Society for Research in Child Development, 28* (3, Serial Number 87).

64. SCHAFFER, H. R. 1966. Activity level as a constitutional determinant of infantile reaction to deprivation. *Child Development 37*, 595.
65. SCHAFFER, H. R., and EMERSON, P. E. 1964. The development of social attachments in infancy. *Monographs of the Society for Research in Child Development, 29* (3, Number 94.).
66. SEARS, R. R., MACCOBY, E. E., and LEVIN, H. 1957. *Patterns of Child Rearing*. Evanston, Illinois: Row, Peterson and Company.
67. SKEELS, H. M. 1966. Adult status of children with contrasting early life experiences. *Monographs of the Society for Research in Child Development, 31,* (3, Serial No. 105).
68. SUOMI, S. J., and HARLOW, H. F. 1971. Abnormal social behavior in young monkeys. In: J. Hellmuth (Ed.), *Exceptional Infant: Studies in Abnormalities*, Vol. 2. New York: Brunner/Mazel.
69. THOMAS, A., CHESS, S., BIRCH, H. G., HERTZIG, M. E., and KORN, S. 1964. *Behavioral Individuality in Early Childhood*. New York: New York University Press.
70. WATSON, J. S. 1966. The development and generalization of "contingency awareness" in early infancy: Some hypotheses. *Merrill-Palmer Quarterly, 12*, 123.
71. WHITE, B. L., and CASTLE, P. W. 1964. Visual exploratory behavior following postnatal handling of human infants. *Perceptual and Motor Skills*, 18, 497.
72. WHITING, J., and CHILD, I. 1953. *Child Training and Personality*. New Haven: Yale University Press.
73. YANG, R. K., and DOUTHITT, T. C. 1974. Newborn responses to threshold tactile stimulation. *Child Development, 45*, 237-242.
74. YARROW, L. J. 1961. Maternal deprivation: Towards an empirical and conceptual re-evaluation. *Psychological Bulletin, 58*, 459.
75. YARROW, L. J. 1967. The development of focused relationships during infancy. In: Hellmuth, J. (Ed.), *Exceptional Infant: The Normal Infant*. New York: Brunner/Mazel.
76. YARROW, L. J. 1963. Dimensions of maternal care. *Merrill-Palmer Quarterly, 9*, 101.
77. YARROW, L. J. 1964. Personality consistency and change: An overview of some conceptual and methodological issues. *Vita Humana, 7*, 67.
78. YARROW, L. J. 1972. Attachment and dependency: A developmental perspective. In: J. L. Gewirtz (Ed.), *Attachment and Dependency*. New York: John Wiley.
79. YARROW, L. J. 1979. Historical perspectives on infant development In: J. D. Osofsky (Ed.), *The Handbook of Infant Development*. New York: Wiley-Interscience.
80. YARROW, L. J., and ANDERSON, B. J. 1979. Procedures for studying parent-infant interaction: A critique. In: E. B. Thoman (Ed.), *Origins of Social Responsiveness*. New York: Erlbaum.
81. YARROW, L. J., RUBENSTEIN, J. L., and PEDERSEN, F. A. 1975. *Infant and Environment: Early Cognitive and Motivational Development*. New York: Halsted Press.
82. YARROW, L. J., GOODWIN, M. S., MANHEIMER, H., and MILOWE, I. D. 1973. Infancy experience and cognitive and personality development at ten years. In: L. J. Stone, H. Smith, and L. B. Murphy (Eds.), *The Competent Infant*. New York: Basic Books.
83. YARROW, L. J., KLEIN, R. P., LOMONACO, S., and MORGAN, G. A. 1975. Cognitive and motivational development in early childhood. In: B. Z. Friedlander, G. M. Sterritt, and G. E. Kirk (Eds.), *Exceptional Infant, Vol. 3*. New York: Brunner/Mazel.
84. YARROW, L. J., MORGAN, G. A., JENNINGS, K. D., HARMON, R. J., and GAITER, J. L. 1978. The conceptualization and measurement of mastery motivation. (Unpublished paper).
85. YARROW, M. R., CAMPBELL, J. D., and BURTON, R. V. 1968. *Child Rearing: An Inquiry into Research and Methods*. San Francisco: Jossey-Bass.

2

THE COGNITIVE DEVELOPMENT
OF THE YOUNG CHILD

M.D. Vernon, M.A., Sc.D.

Emeritus Professor, University of Reading, England

INTRODUCTION

In recent years extensive investigation of the capacities of infants to perceive and react to features of their environment has indicated that they are in no sense passive or responsive only to stimuli which are directly relevant to their needs for food and safety. Even newborns are aware of objects and shapes presented to them which have no such motivational connotations, and exhibit some degree of attention in looking at them, even examining them intently. Nevertheless their early awareness, during what Piaget termed the "sensorimotor" stage (68), is transitory, and they rapidly forget what they have perceived. Moreover, it is essentially fragmentary; impressions are not related and organized into general notions of the nature of the environment. However, as we shall see, such organization begins to develop in a rudimentary form during the second year of life, at Piaget's "preconceptual" stage (67), though its establishment is gradual. Young children do, in fact, begin to acquire concepts during the preconceptual stage, but these concepts are partial and do not operate with regard to many relations between objects, for instance, their numbers, spatial relations, etc. Full conceptual development is not acquired until Piaget's stage of "concrete operations" at five to six years (68).

The investigation of the young child's cognitive development is difficult to perform because findings can seldom be widely generalized, especially in infants. It cannot be assumed that these children, even though they appear to understand and react appropriately in certain particular situations, will also do so in other situations which to the adult appear similar, but for the child are unrelated. Also, in infants responsiveness varies markedly with state and level of arousal. However, in recent investigations the infants studied were usually in a state of quiet alertness. But there are also individual differences in arousal and responsiveness. Consequently, it is difficult to establish general principles of cognition during infancy and early childhood. Although different experimenters have obtained different findings and arrived at varying conclusions as to the nature of these principles, we shall consider some of the data which have been obtained at the sensorimotor and the preconceptual stages.

THE SENSORIMOTOR STAGE IN INFANCY

Direction of Attention

Newborn infants orientate their gaze towards particularly intense stimuli and also pursue moving stimuli with their eyes, especially if these show strong visual contrast to the background (74). Spontaneous scanning of the field of view begins soon after birth, interspersed with steady fixations. By 16 weeks, attention to the field of view has increased to 40 percent of waking time (96). At this age the gaze is directed towards and attention appears to be "captured" and held by the sensorily salient aspects of figures, such as large size, strong contrasts, as with solid black figures on white backgrounds (78), and clearly contoured patterns (11), as well as by salient parts of figures such as the vertex of a triangle (79). But general scanning of the field is random and uncoordinated.

During the second month there is a change in the direction of attention. Scanning becomes more extensive and varied in direction, and includes the peripheral as well as the central area of the field (84, 85). The whole contour of a shape, not merely small segments of it (80), is scanned at eight to ten weeks. The interior detail of more complex figures is not attended to by one-month-old infants, who react only to external features, possibly in a primitive figure-ground discrimination (57); but at four months there are responses to both internal and external features. It would appear that attention, though it is still intermittent, is beginning to be directed towards exploration of the field and towards gaining information as to its nature by perceptual analysis of complex patterns. However, for a time sensorily salient features continue to capture attention from other features. But this is gradually supplemented and eventually replaced by cognitively organized and goal-directed search (98).

Form Discrimination

Capacity to discriminate between forms and patterns has been investigated in numerous experiments in which infants were presented with two stimuli, side by side—usually black and white or coloured patterns. It has then been found that even newborn infants generally prefer to look at one rather than the other, and to spend longer in fixating it with the eyes. They look longer at patterned than at plain fields (27), and at clearly defined than at less clearly defined patterns (60). Thus, it would seem that even in newborn infants there exists some capacity to discriminate different patterns.

Infants also appear at an early age to seek for information in such patterns, that is to say, to make out what they are. Although there is some disagreement between the findings of different experimenters, it would seem that young infants of about three weeks tend to fixate relatively simple patterns, such as four-square check patterns, but by 14 weeks they prefer to examine more complex patterns containing more squares (46). This preference increases with increasing age, with longer fixation of more and more complex patterns containing greater amounts of information. These effects are also related to previous experience; attention is maximally aroused by prolonged exposure to patterns slightly more complex than those which have initially been preferred (40). These patterns, it would seem, stimulated efforts at information processing and assimilation.

That information processing is limited in extent in young infants is shown by the preference of newborn infants for regular and redundant patterns such as check patterns and bull's-eyes rather than irregular patterns such as random lines (30). But at 25 weeks infants look longer at patterns with angular than with straight lines, the former containing more information (77). Infants of six weeks, who have been shown complex objects over a considerable period of time, prefer these familiar objects to novel ones, but infants of eight weeks prefer novel objects (94). Thus it would seem that infants direct their gaze principally towards patterns containing information which they can assimilate, and the capacity to process this information increases gradually from birth onwards.

Identification of Forms

Clearly the infant's understanding of his environment must be very rudimentary insofar as objects are perceived only momentarily and immediately forgotten. Such percepts could produce only a highly fragmented awareness of environmental events. Further, for the identification of objects it is essential that the infant compare what he perceives at the moment with what he has experienced formerly. It is possible, however, that a kind of vague short-term familiarity precedes the establishment of any precise and persistent memory traces of previous experiences.

The early development of memory has been investigated by repeatedly presenting the same stimulus to an infant at short intervals of time. It is then found that the amount of time he spends fixating it decreases with repetition. This habituation indicates that the infant remembers having seen this stimulus before and is no longer concerned with attending to it and discovering what it is like. But if a novel stimulus is then presented, attention recovers and fixation time increases. It has been claimed that habituation is exhibited even by newborn infants, whose fixations decrease with repeated 60-second exposures of a check pattern at 5-10-second intervals (33). Some of these infants show recovery when a different check pattern is subsequently presented (31). However, there are individual differences in habituation and recovery; rapid habituators commonly show greater recovery than slow habituators. These differences may be associated with degree of cognitive development; thus, fast habituators prefer more complex patterns than slow habituators (41). The former also show greater cognitive development at 15 months than do the latter (59).

In these experiments, the intervals between successive presentations of the repeated stimulus are very short, and therefore, familiarity is short-lived. It has been hypothesized that a genuine capacity to encode visual patterns in memory, with assimilation of their structures, does not develop until two to three months (11, 48). Thus, there is no habituation to a coloured geometric shape presented at eight-second intervals at six to eight weeks, but habituation does occur at 10 weeks (95). Recovery to a novel stimulus develops at about the same time (94). But even at four months there was no habituation to a coloured shape or recovery to a novel one when there was a five-minute interval between successive presentations of the habituating stimulus (65).

The amount of recovery also depends on the degree of discrepancy between the initial and the novel stimulus—that is, the magnitude and the obviousness of the change from one to the other. In young infants, recovery is greatest when the discrepancy is large, especially for male infants (32). Female infants respond more to a moderate discrepancy; it has been suggested that they are either more alert or more discriminating than male infants. The most effective type of discrepancy also becomes modified with cognitive development. By 12 weeks, recovery of rapidly habituating infants is maximal to a moderate discrepancy of the novel stimulus, but for slow habituators recovery is greater for the most discrepant stimulus (56). However, when a novel object of a completely different type is presented to infants of seven and a half months, there is no increase in fixation time; that is to say, the novel object was not, for the infant, related to the repeated stimulus (45).

The encoding in memory of visual patterns would appear to assist infants in the direction and control of gaze (11), such that parts of these patterns may be successively fixated in an orderly fashion until critical component parts are finally coordinated to produce a single integrated response (48). It is not entirely clear when infants cease simply to regard the pattern as a whole and begin to differentiate separate elements in it. However, at four months infants habituate to the salient parts of complex patterns and not to the less salient, indicating that they do perceive some parts within the whole (58). At this age infants also are aware of more than one aspect of a form; thus, recovery is greater when a shape changes in both form and colour than when it changes in form or colour alone (19).

There is some evidence from numerous experiments on the response to pictures of human faces that infants begin to acquire rudimentary impressions of the general characteristics of certain classes of pattern. In the early months, infants regard pictures of human faces in much the same way as they regard other patterns, fixating first features of high contrast such as the eyes, (18) and then pictures of increasing complexity (42). At two and a half months there is no discrimination between drawings of faces and drawings with the same features scrambled (50). But thereafter a preference emerges for pictures with increasing resemblance to faces (83). Moreover, smiling, which in early months was indiscriminate, appears as a specific response to pictures of faces, with a maximum response at four months (49). It is hypothesized that at this age infants have acquired a "schema," a general impression of the pictured face as such, which differentiates it from other patterns (53). It cannot be assumed, however, that these infants associate this "schema" with living faces, even though they seem to perceive some similarity between living faces and photographs of them (23).

Identification of Objects

Infants have increasingly more experience of solid objects as their age increases, and they become more interested in observing them and differentiating them from flat surfaces. As early as the third month, infants look longer at a solid sphere with a textured surface than at a flat disc (26). However, infants are not necessarily able to identify objects of particular shapes. Thus, when a cube is instantaneously substituted for a ball, infants under six months do not appear surprised (7).

It seems probable that identification of such a familiar and important object as the mother precedes identification of other objects. Though infants of one month do not appear to look directly at the mother's face and features (55), it has been claimed that, even at two weeks, infants distinguish the mother's face, seen through a peephole, from that of a stranger, and are puzzled that they cannot see her body (7). They also associate the mother's voice with her face and avert their own faces when the voices of the mother and of a stranger are transposed. If the mother's voice is shifted to the left or right of them by a stereospeaker, infants of 30 days become greatly agitated (1). Though it has been claimed that newborn infants look towards a source of sound and hence associate sight and sound, recent evidence has shown that this is not so (17). But it would appear that the coordination between the sight of the mother and the sound of her voice develops at an early age. This coordination soon extends to other objects. Thus, at 15-16 weeks, infants who have been familiarized with the sound made by a particular toy anticipate its visual appearance when its characteristic sound is presented in a new spatial position (54).

The association between different sensory patterns arising from a single object marks a fundamental stage in the development of the concept of objects as such—as entities possessing different sensory attributes which are nevertheless linked together as belonging to the same object. In the second half of the first year, association between visual and tactile sensory patterns becomes increasingly important. By seven months, infants who have learned to discriminate by touch between a complete object and one with a piece cut out of it can make the same discrimination visually (15). The visual and tactile sensory patterns are associated in object identification of a simple kind.

The infant does not have to depend solely on passive observation in learning to identify objects; he also employs his own activities—what he can do with objects. It has been claimed that even one-week-old infants attempt to explore objects manually, by reaching out and trying to touch them—even by reaching for a small ball, with the fingers adjusted to its size, rather than for a large ball at double the distance (6). Moreover, a solid ball is differentiated from the photograph of the ball, to which no reaching movements are made. However, a later experiment has not substantiated these findings. In this study, infants of 6-23 days do not reach for a solid ball any more than for a photograph of it (24). It is not until 24 weeks that a solid object is reached for and touched more frequently than a picture of it (29); at about the same age solid objects are reached for more frequently than are stereoscopically presented virtual objects, that is to say, images of objects (37).

Thus, by 6 months there is a definite discrimination between solid objects which can be touched and handled and flat pictures which cannot. But effective manipulation develops slowly. Thus, not until four to four and a half months is a regarded object roughly grasped if the reaching hand happens to strike it (96). At five months the hand reaches out in a single accurately adjusted movement, opens and then grasps the object. Throughout this period, the object grasped is usually put in the mouth, as a further type of exploration. These developments are expedited by the provision of numerous attractive toys. From five months infants feel objects with their fingers, manipulate them and turn them round in space to look at all sides of them. They also try to discover what they can do with them, and what are the consequences of their actions, by rubbing, banging, striking and dropping them. Thus, they actively coordinate the various sensorimotor patterns arising from these actions in what Piaget termed "schemes"—patterns of perceived actions related to objects, their properties and interrelations (68). At first, these schemes concern single objects, but during the latter part of the first year they may be coordinated when two objects are handled successively (86). These processes are stated by Bruner to characterize the stage of "enactive" memory (13).

The Object Concept

During the latter part of the first year, schemes begin to lead to the acquisition of the object concept—a generalization about the nature and properties of objects or particular groups of objects, covering a number of separate instances. Perhaps the earliest concept relates to objects in general, and the most important feature of this concept is that objects continue to exist permanently, independent of the particular situations in which they are encountered and even when they are not actually visible. But this object concept develops only gradually and is for a considerable period subject to several erroneous and misleading impressions.

In early months infants appear not to be aware that objects maintain their identity irrespective of the particular situation in which they are perceived. At first the infants identify an object with its movements, perhaps because movement is a phenomenon which is perceived at a very early age. Thus when an object is moved in front of an infant, he attends primarily to the movement. At eight weeks infants follow the trajectory of a moving object with their eyes, pause momentarily when it stops and then continue to move along the same trajectory, away from the object (5). Infants of 20 weeks continue to follow the trajectory of an object which passes behind a screen and anticipate its reappearance when it stops for a time behind the screen. They appear upset if it appears earlier than they have expected. But they do not seem to notice if a different object is substituted behind the screen. Thus, at this age, a moving object is identified with its movement, and its other characteristics are relatively unimportant. But after 20 weeks, infants begin to notice if the object changes while passing behind a screen (8). Apparently, discrimination of its other characteristics has begun to develop.

There may also be confusion between the identity of objects and their spatial positions; the object may be identified with a particular location and may change its identity if it changes place (90). This has been demonstrated in experiments in which an object is hidden from sight. Piaget considered that infants under seven to eight months do not realize the continued and permanent existence of objects, since they do not search for them when they are hidden from sight (69). Later experiments have shown that this understanding develops gradually. At seven to eight weeks infants reach for an object if it gradually is covered by a screen, but not if it is suddenly covered (4); at six months they reach for an object partially, but not wholly, covered, even if it is covered only just before their fingers touch it (38). However, at seven and a half months infants are more likely to search for a hidden object they have previously grasped than for one which they have not touched, suggesting that in the former case it has been incorporated in a scheme of action (39).

Failure to search for a hidden object is not due merely to inability to see it. If while an infant is looking at an object, the light is suddenly turned off, he still reaches for it (10). But if it is covered by a transparent cup, so that it can still be seen, infants of 21 weeks are very slow to pick up the cup and grasp the object. It has been argued that infants of this age do not understand the relationship of "inside" (25). Thus, an object seen to be inside another, occupying the same spatial position, no longer retains its initial identity.

The confusion of identity with spatial location has been shown in further experiments on hiding. If a new object is substituted for one hidden in a box and covered by a lid, infants of nine months seem confused when they see the new object, but they do not search for the original object before 12 months (52). Twelve-month-old infants are also confused when, having searched for and found the hidden object in one place, they then have to find it hidden in another place; they tend to look for it in the first place (39). Even when an object which has been obtained from behind a transparent door is put behind another transparent door, infants of one year frequently try to open the former (44). This tendency to search in the initial hiding place would seem to result from an association with the successful actions of the initial search in retrieving the object. It has been found to persist until 16 months, and is thereafter only gradually superseded by ability to search in the actual hiding place (93). This development can to some extent be accelerated by earlier training in tracking moving objects (9). However, not all errors of retrieval are eliminated.

It appears that the concept of an object as having a permanent identity which is associated with its perceived characteristics but independent of the particular situation of the moment may not be acquired until the end of the first year of life or even after. However, the permanent identity of a very familiar and important object such as the mother may be understood much earlier. An infant of eight months searches for his mother, but not for other objects, when hidden behind a screen (2). With the latter, identity may be associated with movement, with spatial location and with the child's actions in relation to the object, particularly when these have been successful in obtaining it. It would appear that before identity of objects is fully conceptualized, it is incorporated in schemes of action, which include the objects' position and movement and the actions which the child has performed with them.

During the second year of life, the child becomes more capable of active exploration as he becomes ambulatory; he also appears to be more capable of obtaining more information by exploration. At 12 months children explore novel rather than familiar rooms, as well as an array of toys rather than a single toy (75). At this age they begin to develop their concepts and to modify their actions in the light of the outcome of their actions. Anticipation of the continued existence of objects develops. Thus they are able to search for a displaced object even when they cannot see how it has been moved (86).

Identity is perceived even at a distance; and they can pull a distant object towards them by means of a string attached to it (87).

It should be noted that in certain recent investigations it has been suggested that the infant's ability to identify objects may be considerably influenced by his interactions with his mother in play and other activities. In early months the infant's spontaneous attention is directed towards his mother to a greater extent than to any other object. But in the second half of the first year, he begins to direct more attention towards other objects and to share activities with objects with the mother. She may draw his attention to objects by handling them, stimulate his interest in investigating them, and assist him by her gestures in performing certain actions, for instance, obtaining an object from behind a barrier. Consequently, the infant may appear capable of exhibiting behaviour relating to object identification and conceptualization at an earlier age when he is with his mother than when he is alone. However, it is not clear whether, or to what extent, his own actual cognitive development is advanced, or whether his existing behaviour is facilitated by the interactive situation. For this reason, no detailed presentation of these findings is included here.*

THE COGNITIVE PROCESSES AT THE PRECONCEPTUAL STAGE

Attention and Perception

The capacity for identifying single objects increases from the age of two years because of improvements in the accuracy of visual exploration and perception. When three-year-old children are familiarizing themselves with shapes and subsequently recognizing these, their eye movements and fixations are clustered at the centres of the shapes (100). Later, the focal features are fixated (21). It is not until six years that eye movements accurately follow the contours of shapes (100). The children then focus fixations on the distinctive features and properties of objects and their interrelations, but not on features irrelevant to information processing (21). The fragmented and relatively undirected exploration of the field of view is replaced by goal-directed search (98), in accordance with the children's expectations as to what they may perceive. At five to six years, attention to detail and subsequent recognition of irregular shapes are facilitated by active exploration and manipulation of these shapes (97).

As this capacity to identify objects increases, perception itself becomes

---

*There is an interesting discussion of these findings in *Studies in Mother-Infant Interaction*, edited by H.R. Schaffer, New York: Academic Press, 1977.

more extensive, more accurate and more selective; that is to say, it covers a wider and more complex field of view, yet concentrates on those aspects and events which supply the most significant information as to the nature of the objects and events appearing in it. It has sometimes been stated that the perceptions of young children are "global," with objects being perceived rather vaguely as wholes and their detailed characteristics not precisely observed. It has been hypothesized that there are three levels of development in form perception (3). At the first, there is a gross discrimination of forms; at the second, a selective perception of certain aspects of whole forms; and at the third, analysis of complex forms into their constituent parts, both the whole and also its details being taken into account. The second level is reached during the period of two to five years. Thus children of four years can match most geometric shapes with fair accuracy (3); at four to five years they can make quite fine discriminations between forms with different numbers of sides (35). But the third level of perception requires what Piaget has termed "perceptual activity," involving "decentration" from prolonged fixation of salient parts of figures, and active exploration and intelligent selection of those features which most significantly indicate the essential structure of the figure (70). This does not develop until about six years. Thus when presented with a figure made up of circles and squares connected to form an irregular sequence, children of five years copy some of the isolated parts but not the whole; this is not reproduced until six years, and then inexactly (81). Again, the extraction of parts from their inclusion within a complex whole is only beginning even at six years (92).

Categorization and Conceptualization

In the second year identification of objects begins to be facilitated by the spontaneous development of the capacity to group objects into categories, such that many objects are no longer recognized as single instances but as members of a class or category of like objects. Consequently, fewer unrelated instances and events have to be remembered. The constitutents of concepts based on these categories are gradually extracted from action schemes and then generalized, both from similar percepts and also from the functional and dynamic properties of the objects which interest young children, namely what they do and what can be done with them (64). For instance, the concept of a ball includes the rolling and bouncing of balls as well as their roundness. But the concept becomes detached both from particular situations, those in which rolling occurs, and from who rolls it. Children learn the names of these concepts at an early age, as we shall discuss below, and can understand these names before they can utter them. When children of 12 and 15 months are asked to take out the balls from a collection of objects, some of which look like balls but do not function like them (for instance, a sphere fixed so that it can rotate but not roll freely) and some which do not look like balls but can roll and bounce (for instance, a cylinder), there are some choices of the former, but the latter are more frequently chosen (64).

Gradually concepts become more closely related to classes of objects of similar appearance, qualities and meanings. When children of 40 months are repeatedly shown sets of pictures either of fruit or of animals, they habituate and cease to show much interest in these (28). There is a recovery of response when entirely novel objects are presented, but rather less recovery with new objects of the same type. This seems to indicate the beginning of discrimination between objects which are entirely different and those which are different instances of the same category.

It has been claimed that the development of concepts subsuming classes or categories of objects with similar properties may be studied by observing how children segregate and group these. They may select particular types of objects in their spontaneous play (82). They may group together objects with common uses or activities or with somewhat superficial similarities of appearance (99). The development of grouping has been investigated by presenting children with heterogeneous collections of objects or shapes and observing how they put these together. Even at 12 months some children, when given collections of beads and clay balls, spontaneously separate one set from the other. With slightly older children, it is more usual to instruct them, for instance, to put things together that are alike. Inhelder and Piaget found that though some children of two to five years do not group at all, others make what are termed "graphic collections" (47), at first in pairs and then in rows of similar shapes. At a slightly later stage, similar shapes might be grouped into patterns and then into quite complex constructions of different shapes. It would appear that the cognitive processes are still dominated by immediate perception of the form characteristics of objects. But later experiments indicate that children of two to five years are very variable in their manner of grouping coloured shapes (22). Some disregard similarity of shape altogether; some group similar shapes together even at two years; some make graphic collections. Among all children, grouping by similarity increases with age.

However, it seems that classification is made by selecting successive instances and putting these together in accordance with such similarities (47). These partial associations are not linked to one another and not all the objects presented are included. They are not thought of as members of mutually exclusive classes within the set, each class being conceptualized as a generalization of common properties. Such classification does not develop until seven to eight years. However, there may be some understanding during this period that there are subsets within a heterogeneous collection of objects, the members of which are meaningfully associated. In the experiments of Inhelder and Piaget, meaningfully related shapes and objects are sometimes put together (47). Thus, a square with a triangle on top of it is called a "house"; a cot is grouped with a baby doll because a "cot belongs with a baby." Children of three and a half years can, when instructed, pick out pictures of "food" and "people" from a miscellaneous collection of pictures of common objects (72). By five years they begin themselves to classify objects in subsets, frequently in terms of their use or function, for instance, "these are for washing" (36, 47).

Even when children are capable of categorizing, they may not be able to select and abstract the characteristics which are relevant and significant for generalization. They may select one particular and obvious characteristic, such as simple shape or bright colour, and neglect all others.

Verbalization and Cognitive Development

When, during the second year of life, children begin to utter words, a high proportion of these are names of objects (12). The child commonly uses one-word sentences to indicate not only that he has observed a particular object, but also that he is commenting on its behaviour and expressing his wishes to obtain it and act on it. Many of the earliest names, for instance, "dog," "cat," "car," "ball," indicate objects that move or change in some way, often relating to the child's own activities (64). He seldom names objects which are static or with which he does not interact. Though these names may initially relate to a single object, they are rapidly generalized to include other objects of similar appearance and function. Even at 18-24 months, children named pictures of familiar objects with variable though characteristic features, such as a "dog," more often than pictures of objects with a single salient feature, such as a "key" (62). Though there were frequent errors in naming the former, such as "lamb" and "horse," it does seem that concept formation was beginning. Naming appears to depend on the emergence and focalizing of concepts, the names being selected from appropriate words in adult speech, and also by asking for the names of objects encountered (25). However, not all concepts are spontaneously named; also, concepts may be formed of relations between objects without these being formulated in language (25).

The understanding of names is linked to the recognition of objects as having a permanent existence. Thus children of 18-24 months who exhibit an understanding of object permanence are more likely than children who do not to look at and manipulate named rather than unnamed objects (73). Some children, however, use their early words less frequently for naming objects than for expressing their own feelings, wishes, etc.; these children have been found to be inferior in the comprehension of words generally (63).

Verbalization, Conceptualization and Memory

From the latter part of the first year children begin to employ "iconic" memory, by means of which objects are represented in imagery, not merely in schemes of action (13). Thus, by the end of the first year infants can recognize and identify toys which they have seen but which have not been embedded in schemes of action (91). However, these imaginal representations are linked to single objects and are often unstable and fragmented. Indeed, even at three years there is a tendency to recognize an object in terms of a single salient characteristic (71). At this age children may be unable to select the significant features to be remembered and to exclude irrelevant features (43).

Iconic memory is gradually reinforced and even replaced by the use of verbalization, at first verbalization of the names of objects. Children of three to four years who are taught to name coloured rectangles subsequently recognize them better than those who are not (16). From four years on, pictures of objects are better recalled by children who have been instructed to name them than by children who have not (34). However, it may be that children do not spontaneously employ internal speech as a "mediational process" in memorizing before the age of five to six years (20). They continue to rely on iconic memory coding, which is only gradually replaced by verbal coding and the interiorization of verbally organized memory to produce a coherent model of the world rather than the scrappy and disjointed models produced by enactive and iconic memory. Visual iconic memory may be adequate for the *recognition* of pictures, even over a period of two weeks (66). But intentional verbal memorization is shown to be effective for *recall* of pictures of objects by children of five to six years (89). Verbal recall and visual recognition are not correlated and appear to be independent processes. Verbal memorization is also greatly facilitated by "rehearsal"—internal repetition of verbal items.

It is particularly in the remembering of conceptualized—that is to say, categorized—items that naming and verbalization are found to be valuable.

It has been claimed that some spontaneous clustering of the names of objects for recall may occur even at two to three years, but it is rudimentary (76). At five years names of pictures of objects belonging fairly obviously to the same category are recalled better than names of unrelated objects (88). Nevertheless, spontaneous voluntary classification of objects for recall is barely beginning at this age. But if such children are instructed as to the categories in which pictures of objects should be placed, the recall of these is facilitated (51). It has been argued that these children possess the ability to recall objects through their category relationships. They do not, however, employ this procedure spontaneously, but only when instructed to do so. Moreover, they quickly abandon the procedure. It would seem, therefore, that categorial encoding is rudimentary at the preconceptual stage.

CONCLUSIONS

We have seen that the cognitive capacities of young children not only develop gradually, but also may be fragmented and illogical during the first few years of life. Young children may have erroneous notions as to the nature of objects in the environment. However, some abilities seem to exist at birth, namely the capacity to attend briefly to and discriminate between simple visual forms and patterns. Though at first attention and discrimination relate mainly to salient sensory characteristics, the capacity to gain information as to the nature of forms and patterns appears restricted at first but improving throughout the first year of life. These forms and patterns are from the first encoded in memory, but initially for very brief durations. Perception also tends to be vague and global in nature, without much differentiation of the constituent parts of forms. Some differentiation and association of parts may arise during the first year of life with particular types of forms, such as pictures of the human face.

The development of memory is facilitated through the acquisition of schemes of action in which objects are remembered by means of the associated sensory patterns from different modes, especially those based on the infant's actions with particular objects. But these schemes are related to the total situations in which the objects are encountered. It is not until about the end of the first year of life that the infant begins to realize that objects have a continuing and permanent identity, deriving from their appearance, behaviour and functions, but independent of any particular situation in which they occur. Further, embedding in schemes of action may persist for longer, until enactive memory is replaced by iconic memory.

Understanding of the environment and knowledge about the objects it contains widen from the second year onwards through: 1) increasingly selective attention towards the distinctive features and essential properties of objects; 2) improved accuracy in perceiving these, though analysis of and concentration on significant details do not become fully effective until the development of perceptual activity at about the sixth year; 3) replacement of action schemes in enactive memory by imaginal representation in iconic memory; 4) conceptualization of objects by abstracting their significant characteristics and generalizing these to classes of objects. This capacity is facilitated by the development of verbalization—in early years by the naming of single objects; later by verbalizing their conceptual relations and encoding these verbally. This verbalization is not employed spontaneously until about the sixth year, although it may operate temporarily at an earlier age when stimulated by instruction.

The earliest conceptual ideas to develop are those concerned with concrete objects, involving their appearance, uses, functions and relationships. These precede more abstract concepts in which certain properties of objects are generalized. It is not until Piaget's stage of concrete operations, at about six years, that children begin to understand that properties such as the number, weight and volume of objects are independent both of their particular characteristics and also of the situation in which they occur. It is important to note that understanding of all these concepts develops gradually; also the child may appear to have grasped them in certain situations and not in others (14). Further, the child does not pass abruptly from one Piagetian stage to the next—from non-comprehension to comprehension—but acquires partial concepts piecemeal over a long period of time. Thus, in early years concepts are not stable, fully integrated and universal, but fragmented, operating on certain occasions but not on others in an uncoordinated manner, such that they may be contradictory and conflicting. A coherent and all-embracing model of the environment is not acquired until later childhood.

REFERENCES

1. ARONSON, E. and ROSENBLOOM, S. 1971. Space perception in early infancy within a common auditory-visual space. *Science, 172,* 1161.
2. BELL, S.M. 1970. The development of the concept of object as related to infant-mother attachment. *Child Devel., 41,* 291.
3. BIRCH, H.G. and LEFFORD, A., 1967. Visual differentiation, intersensory integration and voluntary motor control. *Monog. Soc. Res. Child Devel., 32,* No. 2 (Whole No. 110).
4. BOWER, T.G.R. 1967. The development of object permanence. *Percept. Psychophys., 2,* 411.
5. BOWER, T.G.R. 1971. The object in the world of the infant. *Sci. Amer., 225* (4), 30.
6. BOWER, T.G.R. 1972. Object perception in infants. *Percept., 1,* 15.

7. BOWER, T.G.R. 1977. *A Primer of Infant Development*. San Francisco: Freeman.
8. BOWER, T.G.R., BROUGHTON, J. and MOORE, M.K. 1971. Development of the object concept as manifested in changes in the tracking behavior of infants between 7 and 20 weeks of age. *J. Exper. Child Psychol., 11*, 182.
9. BOWER, T.G.R. and PATERSON, J.G. 1972. Stages in the development of the object concept. *Cognit., 1*, 47.
10. BOWER, T.G.R. and WISHART, J.G. 1972. The effects of motor skill on object permanence. *Cognit., 1*, 165.
11. BRONSON, G. 1974. The postnatal growth of visual capacity. *Child Devel., 45*, 873.
12. BROWN, R.W. 1973. *A First Language*. London: Allen & Unwin.
13. BRUNER, J.S. 1966. On cognitive growth. In J.S. Bruner, R.R. Oliver and P.M. Greenfield (Eds.), *Studies in Cognitive Growth*. New York: Wiley.
14. BRYANT, P. 1974. *Perception and Understanding in Young Children*. London: Methuen.
15. BRYANT, P.E., JONES, P., CLAXTON, V. and PERKINS, G.M. 1972. Recognition of shapes across modalities by infants. *Nature, 240*, 303.
16. BUSH, E.S. and COHEN, L.B. 1970. The effects of relevant and irrelevant labels on short-term memory in nursery school children. *Psychonom. Sci., 18*, 228.
17. BUTTERWORTH, G. and CASTILLO, M. 1976. Coordination of auditory and visual space in newborn human infants. *Percept., 5*, 155.
18. CARON, A.J., CARON, R.F., CALDWELL, R.C. and WEISS, S.J. 1975. Infant perception of the structural properties of the face. *Devel. Psychol., 9*, 385.
19. CARON, A.J., CARON, R.F., MINICHIELLO, M.D., WEISS, S.J. and FRIEDMAN, S.L. 1977. Constraints on the use of the familiarization-novelty method in the assessment of infant discrimination. *Child Devel., 48*, 747.
20. CONRAD, R. 1972. The developmental role of vocalizing in short-term memory. *J. Verb. Learn. Verb. Behav., 11*, 521.
21. DAY, M.C. 1975. Developmental trends in visual scanning. In H.W. Reese (Ed.), *Advances in Child Development and Behavior*, Vol. 10. New York: Academic Press.
22. DENNEY, N.W. 1972. Free classification in preschool children. *Child Devel., 43*, 1161.
23. DIRKS, J. and GIBSON, E. 1977. Infants' perception of similarity between live people and their photographs. *Child Devel., 48*, 124.
24. DODWELL, P.C., MUIR, D. and DI FRANCO, D. 1976. Responses of infants to visually presented objects. *Science, 194*, 209.
25. DONALDSON, M. 1976. Development of conceptualization. In V. Hamilton and M.D. Vernon (Eds.), *The Development of Cognitive Processes*. London: Academic Press.
26. FANTZ, R.L. 1961. A method of studying depth perception in infants under 6 months of age. *Psychol. Rec., 11*, 27.
27. FANTZ, R.L. 1963. Pattern vision in newborn infants. *Science, 140*, 296.
28. FAULKENDER, P.J., WRIGHT, J.C. and WALDRON, A. 1974. Generalized habituation of concept stimuli in toddlers. *Child Devel., 45*, 1002.
29. FIELD, J. 1976. Relation of young infants' reaching behavior to stimulus distance and solidity. *Devel. Psychol., 12*, 444.
30. FRIEDMAN, S. 1972. Newborn visual attention to repeated exposure of redundant *vs.* 'novel' targets. *Percept. Psychophys., 12*, 291.
31. FRIEDMAN, S. 1972. Habituation and recovery of visual response in the alert human newborn. *J. Exper. Child Psychol., 13*, 339.
32. FRIEDMAN, S., BRUNO, L.A. and VIETZE, P. 1974. Newborn habituation to visual stimuli: A sex difference in novelty detection. *J. Exper. Child Psychol., 18*, 242.
33. FRIEDMAN, S., NAGY, A.N. and CARPENTER, G.C. 1970. Newborn attention: Differential response decrement to visual stimuli. *J. Exper. Child Psychol., 10*, 44.
34. FURTH, H.G. and MILGRAM, N.A. 1973. Labeling and grouping effects in the recall of pictures by children. *Child Devel., 44*, 511.
35. GAINES, R. 1969. The discriminability of form among young children. *J. Exper. Child Psychol., 8*, 418.

36. GOLDMAN, A.E. and LEVINE, M. 1963. A developmental study of object sorting. *Child Devel.*, *34*, 649.
37. GORDON, F.R. and YONAS, A. 1976. Sensitivity to binocular depth information in infants. *J. Exper. Child Psychol.*, *22*, 413.
38. GRATCH, G. 1972. A study of the relative dominance of vision and touch in six-month infants. *Child Devel.*, *43*, 615.
39. GRATCH, G. and LANDERS, W.F. 1971. Stage IV of Piaget's theory of infants' object concepts. *Child Devel.*, *42*, 359.
40. GREENBERG, D.J. 1971. Accelerating visual complexity levels in the human infant. *Child Devel.*, *42*, 905.
41. GREENBERG, D.J., O'DONNELL, W.J. and CRAWFORD, D. 1973. Complexity levels, habituation and individual differences in early infancy. *Child Devel.*, *44*, 569.
42. HAAF, R.A. and BROWN, C.J. 1976. Infants' response to facelike patterns: Developmental changes between 10 and 15 weeks of age. *J. Exper. Child Psychol.*, *22*, 155.
43. HAGEN, J.W. 1972. Strategies for remembering. In: S. Farnham-Diggory (Ed.), *Information Processing in Children*. New York: Academic Press.
44. HARRIS, P.L. 1974. Perseverative search at a visibly empty place by young infants. *J. Exper. Child Psychol.*, *18*, 535.
45. HOPKINS, J.R., ZELAZO, P.R., JACOBSON, S.W. and KAGAN, J. 1976. Infant reactivity to stimulus-schema discrepancy. *Genet. Psychol. Monog.*, *93*, 27.
46. HOROWITZ, F.D., PADEN, L., BHANA, K., AITCHISON, R. and SELF, P. 1972. Developmental changes in infant visual fixation to different complexity levels among cross-sectionally and longitudinally studied infants. *Devel. Psychol.*, *7*, 88.
47. INHELDER, B. and PIAGET, J. 1964. *The Early Growth of Logic in the Child*. London: Routledge & Kegan Paul.
48. JEFFREY, W.E. and COHEN, L.B. 1971. Habituation in the human infant. In: H.W. Reese (Ed.), *Advances in Child Development and Behavior*, Vol. 6. New York: Academic Press.
49. KAGAN, J. 1971. *Change and Continuity in Infancy*. New York: Wiley.
50. KOOPMAN, P.R. and AMES, E.N. 1968. Infants' preferences for facial arrangements. *Child Devel.*, *39*, 481.
51. LANGE, G. 1973. The development of conceptual and rote recall skills among school age children. *J. Exper. Child Psychol.*, *15*, 394.
52. LeCOMPTE, G.K. and GRATCH, G. 1972. Violation of a rule as a method of diagnosing infants' levels of object concept. *Child Devel.*, *43*, 385.
53. LEWIS, M. 1969. Infants' responses to facial stimuli during the first year of life. *Devel. Psychol.*, *1*, 75.
54. LYONS-RUTH, K. 1977. Bimodal perception in infancy: Response to auditory-visual incongruity. *Child Devel.*, *48*, 820.
55. MAURER, D. and SALAPATEK, P. 1976. Developmental changes in the scanning of faces by young infants. *Child Devel.*, *47*, 523.
56. McCALL, R.B., HOGARTY, P.S., HAMILTON, J.S.and VINCENT, J.H. 1973. Habituation rate and the infant's response to visual discrepancies. *Child Devel.*, *44*, 280.
57. MILEWSKI, A.E. 1976. Infants' discrimination of internal and external pattern elements. *J. Exper. Child Psychol.*, *22*, 229.
58. MILLER, D.J. 1972. Visual habituation in the human infant. *Child Devel.*, *43*, 481.
59. MILLER, D.J. *et al.* 1977. Relationships between early habituation and later cognitive performance in infancy. *Child Devel.*, *48*, 658.
60. MIRANDA, S.B. 1970. Visual abilities and pattern preferences of premature infants and full-term neonates. *J. Exper. Child Psychol.*, *10*, 189.
61. MOELY, B.E., OLSON, F.A., HALWES, T.G. and FLAVELL, J.H. 1969. Production deficiency in young children's clustered recall. *Devel. Psychol.*, *1*, 26.
62. NELSON, K. 1972. The relation of form recognition to concept development. *Child Devel.*, *43*, 67.

63. NELSON, K. 1973. Structure and strategy in learning to talk. *Monog. Soc. Res. Child Devel. 38*, 1 (Whole No. 149).
64. NELSON, K. 1974. Concept, word and sentence: Inter-relations in acquisition and development. *Psychol. Rev., 81*, 267.
65. PANCRATZ, C.N. and COHEN, L.B. 1970. Recovery of habituation in infants. *J. Exper. Child Psychol., 9*, 208.
66. PERLMUTTER, M. and MYERS, N.A. 1975. Young children's coding and storage of visual and verbal material. *Child Devel., 46*, 215.
67. PIAGET, J. 1951. *Play, Dreams and Imitation in Childhood*. London: Heinemann.
68. PIAGET, J. 1952. *The Origins of Intelligence in Children*. New York: International Universities Press.
69. PIAGET, J. 1955. *The Child's Construction of Reality*. London: Routledge & Kegan Paul.
70. PIAGET, J. 1969. *The Mechanisms of Perception*. London: Routledge & Kegan Paul.
71. PIAGET, J., SINCLAIR, H. and VINH-BANG. 1968. *Epistémologie et Psychologie de l'Identité*. Paris: Presses Universitaires de France.
72. POVEY, R. and HILL, E. 1975. Can pre-school children form concepts? *Educ. Res., 17*, 180.
73. ROBERTS, G.C. and BLACK, K.N. 1972. The effect of naming and object permanence on toy preferences. *Child Devel., 43*, 858.
74. ROSE, S., KATZ, P.A., BIRKE, M. and ROSSMAN, E. 1977. Visual following in newborns. *Percept. Motor Skills, 45*, 515.
75. ROSS, H.S. 1974. The influence of novelty and complexity on exploratory behavior in 12-month-old infants. *J. Exper. Child Psychol., 17*, 436.
76. ROSSI, E.L. and ROSSI, S.I. 1965. Concept utilization, serial order and recall in nursery-school children. *Child Devel., 36*, 771.
77. RUFF, H.A. 1976. Developmental changes in the infant's attention to pattern detail. *Percept. Motor Skills, 43*, 351.
78. SALAPATEK, P. 1968. Visual scanning of geometric figures by the human newborn. *J. Comp. Physiol. Psychol., 66*, 247.
79. SALAPATEK, P. and KESSEN, W. 1966. Visual scanning of triangles by the human newborn. *J. Exper. Child Psychol., 3*, 155.
80. SALAPATEK, P. and KESSEN, W. 1973. Prolonged investigation of a plane geometric triangle by the human newborn. *J. Exper. Child Psychol., 15*, 22.
81. STAMBAK, M. and PÊCHEUX, M.-G. 1969. Essai d'analyse d'activité de réproduction de figures géométriques complexes. *L'Année Psychol., 69*, 55.
82. STOTT, D.H. 1961. An empirical approach to motivation based on the behaviour of a young child. *J. Child Psychol. Psychiat., 2*, 97.
83. THOMAS, H. 1973. Unfolding the baby's mind: the infant's selection of visual stimuli. *Psychol. Rev., 80*, 468.
84. TRONICK, E. 1972. Stimulus control and the growth of the infant's effective visual field. *Percept. Psychophys., 11*, 373.
85. TRONICK, E. and CLANTON, C. 1971. Infant looking patterns. *Vis. Res., 11*, 1479.
86. UZGIRIS, I.C. 1976. Organization of sensorimotor intelligence. In M. Lewis (Ed.), *Origins of Intelligence: Infancy and Early Childhood*. New York: Wiley.
87. UZGIRIS, I.C. and HUNT, J. McV. 1975. *Assessment in Infancy*. Urbana: University of Illinois Press.
88. VAUGHAN, M.E. 1968. Clustering, age and incidental learning. *J. Exper. Child Psychol., 6*, 323.
89. VON WRIGHT, J.M. 1973. Relation between verbal recall and visual recognition of the same stimuli in young children. *J. Exper. Child Psychol., 15*, 481.
90. VURPILLOT, E. 1976. Development of identification of objects. In V. Hamilton and M.D. Vernon (Eds.), *The Development of Cognitive Processes*. London: Academic Press.
91. VURPILLOT, E. 1976. *The Visual World of the Child*. London: Allen & Unwin.
92. VURPILLOT, E. and FLORÉS, A. 1964. La genèse de l'organization perceptive. I. Rôle du

contour et de la surface enclose dans la perception des figures. *L'Année Psychol.*, *64*, 375.

93. WEBB, R.A., MASSAR, B. and NADOLNY, T. 1972. Information and strategy in the young child's search for hidden objects. *Child Devel.*, *43*, 91.

94. WEIZMANN, F., COHEN, L.B. and PRATT, R.J. 1971. Novelty, familiarity and the development of infant attention. *Devel. Psychol.*, *4*, 149.

95. WETHERFORD, M.J. and COHEN, L.B. 1973. Developmental changes in infant visual preferences for novelty and familiarity. *Child Devel.*, *44*, 416.

96. WHITE, B.L. 1971. *Human Infants: Experience and Psychological Development.* New Jersey, Englewood Cliffs: Prentice-Hall.

97. WOLFF, P. 1972. The role of stimulus-correlated activity in children's recognition of nonsense forms. *J. Exper. Child Psychol.*, *14*, 427.

98. WRIGHT, J.C. and VLIETSTRA, A.G. 1975. The development of selective attention. In: H.W. Reese, (Ed.), *Advances in Child Development and Behavior*, Vol. *10*. New York: Academic Press.

99. ZAPOROZHETS, A.V., ZINCHENKO, V.P. and ELKONIN, D.B. 1971. Development of thinking. In A.V. Zaporozhets and D.B. Elkonin (Eds.), *The Psychology of Preschool Children.* Cambridge, Mass.: M.I.T. Press.

100. ZINCHENKO, V.P., VAN CHZHI-TSIN and TARAKANOV, V.V. 1963. The formation and development of perceptual activity. *Sov. Psychol. and Psychiat.*, *2*, 3.

3

STIMULATION AND INFANT
DEVELOPMENT

KATHLEEN A. McCLUSKEY, Ph.D.

Department of Psychology
West Virginia University
Morgantown, West Virginia

and
CHRISTINA M.B. ARCO, Ph.D.

Department of Psychology
State University of New York at Brockport
Brockport, New York

INTRODUCTION

The significance of environmental stimulation during infancy for normal developmental outcome has been dramatically and convincingly reported in the psychological literature in the past 40 years. These data have stimulated the burgeoning of numerous programs and projects designed to facilitate adequate stimulation for populations of infants considered at risk in terms of normal developmental progress. The rationale for these infant stimulation programs is based on a wide variety of research that has shed light on the determinants of human growth and development.

In the past three decades, an abundance of conclusive evidence has demonstrated that, from birth, the human infant is a competent organism ca-

The authors wish to thank Frances Degen Horowitz of the University of Kansas and Sharon L. Foster of West Virginia University for their invaluable assistance in the preparation of this chapter.

45

pable of effectively interacting with the environment. Since initial reports in 1958 by both Fantz (20) and Berlyne (8), the rapidly growing data base on the perceptual capabilities of the infant has supported the notion that the perceptual systems of the human neonate are intact and functional at birth. The young infant can perceive a large number of stimuli in all sensory modalities, can make fine discriminations between similar stimuli, and has definite preferences for certain categories of environmental input (3).

In addition to demonstrating remarkable perceptual sophistication, the young infant appears to be quite cognitively capable. Much of our knowledge concerning cognition in the early stages of development has been based upon the extensive work of Jean Piaget during the past 30 years (59, 60, 61). His outstanding explication of sensori-motor development has been the major impetus for much of the subsequent work in human cognitive processes done by other investigators. His theory suggests that the infant begins life as an organism interacting with the environment through the use of innate reflexes. By the end of the infancy period (24 months), the developing child is capable of using language and solving mental problems rather than merely responding reflexively to external stimuli. This development occurs through the active processes of assimilation and accommodation: The infant is continually exercising and altering his cognitive structures in response to environmental demands. Piaget postulates that this results from the organism's innate need to maintain a homeostatic balance, a state of cognitive equilibrium, with an ever-expanding and changing environment. Thus, Piaget views the infant as an active participant in the developmental course.

Other work demonstrating the competence of the infant has been done in the areas of learning and memory. Early work by Rheingold (68), Lipsitt (54), and Papousek (58) suggested that the infant was capable of learning a large number of behaviors in a variety of contexts. Subsequent work has refined and expanded upon these early findings (73, 82), lending additional support to the contention that the infant is a capable, active being who is in constant interaction and transaction with highly complex physical and social environments (72).

It is quite clear that from the beginning the infant is actively responsive to his environment and is capable of altering both his own actions and many aspects of the environment upon which he acts. The environment itself, or more specifically the stimulation that it provides, is crucial to the normal development of the infant. Numerous studies using infant animals as subjects have demonstrated the deleterious effects of various types of sensory deprivation (39, 40, 48). While laboratory work altering the environment to investigate the effects of stimulus deprivation on human infants is ethically and morally impossible, reports of children raised in barren, sterile environments parallel the findings of the animal studies. Many of these have helped to define the levels and types of stimulation necessary for normal human development.

The importance of minimal amounts of stimulation for normal development was clearly documented by Skeels and Dye (84) and later by Skeels (83) in their investigation of infants raised in a foundling home in the Midwestern United States. Upon admission to this home, the majority of the infants showed no signs of physical or mental retardation. By the time they reached middle school (12-14 years), these same children were displaying such degrees of intellectual retardation that many of them had to be institutionalized in settings designed for residential care of the mentally handicapped. Skeels and Dye attributed this progressive decline in mental functioning to the bleak surroundings in which the children were raised. Although physical and nutritional needs were adequately met, these infants experienced almost no social or sensory stimulation (84). Their physical surroundings were devoid of patterns and color—Skeel describes the infants' housing as strikingly sterile (83). Contact with caretakers consisted of the minimal time needed to change, clean, and feed each baby. Children were seldom removed from their cribs and had little opportunity to interact with other children. The majority of their time was spent alone with no toys or other objects to engage their attention.

In a very controversial experiment, Skeels and Dye arranged to have 13 infants moved from the foundling home to a nearby institution for adult retardates (84). Each child was placed on a separate ward with adult females. The child received much social and sensory stimulation from the patients and staff in the institution. A contrast group of 12 children raised in the foundling home was employed to compare the effects of differential rearing practices on subsequent developmental outcome. The results of the original study and of a follow-up 30 years later dramatically demonstrated the necessity of stimulation for normal development (83, 84). The infants showed marked increases in intellectual functioning during their residence in the institution for retarded adults. In stark contrast was the intellectual development of the 12 infants assessed in the foundling home. These infants showed progressive decline in functioning with age. Most of the infants raised by the retarded adults were adopted into stable families, whereas most of the contrast group continued to reside in the foundling home until they reached adulthood. In his follow-up study, Skeels convincingly reported the stability of the change effected in early childhood: The experimental group all led productive lives, while the majority of adults in the contrast group were either still institutionalized or living marginal existences. While this study has some methodological problems, the evidence it presents suggests the importance of sensory and social stimulation for adequate child development.

Other work which substantiates these findings is that of Spitz, who reported a phenomenon he labeled as "hospitalism" in infants raised in sterile environments without mother figures (86, 87). A high proportion of children he observed displayed severe delays in physical, motor, cognitive, and social development. Spitz attributed these delays to the lack of adequate mothering present in the foundling home he investigated. Similarly, Provence and Lipton reported abnormal development in institution-reared infants on measures of motor maturity, language competence, social reactions, and discovery of body and self (63). These investigators attributed this progressive decline to the non-stimulating environment in which the infants were being raised. It is evident from these reports that there exists a necessity for at least a minimal amount of social and environmental stimulation for the nurturance of normal child development.

The work of ethologists also supports the importance of adequate stimulation during the infancy period. Numerous investigators have reported the existence of critical periods for the establishment of certain behaviors in many species of animals and birds (37). While the data on humans are far from conclusive, there is some indication that certain periods of the developmental continuum may be sensitive periods for the development of specific abilities. Several investigators have found that developmental delays in infants raised in stimulus-deprived environments do not emerge until at least the seventh month of life (93), and in some cases not until the fifteenth month (6). It is possible that the levels of stimulation in deprived environments are sufficient for the younger infant, but as the child becomes perceptually and cognitively more sophisticated, he requires greater stimulation from the environment. Or, alternatively, it is possible that the effects of deficiencies in levels and types of environmental stimulation are cumulative; while significant developmental delays do not emerge until somewhat later, the roots of these deficiencies are established in the interaction between the very young infant and his environment. Either of these hypotheses would imply that a critical or sensitive period exists at approximately the end of the first year, and that if adequate stimulation of a certain level is not provided, the child's development will not progress at its previous rate. There is much evidence to support the progressive decline seen after the age of 18 months in children living in stimulus-deprived homes (27); it appears crucial that sufficient levels of stimulation be provided at this time for continued normal development.

This notion of critical periods may account for the frequently reported findings of the failure of remedial or intervention programs begun when children are four or five years old (12). These failures can be attributed to a variety of factors, among which is the possibility that the programs were initiated too late in the child's development to reverse the effects of a deprived home environment during the early years (9). Stimulation programs designed to offset the deleterious effects of deprived homes may have to be started before the child begins to fall behind a normal developmental course; this may be as early as the first year.

Evidence cited thus far provides preliminary support for the implementation of stimulation programs during early infancy. Infants are active, capable organisms who need certain types and levels of sensory and social stimulation to thrive. In the past 15 years, efforts have begun in the United States to identify infants who have been labeled as either caretaking or reproductive casualties (74). *Caretaking casualties* refer to infants raised in homes considered inadequate for the provision of essential stimulation for normal growth and development. *Reproductive casualties* are those children whose physiological or medical problems may affect their development. Once identified, these children have been provided with enhanced environments to support normal development; then the effects of these early intervention programs have been empirically assessed. This chapter is a review of representative programs aimed at providing interventive stimulation for both of these target populations. Samples of the three approaches to intervention with infants classified as caretaking casualties will be presented in the first section. The second section illustrates types of programs aimed at a variety of reproductive casualties. The final section of this chapter is a discussion of the implications of the methods and outcomes of these stimulation programs, along with some suggestions for future directions in this area.

INTERVENTION WITH INFANTS CLASSIFIED AS CARETAKING CASUALTIES

Early intervention projects which have been implemented with infants classified as caretaking casualties vary with regard to the target(s) of the intervention strategies. Some of the programs have been designed within a *parent-centered* orientation, in that their main goals revolve around changing the teaching techniques, social competencies, and attitudes of primary caregivers. Others have dual *parent-centered and child-centered* aspects with specific goals for both parents and children. Still others are exclusively *child-centered*, focusing primarily upon the developmental course of the child. These programs also vary in the location of program implementation:

Some provide home visitation policies, others combine home visits with center-based sessions for children and/or parents, whereas others use a program center as the single location of program operation. Representative programs of the parent-centered, parent- and child-centered, and child-centered orientations to early intervention will be summarized in the three sections which follow.

Parent-Centered Intervention Programs

Bowlby has aptly captured the essence of the imbalanced input between infant and family at birth (10). He describes the infant as entering a family unit with established codes of attitudes and values based upon genetic endowment, societal variables, and cultural heritage. According to Bowlby, these familial codes will have profound effects upon the young infant's cognitive and socio-emotional development. Because of these pervasive influences, the family unit emerges as a major target for preventive intervention. Moreover, the recent deluge of literature on the extensive social capacities of the young infant confirms the young infant's capacities for perceiving these influences and attests to the early formation of social expectancies and capacities for meaningful social exchanges (80, 90). The reciprocal influences of cognitive and socio-emotional development have been well-documented (61); this reciprocity indicates that anything less than a family or home-centered approach to preventive intervention may be ecologically invalid (12, 41, 76). In addition, the data which reflect the very early development of relatively stable patterns of parental behaviors and expectancies highlight the need for very early family-centered intervention (7, 13, 47).

Merle Karnes and associates (43, 44, 45) and Phyllis Levenstein and co-workers (51, 52, 55) have conducted extensive parent-centered early intervention programs with the mother as the major target of emphasis. These projects included samples of low-income, culturally deprived mother-child dyads; both were directed toward enhancing maternal social competencies and self-esteem as well as a variety of infant developmental areas, including conceptual and language development and social-emotional development.

Mothers were grouped according to infant age and met weekly for two-hour sessions with a parent coordinator. The focus of the meetings was upon enhancement of positive self-regard and demonstration of teaching strategies and stimulus materials. A parent coordinator also visited each home weekly to monitor maternal progress and the child's readiness for new materials.

Two outcome evaluations have been reported for this project. An exploratory test of the effectiveness of this intervention program was conducted with 30 black mother-child dyads from an economically disadvantaged neighborhood. The children ranged in age from three years, four months to four years, three months. This pilot program consisted of 12 weeks of weekly two-hour classes. The evaluation of the program was based upon pre- and post-test measures on the Stanford-Binet Intelligence Test and the Illinois Test of Psycholinguistic Abilities (ITPA). The exploratory data on both of these measures revealed differences between the control and experimental groups and indicated initial success of the program (44).

The second more extensive test of this project was aimed at a younger infant population: 18 mother-infant pairs and two grandmother-infant pairs participated in the 15-month program. The children ranged in age from 13 to 27 months, with a mean age of 20 months. Two control groups were used as bases of comparison to the treatment group. One consisted of 15 culturally disadvantaged infants matched on several demographic variables, the other of six older siblings of the experimental infants for whom pre-intervention test scores were available. Data for all three groups were collected within a three-year period. Evaluation of the program was again based upon pre- and post-test measures on the Stanford-Binet and the ITPA.

Results indicated that for the matched control comparison group, the experimental group was superior on both standardized measures. The experimental group scored 16 points above the controls and 28 points above their siblings on IQ. On the ITPA, the scores for the experimental infants were normal whereas the scores showed a six-month delay for the matched controls and a seven-month discrepancy for the sibling controls (45). On the basis of these data, the parent-centered approach employed in the Karnes project appears to be effective. Unfortunately, no long-term data on the retention of cognitive gains were available for this project, making any statements about its long-term effectiveness impossible.

In contrast to the group meeting procedure for introducing teaching strategies and stimulus materials employed by the Karnes project, Levenstein's intervention program involved semi-weekly home visits by a Toy Demonstrator who modeled play techniques with toys and books called the Verbal Interaction Stimulus Materials (VISM). Toys and books were chosen for their abilities to elicit verbal, cognitive, and motor components of mother-child play. Initially known as Project Verbal Interaction, the program was implemented with five control and six experimental lower-class black mother-child pairs. The subjects were paired on their initial scores on the Peabody Picture Vocabulary Test (PPVT) and were then randomly assigned to experimental and control groups. The intervention consisted of 15 home visits of approximately one-half hour in length over a four-month period. The control group received no contact except for a single home visit. Post-test PPVT scores indicated that the average increase among the experimental subjects was 13.7 points, whereas a mean loss of .4 was demonstrated by the control group (52).

In a broader scale investigation, Levenstein reported significant child cognitive growth as a result of the intervention with a group of 54 mother-child pairs (51). The children ranged in age from 20 to 43 months and were divided into experimental (N = 33), contact control (N = 9), and no-contact control groups (N = 12). The contact control group received approximately 24 home visits by a Toy Demonstrator who brought non-VISM toys to the home. The PPVT and either the Cattell or the Stanford-Binet Intelligence Scales were administered for pre-test and post-test measures. Results indicated that the experimental subjects gained significantly more IQ points than did either control group. On the PPVT, the experimental group scored significantly higher than the contact control group, but not significantly higher than the no-contact control group. In addition, long-term significant differences have been reported between 96 experimental dyads and 55 control dyads when the children were four to six years old. Data from the Stanford-Binet and Weschler Intelligence Scale demonstrated a linear relationship between the quantity of intervention and the follow-up IQ scores. Additional data from experimental and sibling control subjects have shown significant IQ differences favoring the treated children (55). On the basis of the longitudinal data already reported, it appears as though the complete two-year treatment program has been effective in that cognitive gains have been maintained at least into the first grade.

Parent- and Child-Centered Intervention Programs

Two programs which exemplify early intervention programs which combined home visits with parents and center-based stimulation for infants and young children are the Florida Parent Education Infant and Toddler Program (29-33, 35) and the Family Development Research Program (49).

The services provided to lower socioeconomic, culturally disadvantaged families by the Florida Parent Education Infant and Toddler Program consisted of weekly home visits by a paraprofessional and small group experiences twice weekly for children aged two and older. During each weekly visit, the parent educator would introduce a new activity, demonstrate it with the child, and then observe the mother teach the activity. The curriculum included Piagetian tasks from the Uzgiris-Hunt Scales (92), items from the Gesell, Cattell, and Bayley Scales of Infant Development (BSID), and stories of various folklore origins (29, 32). Small group experience was added to the program's services for the older children. It was expected that the children would gain from increased exposure to expressive and productive language activities and would demonstrate overall increments in intellectual performance. It was hoped that parents would both increase the amount of verbal interaction with their children and experience a heightened sense of self-esteem and internal control.

Initially, children were randomly assigned to experimental and control groups. Then, in the second year of the program, one-half of the original experimental group was randomly assigned to a new control group. In the third year of the project, one-half of the children in each group were randomly assigned to the experimental group and one-half were randomly assigned to a control group. New families were also recruited for program participation. Therefore, the effects of both quantity and timing of interventive stimulation could be evaluated. At the end of the first year, the Griffiths Scale was used to assess infant functioning; other assessments given at yearly intervals included a series of tests designed specifically for the project, the BSID, the PPVT, the Stanford-Binet Intelligence Test, and the Caldwell Preschool Inventory (14).

At the 12-month testing, infants whose mothers had been trained in the stimulation activities scored higher on the Griffiths Scales and on the series of tests than did the matched control infants (30). Further longitudinal testing when the children were five, six, and eight and a half years old confirmed the positive effects of this early intervention. Program success was reflected in such measures as standardized test scores and academic progress of the children. Significantly fewer of the experimental children were referred to classes for the educable mentally retarded relative to the control subjects (35).

The impact of this parent education program upon the young child's intellectual functioning and school placement can be largely attributed to the impact made upon familial atmosphere, attitudes, and aspirations. In addition, the data indicate that the timing, the quantity, and the consistency of the parent intervention were major variables. Gordon, Guinagh, and Jester have concluded that ". . .the earlier, the better; the longer, the better; and the more consistent, the better" (33, p. 116).

A second parent- and child-oriented stimulation program was the Family Development Research Program (49). This project was aimed towards those families whose annual income was at poverty level. Weekly home visits by a paraprofessional were made to both expectant mothers and mothers with children in the program. During home visits, the home visitor introduced curriculum materials to the family and stimulated total parental involvement in the program. Parent-centered goals included increments in awareness of health and nutritional needs of children, increased involvement in the course of child development, and enhanced family cohesiveness.

The center-based child-centered stimulation program consisted of three levels based on infant age. The Infant-Fold Center activities were designed for infants six to 15 months of age. Half-day sessions were conducted at the center with a ratio of four infants to one teacher. Piagetian (59) and Erik-sonian (19) influences were incorporated into the infant curricula, which emphasized the development of prehension skills, object permanence, means-end relationships, and sensory experiences. When the children were 18-48 months old, a family style program was implemented in which multi-age infants interacted with each other and with a number of adults. Parents were invited to attend the center and to participate in the ongoing activities.

At age six months, 40 experimental infants scored significantly higher on the Cattell Infant Scale than did 46 no-contact control subjects. However, these IQ differences were not apparent at age 12 months. Twelve-month-old experimental subjects performed significantly better on Piagetian object permanence tasks than did controls. However, these tasks were inherent in the curricula; therefore, apparent intervention success in these abilities could be attributed to training of test-appropriate behaviors. At 36 months, 93 percent of the experimental children were functioning within the average or above average level of intelligence on the Stanford-Binet whereas only 74.4 percent of the control group children were functioning at this level. At 36 months, no significant differences were reported on the ITPA. Assessments of personal-social behaviors with a variety of rating scales and scores from the Inventory of Home Stimulation indicated differences favoring the experimental families.

Child-Centered Intervention Programs

The four child-centered programs selected for inclusion in this chapter have employed an approach to infant stimulation that is very different in focus from those previously presented. Rather than using the parents as teachers, the child-centered approach uses trained personnel to work directly with the infant. Two of these programs, those of Painter (56) and Schaefer and Aaronson (77), have provided structured child tutorial sessions in the home. The Milwaukee Project (25) and the Carolina Abecedarian Project (64) remove the infant from the home for several hours a day and provide a curriculum at an established intervention site. None of these programs includes the infant's parents as integral members of the child's education.

Painter's program was designed as preventive intervention for culturally disadvantaged infants (56). Primary program goals were the acceleration of cognitive and language development. Daily home visits five days per week were provided by tutors for one year. Control subjects from the same population received pre-test and post-test evaluations but no other contact throughout the year. Pre-tests on the Uzgiris-Hunt Scales (92) and other assessments indicated the need for language, symbolic representation, and concept formation enhancement. The intensive tutorial program primarily emphasized the training of language abilities and conceptual understanding.

The subjects of the study were 30 infants between the ages of eight and 24 months whose Cattell scores fell between 80 and 120. Data on 20 of the 30 subjects, 10 experimental and 10 control subjects, were available. Post-test evaluations were made with the Stanford-Binet, the ITPA, conceptual subtests of the Merrill-Palmer Scale of Mental Tests, and other measurements selected specifically for this project. Post-test scores on the Stanford-Binet revealed significantly higher IQ scores for the experimental than for the control subjects; however, only singular subtests of the ITPA and the Merrill-Palmer Scales revealed any group differences. The durability of these higher IQ scores was unknown as no longitudinal data were available on the long-term effects of the tutorial approach.

A more intensive child-centered tutorial program was the Infant Education Research Project (77). This project focused upon home tutoring of infants aged 15-36 months who were members of economically depressed, culturally deprived families. Tutors provided daily weekday visits of one hour when the children were 15-36 months old. Tutoring activities stressed the stimulation of gross and fine motor, sensory, language and cultural experiences. Control subjects from the same population received regular assessments of developmental performance, but no tutoring.

Standardized intelligence tests and scales (Bayley, Stanford-Binet, and PPVT) were administered when the children were 14, 21, 27 and 36 months old. The Infant Behavior Record of the Bayley was also completed for each child. Follow-up tests when the children were four, five, and six years of age have been completed.

At 36 months, the tutored group had attained a Stanford-Binet IQ score of 106; in contrast, the control group was maintaining a relatively stable score of 90 between 21 and 36 months. Significant differences between groups were also obtained from measures of the PPVT and Bayley Infant Behavior Record. Follow-up scores on the Stanford-Binet indicated that only small, insignificant differences were obtained at age six, and that by the end of the first grade no group differences existed.

Ratings of aspects of maternal behaviors with the Maternal Behavior Research Instrument (79) and the Maternal Behaviors with Tutor and Child Inventory (78) were correlated with child behaviors and level of intellectual functioning. Additive effects of these variables were evidenced in that those children who scored highest on the intelligence measures had received tutoring and had experienced positive relationships with their mothers. Schaefer and Aaronson attributed the failure of retention effects to the lack of emphasis upon parental involvement and stressed the need for earlier and continued intervention with the inclusion of parental involvement (77).

Two large-scale projects which have employed primarily child-focused, center-based curriculum have been in progress in the United States since the early seventies. The goal of these centers, like that of other intervention programs, is to intervene with infants who are at high risk for cultural-familial retardation and to prevent the lags in cognitive and intellectual functioning all too frequently observed in these children as they develop.

One of the most extensive and successful of these programs is the Milwaukee Project of Garber and Heber (24, 25, 26). Garber and Heber have determined that a maternal IQ of less than 80 is highly correlated with subsequent mental retardation in offspring; thus 20 infants have been selected for inclusion in this program on the basis of low maternal IQ (25). The program combines vocational rehabilitation for mothers with an intensive infant instructional package beginning at age six months.

For the first six months of the curriculum, the infant spent eight hours a day with a specific caregiver at the center. This caregiver was responsible for only one infant and met caretaking needs, taught a prescribed series of activities, and evaluated the infant's progress. As the child became older, greater exposure to other teachers and children was instituted. At all age levels structured learning tasks were provided for the child. Emphasis was placed upon the development of language, cognition, and motivation and upon the application of these abilities in several contexts (25). Results from extensive assessment of children enrolled in the program and a matched sample of control children indicated superior functioning on several measures from as early as 14 months (24, 25, 26). Language differences as measured by the Gesell Developmental Scales appeared at 14-18 months and continued throughout the program. As early as age three years, some of the measures of language facility indicated a two-year superiority for the experimental infants. On problem-solving tasks, the performance of the intervention group tended to be more rapid and successful; a number of systematic problem-solving strategies were also in evidence, whereas the control children tended to approach tasks more haphazardly. IQ scores assessed with the Stanford-Binet indicated the most impressive gains: The experimental infants scored 10 points higher at 18 months, 34 points higher at 72 months, and approximately 20 points higher at 96 months of age. Many of the control children whose scores continued to decline with age were classified as borderline retarded by the end of the assessment period. Older siblings of the experimental subjects also showed continual decline in IQ scores with increasing age.

The results of this study are impressive. Intensive one-to-one teacher-infant interaction during the first year of life, coupled with a structured learning environment until the child reached school-age, successfully prevented the onset of delays in intellectual and cognitive functioning. Although successful in the exploratory stage, one of the more serious drawbacks of this program is economic. The one-on-one interaction that appears central to this approach would be tremendously expensive unless provisions could be made to utilize mothers of other children in the program to defray some of the cost. While this program has proven to be highly successful in meeting its goals, its usefulness on a widespread basis is questionable.

Another program that has reported successful prevention of decrements in intellectual functioning in high-risk infants is the Carolina Abecedarian Project (64). A current sample of 100 experimental and control infants and children are participating in the program. Selection for inclusion in the program was based upon the High Risk Index (67) which assessed a number of factors such as parental educational level, family income, and retardation in siblings, all of which are correlated with cultural-familial retardation. Infants in the intervention program were matched with control infants on the basis of this index as well as age and sex. Both groups of infants were provided with social welfare services, nutritional supplements and medical care (65). These services were included both as incentives for participation and as controls for these variables in assessing the effectiveness of the curriculum.

Infants began participation in the center-based program when they were six to 12 weeks of age. They attended the center eight hours a day, five days a week. The curriculum goals were designed in the hopes of meeting the complex needs of a high-risk population. With both professional and paraprofessional personnel, the program maintained a four-to-one infant to teacher ratio during the first three years. Using a Piagetian-based curriculum for instruction, coupled with eclectic theoretical approaches to teaching infant adaptive skills, the program emphasized the development of perceptual-cognitive abilities, physical-motor growth, language skills, and social competencies.

Scores on the BSID did not discriminate between the two groups at six and 12 months, but the 18-month test revealed significant decrements among the control infants while the experimental infants maintained normal levels of functioning. Stanford-Binet scores indicated a 10-point superiority for program infants at age 24 months and a 15-point superiority at 36 months. Measures of language ability suggested that the experimental infants had significantly advanced language skills by 30 months (15). Measures of skills related to cognitive and perceptual development also indicated better performances by the experimental infants (66). Assessments of mother-infant interaction indicated no evidence of disruption of the dyadic relationship for these infants who were absent from the home 40 hours per week.

The Carolina Abecedarian Project, like the Milwaukee Project, is still in its exploratory phase. The results of the program to date are promising. Long-term follow-up of these infants and their families will be necessary, however, to assess the long-range effectiveness of programs such as these for preventing developmental declines in high-risk populations (64).

INTERVENTION WITH INFANTS CLASSIFIED AS REPRODUCTIVE CASUALTIES

The intervention research with infants who have been classified as reproductive casualties can be divided into two broad categories: that research conducted with sick, premature or small-for-date infants, and that research conducted with infants who are biologically, physically, and/or mentally handicapped.

Intervention with Sick, Premature and/or Small-for-Date Infants

The sick, premature and/or small-for-date infant experiences an environment in which the types and levels of stimulation are extremely different from those experienced by the healthy, full-term neonate. The medical procedures that must be instituted to insure the survival of these infants mandate these unusual surroundings. Since these infants are already at risk for normal development because of their physical condition, a number of investigators have been concerned that the abnormal stimulation to which these infants are exposed may be contributing further to their subsequent delays in development.

In the late 1960s and early 1970s, a number of reports substantiated the poor developmental prognosis of low-birthweight infants, reporting lower intellectual functioning, delayed motor development, and a myriad of other problems, including language impairment and behavior problems (11,16,70,95,96). While recent reports on developmental outcome have been more optimistic (57,71,91), a great deal of concern still exists about the potentially harmful effects of the long-term intensive care hospitalization that is requisite for survival with this high-risk population. It is not known to what extent reported impairment can be attributed to low birthweight *per se*, and how much can be attributed to environmental factors. Little work has been reported on the effectiveness of providing this population with the types of stimulation experienced by the normal newborn. However, explorations into this area suggest that this may be a promising approach in enhancing positive developmental prognoses.

A number of studies have demonstrated positive effects of the addition of a single type of stimulation to the environment. Katz provided infants born at 28 to 32 weeks gestational age with a tape recording of the mother's voice for 30 minutes daily from the fifth day after birth until the child reached 252 days gestational age. He reported advanced visual, auditory and motor capabilities in this group relative to a control group of similar infants who experienced routine intensive care procedures (46).

A number of investigations have manipulated tactile and kinesthetic stimulation to enhance normal development. Solkoff, Yaffe, Weintraub, and Blase instituted a program whereby five premature infants were given body rubs for five minutes every hour for 10 days. Compared to five control infants, the stimulated newborns showed more rapid weight gain and a higher activity level. While no differences between the two groups were present at six weeks of age, a follow-up assessment eight months after hospital discharge indicated normal, healthy development in all the stimulated infants, and normal development in only one of the five non-stimulated infants (85). Using a similar stimulation procedure, White and LaBarba reported significantly greater weight gains and higher levels of formula intake in a group of six healthy prematures who were provided with tactile stimulation for an hour a day for nine days in comparison with non-stimulated controls (94). Rice taught mothers of 15 premature infants to stroke, massage, and rock their infants in a carefully prescribed manner for 80 minutes a day for the first 30 days the infant was home from the hospital. When the infants were four months of age, the stimulated children showed significantly higher weight gains, stronger reflexes, and high scores on the mental subscale of the Bayley Scales of Infant Development than a matched sample of non-stimulated infants (69).

Powell has further demonstrated the effectiveness of maternal handling and stimulation. In this study of prematures weighing between 1000 and 2000 grams, 24 infants were handled by their mothers and the nursery staff 40 minutes a day until they regained their birthweight and then 20 minutes daily until discharged from the hospital. A second group of 12 infants was not provided with this special handling. Handled infants regained their birthweights more rapidly than non-handled infants, but there were no measurable differences in weight or height at two, four, and six months of age. On the Bayley Scales, significant differences were found favoring the stimulated group at four months on both the mental and motor scales, and at six months on the social behavior record (62).

Two studies have attempted to provide the infant in intensive care with stimulation in a number of sensory modalities. In a pilot study, Wright provided five premature infants with 21 days of eight daily periods of kinesthetic, auditory, tactile and visual stimulation. The stimulated infants gained less weight than the non-stimulated controls, produced less glucocorticoid material, and exhibited stronger rooting reflexes. While the results of this study are far from conclusive, they do suggest that stimulation may be effective (97).

By far the most impressive example of the effectiveness of environmental stimulation on the development of the premature infant is the work of Scarr-Salapatek and Williams. Their stimulation program was begun in the hospital at the end of the infant's first week of life and was continued through the end of the first year. The 15 stimulated infants, who weighed between 1300 and 1800 grams at birth, were provided with auditory, visual and tactile stimulation that was designed to simulate that found in the home as experienced by the healthy newborn. The infants were also removed from the isolette or incubator for eight 30-minute stimulation sessions daily. After six weeks of this stimulation, measures indicated superiority in comparison to the no-treatment controls on amount of weight gained, as well as in reflexive and behavioral development. After these infants were discharged from the hospital, a home-based program was initiated in which the mothers received weekly training sessions on specific activities designed to aid cognitive growth. At the end of the first year, stimulated infants tested significantly higher than the controls on the Cattell Infant Intelligence Scale. This program illustrates the importance of long-term stimulation for premature or sick newborns (75).

While these attempts at systematically stimulating infants who are reproductive casualties because of low birth weight are too diverse to provide conclusive data, they are provocative. With increasingly large numbers of premature infants surviving due to recent advances in medical care, it is crucial that the cognitive and mental development of these infants also be taken into consideration. It appears likely that developmental outcome can be promoted by altering the types of stimulation typically found in newborn intensive care settings to match more closely those to which healthy, full-term infants are exposed.

Intervention with Infants Having Special Handicaps

Early intervention programs with infants and young children who have special handicaps and problems are designed to enhance specific behaviors and developmental processes considered to be at risk for severe delay because of the nature of the handicaps. Selma Fraiberg and associates have been extensively involved with the study of the development of blind infants (21,22,23). Longitudinal work with these children has indicated that blindness often results in complications with adaptive behaviors, gross motor functioning, conceptualization of body and self-image, and intellectual retardation. In addition, the provision of facilitation of parent-infant attachment is often necessary with children with special handicaps, particularly blind infants who lack the capacity to participate in the early social visual communication system which plays such an important role in early parent-infant interaction (21).

The approach of Fraiberg's intervention project was largely parent-centered. Services included home visits made by professionals twice monthly during which time mothers and infants were observed in interaction. De-Carie's Objectal Scale (18) was used to compare blind infant-mother pairs with sighted infant-mother pairs on human object relations and social communication skills. The most important aspect of the intervention was the enhancement of maternal sensitivity to her blind infant's cues and signals which may have been too different from those expected or too subtle for her to read without help. Special emphases were given to aspects of social communicative capacities, use of hands for environmental exploration and communication, coordination of reaching with auditory signals (i.e., ear-hand coordination) and development of locomotor abilities. Reports of case studies indicate the effectiveness of this approach in facilitation of blind infant-mother communication and infant developmental performance (22).

A very special intervention program for hearing-impaired infants and children has been conducted at the Bill Wilkerson Hearing and Speech Center (38). The program has emphasized early detection of and immediate intervention for hearing impairments. These include provision of appropriate amplification equipment and special training for development of residual hearing capacities.

Subjects for this program were infants and young children who had hearing impairments but very few of whom were completely deaf. With amplification equipment, development of residual hearing capacities, and speech reading intervention, these children were taught to adjust to their problem without retardation or language deficits. Infant intervention through parent education was a major thrust of the intervention program which involved parent, infant and staff attendance in a model home environment. In this environment, teachers modeled appropriate stimulation exercises which parents could implement in the course of everyday activities. The Teaching Home was attended by infants aged one month to three years and their parents. In addition to this form of parent-child centered intervention, the program also included an acoustic preschool for children aged three to six years. The preschool consisted of child-centered classes which were attended by nonhearing-impaired children as well as the hearing-impaired children.

As a test of program effectiveness, Liff compared the spoken language abilities of a group of children who had attended the Training Home (median age, two years, three months) with hearing-impaired children who had attended the preschool classes but not the infant program and also with hearing children who were of average achievement level (53). Analyses of utterance complexity indicated that the children who had experienced only preschool intervention scored significantly lower than both the hearing-impaired children who had infant intervention and the hearing children. Longitudinal assessments of school performance indicated that normal, hearing second graders and early intervention hearing-impaired children were relatively equivalent on verbal aspects of the Metropolitan Achievement Test (MAT); however, mathematical subtests differentiated the two groups, with the hearing children scoring significantly higher. Nevertheless, considering the data which indicate that children with severe hearing impairments are often approximately four years retarded, the effectiveness of the early detection and intervention of this program is encouraging.

As victims of the most prevalent kind of severe mental retardation, Down's syndrome infants and young children require special early intervention attention (89). Hayden and Haring have described an early intervention program specifically designed for infants with Down's syndrome which incorporates parental involvement and parent-child-centered classes (36). The primary goal of the program was the acceleration of general development to normal level. The early intervention aspects of the program included Infant Learning Classes for infants aged five to 18 months and Early Preschool Classes for children aged 18 months to three years. Parent training involved group meetings in which teachers modeled exercises appropriate for stimulation of various aspects of development.

The Infant Learning Classes involved parent and infant attendance at weekly meetings in which training sessions for motor and cognitive development were conducted. Positive reinforcement for the attainment of behavioral goals based upon items from the Gesell norms and the Denver Developmental Screening Test was featured in the program. Repeated testings on the Gesell tasks, the Denver Screening Test, and a special checklist of Down's syndrome norms indicated little discrepancy between chronological age and mental age on the Gesell Preliminary Behavioral Inventory. However, since items were drawn directly from the Gesell checklists, these successes could be attributed to direct training of test-appropriate behaviors rather than truly enhanced developmental level.

The Preschool Classes were designed to train parents in more activities for stimulation of language and concept development, self-help skills, and more mature motor functioning. Data from those children who were enrolled only in Preschool Classes indicated the significance of early intervention. Longitudinal research is currently being conducted with these Down's syndrome infants (36).

The Portage Project presented by Shearer and Shearer was an intervention project for infants and young children handicapped in one or more developmental areas (81). In addition to multiple handicaps, project admission was based upon screening scores on a variety of abilities as assessed by the Alpern-Boll Developmental Profile (1). The Portage Project relied heavily upon parental administration of intervention. Assigned to each family was a home teacher who discussed weekly activities to be practiced by the mother-child pairs during the week. Behavioral objectives were constructed weekly, and the home visitor took pre- and post-test measurements of the infant's performance on the specific behaviors.

Cattell and Stanford-Binet measurements were available on the 75 children who were participating in the project. The average gain in mental age made by those children in an eight-month period was 15 months. A study comparing children from the Portage Project with children attending preschool classes for the culturally disadvantaged indicated significantly greater gains in mental age and IQ for the Portage Project children than for the other children. However, differences in the specific deficits, initial levels of functioning, and types of intervention-trained behaviors existed between these two samples. Shearer and Shearer, using the Portage Project children as their own controls, have reported a significant average gain of 18.3 points as assessed by the Stanford-Binet Intelligence Test (81).

Barrera and associates have described an early intervention project with biologically handicapped infants and young children that involved primarily center-based instruction (5). The typical child in the program was approximately 18 months old, with biologically-based severe to moderate retardation in several areas of functioning; there was, however, extreme variance in the cases described.

The intervention setting consisted of a nursery room to which the children came twice weekly for intervention treatment in three of five areas of depressed functioning. The area of greatest deficit was treated according to clinical recommendations. Two of the remaining depressed areas did not receive treatment. In addition to this center-based work with the child, parents were involved in meetings with social workers designed to introduce new activities and to enhance personal growth.

Significant differences between progress on the randomly selected areas in comparison to that on the clinically prescribed area and between progress on the clinically prescribed area in comparison to that on the no-treatment (control) areas were demonstrated. However, the comparison between progress on randomly selected treatment areas and the control area revealed no significant difference. The implementation of a within-subject control design is an improvement upon the use of no-contact control to which comparisons are made for analysis of program effectiveness; this methodology should be expanded to other intervention programs.

Clearly, the themes of family- and parent-centered intervention are predominant throughout this summary of special types of early intervention programs. Parental involvement is not only a more realistic, economical approach to intervention, but also perhaps a more critical feature of the delivery of intervention treatment to children with special problems. These parent-infant relationships may already be at risk because of difficulty of mutual adjustments enhanced by the child's special handicaps (4,34). The necessity for early diagnosis of special problems followed by early family-centered intervention is highlighted by these representative projects.

IMPLICATIONS AND FUTURE DIRECTIONS

The results of these various stimulation programs are provocative. It is evident that the course of developmental outcome can be altered through environmental intervention. These studies have indicated that the intellectual functioning of young children at risk because of inadequate stimulation can be maintained at normal levels, and in some cases, accelerated; that certain types of stimulation are related to weight gains in premature infants, and intensive stimulation of premature infants is correlated with enhancement of normal intellectual development; and that stimulation provided for children with a wide variety of handicaps is beneficial in promoting normal levels of functioning in many behavioral areas. While all the projects reviewed in this chapter strongly suggest the important of widespread implementation of preventive stimulation for at-risk infants, we would like to suggest that clinicians proceed with caution in initiating similar programs. There are *methodological, ecological* and *ethical* issues that warrant consideration before such programs are generally instituted.

Methodological Considerations

A question central to the implementation of these programs is the reliability of the results reported. One of the most prominent weaknesses with all the programs discussed in this chapter is that the evaluations of program effectiveness were designed and implemented as part of the project itself. No outside evaluations were available. The strengths of the results obtained would be greatly enhanced by the inclusion of evaluation data from agents who had no direct investment in the outcome or continuation of the program.

A second methodological problem involves the measurements used to assess the subjects' development. One issue involves the tests employed. While most studies used well-known measures of intelligence such as the Bayley Scales of Infant Development or the Stanford-Binet, other areas of developmental functioning were frequently assessed with far more obscure measures or, in many cases, measures designed specifically for a given project. These unfamiliar measures make outside interpretation of development in areas other than intellectual functioning difficult. It is crucial that the intervention promote all aspects of the child's development, not just the cognitive and intellectual. On the basis of much of the data reported, it is difficult to draw any firm conclusions concerning the enhancement of overall development. A second problem of measurement concerns the repeated testing of the children with the same instruments. It is possible that some of the gains reported have been influenced by the children's increasing familiarity with the tests and the testing situation. While comparison groups of no-intervention children have been included in most projects to control for this possibility, it is conceivable that experimental children were more frequently exposed to the appropriate materials and responses than were controls. Some projects even employed the teaching of standardized test items as part of the curriculum (36,49). The validity of scores obtained under these circumstances is questionable.

Use of inadequate control groups is another methodological flaw present in some of these programs. In order to fully assess the effectiveness of any intervention strategy, adequate control groups must be employed. While most of these projects have included no-treatment comparison children in the design, some projects have used more sophisticated control procedures that provide the basis for a better understanding of the effectiveness of the treatment. The Carolina Abecedarian Project provided control subjects with medical care and nutritional supplements. This controlled for the possibility that the superiority of the treatment group was based solely on their better physical condition (64,67). The inclusion of two control groups in addition to the standard no-contact group in the Mother-Child Home Project also provided stronger data on which to evaluate the effectiveness of the intervention. To insure that group differences were not based merely on contact with the family, weekly contact was made with control group families who were not provided with the curriculum materials and instructions. In addition, analysis of the developmental progress of older siblings who were evaluated prior to the start of the intervention with the target child controlled for possible differences inherent in the experimental families (51,52,55). Examination of control measures is strongly suggested when evaluating the effectiveness of an intervention strategy. Significant differences between treatment and no-treatment groups need to be carefully scrutinized in light of the control measures employed.

Ecological Considerations

The infant is engaged in a continual process of transaction with the components of the environment (72). One of the variables critical to the success of programs such as those presented in this chapter is a complete understanding of the interrelationship between the infant and these many environmental components. A complete analysis of the environmental factors that may be affecting the child, in combination with a program designed to alter the effective portions of the environment, is a requisite for successful intervention.

The intervention done with premature infants has suffered greatly from the lack of ecological analysis (17). Most of the programs implemented extra stimulation without prior analysis of the amount or types of stimulation that might be critical in the development of high-risk newborns. The notion that hospital surroundings are stimulus-deprived has been questioned by Lawson and associates, who have performed an ecological analysis of the environment of the intensive care nursery. Their data indicate that the environment of the sick newborn contains a variety of stimulation in most of the sensory modalities, but that the patterning of this stimulation differs from that found in a home environment (50). For effective intervention with prematures to be undertaken, a more complete understanding of both the premature and its environment is mandatory. The exploratory studies reported here are a beginning, but much refinement is needed before these types of programs can be instituted on a widespread basis. With increasingly large numbers of very small infants surviving, this area of investigation is urgent.

A second area of ecological validity that needs further investigation involves the stimulation programs done with children classified as caretaker casualties (12). In most of the programs developed to encourage normal development, the infant has been the primary target of the intervention. In order to obtain maximum effectiveness, however, the child's environment must be altered, rather than trying merely to alter the child. The long-term stability and durability of change reported by such programs as the Mother-Child Home Project (51,52,55) and the Florida Parent Education Infant and Toddler Program (33) can likely be attributed to the inclusion of the family in the intervention. Unless the child's primary caregiver is the ultimate source of stimulation for the child, the termination of the program may signal an end to the child's continued normal development. Schaefer and Aaronson (78) attributed much of the failure of the long-term effectiveness of their program to lack of involvement by the mother. Emphasis on employing the mother and family as primary agents of change should be central in initiating any programs designed to intervene with infants and children at risk for developmental delay (2,28,42).

Ethical Considerations

The ethical issue of primary importance in initiating these types of programs concerns the families of the children who are the targets for the stimulation. It is critical to the well-being of the child and the family that the child be viewed as a member of a functioning social unit. Treating the child in isolation could have serious negative consequences for all the members of the familial unit. The disruption of this integral part of the child's life will likely do far greater harm to the child's development than could be offset by providing high levels of intellectual stimulation in an attempt to insure academic success. Programs must be designed so that the family unit, rather than a single child, is the target for intervention. The detrimental effects of isolating the child from this all-important social unit may cause irreparable harm for all members concerned.

A second issue for ethical consideration is the attitude of the directors and workers involved with the families and children served by these programs. It is crucial that respect for the familial and cultural traditions of these families be maintained. The goals of these intervention projects should be to provide the families with the support and information they require to provide positive environments for their children; the goals should not include alteration of the values and moral beliefs of the families (88). Intervention programs should have as their sole purpose the enhancement of infant and child development within a family context. Tampering with the culture and social structure of these families could have very dangerous consequences for both the individual families involved and the society at large.

Future Directions

While these projects have contributed greatly to the data base on the effectiveness of environmental intervention, there is still a great deal of research that needs to be undertaken before any firm conclusions concerning the effects of these programs can be drawn.

An area of primary importance is the investigation of the effects the participation of a child in the program has on the other family members. Some work has been reported from the Carolina Abecedarian Project which suggests that mother-child relationships are not disrupted by center-based intervention (67). This relationship is primary in the child's development, and more extensive investigation of any changes or alterations that may occur because of this intervention is needed. Other family members, especially the child's siblings, may also be affected by the child's participation. Positive and negative consequences on other members of the familial unit require study.

Most of the stimulation projects reviewed here have placed primary emphasis on enhancing the child's intellectual and cognitive capabilities. Future programs should focus upon promotion of all aspects of development, rather than just upon those which will affect academic progress. Focusing upon only this single aspect of the child's development to the exclusion of the others is a great disservice to the child.

Our children are our most important natural resource. Every attempt must be made to provide *all* of our children and their families with firm foundations for optimal intellectual and socio-emotional functioning. Widespread implementation of such programs will have strong positive consequences not only for the individuals involved but also for society as a whole.

REFERENCES

1. ALPERN, G. and BOLL T. 1972. *Developmental Profile*. Indianapolis: Psychological Development Publication.
2. AMBRON, S. R. 1977. A review and analysis of infant and parent education programs. In: M. C. Day and R. K. Parker (Eds.), *The Preschool in Action*. Boston: Allyn & Bacon.
3. APPLETON, T., CLIFTON, R. and GOLDBERG, S. 1975. The development of behavioral competence in infancy. In: F. D. Horowitz (Ed.), *Review of Child Development Research*. Chicago: University of Chicago Press.
4. BARNARD, K. E. 1976. Nursing: High risk infants. In: T.D. Tjossem, (Ed.), *Intervention Strategies for High Risk Infants and Young Children*. Baltimore: University Park Press.
5. BARRERA, M. E. C., ROUTH, D. K., PAIR, C. A., JOHNSON, N., ARENDSHORST, D., GOOLSBY, E. L., and SCHROEDER, S. R. 1976. Early intervention with biologically handicapped infants and young children: A preliminary study with each child as his own control. In: T. D. Tjossem, (Ed.), *Intervention Strategies for High Risk Infants and Young Children*. Baltimore: University Park Press.
6. BAYLEY, N. 1965. Comparisons of mental and motor test scores for ages 1-15 months by sex, birth order, race, geographical location, and education of parents. *Child Dev.*, *36*, 397.
7. BELL, S. M. and AINSWORTH, M. D. S. 1972. Infant crying and maternal responsiveness. *Child Dev.*, *43*, 1171.
8. BERLYNE, D. E. 1958. The influence of albedo and complexity of stimuli on visual fixation in the human infant. *Br. J. Psychol.*, *49*, 315.
9. BLOOM, B. S. 1964. *Stability and Change in Human Characteristics*. New York: Wiley.
10. BOWLBY, J. 1969. *Attachment and Loss*. London: Hogarth Press and Institute of Psychoanalysis.
11. BRAINE, M. D. S., HEIMER, C. B., WORTIS, H. and FREEDMAN, A. M. 1966. Factors associated with the impairment of the early development of prematures. *Monogr. Soc. Res. Child Dev.*, *31*, No. 106.
12. BRONFENBRENNER, U. 1974. Is early intervention effective? A report on longitudinal evaluations of preschool programs. Washington, D. C.: Department of Health, Education, and Welfare, Office of Child Development.
13. BROUSSARD, E. and HARTNER, M.S. S. 1971. Further considerations regarding material perception of the first born. In: J. Hellmuth (Ed.), *Exceptional Infant, Vol. 2.: Studies in Abnormalities*. New York: Brunner/Mazel.
14. CALDWELL, B. M., HEIDER, J. and KAPLAN, B. 1966. The inventory of home stimulation. Paper presented at the meeting of the American Psychological Association. New York.
15. CAMPBELL, F. and RAMEY, C. 1977. The effects of early intervention on intellectual development. Paper presented at the biennial meeting of the Society for Research in Child Development. New Orleans, Louisiana.
16. CAPUTO, D. V. and MANDELL, W. 1970. Consequences of low birth weight. *Dev. Psychol.*, *3*, 363.
17. CORNELL, E. H. and GOTTFRIED, A. W. 1976. Intervention with premature human infants. *Child Dev.*, *47*, 32.
18. DeCARIE, T. G. 1963. *Intelligence and Affectivity in Early Childhood*. New York: International Universities Press.
19. ERIKSON, E. 1950. *Childhood and Society*. New York: W. W. Norton.
20. FANTZ, R. L. 1958. Pattern vision in young infants. *Psychol. Rec.*, *8*, 43.
21. FRAIBERG, S. 1974. Blind infants and their mothers: An examination of the sign system. In: M. Lewis and L. Rosenblum (Eds.), *The Effect of the Infant on its Caregiver*. New York: Wiley.

22. FRAIBERG, S. 1976. Intervention in infancy: A program for blind infants. In: E. Rexford, L. Sander, and T. Shapiro (Eds.), *Infant Psychiatry: A New Synthesis*. New Haven: Yale University Press.
23. FRAIBERG, S., SMITH, M. and ADELSON, M.A. 1969. An educational program for blind infants. *J. Spec. Educ.*, 3, 121.
24. GARBER, H. 1975. Intervention in infancy: A developmental approach. In: M. Begab and S. Richardson (Eds.), *The Mentally Retarded and Society: A Social Science Perspective*. Baltimore: University Park Press.
25. GARBER, H. and HEBER, R. 1977. The Milwaukee Project: Early intervention as a technique to prevent mental retardation. In: E. M. Hetherington, and R. D. Parke, (Eds.), *Contemporary Readings in Child Psychology*. New York: McGraw-Hill.
26. GARBER, H. and HEBER, R. 1977. The Milwaukee Project: Indication of the effectiveness of early intervention in preventing mental retardation. In: P. Mittler (Ed.), *Research to Practice in Mental Retardation Vol I: Care and Intervention*. Baltimore: University Park Press.
27. GOLDEN, M. and BIRNS, B. 1976. Social class and infant intelligence. In: M. Lewis (Ed.), *Origins of Intelligence: Infancy and Early Childhood*. New York: Plenum Press.
28. GOODSON, B. D. and HESS, R. D. 1975. Parents as teachers of young children: An evaluative review of some contemporary concepts and programs. Stanford University.
29. GORDON, I. J. 1970. *Baby Learning Through Baby Play*. New York: St. Martin's Press.
30. GORDON, I. J. 1973. Early child stimulation through parent education. In: L. Stone, H. Smith, and L. Murphy (Eds.), *The Competent Infant*. New York: Basic Books.
31. GORDON, I. J. and GUINAGH, B. J. 1974. A home learning center approach to early stimulation. Final report (on Grant No. 5 RPI MHI 6037-06) to National Institute of Mental Health, Department of Health, Education, and Welfare.
32. GORDON, I. J., GUINAGH, B. J., JESTER, R. E. and Associates (1972. *Child Learning Through Child Play*. New York: St. Martin's Press.
33. GORDON, I. J., GUINAGH, B. J. and JESTER, R. E. 1977. The Florida Parent Education Infant and Toddler Program. In: M. C. Day and R. K. Parker, (Eds.), *The Preschool in Action*. Boston: Allyn & Bacon.
34. GREENBERG, N. H. 1971. A comparison of infant-mother interactional behavior in infants with atypical behavior and normal infants. In J. Hellmuth (Ed.), *Exceptional Infant: Studies in Abnormalities*, Vol. 2. New York: Brunner/Mazel.
35. GUINAGH, B. J. and GORDON, I. J. 1976. School performance as a function of early stimulation. Final report (on Grant No. NIH-HEW-OCH-09-C-638) to Office of Child Development.
36. HAYDEN, A. H. and HARING, N. S. 1976. Early intervention for high-risk infants and young children: Programs for Down's syndrome children. In: T. D. Tjossem (Ed.), *Intervention Strategies for High Risk Infants and Young Children*. Baltimore: University Park Press.
37. HESS, E. H. 1970. Ethology and developmental psychology. In: P. H. Mussen (Ed.), *Carmichael's Manual of Child Psychology*. New York: John Wiley.
38. HORTON, K. B. 1976. Early intervention for hearing-impaired infants and young children. In: T. D. Tjossem (Ed.), *Intervention Strategies for High Risk Infants and Young Children*. Baltimore: University of Park Press.
39. HUBEL, D. H. 1967. Effects of distortion of sensory input on the visual system of kittens. *Physiologist 10*, 17.
40. HUBEL, D. H. and WIESEL, T. N. 1970. The period of susceptibility to the physiological effects of unilateral eye closure in kittens. *J. Physiology, 206*, 419.
41. INSEL, P. M. and MOOS, R. H. 1974. Psychological environments: Expanding the scope of human ecology. *Am. Psychologist, 29*, 179.
42. JOHNSON, C. A. and KATZ, R. C. 1973. Using parents as change agents for children: A review. *J. Child Psychol. Psychiat., 14*, 181.

43. KARNES, M. B. and ZEHRBACH, R. R. 1977. Educational intervention at home. In: M. C. Day and R. K. Parker (Eds.), *The Preschool in Action*. Boston: Allyn & Bacon.
44. KARNES, B. M., STUDLEY, W. M., WRIGHT, W. R. and HODGINS, A. S. 1968. An approach for working with mothers of disadvantaged preschool children. *Merrill-Palmer Quarterly, 14*, 173.
45. KARNES, M. B., TESKA, J. A., HODGINS, A. S. and BADGER, E. D. 1970. Educational intervention at home by mothers of disadvantaged infants. *Child Dev., 41*, 925.
46. KATZ, V. 1971. Auditory stimulation and developmental behavior of the premature infant. *Nurs. Res., 20*, 196.
47. KLAUS, M. H., JERAULD, R., DREGER, N. C., McALPINE, W., STEFFA, M. and KENNELL, J. H. 1972. Maternal attachment: Importance of the first postpartum days. *New Engl. J. Med., 286*, 460.
48. KRECH, D., ROSENZWEIG, M. and BENNETT, E. 1962. Relations between brain chemistry and problem-solving among rats in enriched and impoverished environments. *J. Comp. Physiol. Psychol., 55*, 801.
49. LALLY, J. R. and HONIG, A. S. 1977. The family development research program. In: M. C. Day and R. K. Parker (Eds.), *The Preschool in Action*. Boston: Allyn & Bacon.
50. LAWSON, K., DAUM, C., and TURKEWITZ, G. 1977. Environmental characteristics of a neonatal intensive care unit. *Child Dev., 48*, 1633.
51. LEVENSTEIN, P. 1970. Cognitive growth in preschoolers through verbal interaction with mothers. *Am. J. Orthopsychiat., 40*, 426.
52. LEVENSTEIN, P. and SUNLEY, R. 1968. Stimulation of verbal interaction between disadvantaged mothers and children. *Am. J. Orthopsychiat., 38*, 116.
53. LIFF, S. 1973. Early intervention and language development in hearing impaired children. Unpublished Master's Thesis, Vanderbilt University.
54. LIPSITT, L. P. 1963. Learning in the first year of life. In: L. P. Lipsitt and C. C. Spiker (Eds.), *Advances in Child Development and Behavior*. New York: Academic Press.
55. MADDEN, J., LEVENSTEIN, P. and LEVENSTEIN, S. 1976. Longitudinal outcomes of the mother-child home program. *Child Dev., 47*, 1015.
56. PAINTER, G. 1969. The effect of a structured tutorial program on the cognitive and language development of culturally disadvantaged infants. *Merrill-Palmer Quarterly, 15*, 279.
57. PAPE, K. E., BUNCIC, R. J., ASHBY, S. and FITZHARDINGE, P. M. 1968. The status at two years of low-birth-weight infants born in 1974 with birth weights of less than 1,0001 grams. *J. Pediat., 92*, 253.
58. PAPOUSEK, H. 1967. Experimental studies of appetitional behavior in human infants and newborns. In: H. W. Stevenson, E. H. Hess, and H. L. Rheingold (Eds.), *Early Behavior: Comparative and Developmental Approaches*. New York: Wiley.
59. PIAGET, J. 1952. *The Origins of Intelligence in Children*. New York: International Universities Press.
60. PIAGET, J. 1970. Piaget's theory. In: P. H. Mussen (Ed.), *Carmichael's Manual of Child Psychology*. New York: Wiley.
61. PIAGET, J. and INHELDER, B. 1969. *The Psychology of the Child*. New York: Basic Books.
62. POWELL, L. F. 1974. The effect of extra stimulation and maternal involvement on the development of low-birth-weight infants and on maternal behavior. *Child Dev., 45*, 106.
63. PROVENCE, S. and LIPTON, R. C. 1962. *Infants in Institutions*. New York: International Universities Press.
64. RAMEY, C. T. 1977. Program characteristics of the Carolina Abecedarian Project. Paper presented at the biennial meeting of the Society for Research in Child Development. New Orleans, Louisiana.
65. RAMEY, C. T. and CAMPBELL, F. A. 1977. Prevention of developmental retardation in high risk children. In: P. Mittler (Ed.), *Research to Practice in Mental Retardation: Volume I, Care and Intervention*. Baltimore: University Park Press.

66. RAMEY, C. T. and SMITH, B. J. 1977. Assessing the intellectual consequences of early intervention with high risk infants. *Am. J. Ment. Defic.*, *81*, 318.
67. RAMEY, C. T., COLLIER, A. M., SPARLING, J. J., LODA, F. A., CAMPBELL, F. A., INGRAM, D. L. and FINKELSTEIN, N. W. 1976. The Carolina Abecedarian Project: A longitudinal and multidisciplinary approach to the prevention of developmental retardation. In: T. D. Tjossem (Ed.), *Intervention Strategies for High Risk Infants and Young Children.* Baltimore: University Park Press.
68. RHEINGOLD, H. L. 1956. The modification of social responsiveness in institutional babies. *Monogr. Soc. Res. Child Dev.*, *21.*
69. RICE, R. D. 1977 Neurophysiological development in premature infants following stimulation. *Devl. Psychol.*, *13*, 69.
70. RUBIN, R. A., ROSENBLATT, C., and BALOR, B. 1973. Psychological and educational sequelae of prematurity. *Pediatrics*, *52*, 352.
71. SAINT-ANNE DARGASSIES, S. 1977. Long-term neurological follow-up study of 286 truly premature infants I: Neurological sequelae. *Devl. Med. and Child Neurol.*, *19*, 462.
72. SAMEROFF, A. J. 1975. Early influences on development: Fact or fancy: *Merrill-Palmer Quarterly*, 21, 267.
73. SAMEROFF, A. 1972. Learning and adaption in infancy: A comparison of models. In: H. W. Reese (Ed.), *Advances in Child Behavior and Development.* New York: Academic Press.
74. SAMEROFF, A. J. and CHANDLER, M. J. 1975. Perinatal risk and the continuum of caretaking casuality. In: F. D. Horowitz (Ed.), *Review of Child Development Research.* Chicago: University of Chicago Press.
75. SCARR-SALAPATEK, S. and WILLIAMS, M. 1973. The effects of early stimulation on low-birth-weight infants. *Child. Dev.*, *44*, 94.
76. SCHAEFER, E. S. 1976. Scope and focus of research relevant to intervention: A sociological perspective. In: T. D. Tjossem (Ed.), *Intervention Strategies for High Risk Infants and Young Children.* Baltimore: University Park Press.
77. SCHAEFER, E. S. and AARONSON, M. 1977. Infant educational research project: Implementation and implications of a home tutoring program. In: M. C. Day, and R. K. Parker (Eds.), *The Preschool in Action.* Boston: Allyn & Bacon.
78. SCHAEFER, E. S. and AARONSON, M. 1966. Mother's behavior with tutor and child during tutoring sessions, unpublished data.
79. SCHAEFER, E. S., BELL, R. Q. and BAYLEY, N. 1959. Development of a maternal behavior research instrument. *J. Genet. Psychol.*, *95*, 83.
80. SCHAFFER, R. 1977. *Mothering.* Cambridge: Harvard University Press.
81. SHEARER, D. E. and SHEARER, M. S. 1976. The Portage Project: A model for early childhood intervention. In: T. D. Tjossem (Ed.), *Intervention Strategies for High Risk Infants and Young Children.* Baltimore: University Park Press.
82. SHEPPARD, W. C. and WILLOUGHBY, R. H. 1975. *Child Behavior: Learning and Development.* Chicago: Rand McNally.
83. SKEELS, H. M. 1966. Adult status of children with contrasting early life experiences. *Monogr. Soc. Res. Child Dev.*, *31.*
84. SKEELS, H. M. and DYE, H. B. 1939. A study of the effects of differential stimulation of mentally retarded children. *Proc. Addr. Am. Ass. Men. Defic.*, *44*, 114.
85. SOLKOFF, N., YAFFE, S., WEINTRUB, D. and BLASE, B. 1969. Effect of handling on the subsequent development of premature infants. *Devl. Psychol.*, *1*, 765.
86. SPITZ, R. A. 1946. Hospitalism: A follow-up report. *Psychoanal. Study Child.*, *2*, 113.
87. SPITZ, R. A. 1945. Hospitalism: An inquiry into the genesis of psychiatric conditions in early childhood. *Psychoanal. Study Child.*, *1*, 53.
88. SROUFE, L. A. 1970. A methodological and philosophical critique of intervention-oriented research. *Devl. Psychol.*, *2*, 140.
89. STEIN, L. A. and SUSSER, M. W. 1971. Changes over time in the incidence and prevalence

of mental retardation. In: J. Hellmuth (Ed.), *The Exceptional Infant: Studies in Abnormalities*, Vol. 2. New York: Brunner/Mazel.
90. STERN, D. 1977. *The First Relationship: Infant and Mother*. Cambridge: Harvard University Press.
91. THOMPSON, T. and REYNOLDS, J. 1977. The results of intensive care therapy for neonates. *J. Perinatal Med.*, 5, 59.
92. UZGIRIS, I. and HUNT, J. McV. 1966. An instrument for assessing infant psychological development. Unpublished manuscript, University of Illinois.
93. WACHS, T. D., UZGIRIS, I. C. and HUNT, J. McV. 1971. Cognitive development in infants of different age levels and from different environmental backgrounds: An exploratory investigation. *Merrill-Palmer Quarterly, 17*, 283.
94. WHITE, J. L. and LaBARBA, R. C. 1976. The effects of tactile and kinesthetic stimulation on neonatal development in the premature infant. *Devl. Psychobiol., 9*, 569.
95. WIENER, G., RIDER, R. V., OPPEL, W. C., FISCHER, L. K. and HARPER, P. A. 1965. Correlates of low birth weight: psychological status at six to seven years of age. *Pediatrics, 41*, 434.
96. WIENER, G., RIDER., OPPEL, W. C. and HARPER, P. A. 1968. Correlates of low birth weight: psychological status at eight to ten years. *Pediat. Res., 2*, 110.
97. WRIGHT, L. 1971. The theoretical and research base for a program of early stimulation, care, and training of premature infants. In: J. Hellmuth (Ed.), *Exceptional Infant: Studies in Abnormalities*. Vol. 2. New York: Brunner/Mazel.

4

DEVELOPMENTAL TESTING OF THE INFANT AND YOUNG CHILD

JANE V. HUNT, PH.D.

and

DOROTHY H. EICHORN, PH.D.

Institute of Human Development
University of California, Berkeley

VALUE OF EARLY DEVELOPMENTAL TESTING

Assessment of Developmental Delay

The clinician whose practice includes infants and very young children often is reluctant to rely entirely on clinical impressions and may desire a more formal assessment of developmental status. This is true when *developmental delay is suspected* or when the importance of delay is in question. Because the pace of normal development is especially rapid during the early years, behaviors that are normal in a very young infant may represent distinct delay when encountered in the older infant or child. For example, retardation of only three months in the nine-month-old infant or of eight months in the two-year-old represents one-third of expected developmental progress. Such developmental delays are difficult to determine reliably without a formal assessment, yet they may be diagnostically significant. Abnormal delays are always worrisome and are sometimes associated with

The authors wish to thank Donya Harvin, who reviewed the manuscript and contributed to the clinical comments included in it.

permanent mental retardation; they may also signal special areas of dysfunction in need of further evaluation and/or early intervention.

Interpretation of Delay

The significance of a generalized delay may depend upon other factors, such as the intactness of sensory or motor functions, physical health, or a history of premature birth. Allowances must be made for special circumstances or disabilities. Cultural factors may exert specific effects on development, e.g., the effect of bilingualism on language development. Clearly, the determination of a developmental level is not the only consideration. *The interpretation of the assessment is of equal importance.*

Interpretation of a young child's level of abilities is always done by comparing his performance with some reference group. When a clinical impression is used, the reference group is the clinican's previous experience with children of the same age. When a test is used, *the reference group is the population on which the test was standardized.* The choice of tests and the interpretation of results is made with the reference group in mind. For example, one may legitimately ask how a blind baby compares in development with sighted babies of the same age, and so use a developmental test standardized on sighted infants. One could not, however, legitimately interpret the results in the same way as one would for a sighted child. Particularly, any assumption that developmental delay suggested intellectual impairment would be suspect. In interpreting test results, particularly when inferring that significant developmental delay may represent underlying intellectual disability, we should keep in mind that *the more atypical the child in comparison with the reference population, the less valid the assessment.* This point is not always obvious. For instance, we certainly would not judge the blind child on the basis of visual skills, but can we assume that other abilities, such as walking or talking, are not delayed in blind babies with normal intelligence? Such questions require comparisons with both blind and sighted infants.

Assessment of Relative Abilities

Developmental testing may be desired at times when the general level of delay is not at issue. For example, one may want to evaluate a young handicapped child primarily to determine relative levels of functional competency and disability. Such a *developmental profile* may be of great benefit in counseling parents and arranging for educational placement. Intervention efforts are likely to be enhanced by this method of assessment. A true differential diagnosis, such as the determination of the degree of mental retardation in a multiply handicapped infant or young child, may be made more easily (and often with more validity) by observing the child's progress in an appropriate intervention program.

Diagnostic Assessment

In other cases, a *differential diagnosis* may be of primary importance. This is true when presenting symptoms can be caused by diverse etiologies or when multiple causes are suspected. One example that is frequently encountered is the three-year-old child who has not developed speech. Possible causes include deafness, mental retardation, expressive aphasia, emotional disturbance, or some combination of problems. In some cases, the delay is unusual but the child is normal and speech develops at a later age. The differential diagnosis is important for prognosis and adequate treatment. In such cases, a *battery of tests* may be required to determine underlying disabilities. Without formal assessment, less obvious contributing factors may go unnoticed.

In pediatric settings, developmental evaluations may provide reassuring information to the young or over-anxious parent who observes differences between the accomplishments of her child and those of his age peers.

Summary

To summarize, indications for developmental evaluations in infancy and early childhood are varied. They include the need to determine the child's current level of development and to relate that finding to an appropriate reference group; to explore the strengths and weaknesses of a disabled child, whether or not there is generalized delay; and to determine a differential diagnosis when presenting symptoms may have varied etiology.

ORIGINS OF CONTEMPORARY TESTS

There are a number of tests and assessments for infants and young children currently available to the clinican. These differ in format and purpose. Some are designed to be given by an expert tester and, at the other extreme, some require only a few minutes of parent interview. We cannot discuss which are "good" tests without first considering "good for what?" Which ones are most appropriate for general use? Which are particularly suited to special situations?

The choice is determined primarily by the purpose of the developmental assessment, but it is also controlled in practice by the time available for testing and the level of experience of the examiner. Three general types of developmental tests are available: those that provide an assessment of the infant or young child's general developmental level for tasks associated with normal intellectual growth; those that provide a comparison of different abilities in the same child; and those that measure specific and discrete functions. A brief consideration of the origins and development of these measuring instruments may provide some perspective.

Tests of General Intelligence

The general intelligence testing movement came about largely through the work of Alfred Binet who, early in this century, developed a test to identify those school children in Paris who would benefit from special education for the retarded. The mental abilities that interested Binet were the *complex mental functions* such as comprehension, reasoning, and judgment. He specifically rejected the use of simpler functions, such as sensory capacity and body measurements, to determine intelligence, despite a strong movement at the time in Germany and America emphasizing these characteristics in intelligence testing (3). His view prevailed when the tests of others failed to identify intellectual status. Two important concepts were carried along with this movement. First, Binet and his followers assumed that general intelligence was made up of major components that could be *tapped in a variety of ways*, so test items at different ages were varied and specific content was not considered. Second, considerable emphasis was placed on *language*, as it appeared to provide easiest access to the child's complex mental abilities.

Interest in intelligence tests became widespread in the first decade of the century and testing of school-age children was common. The standard score or *Intelligence Quotient* (IQ), the ratio of mental age to chronological age, was widely accepted as a measure of general intelligence and even as a measure of the *intellectual potential* of the child. That is, many assumed that the child's IQ was a direct reflection of his innate intelligence and that it would remain constant. As interest in *preschool children* developed in the 1920s, downward revisions of the original Binet test were constructed. In general, these tests consisted of items focusing on the same abilities that Binet considered basic to general intelligence.

At the same time, other investigators were studying the *development of infants*(Buhler in Vienna and Gesell, Fillmore, Shirley, and Bayley in America (3). Infant tests were constructed by these investigators and by others who studied their work, e.g., Cattell and Griffiths (16). Because these tests also incorporated the concept of a mental or developmental age that could be compared with chronological age, they were used to generate a standard score of the IQ type. Often, a tacit assumption was made that such a score would give an early measure of innate intelligence. Test items reflected a broad range of infant abilities at each age. In general, the infant tests measured the progressive competence of infants, exemplified by the acquisition of specific skills and an increasing comprehension of the social and inanimate environment.

Longitudinal studies of normal infants, such as those of Shirley and Bayley begun in the late 1920s, showed that infants were not constant in their "IQs" during the first year of life and it was not unusual for infants to show wide fluctuations in their performance levels at different ages. Bayley continued to follow her group and found the same tendency toward individual differences in rate of mental growth during childhood, although relative IQ status within the group became increasingly stable after two years of age. She also reported that *total scores on the infant tests were not generally predictive* of later Standford-Binet IQ for these normal children. This finding was replicated by others (see 11). It became clear that general precocity during infancy was not necessarily predictive of high IQ later, nor did slower normal development in infancy necessarily predict subsequent lower IQ.

The lack of prediction from infancy posed problems for those who believed that intelligence tests measured intellectual potential, for they also assumed that this potential should be present from birth. At the same time, Wellman reported that *environmental effects produced IQ changes* in preschool children, a finding that led to a great controversy (see 3). However, a number of subsequent studies yielded similar findings on the importance of environmental variables, and the myth of the immutable IQ was shattered. The result was a research climate favorable to investigations of the nature and determinants of intelligence, as well as to further refinement, analysis, and standardization of general intelligence tests.

Tests of Multiple Abilities

The range of human abilities and their individual differences have intrigued psychologists since the turn of the century. Despite the popularity of Binet's views, others regarded general intelligence as a construct, recognizing that individuals can show marked variation in specific intellectual abilities. Notable among these was David Wechsler, who addressed himself to the issues and problems of measuring *multiple abilities* and published a detailed analysis of his methods and results in 1935. He wrote, "Human beings differ from each other not so much with respect to the kind of abilities and traits which they possess (but rather in) the degree to which they possess them'' (19). He devised intelligence tests for adults and children that were composed of a number of subtests. He also included performance tasks not found in Binet's tests. But the unique feature of Wechsler's tests was the *systematic assessment of a number of abilities at all ages.* (In the general intelligence tests no such systematic arrangement was included because it was believed that general intelligence could be tapped in interchangeable ways.) His subtests could be compared with each other and a profile of abilities for the individual could be developed. Wechsler provided for a separate Verbal IQ and Performance IQ, as well as an overall IQ.

Wechsler has not constructed tests for children below four years of age, but his concept of testing multiple abilities was shared by others interested in preschool intelligence. In 1931, Stutsman (17) reviewed a number of studies that described the performance of preschool children on varied intellectual tasks. For example, a scale for ages two and a half to five and a half that measured ability in completions, arithmetic, vocabulary, and directions was published in 1927 by K. S. Cunningham, a student of E. L. Thorndike at Columbia Teachers College. In 1924, researchers at the University of Iowa Child Welfare Research station working with B. T. Baldwin published data on preschool children's performance on a range of tasks including form discrimination, vocabulary, color sorting, and picture memory. None of these tests of multiple abilities found its way into general use, whereas tests of general intelligence for preschool ages multiplied.

Tests of multiple abilities are difficult to construct, in part because of statistical problems related to the reliability of the separate components. Preschool tests present special problems because of the rapidly changing capabilities of very young children. More recently, McCarthy (15) standardized and published a test of multiple abilities for ages two and a half through eight and a half containing 18 tests grouped into subscales of verbal, perceptual-performance, quantitative, memory, and motor abilities. The first three scales are combined to yield a standard score of the IQ type.

Some of the earliest *infant tests* were specifically designed to assess the comparative development of different abilities. The *Gesell Developmental Schedules* (13) for ages two through 36 months, the product of extensive research by Arnold Gesell in the 1920s and 1930s, were not designed as a general test. These scales examine adaptive, gross motor, fine motor, language, and personal-social development. The use of the DQ (Developmental Quotient), a ratio score based largely on the mental age equivalent of the *adaptive* scale, has come into general use. The *Brunet-Lezine Test*, similar in construction to the Gesell schedules, is widely used in Europe for ages one through 30 months. The *Griffiths Mental Development Scale*, standardized in the 1950s on British infants aged two weeks to two years, is organized in a similar manner. These scales have been reviewed by Honzik (11).

Tests of Specific Abilities

An interest in some specific aspects of intellectual performance predates the development of Binet's general tests and the composite tests of multiple abilities. The German emphasis on the psychology of sensation and perception promoted an interest in *individual differences in specific abilities*, in contrast to an emphasis on general performance and average mental age found in the IQ testing movement.

Performance tests of various kinds were devised, sometimes to investigate special populations (2). Seguin's formboard was designed to train sensory and motor skills in mentally retarded children. (Seguin established perhaps the earliest training school for the retarded in 1837.) Healey, a pioneer in psychological work with delinquent children, devised a series of performance tests in 1911 as a necessary supplement to the highly verbal Binet tests. Other investigators also emphasized non-linguistic abilities in studies of immigrants to America who did not speak English. When the preschool scales of general intelligence were developed, many of these performance tasks were adapted and incorporated, including figure drawing (copying shapes), block building, puzzles, formboards, and pegboards; where possible, such performance tasks were also incorporated into infant assessments. At present there are few standardized tests of specific performance abilities available for use with very young children. For the older preschool child (age two and a half and above), the Beery Test of Visual-Motor Integration (Follett Publishing Co., Chicago, 1967) has been used frequently to assess development of visual perception, motor coordination, and especially, the *integration* of the two processes, as its name implies.

Language development has received special attention, sometimes as an outgrowth of special theoretical interests and at other times as a presumed quick indicator of general intelligence. An example of the latter category is the development of *vocabulary tests* to measure general intelligence. Among those that include children of preschool age, one of the best known is the *Peabody Picture Vocabulary Test*, published by Doll in 1959. This test requires no speech of the child, who points to the correct picture in an array as the object or action depicted is named. (The specific ability measured is *recognition of words*, although both a "language age" and an "IQ" are scored.) A more sophisticated test of language abilities is the *Illinois Test of Psycholinguistic Abilities*, first published by Kirk in 1961 for ages two through 10 years. This test provides a profile of *receptive and expressive* abilities, as well as some measures of related non-language abilities. At present, a number of language research instruments are in use that may ultimately be refined into tests.

Concept development has been the focus of many recent studies of intelligence in the infant and young child, following the seminal work of Jean Piaget. A recently published infant study by Uzgiris and Hunt (18) presents six ordinal scales measuring constructs, such as the development of visual pursuit and the permanence of objects, means for obtaining desired environmental events, vocal and gestural imitation, and the like. The specific behaviors observed are similar to those found in the standard infant tests of Bayley and Cattell, but the organization and interpretation of the tests are different. According to the authors, "Where traditional tests have presumed competency and intelligence to be based, for the most part, upon a unitary ability, we have presumed that competence is based on a hierarchical organization of a number of abilities and motive systems with several relatively independent branches" (18, p. 15). At present these authors have provided this assessment for research purposes rather than clinical use. Concept development in preschool children is a very active focus of current research, and assessments for these ages are emerging. For example, Swanson has developed the *Conceptual Behavior Battery* for ages approximately three to seven years to measure conservation of number, judgment of quantity relationships, and the Piagetian concept of seriation (see 12).

Measures of social competence are of interest to clinicians, educators of exceptional children, and others concerned with the child's ability to function adequately in the home and school environment. This ability is not the same as Binet's concept of general intelligence (which emphasizes complex mental functions), and the two may not always be highly correlated. The appraisal of practical or social intelligence is often important, as when institutionalization of the mentally retarded child is at issue. Such an appraisal of the normal preschool child may be helpful in advising and guiding parents and in planning educational programs.

The *Vineland Social Maturity Scale*, first published by E. A. Doll in 1936, has been widely used to estimate social maturity, as judged by the child's self-help skills, communication, locomotion, and socialization. A refined and expanded inventory for use with preschool children was published in 1966 (6); a version for blind preschool children was developed by Maxfield and

Buchholz in 1957 (14). A new scale for infants and preschool children was introduced by Alpern and Boll in 1972 (1).

The information used to score these scales is obtained primarily by interviewing a parent or caretaker and includes items not readily observed in a test situation, such as skills in toileting, bathing, dressing, and eating. Other items are related to a general level of understanding appropriate to functioning in the child's own milieu, such as the ability to avoid common hazards and the ability to observe rules and proprieties expected in the child's cultural group. Obtaining information by report rather than by direct observation is both a strength and weakness of such scales. It permits assessment of important practical skills not represented in IQ tests, but the reliability of the reporter is an important issue in evaluating the obtained results. Scores are typically reported as "social age" and are sometimes used as an estimate of "mental age" for children who cannot be tested with conventional intelligence tests.

In summary, few tests of perceptual-motor skills and language abilities have been developed for use with infants and preschool children that meet rigorous psychometric criteria of validity and reliability. The earlier interest in differential ability testing gave way to the development of general intelligence tests. Tests of multiple abilities usually were constructed to give scores from combined subtests, although they allow for some within-child comparisons. A renewed interest in the differential abilities of infants and young children is evident. This interest is indicated by the diversity of special research instruments now in use (see 12). New tests are appearing that reflect a renewed interest in social intelligence. Given current interest in concept development, we predict the emergence of new clinical tests to measure these functions.

THE EXAMINER

The primary consideration in any proposed testing of infants and preschool children is the competence of the examiner. A good understanding of the behavior of infants and preschool children is a prerequisite to successful testing at these ages. Performance on tests is markedly affected by the skills of the examiner in guiding behavior to desired goals and in maintaining the interest and cooperation of the child. Also, the examiner must be well trained on the specific test(s) being considered. Any test that includes direct observations of behavior requires specific training in the details of administration and scoring of the test in question. Unless the test is administered and scored exactly and the child's best performance is elicited, test results cannot be interpreted with any confidence.

Some tests are easier to learn than are others. *Screening tests*, for example, are usually simpler to administer and score than are more intensive tests. Often screening tests are standardized using examiners who are not testing experts, although these examiners were carefully trained on the specific screening instrument. Such tests can be useful when their limitations are respected. Their intended purpose is to *detect individuals who will benefit from a more thorough evaluation*, so the user must be wary of overinterpreting test scores. A competently administered screening test is appropriate in situations where the examiner is not expected to be proficient on more complex tests.

A number of *short or "quick" tests* are available to estimate the development of infants and preschool children. The appeal of such tests is that they can be used when time constraints preclude giving a more general test. Unlike true screening tests (which are designed to make only broad distinctions), the short test may generate an IQ or mental age, but scores are based on few items at each age level. Such tests present a number of administrative and interpretive problems. Generally, the more time the examiner spends with the child in a structured behavioral observation, the more reliable the results will be. In a more detailed examination, a wider range of behaviors can be evaluated, scoring is not as dependent on any particular item, and shy or inhibited children will reveal more of their typical behavior if given adequate time to adapt to the situation. Because of the problems inherent in short tests, only highly skilled examiners can be expected to use them effectively.

Some developmental assessments are scored wholly or in part from *parent interviews*, thus avoiding or reducing direct interaction with the infant or child. Special skills are needed to elicit parental descriptions of behavior because the scores obtained rely on their perceptions, which may be biased. One potential source of error is an overestimation of development by an anxious parent. The interviewer must make a judgment as to the reliability of the information obtained by the interview and try tactfully to ascertain the true state of affairs.

Experienced examiners often develop preferences for specific tests, usually because familiarity allows for more valid *interpretation* of individual performance. Some tests have become increasingly familiar to a range of professionals working in interdisciplinary settings and are preferred because test results are easily communicated. For example, most professionals today have some sense of the implications and limitations of a reported Stanford-Binet IQ. However, misinterpretation of test results is a hazard that deserves emphasis. Is the IQ derived from a short test comparable to that of the Stanford-Binet? How much importance can be attached to subtest differences in tests of multiple abilities? Test selection must be accompanied by some consideration of the competence of those who will be interpreting and applying the test data.

Developmental tests provide a standard situation for observing certain abilities of the infant and young child. They afford a valuable opportunity to observe general behavior patterns (i.e., stability of attention, frustration tolerance, modes of social interaction). They also provide scores that can be used for comparative purposes. The score is basically a *comparison of the child with the standardization population* of that test at that age. We may examine a child's developmental progress by comparing his scores with the standard across age or we may compare the scores of different groups of children. Not all test scores are useful for all purposes.

The most familiar scores are those that are reported as *mental age* (or other age equivalents) or as *standard scores*, such as the IQ. The standard score is designed to eliminate age differences. For example, an IQ of 100 is considered average at each age. Early versions of the Binet tests provided for a *ratio IQ*, calculated as mental age/chronological age X 100. Thus, if an eight-month-old infant earns a score equivalent to eight months of age, his standard score is 100; if he earns a score equivalent to four months of his age his score is 50. In principle, a ratio IQ can be calculated at any age.

The *standard deviation IQ* has replaced the ratio IQ in the current Stanford-Binet and is now widely used in other tests. Scores are based on the standard deviation, or the spread of raw scores at each age. (Raw scores represent the actual number of test items passed.) The standard deviation IQ makes it possible to determine just how abnormal a score is in relation to the standard and to compare performance more exactly from one age to another. For example, on the Stanford-Binet, the McCarthy scales, and the Bayley scales, a score of 84 is exactly one standard deviation below the mean for any age; the IQ range is set at 16 points for each standard deviation. The advantage of the standard deviation score is that it corrects for the observed variations from age to age in the range of raw scores.

Many tests give *age equivalents*, such as mental age, social age, or language age. If the test is well constructed, the age equivalent can be very useful in assessing the infant or child. Caution must be used in interpreting such an age score in instances where the child's performance is erratic, with an unusually wide range of successes and failures across age levels. In such a case, the age equivalent is an approximation but the child's performance is not typical for the age.

Some tests provide *subscale scores* that permit within-child comparisons of different abilities. Subscale scores are often less dependable, and comparisons among them are often less meaningful than the total score. This information is typically provided in the test manual and can be evaluated. In general, less reliance can be placed on subscale differences than on the test as a whole.

A few developmental assessments do not provide any interpolated scores and only *raw scores* are available. Such assessments are not suitable for general clinical use but are frequently used for research purposes. The Brazelton Neonatal Assessment Scale, for example, does not provide a score but permits comparisons among infants and, more importantly, among groups of newborn infants who may be expected to differ for theoretical reasons. The cognitive scales of Uzgiris and Hunt are also designed to allow comparisons between infants or groups of infants. In the hands of experienced clinicians, such observations can be revealing. We may anticipate that standardized tests based on these research instruments will be forthcoming.

TEST CONSTRUCTION

Certain criteria distinguish tests with general usefulness from those of unproven merit. Most tests in wide use today had their origins as research instruments, and new tests can be expected to appear as the product of current and future research. Before a research instrument becomes a useful test, several steps must be taken.

Standardization

The number or kind of infants or children studied usually must be expanded to provide a representative group. For example, if the pilot research was with infants of one sex, race, social class, or locality, sampling is extended so the normative data are based on a broader population. For some of the major general tests of intelligence (*Stanford-Binet Intelligence Scale, Wechsler Preschool and Primary Scale of Intelligence, McCarthy Scales of Children's Abilities, Bayley Scales of Infant Development*), standardization was based on a nationwide sampling within the United States. Stratified sampling according to a number of characteristics, e.g., social class, race, occupation, and community size, reflected the most recent census data at the time. This procedure does not, of course, lead to the conclusion that there is necessarily an "average" American infant or child, but it does tend to eliminate idiosyncrasies arising from specific subsamples. In contrast, the *Peabody Picture Vocabulary Test* was standardized in the area of Nashville,

Tennessee. Although the sample was large—approximately 4,000 white children, with about 100 at each half-year age interval in the preschool ages—the regionalization of the standardization has been of some concern, prompting several comparative studies in other localities.

Some of the infant and preschool tests in use today were standardized several decades ago. Perhaps the reader will be surprised to learn that the *date of test standardization* appears to exert an effect on the average score and the distribution of scores at all ages, from infancy through adulthood. Comparisons of recent with earlier data show that, in general, contemporary samples score higher than did their age counterparts when the tests were first standardized. Exact differences vary according to the test in question, chronological age, and intellectual level.

For example, the Stanford-Binet Intelligence Scale was restandardized in 1972 by testing new groups of children at each age, and results were compared with those obtained for the 1937 sample. Higher scores were found at all ages, but the effect was most marked at preschool ages (two through four and a half years), where the average IQ had risen from 100 to 110-111. The scores of the restandardization sample were adjusted so that the average once again equalled an IQ of 100, and these data were published as the 1972 revision. When the appropriate tables are consulted, one finds that the IQ of 100 no longer approximates the mental age/chronological age ratio; for example, an IQ of 100 at three years of age is equivalent to a mental age of three years and six months on the test. This change tells us that the average three-year-old now performs at a level that is advanced by six months when compared with the average three-year-old tested in 1937.

Similarly, the age placements of specific items in the current *Bayley Scales of Infant Development* are typically some months higher than are the age placements of the same items in the older infant tests such as the *Gesell Developmental Schedules*. The reader is left to ponder the causes and implications of the increased precocity of infants and young children.

Reliability

Is the test so constructed that the child will perform at approximately the same level if he is retested after a few days? *Test-retest reliability* reveals how well the test is measuring some stable behavior of the child. The stability of the test score over a short time interval is expressed as a coefficient of correlation between scores. When a test has separately scored components, some may be less reliable than others on retesting.

How consistent is the test in what it measures? *Internal consistency*, the consistency of the individual's performance on different portions of the same test, is another aspect of reliability. In this instance, the correlation coefficient is derived from a single test administration. For general IQ tests, internal consistency is usually reported as split-half reliability, comparing the individual's performance on two halves of the same test. Items within a subtest can also be examined in the same manner, and a method is available to examine the reliability of a composite group of tests.

Once a reliability coefficient has been determined, we can ask a hypothetical question: If the child could immediately retake the test many times (ruling out the effects of practice and fatigue) how much would his scores on the test vary? *The standard error of measurement,* which is a function of the reliability coefficient and the spread of test scores, provides an estimate. This measure gives a "band of error" that is useful in interpreting an individual's score. A small standard error of measurement for a test means that an earned score is close to the individual's expected or "true" score, a statistically derived hypothetical value.

If two examiners give the test to the same infant or child, will they get the same results? *Inter-rater reliability* is often reported for tests, based on having more than one examiner score the same test performance. If inter-rater reliability is high, the kinds of behavior being scored and the scoring system are considered sufficiently objective.

Validity

How do we know what a test measures? How well does it do so? Validity is a primary concern of test selection. The potential user must be wary of accepting "face validity" for any test without examining the evidence that the test meets more stringent criteria of validity.

Binet designed his original intelligence test for the practical purpose of identifying mentally retarded children prior to school enrollment. To the extent that he was successful, as judged by educational criteria, the test had *concurrent validity,* i.e., agreement was found between the test and an independent estimate of the same trait. Because Binet believed that intelligence must be measured by testing higher mental functions, he selected items that he believed would tap those functions to give the test *content validity.* As the Binet tests became increasingly popular for use with normal children, it was noted that they had *predictive validity* for subsequent school performance. The assumption that the tests measured innate intelligence was vigorously attacked by those who demonstrated that the IQ could be changed by experience. This was an attack on *construct validity* or the extent to which a test measures a theoretical construct.

Most of the major infant and preschool tests in general use have been examined for *construct validity*, either during test development or through subsequent research. The major criterion employed in test development has been *age differentiation*, with scores increasing systematically across age. For example, in the development of the Bayley scales, each item was ordered according to age; the age placement of each item was determined by finding the age at which 50 percent of the standardization sample passed the item. Average total scores for each age were then computed. Depending on the theoretical constructs of the test originator, a new test might or might not be expected to show high *correlations with other existing tests*. When subscales are combined to give a general score, as is the case with the McCarthy scales and some other preschool tests, the *correlations between subscales and total score* are examined during test construction. A subscale that has a low correlation with the total score is usually either eliminated or relegated to a separate scoring system. Construct validity has also been examined by subjecting test items to *factor analysis* or *cluster analysis* to find the psychological traits represented in the test.

The problem of *predictive validity* for infant tests is well known. With the exception of some handicapped infants, total test scores during the first year do not predict subsequent childhood performance on intelligence tests, even when the best standardized tests are used. The value of infant tests is in describing current status. Some infant tests are predictive over short intervals of a few months, particularly when scores are derived from the standard deviation or range of normal scores at each age. Some research evidence suggests that certain components of infant tests, such as clusters of specific test items, may be more predictive than total scores. Further investigations and refinements may lead to more predictive tests for clinical use. Test scores become increasingly predictive during the preschool years and users should examine preschool tests for this validity criterion.

The best *screening tests* are validated by determining their usefulness in detecting infants and young children who require more extensive evaluation. This task is done in two steps. First, screening results are compared with concurrent performance on a standardized test; then the incidence of false positive and false negatives yielded by the screening is determined. The *Denver Developmental Screening Test* (8) is an example of a screening instrument which has been subjected to this process (concurrent validity was assessed by performance on the Bayley scales). Scoring procedures were then modified to reduce the rate of false identifications from screening.

Short tests usually are designed as a substitute for more extensive tests. For them, the most important validity measure is *concurrent validity* with other tests. Testers should be extremely hesitant to use a short test unless high validity has been demonstrated for a representative normal sample. Spuriously high correlations are sometimes reported; these can be expected if the range of intelligence is very great (for example, when both retarded and normal children are included in the score comparisons) or if the age range used in the score comparisons is very broad (within-age comparisons are more meaningful). The *Quick Test* of Ammons and Ammons is a well-known short test for ages two years to adults. Typical of many other short tests, it has moderate validity when compared with Wechsler test performance of older children and adults but is largely unproven for use with preschool ages (see 7).

Rating scales based on parents' report of behavior can also be validated by *comparisons with observed behavior*. For example, Alpern and Boll (1) reported an overall agreement of 84 percent between scores by interview and scores by direct testing with appropriate portions of the *Developmental Profile*. However, these investigators cautioned that the mothers they interviewed for this purpose may not have been comparable to a clinic population because they were not anxious about their children. Rating scales can also be *derived from more extensive instruments* or research data, and then validated against them. This procedure was used by Carey (5) in developing an interview with mothers about the temperament of infants and by Knobloch and Pasamanick in developing a questionnaire version of the *Developmental Screening Inventory* (13).

APPROPRIATENESS

The *purposes of testing* and the *characteristics of the clinical population* of infants and young children are important considerations in test selection. The user must consider whether or not the test can be administered, scored, and interpreted in a standard manner. If not, what modifications must be made? How interpretable are the results? Is the test useful or possibly misleading in assessing development?

The test score is not valid if the procedures for test administration or scoring are violated. The standardization of tests to determine both the age placement of items and the normal range of total scores *depends upon specificity* for the materials used, the instructions given, the number of trials allowed, and so on. If the examiner alters specific aspects of some test items to make them more "fair" or "appropriate" for an individual child, the value of the item in a cumulative raw score is lost. The cumulative score is also meaningless in instances where many items are omitted in determining the score. In either situation, the test has been made idiosyncratic. In the hands of a good diagnostician, the observation of performance under these individualized conditions may provide useful clinical information about development. However, the results of such adaptations should not be reported as a score.

If the infants or young children being examined have significant sensory or motor handicaps, the standard test is inappropriate. Standard infant tests are heavily weighted with items that require sensori-motor skills to demonstrate the infant's understanding and mastery of his environment. When an infant with sensory or motor handicap is assessed on such a test, little may be learned about his understanding. For example, if he cannot physically remove the covering from a covered toy, we cannot know whether or not he has developed the concept of object permanence. The test therefore lacks construct validity as an assessment of the current developmental status of the infant.

In other instances, the infant or child with a physical or sensory handicap may be capable of performing some tasks (as when subscale performance is examined using the Griffiths or Gesell scales), but the handicap may have limited his experience and depressed his developmental progress compared with normal children. Such comparisons may be useful, but the resulting lower score may not be predictive for the preschool child. Special tests are available for handicapped populations, such as the Hayes-Binet for the blind, and the user can acquaint himself with the reliability and validity of such tests for use with handicapped populations.

When a handicapped child is evaluated on a standard test, the examiner may tend to over-interpret any successes, giving the child the benefit of the doubt. This practice may be misleading and fail to uncover significant intellectual disabilities. Handicapped children, such as those with cerebral palsy, may have a variety of more subtle problems, for example, defects of visual perception or tactile sensitivity. Standard tests are not designed to detect these problems and they may go undiagnosed without special evaluation. The developmental assessment of Else Haeussermann (10) is specifically designed to assess the intellectual capacities and functional abilities of multiply handicapped preschool children. The determination of subtle functional abnormalities may alter the examiner's perceptions of the child's intellectual capacities and suggest appropriate remedial efforts.

In summary, the appropriateness of a test depends very much on the match between the child being evaluated and the characteristics of the population used in test standardization. If the question is, "How does the child compare with the norm?", then the standard tests may be appropriate even when the environmental experience of the child is known to be grossly deviant from the standard. However, such a comparison is not meaningful if the child has a handicap that makes him incapable of performing the tasks that are used to assess his comprehension. Scores from standard tests should not be reported if the test has been altered to fit the special needs of the child; the standard properties of the test have been lost and the resulting score is not valid. It may be meaningful to report the age equivalent for specific abilities that are available for assessment. A better approach to the assessment of the child with physical or sensory handicap is the use of a special test with normative data that are appropriate. A differential diagnosis requires the examiner to assess a variety of functions that may be abnormal in the handicapped child.

COMPARISONS AMONG TESTS

General Considerations

An evaluation of all the mental tests available for infants and preschool children is beyond the scope of this review. The specific merits of individual tests depend largely upon the requirements of individual users, including the skills of examiners, the population being examined, and the questions being posed. Some generalities can be stated:

1) In selecting any developmental test, *features of test construction* should be considered, including standardization, reliability, and validity. Such considerations apply not only for the widely accepted general tests, but also for *any* test. In fact, as we have noted, screening tests, short tests, and interviews have intrinsic problems that make such aspects of test construction especially important.

The user may be willing to consider certain tests that are in a transitional stage between research use and standardization. Few well-constructed infant and preschool tests to measure specific abilities exist, but some promising ones are currently in research use. The authors of such tests may be soliciting some clinical experience with these new instruments in order to reach a larger population. Certainly such an effort may be more justifiable than continuing the use of outdated or unsatisfactory tests.

2) Any test should be constructed so that it can be *administered and scored objectively*. Tests that rely heavily on subjective judgments are difficult to evaluate, and inter-rater reliability is certain to be low. The examiner must take responsibility for acquiring the training necessary to achieve reliability on objective tests. Even screening tests require the user to be trained to criterion, and each test has fine points of administration and

scoring that must be learned. In addition, the examiner must gain experience with infants and young children before tests can be given reliably. Experience with older children does not necessarily qualify an examiner to work with younger ages.

3) Any test must be *interpretable to those using the information* derived from it. Reliability and validity data from the test standardization and from research with special populations often are helpful in evaluating the meaning of test scores. The meaning of subscale scores and their comparisons must also be clearly presented. One recurrent problem in interpreting scores is the assumption that standard scores, such as the IQ, or age equivalents, such as the mental age, are comparable and interchangeable from test to test. Score comparability among tests cannot be assumed without specific evidence for such concurrent validity. The user should also examine the content of tests to see which abilities are included and omitted. Short tests that rely on very few items for scores require special scrutiny and cautious interpretation.

SOURCES OF FURTHER INFORMATION

The particular characteristics of each test can be investigated in detail through published sources. The potential user can use these sources to determine tests best suited to specific needs.

Test Manuals

The American Psychological Association (9) has published standards for psychological tests and manuals. The standards include statements of the purposes and applications recommended, qualifications required to administer the test, data on reliability and validity, and a description of the sample of children used in deriving test scores. The test manual is a primary source of information. Where the manual is inadequate, the potential user should be alert to the possibility of inadequate test criteria.

Test Reviews

Tests are reviewed and compared in published reference works. The best known reference is the *Mental Measurement Yearbook* series edited by Buros (4). Now in its eighth volume, this work is a compendium of all known tests in the English language. Included are reviews that provide critical and comparative information not available in a test manual. Lists of references to research studies are also provided and may be of clinical interest.

A recent review of pediatric screening tests edited by Frankenburg and Camp (7) includes discussions of many *screening tests* and *short tests* of early mental development currently in use. The reader may also be interested to learn about *new test instruments* now being used for research purposes that are becoming available for more general use. Many of these are described in an extensive recent survey by Johnson (12) of tests and measurements in child development.

SUMMARY

Perhaps the reader anticipated a more didactic compilation and review of infant and preschool tests than we have provided. Many adequate tests have not been mentioned, whereas some of those discussed do not meet all criteria for good test construction. Specific tests have been cited primarily for illustrative purposes. Our intent has been to acquaint the reader with the important issues to be considered in selecting tests and to provide some guides for making test comparisons. In particular, we tried to indicate to interested professionals who are not themselves psychometricians that the interpretation of test scores is not a mystery and that test selection can be based on objective criteria.

REFERENCES

1. ALPERN, G.D. and BOLL, T.J. 1972. *Developmental Profile.* Indianapolis: Psychological Development Publications.
2. ANASTASI, A. 1968. *Psychological Testing* (Third Edition). New York: Macmillan.
3. BROOKS, J. and WEINRAUB, M. 1976. A history of infant intelligence testing. In M. Lewis (Ed.), *Origins of Intelligence: Infancy and Early Childhood.* New York: Plenum Press.
4. BUROS, O.K. 1978. *The Eighth Mental Measurements Yearbook.* Highland Park, N.J.: Gryphon Press.
5. CAREY, W.B. 1972. Measuring infant temperament. *Journal of Pediatrics, 81,* 414.
6. DOLL, E.A. 1966. *Preschool Attainment Record: Research Edition.* Circle Pines, Minn.: American Guidance Service, Inc.
7. FRANKENBURG, W.K. and CAMP, B.W. 1975. *Pediatric Screening Tests.* Springfield: Charles C Thomas.
8. FRANKENBURG, W.K., DOBBS, J.B., and FANDAL, A.W. 1970. *Denver Developmental Screening Test.* Denver: LADOCA Foundation.
9. FRENCH, J.W. and MICHAEL, W.B. 1966. *Standards for Educational and Psychological Tests and Manuals.* Washington, D.C.: American Psychological Association, Inc.
10. HAEUSSERMANN, E. 1958. *Developmental Potential of Preschool Children.* New York: Grune & Stratton.
11. HONZIK, M.P. 1976. Value and limitations of infant tests: An overview. In M. Lewis (Ed.), *Origins of Intelligence: Infancy and Early Childhood.* New York: Plenum Press.
12. JOHNSON, O.G. 1976. *Tests and Measurements in Child Development: Handbook II.* San Francisco: Jossey-Bass.

13. KNOBLOCH, H. and PASAMANICK, B. 1974. *Gesell and Amatruda's Developmental Diagnosis* (Third Edition). Hagerstown: Harper & Row.
14. MAXFIELD, K.B. and BUCHHOLZ, S. 1957. *A Social Maturity Scale for Blind Preschool Children: A Guide to its Use.* New York: American Foundation for the Blind.
15. McCARTHY, D. 1970. *McCarthy Scales of Children's Abilities.* New York: The Psychological Corporation.
16. STOTT, L.H. and BALL, R.S. 1965. Infant and preschool mental tests: review and evaluation, *Monographs of the Society for Research in Child Development,* 30 (3), Serial No. 101.
17. STUTSMAN, R. 1931. *Mental Measurement of Preschool Children.* Yonkers: World Book Co.
18. UZGIRIS, I.C. and HUNT, J.M. 1975. *Assessment in Infancy: Ordinal Scales of Psychological Development.* Urbana: University of Illinois Press.
19. WECHSLER, D. 1952. *The Range of Human Capacities* (Second Edition). Baltimore: Williams & Wilkins.

5

PLAY IN THE UNDER-FIVES: FORM, DEVELOPMENT AND FUNCTION

CORINNE HUTT, B.SC., D. PHIL.

Reader in Psychology,
University of Keele, England

CONCEPTS OF PLAY AND CHILDHOOD

Play in childhood has assumed such significance in recent years that it is difficult to imagine that there were times historically, or places culturally, where children did not play. However, opportunities and facilities for play assume that cultures and societies acknowledge the concept of *childhood*, a period of life during which children are relatively free and unconstrained, unbeset by pressures for survival and unhampered by the chores of existence. Surprisingly, this concept of childhood is fairly recent.

Concepts of Play

Notions of play are inextricably intertwined with the concept of childhood. No culture or society that does not value one can value the other. Thus, even two decades ago, children playing in rural Egypt had to move away on the approach of adult males lest they be scolded or have something thrown at them. Nyansongo children in Kenya received little parental affection and

The preparation of this chapter was made possible by the generous support of the Department of Education and Science. U. K.

were vigorously caned for their misdemeanours; their frivolous "play" activities were firmly discouraged (68).

Even in societies less beset by the exigencies of survival and permitting some non-utilitarian activity, miniature replicas and playthings that were fashioned were not used for play. Feitelson (33) refers to Wiener's observations in Katanga where many dolls were forbidden to children; similarly "playthings" created by New Mexican children out of clay or wood were generally placed on shelves to be admired but never handled (12).

In other cultures play activities occupy a brief transitory period and merge almost undetectably into adult routines like the pegging out of goats by Tallensi boys (35) or the fetching of water by Kamban girls (80) or farming and cooking among the Rajputs (77).

In Western Europe an alternative view of childhood was emerging in the 18th century (17): Blake and Wordsworth eulogised the innocence and beauty of childhood, and Dewey and Rousseau emphasised the distinctive educational potential of childhood.

Partly as a reaction to the repressive attitudes of earlier times, partly as a result of their own early experience and convictions, humanitarian educationists like Pestalozzi and Froebel urged, in the earlier part of this century, that children should have the liberty and opportunity to develop their spirit. Since this development was to be through their free and unfettered activities, children's play became invested with almost poetic qualities: "Play then, is the highest expression of human development in childhood, for it alone is the free expression of what is in the child's soul. It is the purest and most spiritual product of the child, and at the same time it is a type and copy of human life at all stages and in all relations . . ." (38A). An instinctive ineluctable quality was ascribed to play: "No one needs to teach a child to play . . . Nature plants strong play propensities in every normal child to make sure that certain basic needs of development will be satisfied" (40, p. 15). There then became little of children's behaviour that was not "play," and Lowenfeld (70) made this explicit: "Since all activities of children other than lessons, eating, and sleeping seem to the watching adult to have no serious purpose, a description of them as play appears apt and fitting . . . (p. 39)."

Such an over-inclusive use of the term "play," however, is unhelpful both theoretically and pragmatically. If all children's activities are to be thought of as play, it then becomes imperative to distinguish between different forms of play—forms which may be motivationally and functionally quite distinct. Moreover, implicit in such a comprehensive use of the term is a dismissal of any serious endeavour on the part of the child, since most authors are agreed that play is spontaneous, has no specific goals and is engaged in for its own sake.

For the present, it would be helpful to be guided by the distinction made by Dearden (19): Most of an adult's activities are serious, he argues, in that they further some purpose or fulfill some obligations, whereas

> play is neither the pursuit of purposes dictated by common prudence, nor is it the fulfilling of the obligation to anybody . . . a child at the sink, for example, may or may not be playing, depending on how he regards his activity. If he does as he pleases, then he is playing . . . Play is a non-serious and self-contained activity which we engage in just for the satisfaction involved in it (p. 81).

Thus, while not precluding serious activity for children, Dearden nevertheless makes the useful distinction between activity which is constrained and that which is not. Reardon (88) adds the important point that in play the player has potential control of the situation (falling down is fun if you mean to) and can stop when he wishes to. Above all, play is *fun* and, like virtue, is its own reward.

PLAY AS MOTOR ACTIVITY

The earliest manifestations of play occur as physical movements of the infant. At a few weeks of age a baby will throw or kick its limbs, clench its fists, roll its head, not simply in an instrumental manner, in order to achieve some goal, but simply, it seems, for the "satisfaction" of executing the action. There is a "mass action" quality to motor activity initially: Arms, legs and body move without much coordination; hands, and even toes, may find their way to the mouth. With increasing age, movements become less generalised and more specific, more coordinated and somewhat more restrained. When an object is presented, the infant will probably swipe at it, but typically with a clenched fist (123).

Activity in Perceptual Development

Hand and eye require to be coordinated before an effective grasp can be made. The Russians saw motor activity as playing a crucial role in perceptual development. Zaporozhets (124), for instance, considered that the hand taught the eye by making contact with the object and tracing its contours, development of object perception resulting from the interaction between orienting movements of the hand and eye. Although there is little experimental support for the motor copy theory of perceptual development (41), this view is very similar to that of Piaget. Space is perceived by the child only in relation to himself and his activity; near or reachable space becomes differentiated with practice and, as the child's sensori-motor activities are extended and elaborated, his phenomenal space enlarges.

The significance of active movements and "movement-produced sensory feedback" in perceptual development has also been argued by Held (48). Passive movements such as having one's limb moved are inadequate for perceptual learning; the immature animal or human requires the proprioceptive feedback from its active movements (reafference) to be matched against an internal copy of the executed movement. Held and Hein (50) showed that if young kittens were precluded from having active commerce with their environment by being moved passively through it, they subsequently exhibited visuo-spatial difficulties as in reaching and paw-placement. Reafferent stimulation from active movements are thus necessary for the developing organism to build a stable model of its perceptual world.

The necessity for adequate opportunity for motor play was implicitly reiterated by Routh et al. (95) with their demonstration of the relatively high activity levels of three-year-olds. This high activity was manifested by high locomotor scores in the experimental situation as well as by restlessness during TV watching, mealtimes etc. The two types of measure were independent, but marked decreases in activity were obtained on both from the ages of three to five years.

Practice Play

Piaget (86) sees the genesis of play in the sensori-motor acts of infancy, beginning with the primitive reflex actions, and leading through the circular reactions to combinational activities. Primitive play, in fact, is almost identical with sensori-motor behaviours, with one principal difference—the motor skill, whether it is sucking, grasping or kicking, has already been acquired and is then practised for no other purpose than the fun of it, or what Buhler (9) referred to as "funktionlust," functional pleasure. As Millar (78, p. 107) says, "Trying to touch a rattle, or to make it swing is not play. Doing it repeatedly when the skill is already within the child's capacity, when it achieves no new perception, and serves no serious purpose, is play." A baby may take a swipe at a mobile hanging above its cot, but then the action of swiping itself may take precedence and the child will repeat the arm movement over and over again, laughing and chuckling all the while.

These types of rehearsal or practice play are the first to appear in childhood. Piaget regards them as the most labile forms of play since they appear with each new acquisition and then wane or disappear. During such play it is the process of assimilation which predominates, i.e., the child incorporates information in accordance with his existing schema. He is relatively unconstrained by the demands of reality and might even distort reality to suit his own needs. This indifference to reality is well illustrated by some of the play patterns characteristic of six-month-olds.

In a study of attention in the first two years of life, we examined children's exploration of and play with novel and familiar toys, when they were six months, then when they were 12 months and again when they were 24 months (58). At six months there were clearly a number of manual skills that the infants were practising, like grasping, scratching, banging and mouthing, and they performed these quite indiscriminately and irrespectively of the nature of the objects and toys which they were handling; the table surface was scratched, so was a yo-yo, as well as the body of a squeaky giraffe; or a drum-rattle was banged, as was a little truck and the yo-yo. Buhler (10) remarked that it was not until about 18 months that her group of children noticed that they produced different effects upon different materials and responded accordingly. Thus, during such practice play it is the *stimulus*, rather than the object of the action, that is important. Although the "autotelic" quality of such play may be evident, the ludic quality very often is not. We found it very difficult at this age to distinguish when such activities might legitimately be called playful and when they might be exploratory, since the child would look serious or absorbed while performing them. Not until they were much older did the children consistently provide behavioural "markers" of enjoyment or having fun.

During the performance of such activities the infant, even when lying in his cot, may find that he makes things happen: Kicking his cot may make a mobile move or a rattle shake; hitting an object may make a noise. There seems to be an instinctive preference for movements and actions which are followed by such contingent events and such actions tend to be repeated over and over again. This is Piaget's secondary circular reaction, involving procedures to make interesting sights and sounds last. Even severely mentally retarded infants will repeat actions to reproduce an effect; moreover, when certain knobs on a "play-panel" controlled the onset of chimes while others did not, the severely retarded infant manifested a distinct preference for the sound-contingent stimulus by showing a discriminatory performance (38).

Physical Competence Through Play

The protracted engagement in and rehearsal of such physical activities

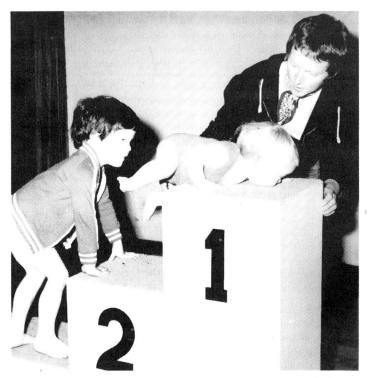

FIGURE 1. A one-year-old levers himself with chin and hand on to a high step in the gymnasium.

inevitably result in increasing agility, dexterity, sense of balance and body image. With increasing age the motor skills that are practised are naturally more complex, but the very rehearsal of these improves performance. During the process of acquiring skills, like riding a bicycle or scooter, walking on stilts etc., children appear to be in deadly earnest and serious in intent and will very probably not admit to be "playing." It is only when they have acquired the skill that they begin to enjoy exercising it. Having watched our son, at five years of age, completing one dizzy figure-of-eight route after another on his cycle and expending much energy doing so, we inquired whether he regarded the activity as play. "Now it is," was his reply, "but it was jolly hard work when I was learning to do it."

As children develop their physical skills, they derive great enjoyment from practising them and, as they do so, they become increasingly self-confident. Children under five years of age do not usually have the oppor-

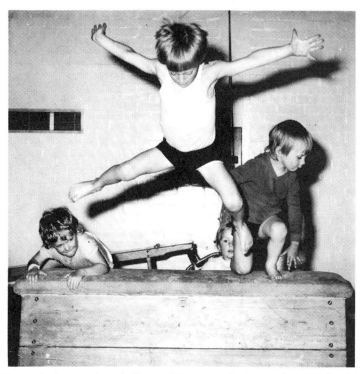

FIGURE 2. A two-and-one-half-year-old strives to climb on to the box (left) while a three-and-one-half-year-old has done so effortlessly (right) while the boy in the centre "plays" at jumping.

tunity to use gymnasium apparatus and are apprehensive when first exposed to it. A gym-class for preschoolers run in the University Department of Physical Education has enabled children to acquire new skills relatively quickly and to extend their capacities to a degree hitherto not thought possible for such young children. Infants under a year have difficulty climbing stair steps and it is at about 13 months that they pull themselves up stairs (103A). Yet the one-year-old infant in Figure 1 is climbing an exceptionally high step without a trace of diffidence; this infant is using the upper half of his body (head or chin and arms and hands) as a fulcrum to lever himself up, while the older child (left, in Figure 2) uses arms and hands with some help from the legs. The still older child of three and a half years (right, Figure 2) has used mainly knees and feet with some support from his hands to climb on to the box. This sequence illustrates the increasing proficiency

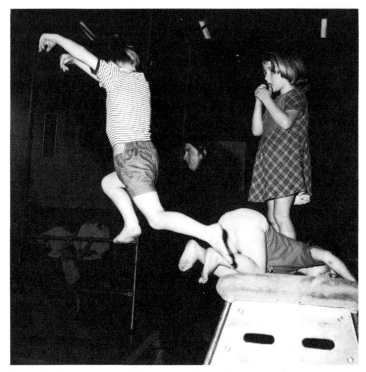

FIGURE 3. An inexperienced three-year-old clambers on to the box, using the patterns of a younger child.

with age in a skill like climbing. A relatively inexperienced but older child still resorts to the "immature" pattern (Figure 3).

Jumping from a higher to a lower level begins at two years of age but it is not until four or five years of age that most children can do this proficiently (45). Note the three-year-olds in Figures 2 (centre) and 3 (left). Walking down a narrow incline is again a skill the young child has difficulty acquiring; similarly the two-year-old balancing and swinging on the bars initially needs his mother's help (Figure 4) while his three-year-old sister swings serenely (Figure 5). What is impressive about this gym class for the under-fives is how much the children enjoy the opportunity for exercising their skills—anyone who doubts that this is physical play is soon convinced by the whoops and shrieks of enjoyment and the peals of laughter. The rapid growth of confidence that such mastery of play confers upon the children enables them to extend their powers and to achieve a degree of physical proficiency that is surprising to the naive adult.

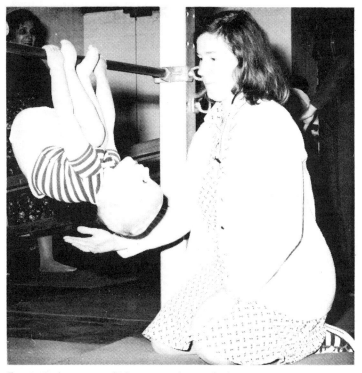

FIGURE 4. A two-year-old learns to swing on the bars.

On the basis of the theory that physical activities skipped in the earliest years may keep the upper levels of the brain from functioning fully, "remedial" programmes of physical activities were instituted in two schools for disadvantaged children; both reported considerable progress in academic learning, physical competence, and poise (12).

However, such play, even though carried out in a group context, is predominantly solitary. That is, the children are concerned with doing their own thing. They may play alongside one another, or wait their turn on a piece of apparatus, but they do not cooperate in their play; they do not play collectively. Physical play which is essentially social does not appear until the age of five years or so. This type of play is generally referred to as *rough-and-tumble* play: It is a heterogeneous collection of physical activities like chasing, wrestling, rolling, pushing, etc. Its distinctive characteristic is that it involves two or more children, but it is more idiosyncratic and spontaneous than any game. Another notable feature of rough-and-tumble play

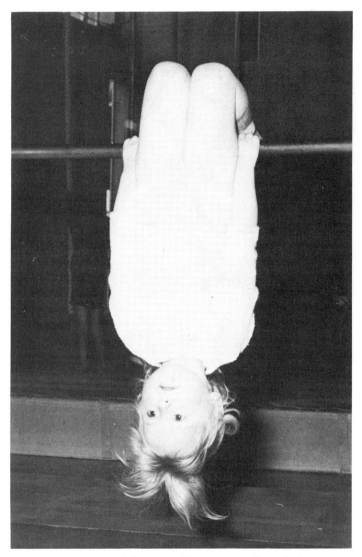

FIGURE 5. An experienced three-year-old swings serenely on the bar.

is that it occurs only among children who know each other well and most commonly among siblings. It seems that the intimate physical contact that is involved in much rough-and-tumble play requires that the participants be familiar and relaxed with each other.

PLAY AS THE PROVISION OF SENSATION

From what has been said in the previous section it will be seen that the motor play of the young child also serves to provide him with much varied sensory stimulation. While waving his arms, he brings his hands into his visual field, whereupon he can inspect them, learn how they look when he moves them, clasp them, reach out and so on. In fact, before the hands can be used to perform an instrumental or manipulative function, they must be studied and examined until they are totally familiar. Kittens were prevented from seeing their paws by a wide collar worn round their necks (47); although these animals could look around and walk freely, they could not see their limbs. When the collars were removed, the animals were unable to place their paws accurately on the solid parts of a slatted surface. In another experiment, Held and Bauer (49) reared monkeys in an apparatus which allowed them to move their limbs freely but not to see them; they were even conditioned to extend their arms upon sight of a feeding bottle. After 34 days, an arm was exposed and visually guided reaching was tested: When the feeding bottle was presented, arm extension occurred right away, but the reaching stopped as soon as the hand came into the monkey's view, whereupon the animal proceeded to gaze intently at it while moving it about. Reaching for objects only became accurate when the monkey stopped studying its hand and glanced between hand and target instead. Thus the many, apparently aimless, movements and thrashing about of the infant actually provide him with both visual and proprioceptive information about his body in relation to his environment—information which it is necessary to integrate before an image of a stable environment can be built up. Sustained hand regard is followed by alternate glances between object and hand; next, the hands are clasped in the mid-line and observed, an activity which integrates tactual and visual information and which facilitates visually guided reaching. Such visuo-motor development was found to be more rapid in a varied rather than a monotonous sensory environment.

Need for Sensory Variety

The early play of infants also ensures the provision of varied sensory input. Reduction of sensory input is distinctly unpleasant for the individual who is awake and striving to remain alert. Studies of sensory deprivation have, in fact, shown that adults would often prefer to receive electric shocks than be subjected to protracted periods of no sensory stimulation (125). The whines and complaints of bored children in a doctor's waiting room or on a train are further testimony to the need for varied sensory stimulation. We found, much to our surprise, that normal children between the ages of three and five years became as distractible and hyperactive as brain-damaged children in a playroom devoid of play materials and equipment (63). As soon as even one toy was introduced, the attention spans of normal children increased markedly.

To the immobile infant, for whom such stimulation is perforce restricted, play activities are an essential means of ensuring adequate perceptual input of a varied kind. One is reminded of the amusing anecdote provided by Millar (76): A girl of four, when told not to fidget with the crockery on the table, replied that her arm would get bored if she stopped!

Perceptual Salience

Infants and young children also attend more to certain stimuli and objects than others. Stimuli which are novel, complex, incongruous and unexpected have a greater salience than ones which are familiar, simple, banal and predictable. From a very young age, differential attention to novel stimuli is very evident (28, 97) and by the age of four years children will exercise themselves in order to view pictures that are novel rather than ones they have seen before (59).

Play activities, then, are an essential avenue of sensory input, affording the child who cannot walk or cannot talk valuable feedback concerning its sensori-motor capacities, while at the same time serving the complementary function of facilitating the development of motor skills like prehension, reaching and dexterity.

MANIPULATIVE PLAY WITH OBJECTS OR TOYS

Anything is a toy if I choose to describe what I am doing with it as play.—Garth Evans.

For children, all objects have play potential; thus no distinction is made between objects and toys. Manipulative play presupposes that a number of perceptuo-motor skills have already been acquired. As Garvey (39) comments:

> . . . play with objects requires the achievement of visually directed grasping and adequate eye and hand coordination so that the child can pick up, hold and turn objects. Such play further depends on the achievement of "object permanence," which is the understanding that an object continues to exist even though it is temporarily out of sight. It also requires some differentiation of action patterns . . . the ability to perform different actions with an object (pp. 44-45).

Not only does the young infant attempt to grasp whatever comes into view, he closely inspects anything he has grasped. Furthermore, anything that is grasped is also likely to find its way into the mouth: Action patterns are as yet undifferentiated and when the infant strives to reach an object the mouth involuntarily opens, and similarly what is grasped in the hands is also very often orally explored.

Individual Patterns

Even at the early age of six months, we see that infants have characteristic patterns of playing with objects. Some infants, when presented with an object, are quick to grab it and manipulate it (58). Such *grabbers* not only engage in a variety of manipulatory explorations of the object but also readily put it in their mouths. Other children, whom we call *lookers*, are much more concerned with visual inspection of the object and seem less keen on manipulations which require taking the object close to the body. These characteristic patterns do not appear to have a particular significance for later activity and exploration since by the age of two years any differences in these respects have disappeared. However, it may be that what is salient in the environment for the *lookers* and *grabbers* in early life is rather different, and we find some indication of this in the fact that colour is much more readily discriminated by *lookers* than by *grabbers*. Similar findings have recently been obtained by other observers working with 12-19-month-old infants:

> Competent children approach their world in different ways. Some children seem to discover and search mainly through hand exploration, a manual movement pattern. They seem manually oriented to searching. A number of children seem to be active doers in play and follow a gross movement pattern . . . some children search through a visual regarding pattern, others through a locomotion pattern . . ." (51, p. 89).

As the infant acquires the capacity for prehension, gross manual movements like hitting, swiping, shaking, banging, scratching and waving are replaced by more complex movements of the hands and fingers. Visual attention is more sustained, though movement, colour and the other attributes of stimuli already mentioned still remain salient. In the second six months of life, throwing and dropping of objects and toys often become prominent play patterns. In many instances, these behaviours are an indication of the infant's lack of attention since, being immobile, he is unable to provide novel stimulation himself. A detailed study of the much-maligned activity of dropping in two seven-month-old infants (55, 65) indicated that while novel objects, however ordinary (e.g., jelly packets, ball of crumpled cellophane, toothbrush) were being manipulated, drops were infrequent; correspondingly, the span of manipulation was greater the more novel the object. Although drops did tend to increase with tiredness, this tendency was minimal in comparison with the effect of boredom. Thus, by dropping his toys, the relatively helpless infant is signifying to his caretaker that the particular object has no further interest for him at that moment and requesting that she provide some better alternative.

Developmental Sequences

In playing with objects, young infants are often impeded by their inability to let go of one object in their hands while reaching for or picking up another. As a result they often lose both! The six-month-infant cannot hold or manipulate two toys simultaneously; he can grasp with both hands an object in the mid-line or pick up with one hand and transfer to the other and manipulate with both hands. But hand use is not differentiated even by the age of 11 months and at this age a common pattern of play is the use of an object as an extension of the hand. Thus, when placing blocks on one another, nesting cups in each other or putting rings on a stick, the child will place the block, cup or ring and immediately withdraw it and repeat the movement without letting go of the particular object. It seems very much that a "block in the hand is worth two on the table" at this stage!

Reporting the results of a detailed study of the manipulative play of nine-to 24-month-olds, Rosenblatt (93, p. 34) made the surprising observation that "the young infant does not know intuitively how to play with objects," implying that there are certain responses which may more legitimately be regarded as "play" than others. Unfortunately, such an observation, referring as it does to the undifferentiated actions of the young infant, may tend to obscure the nature of the developmental sequence which Rosenblatt charts extremely well.

At nine months manipulative responses are largely undifferentiated and stereotyped; *indiscriminate* responses account for 50 percent of the responses to novel toys; *investigative* behaviour also figures prominentaly but *appropriate* behaviour (that which acknowledges the function of properties of the object) hardly at all. By 13 or 14 months, however, indiscriminate responses have almost disappeared and appropriate responses are the most evident.

In terms of the *type* of play activity, the predominant pattern between 12 and 18 months consists of sensori-motor play with a single toy. By 15 months, representational or "pretend" play has made its appearance, e.g., pushing a car, dialing a toy telephone, or "drinking" out of a cup. By 18 months several toys are used in combination in this manner. *Sensori-motor* activities with more than one toy at a time virtually disappear after 12 months, suggesting, as Rosenblatt (93) remarks, "that once the infant is able to deal simultaneously with several toys he is more likely to develop schemes for relating them in a meaningful, representational way (p. 36)." Rosenblatt also notes that development in play behaviour, i.e. the shift from simple to complex play routines, the decline in indiscriminate activity and corresponding increase in appropriate behaviours, is related to other cognitive abilities:

> Children who were early language learners demonstrated less mouthing and more social play even at nine months, and the power and range of significantly related variables increased over time. The most significant of these behaviours tended to be a greater amount of appropriate play, representational play, variety of responses, and amount of gesture and imitation in the mother-infant play sessions (p. 39).

The further development of manipulative strategies in the first three years of life is nicely illustrated by Greenfield, Nelson and Saltzman (44). They provided children with five nesting cups, which were placed before them individually; the children were given no specific instructions but the experimenter demonstrated the seriation strategy, i.e. nesting the cups starting with the smallest in the next size, these two in the third largest and so on. The child was then told to "play with the cups." On one trial the child was handed the smallest cup at the outset, on the next, the middle-sized, and on the third the largest cup. A strategy consisted of one or more moves, each involving the placement of an "acting" cup onto or into a stationary one. The most elementary strategy was *pairing*, where one cup was placed in or on another; very often the child would immediately remove the cup and place it on another and so on. This was the strategy predominantly used by the 11- to 12-month-old infants. In a slightly more complex strategy, the *pot method*, the child would form a nest or pile of three or more cups by moving one cup in/on to another and then another in/on to it, so that the stationary cup would serve as a pot into which the "acting" cups were put. Between the ages of 16 and 32 months this was the dominant strategy employed. The most sophisticated strategy, the *subassembly method*, involved placing one cup in another and these two together in a third and so on, the distinctive feature about this method being that a cup could have a dual role, being a stationary cup on one move and an "acting" cup on another. This strategy was not consistently in evidence until the age of three years, although it did make an appearance at around two years. The authors draw and develop the analogy between the development of these combinational action sequences and the development of linguistic structures, their concern being with the rules governing hierarchical organisation in each domain.

The strong tendency for the young child to use an object as an extension of its hand and not to differentiate its actions according to what is being held was revealed in the insistence on *pairing* even when given the biggest cup first—putting this down and picking up a smaller one to put in it was an impossible exercise. By this age, size and contiguity appear to replace colour as salient attributes of manipulable objects. The one- and two-year-olds always selected first those cups which were nearest to their active hand. Even two-year-olds have great difficulty bypassing a nearer object in order to reach a farther one, despite being cued by verbal signals.

Although by the age of three years children are able to order objects of different size into an increasing or decreasing series, younger children have a binary conception of size (44): One is "biggest" and the others are "little." Similarly, children younger than three have a binary conception of number—"one" versus "many." Only at preschool age do gradations come to be appreciated.

As the child's manual dexterity and coordination improve and as he gains independence through his mobility, materials and ordinary objects around the house acquire importance in play. Miniature replicas like toy cars, which can be pushed and "brummed" now become less attractive and spools of thread, cardboard boxes, saucepans, wooden spoons—objects which have a multiplicity of uses—are preferred. *Structural* complexity is replaced by *functional* complexity as the principal requirement of playthings. In other words, it is not the complexity of the design or appearance of the object that is important, but what a child is able to do with it. "A rubber ball is an extremely simple object," as Chance (15) says, "but it has a good deal of functional complexity: It can be bounced, rolled, thrown, chewed, squeezed, hit with a bat, spun around, tossed in the air. And the child's use of the rubber ball almost certainly teaches him more about the laws of physics than he would learn from watching Superman leap tall buildings in a single bound."

Chiefly for this reason, materials like sand, water, clay, plasticine and dough become important after the age of two years. The versatility of these materials is self-evident: The properties of the materials may be changed by relatively simple modifications like the addition of water to sand or the addition of dye or paint to water; the introduction of different ancillary equipment enhances and extends the use of the material, as when pipes and hoses in the water bucket or trough permit activities different from those with cups, jugs and bottles. Because the three- or four-year-old is manipulatively more adept than his younger counterpart, he can combine a variety of motor skills—he can pour and measure, or fill and empty, or roll and pat and lump; he can also use materials inventively, imaginatively and productively. Not only does such manipulative play extend the sensori-motor skills of the young child but also, in a more general way, it facilitates cognitive skills, as we shall see later.

Play with constructional toys like Lego, Meccano, and erector sets, which embody principles of both design and inventiveness, also become favoured activities of the three and four-year-old. So do puzzles, jigsaws and other problems which have an explicit goal of *solution*. These activities test higher level cognitive abilities; they require facility in, and manipulation of, two or more conceptual domains, such as evaluating size and shape or distance and movement. The attraction of such problems and tasks lies largely in the fact that they test the limits of the child's skill and capacity but do not exceed them, so that the child acquires a sense of mastery. Even older children derive more pleasure from solving a difficult problem rather than an easy one (46).

EXPLORATION AND PLAY

From the latter part of its first year, exploration is the predominant activity of the young child. As soon as he is mobile, he investigates the commonest of fixtures with the greatest avidity—plugs, switches, faucets, holes, and fluff all have the greatest attraction, and the harassed caretaker complains that he is "into everything." But most things *are* new to him and, driven by his innate curiosity (Pavlov, after all, termed the orienting reflex the "what-is-it" reflex), the young child has to investigate and explore it all. Because of this basic need to explore, stones and earthworms may be calmly eaten, beads and sticks pushed in noses or ears, or mud and sludge licked and sniffed. A detailed study of 84 infants by Uzgiris (120) attests to the significance of exploration, which she terms "examining":

> In examining, the infant no longer keeps the object stationary while looking at it; contrariwise he turns it around, pokes at it, feels its surface, manipulates its parts while observing the object and the effect of his manipulations on it. The appearance of the schema of examining represents a turning point in the infant's interactions with objects . . . Once the examining schema appears, it remains quite prominent in the infant's repertoire, especially in relation to objects which are relatively novel to him (p. 324).

In fact, examining remains the principal mode of interaction with objects presented to the child throughout the second year of life, and we may surmise, for the next few years.

Similar findings were obtained by White and Watts (120) in a study of children in their own homes—during the first two years of life. The ultimate objective of their study was an attempt to distinguish the salient experiences in the homes of children who developed well from those who proceeded to develop less well. Irrespective of whether a child was developing well or poorly, during the ages of one and two years he spent far more time oriented towards interactions with the physical environment than he did trying to affect people. In other words, non-social activities occupied far more of the child's time (89.4 percent for one-year-olds and 82.3 percent for two-year-olds) than did social ones, and of these, visual inspection and exploration were the most prominent activities.

Thus, exploration is the principal activity through which latent learning takes place, i.e., learning which is not reinforced or rewarded and which has no direct consequences for the child; it is the manner in which young children acquire information about their physical environment and, subsequently, about their social one. Exploration continues until the child feels he has learned the properties of the object being explored, whether this is objectively so or not. In the young infant exploration is chiefly visual, but by the age of eight months concentrated manipulation takes place and little time is lost looking around (71). At 12 months, exploration overrides many other attractions and may be sustained for long periods of times; as McCall says, the tempo of exploration becomes "denser and richer."

The opportunity to explore is one of the few conditions which will induce a young child to enter an unfamiliar environment or to leave the security of his mother (89, 90). Furthermore, when confronted with a new toy and a stranger, infants of nearly a year readily approached and explored the toy while showing less interest in the person (22). Investigation and exploration of toys also take precedence over interaction with peers in toddlers (6, 79). In the presence of peers, such play often leads to appropriation of the object, and the child's acquisitive propensity precludes any but hostile encounters—how familiar are the words "That's mine . . . *mine*!" The interest in exploration, on the other hand, can facilitate rudimentary social exchanges, even though the primary focus of attention remains the inanimate object:

> . . . the simultaneous explorations of common objects by two or more children provides opportunities to gain more understanding of their

peers . . . The formation of object-centred contacts is attributed more to the interest each child has invested in some activity with an object than to his curiosity concerning the behaviour of his age mates. For example, the engagement of child A with an object creates an interesting display that attracts the attention of another child and prompts his approach. Both children focus their attention on the same object and both act on it in nearly identical fashion. Yet because each one's interest is invested in the object itself, neither child recognises the effects of his own actions on the behaviour of the other child.

A cluster at the play group's toy train engine exemplifies an object-centred contact . . . Basically, one child discovers the engine, squats down, and makes the engine's whistle sound repeatedly. All other children in the room immediately toddle over to the engine and either sound the whistle or manipulate the steering handle, an action introduced by a second child. During the 68 seconds that several children are at the train, three children never look at their peers' faces and the other two children look only once or twice, and get no responses to their looks (79, p. 229).

Distinctions Between Exploration and Play

Although exploration is commonly regarded as play, and colloquially this may make sense, much of it is serious, concentrated activity which should be distinguished from more playful behaviours. The need to do so was emphasised by the results of studies of exploration in over 100 three- to five-year-old children. For these studies a completely new toy was designed so that by moving a lever children could produce lights or sounds (with a buzzer and a bell) or clock up counters; thus the toy provided novelty as well as allowing varying levels of complexity (53). When children were allowed to play with the toy on six successive occasions, an interesting sequence of behaviours emerged. First the child would approach and inspect the toy, then investigate it by touching, feeling and manipulating the lever; once he found out some of the features and properties of the toy he strove to reproduce this very active manipulation, using the toy all the time quite appropriately and with what Bronson (5) calls "functional fixity." Having learned the properties of this new toy, the child would then proceed to use it "playfully" and often inappropriately, in its functional sense, like climbing on it. The child appeared no longer to ask "what does this *object* do?" but "what can *I* do with this object?"—the emphasis shifted from inquiry to invention. Behaviourally, this transition was most marked: During the exploration the child was intent and attentive, looking closely at what he was doing but during the latter playful activity he was quite relaxed and at ease. The information and knowledge acquired during exploration were now being used in play: While exploration had been *assimilatory*, play was *expressive*. Exploration was also obligatory in that all children engaged in it and in much the same manner, while play was optional and idiosyncratic. There was no predicting how a child would play with the toy once he had explored it—one might sit on it and get the panda to "shoot" the lever, another might use the lever as a pop-singer's microphone. A formal analysis of these two classes of behaviour has shown exploration to be more constrained and systematically organised while play has a more flexible structure, this difference being interpreted in terms of the functional significance of the two behaviours (52).

Other findings that emerged from these studies were that when no sights or sounds were contingent upon the children's movements they lost interest in the toy fairly quickly and that the amount of play the children engaged in with the toy depended both on its complexity and how recently it had been played with. In other words, when play sessions occurred twice a day, the toy was *played* with far less than if they had occurred every other day (54). But a similar effect was not observed for exploration, suggesting that the rate at which a child *explores* and acquires information from a particular aspect of its environment is a function of the informational complexity of that aspect as well as the cognitive capacity of the child, other factors making only a marginal difference; on the other hand, the rate or extent to which the child *plays* with that particular source depends upon a number of adventitious factors, such as how often he has encountered it, for how long, his mood state, his inventiveness and so on.

Implications for Learning

Thus, it may be seen that a distinction between exploration and play may be made on several grounds. Far from being an academic exercise, it becomes imperative to do so when one considers the implications for learning. We found that if children engaged in playful activity with this toy prematurely, i.e., before they had learned all there was to know about it, they were likely not to acquire any further information during their play (57). For instance, a boy, having found the bell and incorporated it in a game in which he ran around the room filling a truck and ringing the bell twice each time he passed the toy, failed in the end to find out about the buzzer. Involvement in the playful activity—"doing his own thing"—precluded his learning any more about the other properties of the toy. Only if, in the course of his play, he chanced upon another feature of the toy would he

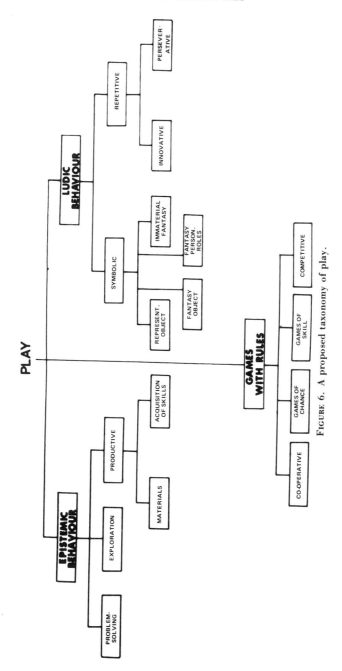

FIGURE 6. A proposed taxonomy of play.

stop and investigate further; learning in this playful phase then was very much a matter of happenstance. The child commenced play when he *thought* he had learned all about the unfamiliar toy and therefore the fact that, objectively, he had more information to glean was immaterial. The assumption that "children learn through play" may be an unjustifiable and hazardous one.

In order to formalise the distinctions in the motivation and function of exploration and play which have been discussed so far, a taxonomy has been developed (60) which opposes *epistemic* behaviour to *ludic* behaviour (see Figure 6). Briefly, the former refers to activities which are concerned with knowledge and information and the latter to those which are playful and fun. These categories differ first in their focus of attention, epistemic behaviour being cued by an external source of stimulation whereas ludic behaviour lacks such a specific focus. Secondly, while epistemic behaviours are relatively independent of mood state, ludic behaviour is highly mood dependent—the child plays because he wishes to and simply for the fun of it; if he is anxious it is hardly reasonable to expect him to "have fun." Thirdly, there are constraints imposed upon epistemic behaviour which stem from the nature of the focus of attention, whereas any constraints in ludic behaviour are only those which the child imposes upon himself. These two major categories may be further subdivided and reading from left to right of the classification we may note a progression from the most task- or work-like activities to those which are least constrained and most idiosyncratic. The classification is elaborated further and related to dimensions of physiological arousal and to cognitive domains in another publication (61).

Exploration and Handicap

We have already mentioned that play, unlike exploration, is affected by a variety of factors. Thus, children with brain damage and those diagnosed as autistic engaged in exploratory activity in a similar situation but failed to manifest any playful behaviour (55A, 56). The reasons were quite different for the two groups: the brain-damaged children failed to retain the information they acquired through exploration from one session to the next, so that on each occasion they would need to investigate the toy anew, their cognitive limitations permitting only a very gradual decline of exploratory activity over time; the autistic children, on the other hand, showed a long latency to explore, but once they had done so, they then left the toy and invariably returned to a stereotypic form of activity, their internal state of high arousal precluding a relaxed and unrestrained activity like play (56).

SYMBOLIC PLAY

Symbolic play is quintessentially human. It involves, as its characteristic ingredient, the element of pretence, the use of "as if"; it reflects the origin of representation and symbolisation. This form of play may be referred to by many other synonymous terms: While Piaget (86) and Sutton-Smith (113) prefer the use of symbolic, others have called it socio-dramatic play (108), imaginative or make-believe play (105), thematic play (34), fantasy play (67, 109) and pretend play (30, 39).

Symbolic play is generally evident from the age of 18 months, when a child may "comb" her hair, eat an imaginary sweet or "drink" from a cup. As Piaget (86) says, "Symbolic play implies representation of an absent object. The symbol can be incorporated into sensori-motor practice whereupon it subordinates it. In the pretence of going to sleep for instance, the actions themselves may become extremely complicated, ritualised or distorted but they are all integrated in the symbolic act of sleeping." Symbolic play may involve many different imaginary constituents: Two objects may be used "as if" they were something else, e.g., a chair as a truck, or a cloth as a baby; the child may play the role of another, be it mother, engine driver or policeman; or the whole incident may be imaginary as when a child talks to an imaginary companion or feeds a non-existent animal. At its simplest level, replicas and miniatures may be used in the conventional manner, i.e., representationally.

Are animals then capable of engaging in symbolic play? Is a kitten who chases after a ball of wool, patting or "teasing" it when it stops, involved in pretend play? Piaget (86, p. 82) would answer in the negative since he sees a distinction between the symbolic play of humans and the incomplete actions which are often regarded as play in young animals—"Kittens which fight with their mother and bite without hurting her are not 'pretending' to fight, since they do not know what real fighting is . . ."—but he does acknowledge that this might be a preparatory stage for representational symbols. Since young animals are clearly capable of playing with objects "as if" they were something else, we may have to concede that this constitutes a rudimentary form of symbolic (representational) play; what children can do, however, is to develop multiple "as if" roles and functions for the same people and objects and integrate and organise these in some thematic form. The child, unlike the animal, is not constrained by the structural properties of his materials in implementing his fantasy, nor by any limits of reality: "Let's pretend that we're not pretending" will tax one's reflexive powers in any literal context.

Developmental Stages

Symbolic play increases in frequency during the first few years, reaching a peak at around four to five years, but within this period there are clearly discernible developmental stages:

> At about 12 months of age, pretending involves a familiar and well-practised behaviour detached from its customary context: the child tilts his head back as he drinks out of an empty cup, or closes his eyes pretending to sleep without actually doing so. In these early forms, the materials are typically ordinary household objects, while the behaviours are notable because the child enacts acting or sleeping in the absence of any apparent desire for food or sleep. By 18 months of age, pretend play begins to acquire two new characteristics. First, the focus shifts from self to other: the child might pretend to feed his mother, a doll or a toy animal . . . Second, between 20 and 26 months, pretending becomes increasingly independent of the features of the immediate situation: an inanimate object (doll or stick) might be treated as if it were animate, and a great many things might be treated as cups, spoons or beds . . . (30, p. 291).

The question arises as to whether the young child is constrained by the physical properties of the prop in using it as a substitute for the real thing. In other words, how much does an object have to satisfy the criteria of "cupness" to be placed in the child's class of "drink-from-ables"? This is an important question since it relates to an aspect of cognitive development. It shows us whether the child is matching for structural equivalence (i.e. roundness, hollowness, handle, etc.) or has passed on to the stage of functional equivalence.

Fein (30) looked at the substitutions that two-year-old children commonly made in their pretend play, paying particular attention to the transformations that were required by these substitutions. For example, drinking from a shell requires more transformation than drinking from a more prototypical beaker; or feeding a toy horse with a leaf would require two transformations—one from the inanimate to the animate and the other from one inanimate object (realistic) to another (functional). Fein predicted that children of this age would find more than one substitution difficult. Her results showed that, in a standard situation, pretending was more likely (in 93 percent of two-year-olds) when the objects were prototypical, e.g., a toy horse was fed when the horse was horselike and the cup cuplike. When less realistic substitutions were offered, the likelihood of pretence dropped; it dropped even further if two such substitutions were offered simultaneously, as when it was suggested that the child should feed a metal horse shape with a clam shell. These results were a clear demonstration that, for the young child, still learning the features of its environment and forming schema, too great a departure from reality is difficult to assimilate; thus, imaginative play was most readily facilitated by miniature replicas. Interestingly, even when adults modeled the pretence play, very few children were able to imitate when the modeling involved less prototypical toys and when more than one substitution was required. This finding supported Piaget's assertion that imitation, even when it involves representation and mental image, only occurs when the schema is well rehearsed and established, and refuted El'Konin's (25) argument that a child's imaginative play will be facilitated by the imitation of a playful adult.

In a subsequent study, Fein et al. (31) found that two-year-old girls engaged more readily in pretend play, even with less prototypical toys, than did boys, and related this finding to girls' relative superiority in other symbolic activities such as language.

With increasing age, the preference for highly structured and prototypical toys decreases (85, 87) and, as we saw earlier, functional complexity becomes a more important attribute than structural similarity. Children show a greater variety and flexibility in their fantasy themes when playing with less realistic toys. Children who showed a high disposition for fantasy play showed an even greater preference for unstructured toys than those with a low disposition for such play (87).

Symbolic play is initially solitary and only later becomes social. Even between the ages of three and five years, cooperative role-playing was a relatively rare occurrence (100), whereas solitary fantasy, particularly among boys, or "interactive" fantasy, where children enacted roles without necessarily reciprocally relating or developing a theme, was much more common. Here, again, four-year-old girls engaged in more cooperative role-playing than boys, presumably as a result of their social propensities and linguistic competence.

Content of Fantasy

The content of symbolic play also changes with age. The earliest themes to appear are domestic ones with Mother and Baby perhaps the commonest. Mothers and Fathers, Husbands and Wives, Teachers and Pupils are followed at the age of three years by what Garvey (39) calls *character* roles—Doctors, Nurses, Policemen, Cowboys, etc. Later still emerge the *fictional* roles, in contemporary society mostly taken from television, such as Batman, Dr. Who, Six-Million-Dollar Man.

Sherrod and Singer (103) consider symbolic play to be dependent on several abilities: the ability to form images; the capacity to store and retrieve the images already formed; the ability to build a store of such images; and skill in recombining, integrating and generally divorcing them from reality. Symbolic play then must reflect the content of the child's own experiences, and it is for this reason that domestic and family themes occur earliest and predominate in the fantasy play of young children. Even at nursery school, the doll-corner is usually the favourite location (43) and Mother and Father are the commonest role portrayals (27, 73) in imaginative play. Knowledge of these roles is extensive and hence the children are able to develop and elaborate them in a manner they cannot with fictional roles. Girls and boys also choose roles which are sex-appropriate—boys will less readily play the part of mother or nurse and girls that of engine-driver, largely because in their experience this is how it has been. A girl's knowledge of a mother's role is far more extensive than a boy's knowledge of his father's. This difference is nicely illustrated by the following story: A boy and girl were playing "home" and being mother and father respectively; the girl busied herself doing a great many things—sweeping, washing, ironing, telephoning, baking and so on; the boy got on his tricycle, rode to the back of the house, reappeared five minutes later, kissed the girl saying "Hallo love," lay down on the couch and "went to sleep"! The little boy had little information about a father's role other than what he observed in the home and therefore little basis upon which to develop the role in play. It is hardly surprising that girls spend 75 percent of their fantasy-play time in house-play as opposed to the boys' 30 percent (73).

Similar restrictions in role enactment are observed in the portrayal of television characters like the Six-Million-Dollar Man or Batman, where supplementary information about the character's attributes or potential is lacking. After all, to the young child, the attribute "bionic" only means that it enables a character to run fast slowly or to heave monumental weights—no other features are explained in a manner readily assimilable by the four- or five-year-old. Thus, portrayal of these characters becomes stereotyped, perseverative and essentially mimetic.

The richness and complexity of symbolic play reflect directly the richness and complexity of a child's experience. It is partly for this reason that disadvantaged children show little fantasy play (34, 92, 108). But perhaps more important is the fact that such children are often linguistically disadvantaged and are observed in situations with which they are unfamiliar and in circumstances in which they are ill at ease, all of which would militate against the manifestation of fantasy play. Feitelson has also suggested that the paucity of toys and playthings in disadvantaged homes may lead to the lack of flexibility and inventiveness in the use of objects.

Social-class differences in the amount and quality of fantasy play have recently been reported (110, 119), though studies of our own have failed to show differences between children in nursery schools and those in day-care centres in the frequency of such play (64). It is difficult to know to what specific factors such differences may be ascribed, but Singer's (105) interpretation offers some suggestion: Fantasy play, he claims, is potentiated by, first, a close identification and frequent interaction with a parent who is sympathetic and supportive in such play and, secondly, some opportunities for privacy so that the child might reprocess and integrate his experiences.

Historical and cultural changes in the content of symbolic play also attest to the fact that such play constitutes the child's endeavours to assimilate his experiences in accordance with his schemas. In contemporary symbolic play, planes and cars have supplanted ships and horse-drawn coaches, Star War heroes and gangsters have supplanted handsome princes and witches. What is salient in a child's experience is immediately and invariably incorporated in his play. Opie and Opie (82) recall that children in Berlin, shortly after the building of the Wall, were shooting at each other across miniature walls and that children at Auschwitz even played "going to the gas chamber." On the other hand, girls in Taleland play house by grinding sand (millet) between two small stones or make dolls out of sticks of wood and carry them on their backs with the support of a cloth wrapping, while boys gather sand and pretend to make a yam mould or pretend to be hunters chasing younger children who walk on all fours in imitation of antelopes or water buffaloes (35).

Sometimes, however, the attempts at assimilation of new experience may go awry, when the disjunction between experience and schema is too great. A humorous illustration is provided by Singer and Singer (107): A four-year-old boy is playing alone on the kitchen floor at home; he has lined up a large number of toy soldiers and plastic cowboys and the mother, seeing them, asks "What are you doing with all your soldiers and cowboys lined up like that?" "I'm getting all my guys ready. We're going to rescue Daddy," he replies. "Why?" asks the mother. The boy replies, "I heard you talking on the telephone and you said that Daddy was 'all tied up' at work."

Through the Looking-glass of Symbolic Play

Since symbolic play lies in the expressive domain, it gives adults access to biographical, motivational and emotional information about the child, information that may not be readily available in conventional contexts. Child psychotherapists, as Lowenfeld (70) so graphically describes, have long made use of such information in working with disturbed or maladjusted children. In the past the utility of such data has been appreciated only in the social and emotional areas of development. A recent study, however, has revealed that such analyses of symbolic play may also inform us about the cognitive skills of the young child. This study in particular was initiated by the general observation that three- and four-year-old children in day-care centres commonly engaged in rather infantile speech, whereas when they were involved in fantasy play they appeared to use more elaborate speech.

Many of the children in the five day nurseries we studied would be classified as disadvantaged on family and socioeconomic criteria. Their general linguistic retardation therefore was not a matter of special concern, though many of them frequently used two-word utterances or "baby words." An analysis was made of 30 utterances recorded during their fantasy play. A syntactic analysis of the speech was carried out using the following measures:

1) Mean length of utterance (MLU): the mean number of morphemes per utterance, an utterance being distinguished by intonation, pauses etc.
2) Type-token ratio (TTR): a measure of lexical diversity expressed as a ratio of the number of different word types occurring in a sequence of 200 words (tokens).
3) Number of adverbs in the 30 utterances.
4) Number of modal auxiliary verbs: auxiliary verbs which refer to the likelihood, possibility, etc. of the event in the main verb, e.g. *can, must, would, may*.

The results (Figure 7) showed that on all four measures the children scored higher during fantasy play sessions and three of these differences were significant. In other words, these children were displaying a greater competence in their language usage than could be discerned from their ordinary speech. It was striking that such young children could be almost "bilingual," having the ability to use two different speech codes; furthermore, their *performance* in everyday speech gave little clue as to their *competence*, i.e., knowledge of the rules that apply to the syntactic structure of language. As sociolinguists like Bernstein (4) have frequently pointed out, linguistic codes are realisations of the social structures and dependent upon the context: Where children are free from constraint in expressing their thoughts, ideas, experiences, the language used is correspondingly unconstrained. In this manner, then, symbolic play serves as a looking-glass through which the percipient adult may be granted access to the inner world of the child.

LANGUAGE

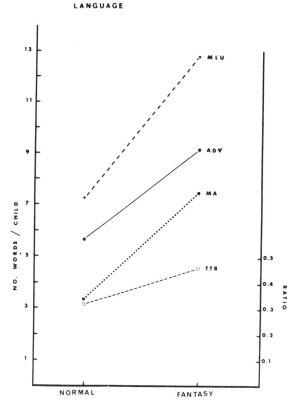

FIGURE 7. Scores on measures of syntax during normal conversation and during fantasy-play.

PLAY WITH LANGUAGE

Play with language can take one of two forms, just as in the case of more tangible material: It may be *exploratory* when the child is trying to find out how his language works, what words and phrases really mean, how literal idioms and metaphors are used; or it may be *ludic* as when the child repeats and rehearses what he has already learned or deliberately tries to flout rules and conventions as in punning or nonsense verse, or places "unacceptable" variations on conventional language. Examples of the former type of play are illustrated by the girl who asked, "Since there is running water, is there sitting water?" (39) or by the boy who, on being told by his mother not to pick fights, replied, "Oh, Mommie, what can I do when the fight just crawls out of me?" Examples of the latter type of language play are much more common, and are often more interesting since once again they give us an insight into the kind of skills the children are rehearsing and consolidating.

Play with sounds appears early in infancy when babbling takes place. Repetition of syllables is the commonest forms, e.g., da-da, goo-goo, and repetitive rhythmic vocalisations are natural accompaniments of states of pleasure. A little later onomatopoeic sounds are repeated, e.g., beep-beep, brmm-brmm. Sounds like tongue-clicking or nasal rasping can give pleasure, as can nonsense syllables:

> da ti di
> do di da
> di do da di go bo di
> di do da di go bo di (39)

A two-year-old chanted this as he was being undressed:

> Nolly lolly, nolly, lolly, nilly, lolly, sillie Billie, nolly lolly (14).

The recordings and analyses made by Weir (121) of her two-year-old son's monologues as he prepared to sleep are beautiful illustrations of a child's play with all aspects of the linguistic system, ranging from sound play and enumeration:

> One two three four
> One two
> One two three four
> One two three
> Anthony counting
> Good boy you
> One two three

to pronominal substitution:

> I go up there
> I go up there
> I go
> She go up there

Sound play occupies a significant place in the young child's experience with linguistic structures. As Sanches and Kirshenblatt-Gimblett (99) point out:

It is not accidental that in children's verbal play rhythmic, highly phonologically patterned gibberish should be employed to a much greater extent than in the traditional verbal act productions of adults who prefer nonsense which is syntactically determined. Gibberish is purely phonologically motivated and depends for its appeal upon the fact that phonology, as compared with semantics and syntax, is far more highly developed in the child's language. For example:

> Inty minty tibbety fig
> Deema dima doma dig
> Howchy powchy domi nowday
> Hom tom tout
> Out goes you (p. 92).

Rhyming, punning and word-play are popular pastimes of older children and ritual recitations are frequently heard in the playgrounds (81). Chukovsky (16) describes how "the more palpable the nonsense," the greater the pleasure the child derives:

> The cook rode on a rickety van
> Harnessed to a frying pan.

"The rooster miaows" caused the utmost hilarity even in a two-year-old.

As the child becomes more proficient in the rules and use of his language, his play becomes more sophisticated; puns and riddles like this one

> Q. What did Tene-see?
> A. The same thing Arkan-saw.

do not appear until late childhood. Cazden (13) makes the important point that language can have two functional attributes: It can be *transparent*, when the speaker, listener or reader is not paying attention to the words themselves but only to their meaning, or it can be made *opaque* when the language itself becomes the focus of attention. Thus, in the first case, it may not matter whether the word "hasty," "speedy" or "quick" was used, whereas in the latter case it would. Children can only be playful with the known and familiar; they must therefore become proficient in the utilitarian or communicative function of language before they are able to use it in the ludic mode. As Sanches and Kirshenblatt-Gimblett (99) point out, the child's concern shifts from phonological to grammatical to semantic and finally to the sociolinguistic level of language—reflecting an exercise in whatever linguistic structure the child is currently mastering.

Mother-Infant Play

The earliest manifestations of social play in the infant are with its mother. As the mother changes her infant's diaper she may lean over and blow gently on his face and after several repetitions the infant coos or laughs. Here, repetitions and the anticipation of a predictable response are what cause merriment.

Social play has four characteristics: mutual involvement with another (others), turn alternation, repetition, and non-literality (94). At its most elementary level it seems that repetition is a sufficient condition for fun. Call (11) describes the involvement of infants as young as two months in the Cough Game:

> It begins when the baby coughs spontaneously, and the mother, out of empathy or experimentation, imitates him. At first her cough and smile only arouse the baby's attention, but eventually he coughs in return, starting an exchange of coughs and smiles that delights the infant totally and makes him laugh.
> At a later stage the baby initiates the game himself by coughing and smiling when the mother is not expecting it . . . The cough game is a source of endless amusement for the baby, and it can be repeated many times, initiated by baby, mother, or anyone who learns the rules (p. 34).

Rules and conventions are indeed inherent in social play. If mutual involvement is to be sustained it is necessary for the partners to acknowledge the rules which govern that involvement. In infancy it is usually the mother who takes the initiative in play with her child and Stern (112) has described the many subtle ways in which she may control and facilitate the child's enjoyment.

The mother's face soon becomes the most salient visual stimulus for the infant and she uses it to good effect in stimulating play: She raises her eyebrows, opens her mouth, exaggerates other features, invariably accompanying them by vocalisations which change pitch or intensity. If these events are contingent upon an action of the infant, the glee is doubled. The child's capacity for sustained involvement is severely limited, so the mother carefully monitors the responses of her child and titrates her behaviour accordingly. Where a mother fails to do this, thereby overstimulating or tiring the child, the play ceases as the child becomes unresponsive. Mothers also modify the types of games they initiate, moving from sensory games with young infants to those involving greater motor activity with older ones (18).

Peek-a-boo is probably the commonest game that adults play with young children. In an analysis of this game in infants between seven and 17 months of age, Bruner and Sherwood (8) demonstrated that children were able to abstract and learn the governing rules: initial contact, disappearance, reappearance and re-established contact. Once these were learned, the children incorporated their own variations. With increasing age, children were more likely to take the initiative and to impose upon the game their own innovations and distortions.

Developmental Sequence

Much of a young child's play is solitary with respect to its peers. The involvement of the mother in many forms of play (21) bears greater testimony to the mother's concern and interest than to the child's reciprocity. We have already seen from the studies of Bronson (6) and Mueller and Lucas (79) that one-year-olds interact little when playing except to retain or appropriate possessions. During their second year of life, however, children begin to show a greater interest in their peers, showing and offering their toys, smiling and gesturing and even attempting to engage in some interactive play (23).

Parten (84) outlined a sequence of six social play categories for preschool children: unoccupied behaviour, solitary play, onlooker behaviour, parallel play, associative play and cooperative play. She found that two-year-olds engaged mostly in solitary play, two-and-a-half-year-olds in parallel play and four-year-olds in associative play. Because of this observed age-dependence there has been a tendency to regard solitary play as less "mature" than associative play. Barnes (2) found much less associative and cooperative play among three- and four-year-olds than did Parten and argued that young children of the 70s were less skilled in organising and negotiating effective participation. However, Moore et al. (78) found no evidence to support the notion of solitary play as immature—on the contrary it was generally associated with task-oriented and educationally significant activities. From a study in which they examined these play categories in different social classes, Rubin et al. (96) conclude:

> It is our contention that parallel, and not solitary, play is indicative of the least mature level of a social-cognitive play hierarchy for three- and four-year-olds. Thus children who play by themselves may purposively wish to "get away from it all," while those who play beside others may desire the company of other children but may not be able to successfully take their points of view in order to play in an associative or cooperative manner (p. 418).

Games

As other forms of play decline in later childhood, they are replaced by games, the characteristic features of which are explicit rules and conventions. Piaget (86) believes that much can be learned about the child's understanding of morality by observing his acceptance of and adherence to the rules and sanctions pertaining to games. Games may be cooperative or competitive; they may be games of chance or games of skill. Sutton-Smith (114) has argued cogently that games are functionally related to culture and patterns of child-rearing. He argues that games do not exist randomly in the structural fabric of society but are there for a cultural purpose, as systems for the socialisation of conflict and power (116). Thus, more complex cultures have more complex games, an important feature of the latter lying in the opportunity it affords the players for *reversibility*—of roles (as in hide-and-seek), of intentionality (to play or not), of social control (adults versus children, boys versus girls), of rules (innovation and violation). Thus, involvement in games enables the child to enact roles and perform responses he would otherwise be unable to, and Sutton-Smith argues that this leads to increased flexibility in behaviour together with increased autonomy and confidence (117).

For Mead (74), on the other hand, play and games were clearly differentiated insofar as they have different functions in relation to the development of self: Play permits the child to take on various social roles and thereby mould his character, but in games the child must be able to understand and take on the role of everyone else—he must be able to be batsman and bowler. It is the involvement in games therefore that is the natural antecedent of the child's becoming "an organic member of society."

FUNCTIONS OF PLAY

Perhaps the most refractory problem in the analysis of play is the ascription of functions to it. If, for reasons of elusive criteria or conceptual convenience, we use the term in its comprehensive, and often loose, sense, then we must accept that almost any function may be attributed to the behaviour, without danger of contradiction or without necessarily furthering our understanding. Thus, any discussion on the "functions of play" is a hazardous exercise and may only be undertaken with the caveat that different forms of play are clearly distinguished. No single function may be ascribed to all play, nor may the function proposed for one type of play be generalised to another.

Classical theories of play have been well reviewed elsewhere (26, 76, 105) and will not be discussed here. Attention will rather be given to those theoretical positions which have most to say about the play of young children and more generally about the role of play in development—both of the individual and the culture.

Emotional Catharsis

"Play," said Klein (66), "is a flight from reality." The forms of play that psychoanalytic theorists were primarily concerned with were symbolic. It is assumed that, operating according to the pleasure principle, children reenact, transform or reconstitute their experiences in accordance with their wishes, needs and desires. Three interrelated functions have been ascribed to children's fantasy play. First, play, being removed from the constraints of reality, is seen as a vehicle for the release of emotional tension. In the face of conflict, frustration and denial in reality, a child can obtain wish-fulfillment and satisfaction through play. The fears and anxieties that a child has are projected into the fantasy play and are thereby divested of their traumatic character; the originally emotional experiences become neutralised, so to speak.

Secondly, in playing out such experiences, the child is assumed to achieve some mastery over a situation in which he was previously impotent; he changes his role from a passive recipient (e.g., at the dentist's) to an active manipulator. And thirdly, in re-enactment of this sort the child becomes increasingly able to identify with the all-powerful adult whose capacities and competence he envies. In Freud's words:

> It is clear that in their play children repeat everything that has made a great impression on them in real life, and that in doing so they abreact the strength of the impression and, as one might put it, make themselves master of the situation. But on the other hand it is obvious that all their play is influenced by a wish that dominates them the whole time—the wish to be grown up and do what grown up people do (37, p. 16).

In considering these functions of play, it is obligatory for us to consider the mechanisms whereby the postulated effects are achieved. Freud suggests that emotional tensions are dissipated through abreaction, but this process only works therapeutically when used in a systematic manner and it is difficult to see how the somewhat haphazard play of hospitals, doctors, etc., would cancel trauma associated with them. Is a child who plays at being in the dentist's chair, or being the dentist for that matter, less anxious when visiting the dentist than a child who has had the dental routine explained to him?

The notion that play with substitute objects and materials aids in the resolution of psychosexual conflicts is difficult to accept in the absence of any explication of the process, e.g., how exactly does play with water and sand aid in the toilet competence of children in the anal stage? Empirical evidence in support of these views is at best equivocal. Opportunities for aggressive play, for example, failed to reduce the amount of aggression displayed in real contexts (26, p. 55). Findings by Gilmore (42) that children in the hospital engaged in play with hospital-type toys more than non-hospitalised children has been interpreted as evidence in support of the cathartic position but it could be as well argued that the toys were chosen for their salience rather than for their association with anxiety.

Similar questions may be raised concerning the child's achievement of mastery through the fantasy situation, where no constraints or sanctions apply. It is difficult to see how the child who is spanked nullifies this or achieves ascendance in the parent-child context by spanking her doll. Moreover, many of the interpretations required by this view of play far transcend the evidence:

> The very fact that the little girl plays with dolls at all—which the mother takes to be such a sweet and natural act of imitation—is in the child's unconscious an aggression against the mother. It is an aggression in that it is a way of saying "It is I who should have the children, not you" . . . it is a way of saying "Mother, you are no longer necessary; I am a big lady now, and it is I who should have the long dresses and babies, not you; you can be dispensed with (75, p. 68).

If fantasy play does in fact ameliorate tension and mitigate conflict, it is unlikely that this occurs at a purely affective level, as Freud supposed. Cognitive mechanisms must inevitably be implicated. One such example is suggested by Gould (43): "The child's ability to verbalise affective stresses and dilemmas symbolically in fantasy scenes tends to effect some psychological distance from terror or rage that might otherwise be expressed in behaviour symptoms (p. 162)." Piaget (86, p. 136), too, speaks of "symbolic games of liquidation" where the "pain" of an anxious event becomes bearable through assimilation to the *whole* activity of the ego.

Activity and Learning

As we have already noted from earlier discussions, sensori-motor play serves multifarious functions. It aids manual skills like prehension and dexterity and gross motor skills like balance and coordination; it enables the young child to build a stable percept of its environment, facilitates the acquisition of object permanence and ensures provision of varied sensory input during development.

But sensori-motor activity also facilitates more complex forms of learning and serves as the basis for the development of cognitive skills. Piaget was the first to stress the importance of action in intellectual development, and actions are the base of his central constructs viz. *operations*: "to know an object is to act upon it." Operations are interiorised actions and are concerned with modifying and transforming the objects of knowledge. Thus, the child actively manipulates and transforms substances before he can acquire the concepts of weight and volume; he counts and measures, he orders objects in a series. These sets of actions modifying the object enable the child to get at the structures of the transformations. As Piaget (86) exhorted teachers:

> Teaching means creating situations where structures may be discovered; it does not mean transmitting structures which may be assimilated at nothing other than a verbal level. Children can learn better by doing things than by being told about them . . . The subject must be active, must transform things, and find the structure of his own actions on the objects (20, p. 3).

An illuminating example of the young child's need to *learn-through-action* is provided by Farnham-Diggory (29). She presented children with blocks arranged in the order shown in Figure 8. The dot cards were placed in scrambled order, face up, and the child was asked to "put the cards with the blocks, the way they are supposed to go." While five-year-olds did this with ease, it proved to be a difficult task for four-year-olds. They could well appreciate that one card had more dots than another and one block more area than another, but they could not match the two: they could not see that a greater-than or more-than relation in one dimension was equivalent to a greater-than relation in another dimension. Children were then rehearsed with verbal cues—to point and say, "This is more than that," or "this is big and this is little," but, although they did this perfectly with each series individually, they were still unable to do the matching. What *did* help, however, was an acting out of these differences as when the children took a small step for the small block and a giant stride for the big block and similarly for the dots. This study elegantly exemplifies the reliance the four-year-old places on action and doing in order to consolidate the bases for more abstract skills.

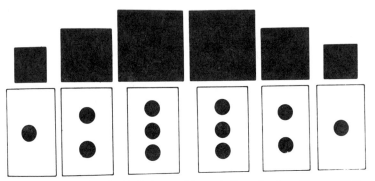

FIGURE 8. Stimuli for the block-dot matching task (from Farnham-Diggory, 1972).

Similarly, in the development of symbolic representation, actions directed towards the self are represented earlier than actions directed to the external world, i.e., pretending to brush one's teeth is easier for a three-year-old than pretending to cut a loaf of bread (83). Moreover, the first representations involve use of the child's body parts rather than symbolic objects—in other words, a child will use his finger *as* a toothbrush rather than pretend to be holding one, indicating again that the origin of symbolic representation lies in the child's own action patterns and only later are other features of the environment represented in this way.

In learning to speak, children learn action words earlier than words relating to static features. Bates et al. (3) give examples of words arising as *part* of actions before they are used to *represent* the actions. Children comprehend adult speech chiefly by mapping meanings on to actions, relations, displacements, etc. that they themselves have experienced (24). Sinclair (104) makes perhaps the strongest theoretical exposition of the parallels between sensori-motor intelligence and language: She argues that the structural constituents of sensori-motor action have their direct equivalent in language, that the pervasive property of language, viz. recursivity, also pertains to action-schema and that this equivalence makes linguistic competence highly probable:

> . . . the child possesses a set of coordinations of action-schemes which can be shown to have certain structural properties which will make it possible for him to start comprehending and producing language. These same structural properties will later develop into the interiorised logical operations (p. 127).

Arguing in a somewhat different vein, Bruner (7) has said that play provides opportunities for trying out, rehearsing and combining action routines, thus facilitating "combinatorial flexibility." He argues that it was just such activity that enabled the higher primates to evolve tool use. In play, children and young animals are abstracting general rules and principles about their experiences rather than learning specific information, and thus active play aids problem-solving. In support of his argument he offers the results of an experiment with colleagues (118), where three- and four-year-old children were given the opportunity of playing with sticks and clamps before using them to solve a problem. Children who had played with the clamps did better than children who had been given instruction in how to use the clamps but no better than those who had observed a complete solution by an adult. Thus, although we do not know that play always leads to the most efficacious solutions, we may be sure that it helps such solutions. As Sylva et al. conclude, ". . . the effect of prior play seems to be not only in combinatorial practice, but also in shifting emphasis in a task from ends to means, from product to process (p. 256)."

Play and Social Skills

Perhaps the strongest proponents of play as a socialising agent in a child's development are anthropologists. Fortes (35) remarked that "play is the paramount educational exercise of Tale children" and argued that in play a child rehearsed his skills, interests and obligations, making experiments in social living without having to pay the penalty for mistakes. Students of many cultures have regarded the mimetic play of young children as an important transitional stage in their acculturation, and games, too, are seen to be models of cultural activities—games of strategy are related to mastery of the social system and games of chance to mastery of the supernatural (102).

Others have argued that engagement in social play, as in any other social encounter, enables the child to learn social rules more easily and to understand the view of the other. Smilansky (108) found that training disadvantaged children to play imaginatively increased their prosocial behaviours and reduced their aggression. Such play-training has also been shown to increase empathy and resistance to temptation (98). Although a number of socially advantageous effects associated with imaginative play have been described by Sherrod and Singer (103), it must be remembered that these effects are correlated and not causal, and we have little idea of what mechanisms are involved. Furthermore, many of the effects reported were results of training programmes and it is possible that it is close involvement with adults in the programme rather than the play *per se* that is the critical factor (111). The importance of *playfulness* for many aspects of development has been well demonstrated by Liebermann (69).

Play as Arousal-modulation

In proposing functions for play, it must not be overlooked that the play activities of young children and young animals have much in common. Hence, explanation of play in wholly psychological terms may not be entirely adequate. Two recent theories have endeavoured to place play in a more biological context, using the psychophysiological construct of arousal which refers to the alertness and activation of the organism.

For each individual there is an optimal level of arousal; both over-arousal and under-arousal impair performance. Arousal level is varied by the amount and rate of stimulus input. These two notions were originally combined by Schultz (101) to formulate a drive for sensory input to maintain optimal arousal and called *sensoristasis*, a process equivalent to homeostasis:

> Sensoristasis can be defined as a drive state of critical arousal which impels the organism (in a waking state) to strive to maintain an optimal level of sensory variation. There is, in other words, a drive to maintain a constant range of varied sensory input in order to maintain cortical arousal at an optimum level (p. 30).

Ellis (26) has used this drive of sensoristasis to explain play: Play, he argues, is stimulus-seeking behaviour, motivated by the sensoristatic drive, and requiring no external reinforcement other than the sensory input itself. Thus, play is more common in the young of a species, in domesticated rather than wild animals, in industrialised as opposed to subsistence communities—all of which share circumstances where time and effort are not pre-empted by the demands of survival. However, not all stimulus-seeking behaviours are play.

The other theory is similar in many respects to Ellis', particularly in its use of the construct of arousal, but conceives of play as a *neural primer*, operating to keep neural centres alert and active in the absence of adequate stimulation (60, 61). But play, in the form of exploratory and other epistemic behaviours, also functions to modulate arousal, when sensory input is high. In addition, pure ludic activity is seen as "time out" for the nervous system: During such playful play the nervous system is offered respite from processing information to engage in recuperative activity, and at a psychological level to consolidate already assimilated information (62). This formulation takes account of the paradox that ludic activity is low in the motivational hierarchy and may be inhibited by almost any other drive-state.

Play and Culture

Play and games are seen by many to reflect the structure and organisation of the societies in which they occur. This view is best exemplified and most originally developed by Sutton-Smith (114) in his *The Two Cultures of Games*, where he contrasts *ascriptive* game cultures and *achievement* game cultures. Ascriptive game cultures typically are seen in communities where the family is extended rather than nuclear and the child has no privacy; the group is dominated by powerful individuals and respect for authority is unilateral rather than reciprocal. In such groups, play is essentially imitative and representative rather than imaginative or innovative; it is mainly object-related and generally solitary or parallel—when it is social it is hierarchical in the sense that one child is boss.

In achievement game cultures, on the other hand, the family is nuclear but more egalitarian and involved in dialogue and negation, and play is imaginative and collective; there is less emphasis on status games and more on achievement games, less aggression in play and in late childhood a shift in preference for individual pursuits (e.g., fishing and cycling) from more formal games like basketball and football. Sutton-Smith relates these differences in play to the culture, social structure and child-rearing practices, arguing that playfulness, autonomy and flexibility are encouraged when cultural roles are not strictly prescribed and when the individuals have to be prepared for new and unexpected situations.

Play can reflect social adaptation as much as individual adaptation, a fact nicely illustrated by the play of refugee Vietnamese children in San Francisco (91): These children chose play forms which were highly structured and rule-governed as opposed to their American peers who engaged in much more spontaneous play. The children who were in an alien society in the midst of much unfamiliarity relied on the game's structure to clarify and define their position in relation to the other players, whereas their socially secure peers were able to transcend social rules or to violate them, simply for the fun of it—they were free to "play with play."

It is interesting, too, that cultures maintain "traditions" in the manufacture of play materials. Nesting eggs are common in Russia, brightly painted wooden horses in Sweden, shadow puppets in Indonesia and miniature cars in Western Europe (36). In fact, national traits have been linked, not entirely frivolously, to the types of playthings and materials used: The large wooden toys of the United States are associated with relaxed and cooperative play and traits of confidence and curiosity; the unstructured materials and innovative playgrounds of Scandinavia are linked with drive and creativity; the didactic toys of the Dutch are linked to an emphasis on problem-solving and the miniature toys of Britain, especially soldiers, to the propensity for colonialism! (12).

SUMMARY

In this review of the young child's play, an attempt has been made to describe the manifold varieties of play and to trace the developmental patterns of play in the maturing individual. The development of play has been considered in the context of the perceptual and motor development of the child, and we have seen how the initially undifferentiated actions of the young infant give way to more distinct and organised sequences. Intention and meaning become evident, soon to be followed by symbolic thought and play. Revealed in his play we see the child's competencies, his wishes, his anxieties, his social aptitude. The important fact remains that in play the child is master; the player calls the tune. What we, as adults, must ensure is that the child does not lose his enjoyment in play lest his adulthood be dreary and dull.

REFERENCES

1. AMMAR, H. M. 1954. *Growing up in an Egyptian Village*. London: Routledge & Kegan Paul.
2. BARNES, K. 1971. Preschool play norms: a replication. *Dev. Psychol.*, 5, 99-103.
3. BATES, E., CAMAIONI, L. and VOLTERRA, V. 1975. The acquisitions of performatives prior to speech. *Merrill-Palmer Quart.*, 21, 205.
4. BERNSTEIN, B. 1971. *Class, Codes and Control*. Paladin.
5. BRONSON, W. C. 1973. Competence and the growth of personality. In: K. J. Connolly and J. S. Bruner (Eds.) *The Growth of Competence*. New York: Academic Press.
6. BRONSON, W. C. 1975. Developments in behaviour with age-mates during the second year of life. In M. Lewis and L. A. Rosenblum (Eds.) *Friendship and Peer Relations*. New York: Wiley.
7. BRUNER, J. S. 1976. Nature and uses of immaturity. In J. S. Bruner, A. Jolly and K. Sylva (Eds.) *Play: Its Role in Development and Evolution*. Harmondsworth: Penguin Books.
8. BRUNER, J. S., and SHERWOOD, V. 1976. Peek-a-boo and the learning of rule structures. In J. S. Bruner, A. Jolly and K. Sylva (Eds.) *Play: Its Role in Development and Evolution*. Harmondsworth: Penguin Books.
9. BUHLER, K. 1930. *The Mental Development of the Child*. New York: Harcourt.
10. BUHLER, C. 1935. *From Birth to Maturity: An Outline of the Psychological Development of the Child*. London: Kegan Paul.
11. CALL, J. D. 1970. Games babies play. *Psychology Today*. Jan., 1970.

12. CAPLAN, F., and CAPLAN, T. 1973. *The Power of Play*. New York: Doubleday.
13. CAZDEN, C. B. 1974. Play with language and metalinguistic awareness: One dimension of language experience. *Int. J. Early Childhood*, *6*, 12.
14. CAZDEN, C. B. 1976. Play with language and metalinguistic awareness: One dimension of language experience. In: J. S. Bruner, A. Jolly and K. Sylva (Eds.) *Play: Its Role in Development and Evolution*. Harmondsworth: Penguin Books.
15. CHANCE, P. 1978. *Play and Learning*. New Brunswick, N.J.: Johnson & Johnson Ltd.
16. CHUKOVSKY, K. 1963. *From Two to Five*. Univ. California Press.
17. COVENEY, P. 1967. *The Image of Childhood*. Harmondsworth: Penguin Books.
18. CRAWLEY, S. B., ROGERS, P. P., FRIEDMAN, S., IACOBBO, M., CRITICOS, A., RICHARDSON, L., and THOMPSON, M. A. 1978. Developmental changes in the structure of mother-infant play. *Dev. Psychol.*, *14*, 30.
19. DEARDEN, R. F. 1967. The concept of play. In: R. S. Peters (Ed.) *The Concept of Education*. London: Routledge & Kegan Paul.
20. DUCKWORTH, E. 1964. Piaget rediscovered. In: R. E. Ripple and V. N. Rockcastle (Eds.) *Piaget rediscovered*. Ithaca: Cornell Univ. School of Education.
21. DUNN, J., and WOODING, C 1977. Play in the home and its implications for learning. In B. Tizard and D. Harvey (Eds.) *Biology of Play*. London: Heinemann.
22. ECKERMAN, C. O. and RHEINGOLD, H. L. 1974. Infants' exploratory responses to toys and people. *Develop. Psychol.*, *10*, 255.
23. ECKERMAN, C. O., WHATLEY, J. L. and KUTZ, S. L. 1975. Growth of social play with peers during the second year of life. *Dev. Psychol.* *11*, 42.
24. EDWARDS, D. 1973. Sensory-motor intelligence and semantic relations in early child grammar. *Cognition*, *2*, 395.
25. EL'KONIN, D. 1966. Symbolics and its function in the play of children. *Soviet Education*, *i*, 35.
26. ELLIS, M. J. 1973. *Why People Play*. Englewood Cliffs, N.J.: Prentice-Hall.
27. EMMERICH, W. 1959. Parental identification in young children. *Genetic Psychol. Monogr.*, *60*, 257.
28. FANTZ, R. L. 1964. Visual experience in infants: decreased attention to familiar patterns relative to novel ones. *Science*, *146*, 668.
29. FARNHAM-DIGGORY, S. 1972. The development of equivalence systems. In S. Farnham-Diggory (Ed.) *Information Processing in Children*. New York: Academic Press.
30. FEIN, G. G. 1975. A transformational analysis of pretending. *Dev. Psychol.*, *3*, 291.
31. FEIN, G. G., BRANCH, A. R. and DIAMOND, E. 1977. Materials and persons: Some influences on the pretend play of two-year-olds. Unpublished paper.
32. FEITELSON, D. 1972. Developing imaginative play in pre-school children as a possible approach to fostering creativity. *Early Child Development & Care*, *1*, 181.
33. FEITELSON, D. 1977. Cross-cultural studies of representational play. In B. Tizard and D. Harven (Eds.) *Biology of Play*. London: Heinemann Medical Books.
34. FEITELSON, D. and ROSS, G. S. 1973. The neglected factor—play. *Human Dev.*, *16*, 202.
35. FORTES, M. 1970. Social and psychological aspects of education in Taleland. In J. Middleton (Ed.) *From Child to Adult*. New York: Natural History Press.
36. FRASER, A. 1972. *A History of Toys*. London: Spring Books.
37. FREUD, S. 1955. Beyond the pleasure principle. In J. Strachey (Ed.) *The Standard Edition of the Complete Psychological Works of S. Freud*. Vol. 18. London: Hogarth Press.
38. FRIEDLANDER, B. Z., McCARTHY, J. J. and SOFORENKO, A. Z. 1967. Automated psychological evaluation with severely retarded institutionalized infants. *Amer. J. Ment. Defic.*, *71*, 909.
38A. FROEBEL, F. 1895. *Pedagogies of the Kindergarten*. London: Appleton (Translated by J. Jarvis).
39. GARVEY, C. 1977. *Play*. London: Fontana/Open Books.

40. GESELL, A. L. and ILG, F. L. 1946. *The Child from Five to Ten*. London: Hamilton.
41. GIBSON, E. J. 1969. *Principles of Perceptual Learning and Development*. New York: Appleton.
42. GILMORE, J. B. 1966. The role of anxiety and cognitive factors in children's play behaviour. *Child. Dev.*, *37*, 397.
43. GOULD, R. 1972. *Child Studies Through Fantasy*. New York: Quadrangle Books.
44. GREENFIELD, P. M., NELSON, K. and SALTZMAN, E. 1972. The development of rulebound strategies for manipulating seriated cups: A parallel between action and grammar. *Cognitive Psychol.*, *3*, 291.
45. GUTTERIDGE, M. V. 1939. A study of motor achievements of young children. *Arch. Psychol.* No. *244*.
46. HARTER, S. 1974. Pleasure derived by children from cognitive challenge and mastery. *Child Dev.*, *45*, 661.
47. HEIN, A. and HELD, R. 1967. Dissociation of the visual placing response into elicited and guided components. *Science, 158*, 390.
48. HELD, R. 1963. Plasticity in human sensory-motor control. *Science, 142*, 455.
49. HELD, R. and BAUER, J. A. 1967. Visually guided reaching in infant monkeys after restricted rearing. *Science, 155*, 718.
50. HELD, R. & HEIN, A. 1963. Movement produced stimulation in the development of visually guided behaviour. *J. Comp. Physiol. Psychol. 56*, 872.
51. HENDRICKSON, N. J. and HANSEN, S. L. 1977. Toddlers: competence and behaviour patterns. *Child Study Journal, 7*, 79.
52. HUGHES, M. M. 1978. Sequential analysis of exploration and play. *International Journal of Behavioural Development, 1*, 83.
53. HUTT, C. 1966. Exploration and play in children. *Symp. Zool. Soc., 18*, 61.
54. HUTT, C. 1967a. Temporal effects on response decrement and stimulus satiation in exploration. *Brit. J. Psychol., 58*, 365.
55. HUTT, C. 1967. Effects of stimulus novelty on manipulatory exploration in an infant. *J. Child Psychol. Psychiat., 8*, 241.
55A. HUTT, C. 1968. Exploration of novelty in children with and without upper CNS lesions and some effects of auditory and visual incentives. *Acta Psychologica, 28*, 150-160.
56. HUTT, C. 1969. Exploration, arousal and autism. *Psychol., Forsch. 33*, 1.
57. HUTT, C. 1970. Specific and diversive exploration. In: H. W. Reese and L. P. Lipsitt (Eds.) *Advances in Child Development and Behaviour*, Vol. 5, New York: Academic Press.
58. HUTT, C. 1974. Behavioural and heart rate responses to novelty at 6 months and 1 year. *Bull. Brit. Psychol. Soc., 27*, 167.
59. HUTT, C. 1975. Degrees of novelty and their effects on children's attention and preference. *Brit. J. Psychol., 66*, 487.
60. HUTT, C. 1979a. Towards a taxonomy of play. In: B. Sutton-Smith (Ed.) *Play and Learning*. New York: Gardner Press.
61. HUTT, C. 1979b. *Play—Contemporary Theory and Research*. New York: Wiley, in preparation.
62. HUTT, C. and HUTT, S. J. 1978. Heart rate variability: the adaptive consequences of individual differences and state changes. In: N. Blurton-Jones and V. Reynolds (Eds.) *Human Behaviour and Adaptation*. London: Taylor & Francis.
63. HUTT, C., HUTT, S. J. and OUNSTED, C. 1965. The behaviour of children with and without upper CNS lesions. *Behaviour, 24*, 246.
64. HUTT, C., TYLER, S. and FOY, H. 1979. *Play, Exploration and Learning*. (In preparation).
65. HUTT, S. J. and HUTT, C. 1970. *Direct Observation and Measurement of Behaviour*. Springfield, Ill.: Charles C. Thomas.
66. KLEIN, M. 1927. Criminal tendencies in normal children. *Brit. J. Med. Psychol., 7*, 177.

67. KLINGER, E. 1971. *Structure and Functions of Fantasy*. New York: Wiley.
68. LEVINE, R. A. & LEVINE, B. B. 1963. Syansongo: a Gusii community in Kenya. In B. B. Whiting (Ed.) *Six Cultures*. New York: Wiley.
69. LIEBERMANN, J. N. 1977. *Playfulness—Its Relationship to Imagination and Creativity*. New York: Academic Press.
70. LOWENFELD, M. 1935. *Play in Childhood*. London: Gollanz.
71. McCALL, R. B. 1974. Exploratory behaviour and play in the human infant. *Monogr. Soc. Res. Child Dev*. No. 55, vol. *39*.
72. MARSHALL, H. and HAHN, S. C. 1967. Experimental modification of dramatic play. *J. Pers. & Soc. Psychol*., *5*, 119.
73. MATTHEWS, W. S. 1977. Sex role perception, portrayal, and preference in the fantasy play of young children. Paper to SRCD meeting, New Orleans, March 1977.
74. MEAD, G. H. 1934. *Mind, Self and Society*. Chicago: Univ. Chicago Press.
75. MENNINGER, K. 1942. *Love against Hate*. New York: Harcourt.
76. MILLAR, S. 1968. *The Psychology of Play*. Hamondsworth: Penguin Books.
77. MINTURN, L. and HITCHCOCK, J. T. 1963. The Rajputs of Khalapur, India. In B. Whiting (Ed.) *Six Cultures*. New York: Wiley.
78. MOORE, N. V., EVERTSON, C. M. and BROPHY, J. E. 1974. Solitary play: Some functional considerations. *Dev. Psychol*., *10*, 830.
79. MUELLER, E. and LUCAS, T. 1975. A developmental analysis of peer interaction among toddlers. In M. Lewis and L. A. Rosenblum (Eds.) *Friendship and Peer Relations*. New York: Wiley.
80. NZIOKI, J. M. 1967. Thorns in the grass: the story of a Kamba boy. In L. K. Fox (Ed.) *East African childhood: Three versions*. O.U.P.
81. OPIE, I. and OPIE, P. 1959. *The Lore and Language of School Children*. O.U.P.
82. OPIE, I. and OPIE, P. 1969. *Children's Games in Street and Playground*. O.U.P.
83. OVERTON, W. F. and JACKSON, J. P. 1973. The representation of imagined objects in action sequences: a developmental study. *Child Dev*., *44*, 309.
84. PARTEN, M. B. 1932. Social participation among pre-school children. *J. Soc. Abnorm. Psychol*., *27*, 243.
85. PHILLIPS, R. 1945. Doll play as a function of the realism of the materials and the length of the experimental session. *Child Dev*., *16*, 145.
86. PIAGET, J. 1951. *Play, Dreams and Imitation in Childhood*. London: Heinemann.
87. PULASKI, M. A. 1973. Toys and Imaginative play. In: J. L. Singer (Ed.) *The Child's World of Make-believe*. New York: Academic Press.
88. REARDON, D. F. 1974. The plight of free play. In L. M. Shears and E. M. Bower (Eds.) *Games in Education and Development*. Springfield, Ill.: Charles C Thomas.
89. RHEINGOLD, H. L. and ECKERMAN, C. O. 1969. The infant's free entry into a new environment. *J. Exptl. child Psychol*., *8*, 271.
90. RHEINGOLD, H. L. and ECKERMAN, C. O. 1970. The infant separates himself from his mother. *Science*, *168*, 78.
91. ROBINSON, C. E. 1977. The uses of order and disorder in play: an analysis of Vietnamese refugee children's play. *Assoc. Anthrop. Study Play Newsletter*, *4*, 9.
92. ROSEN, C. E. 1974. The effects of sociodramatic play on problem-solving behaviour among culturally disadvantaged preschool children. *Child Dev*., *45*, 920.
93. ROSENBLATT, D. 1977. Developmental trends in infant play. In B. Tizard and D. Harvey (Eds.) *Biology of Play*. London: Heinemann.
94. ROSS, H. S., GOLDMAN, B. D. and HAY, D. F. 1976. Features and functions of infant games. Paper to the Annual Meeting of *Canad. Psychol. Assoc*., Toronto, June 1976.
95. ROUTH, D. K., SCHROEDER, C. S. and O'TOUMA, L. A. 1974. Development of activity level in children. *Dev. Psychol*., *10*, 163.
96. RUBIN, K. H., MAIONI, T. L. and HORNUNG, M. 1976. Free play behaviours in middle-class and lower-class preschoolers: Parten and Piaget revisited. *Child Dev*., *47*, 414.

97. SAAYMAN, G., AMES, E. W. & MOFFETT, A. 1964. Response to novelty as an indicator of visual discrimination in the human infant. *J. Exp. child Psychol.*, 1, 189.

98. SALTZ, E., DIXON, D. & JOHNSON, J. 1977. Training disadvantaged preschoolers on various fantasy activities: effects on cognitive functioning and impulse control. *Child Dev.*, 48, 367.

99. SANCHES, M. and KIRSHENBLATT-GIMBLETT, B. 1976. Children's traditional speech play and child language. In: B. Kirschenblatt-Gimblett, (Ed.) *Speech play*. Univ. Pennsylv. Press.

100. SANDERS, K. M. and HARPER, L. V. 1976. Free-play fantasy behaviour in pre-school children: Relations among gender, age, season, and location. *Child Dev.*, 47, 1182.

101. SCHULTZ, D. D. 1965. *Sensory Restriction: Effects on Behavior*. New York: Academic Press.

102. SCHWARTZMAN, H. 1976. The anthropological study of children's play. *Annual Rev. Anthropol.*, 5, 289.

103. SHERROD, L. and SINGER, J. L. 1977. The development of make-believe play. In J. Goldstein (Ed.) *Sports, Games and Play*. Hillsdale, N.J.: Erlbaum.

103A. SHIRLEY, M. M. 1933. *The First Two Years*. Vol. 1. *Postural and Locomotor Development*. Minneapolis: University of Minnesota Press.

104. SINCLAIR, H. 1971. Sensorimotor action patterns as a condition for the acquisition of syntax. In: R. Huxley and E. Ingram (Eds.) *Language Acquisition: Models and Methods*. New York: Academic Press.

105. SINGER, J. L. 1973. *The Child's World of Make-Believe*. New York: Academic Press.

106. SINGER, J. L. 1977. Imagination and make-believe play in early childhood: some educational implications. *J. Mental Imagery.*, 5, 211.

107. SINGER, J. L. & SINGER, D. G. 1976. Imaginative play and pretending in early childhood: some experimental approaches. In A. Davids (Ed.) *Child Personality and Psychopathology: Current Topics*, Vol. 3. New York: Wiley.

108. SMILANSKY, S. 1968. *The Effects of Sociodramatic Play on Disadvantaged Preschool Children*. New York: Wiley.

109. SMITH, P. K. 1977. Social and fantasy play in young children. In B. Tizard and D. Harvey (Eds.) *Biology of Play*. London: Heinemann Medical Books.

110. SMITH, P. K. and DODSWORTH, C. 1979. Social class differences in the fantasy play of preschool children. *J. Genetic Psychol.*

111. SMITH, P. K. and SYDALL, S. 1978. Play and non-play tutoring in preschool children: is it play or tutoring which matters? *Br. J. Educ. Psychol.*, 48, 315.

112. STERN, D. N. 1974. The goal and structure of mother-infant play. *J. Amer. Acad. Science*, 13, 402.

113. SUTTON-SMITH, B. 1966. Piaget on play: A critique. *Psychol. Rev.*, 73, 104.

114. SUTTON-SMITH, B. 1972. The two cultures of games. In: *The Folkgames of Children*. Austin: Univ. Texas Press.

115. SUTTON-SMITH, B. 1973. Das Spiel als Mittler des Neuen. In: A. Flitner (Ed.) *Das Kinderspiel*. The Hague: Mouton.

116. SUTTON-SMITH, B. 1974. Toward an anthropology of play. *Assoc. Anthropol. Study of Play Newsletter*, 1, 8.

117. SUTTON-SMITH, B. 1976. Current research and theory on play, games and sports. In: T. T. Craig (Ed.) *The Humanistic and Mental Health Aspects of Sports, Exercise and Recreation*. American Medical Association.

118. SYLVA, K., BRUNER, J.S. and GENOVA, P. 1976. The role of play in the problem-solving of children 3-5-years-old. In J. S. Bruner, A. Jolly and K. Sylva (Eds.) *Play: Its Role in Development and Evolution*. Harmondsworth: Penguin Books.

119. TIZARD, B., PHILPS, J. and PLEWIS, I. 1976. Play in pre-school centres—II. Effects on play of the child's social class and of the educational orientation of the centre. *J. Child Psychol. Psychiat.* 17, 265.

120. UZGIRIS, I. C. 1967. Ordinality in the development of schemas for relating to objects. In J. Hellmuth (Ed.) *The Exceptional Infant* Vol. I, *The Normal Infant*. New York: Brunner/Mazel.
121. WEIR, R. 1962. *Language in the Crib*. The Hague: Mouton.
122. WHITE, B. L., HELD, R. and CASTLE, P. 1967. Experience in early human development: observations on the development of visually directed reaching. In: J. Hellmuth (Ed.) *Exceptional infant*, Vol. I, *The Normal Infant*. New York: Brunner/Mazel.
123. WHITE, B. L. and WATTS, J. C. 1973. *Experience and Environment*. Englewood Cliffs, N.J.: Prentice-Hall.
124. ZAPOROZHETS, A. V. 1965. The development of perception in the pre-school child. In P. H. Mussen (Ed.) *European Research in Child Development. Monogr. Soc. Res. Child Dev.*, *30*, Serial No. 100, 82.
125. ZUBEK, J. P. (Ed.) 1969. *Sensory Deprivation: Fifteen Years of Research*. New York: Appleton-Century-Crofts.

6

MATERNAL AND PSYCHOSOCIAL
DEPRIVATION

INGEBORG KRIEGER, M.D.

Professor, Department of Pediatrics,
Wayne State University, School of Medicine;
Director, Nutrition and Metabolism Service, Children's Hospital of
Michigan, Detroit, Michigan

The maternal deprivation syndrome (MDS) (1, 40) is characterized by growth failure, developmental retardation, and affective abnormalities which develop in an adverse environment and improve after removal from it. The patients are, as the term indicates, infants who are dependent on their mother or caretaker for nurture. This syndrome has also been called emotional (42) or sensory (28) deprivation, and environmental retardation (7). By contrast, the term psychosocial dwarfism (PSD) (48) has been used to single out patients with a disorder that also causes abnormalities of growth, intelligence, and affect, but these patients demonstrate in addition unusual behavior, like garbage eating, polydipsia, night wandering, tempers, and self-abusiveness (42, 46). All described patients have been at least two and generally more than three years old.

It is not known whether the two syndromes represent a biological continuum or different entities caused by a different environmental insult. Physical characteristics do not distinguish the two syndromes and differences in abnormalities of behavior may reflect merely differences in maturation. Deficient growth hormone (GH) release is the only finding in PSD which—given current knowledge of pituitary function—cannot be explained by the difference in age or duration of disease.

The growth-retarding environment has not been adequately studied and it is quite possible that psychic insults which delay intellectual development and distort affect and behavior are different in the two syndromes. It appears that in some cases neglect and sensory deprivation play a greater role, while in other cases evidence of physical abuse shows that punitive interaction is a predominant characteristic of the environment. The role of undernutrition in the pathogenesis is not understood.

CLINICAL MANIFESTATION

Growth failure is the most obvious feature of these syndromes and the one which usually leads to the detection. Weight is generally more severely affected than height in MDS. By contrast, older patients with PSD may be proportionate or even obese (5). However, children in the two-to-five-year-old age group tend, like infants with MDS, to be underweight for their height (22, 27), and even those who are proportionate at the time of first contact may have been malnourished in infancy—as is indicated by the few cases for which documented earlier measurements are available (24, 42). Bone age, which generally corresponds to height age, is delayed unless the patient is very young and the duration of the insult short. Twenty patients over three years of age studied by the author (24) had a mean chronological age of 51 months, a mean height age of 22 months, and a mean bone age of 24 months. The characteristic appearance of infantilism is due to skeletal proportions and facial features which are appropriate for height.

Onset of growth failure appears to be at or very soon after birth in MDS. In contrast, records of previous weight measurements, which could be obtained in 10 of 20 cases of PSD, showed that onset was between six and 18 months in all but two cases (24). This may be indicative of later onset for patients with PSD, in general, compared to MDS.

Motor and language development is slow in both groups. Deprived infants and children do mature eventually, as they acquire motor skills which allow them to venture beyond their mothers' sphere. As they come into contact with more people, they may be subjected to modifying influences, so that some manifestations can improve spontaneously.

Speech and language are affected in PSD. Articulation is poor and some children refuse to talk altogether. Flirtatious nonverbal communication of some older patients suggests an ability for higher function that is not reflected by their language performance. A watchful look, termed "radar gaze," has been described in infants (34) which also belies the degree of retardation evidenced by standard intelligence tests.

Affect and behavior are abnormal in both MDS and PSD. Infants are

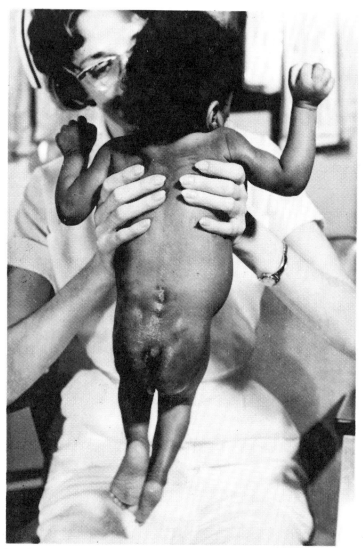

FIGURE 1. Thirteen-month-old infant with maternal deprivation syndrome, showing linear growth failure (height age four months), malnutrition (weight age one month), infantile posture, and physical evidence of neglect (decubitus ulcers and diaper rash).

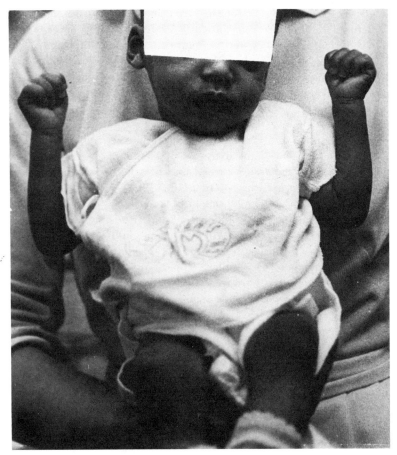

FIGURE 2. The same infant three weeks later, after having gained 1790 gm. The infantile posture was still maintained in the sitting position for periods throughout the day, but gradually disappeared during the next two weeks.

generally withdrawn and apathetic. They do not reach out with their hands to explore and actively seek attention, assert themselves, cry or fight. Thus, they may appear to be autistic; yet when held they do respond to body contact, cling, and seem to enjoy being held, which is not compatible with autism. Since they are undemanding, they are considered "good babies." They also do not usually cry for food. They can be passed around to anyone willing to hold them, seemingly fearless of strangers. Although these infants withdraw, they find ways to amuse themselves through repetitive motions, such as rocking. Autoerotic behavior takes more vehement forms in older patients, who may have scars on the forehead from repetitive head banging.

Patients with PSD are intermittently withdrawn and depressed; during episodes of depression they may be anorexic. Although they may appear to be affectionate, likable, and very well behaved, closer examination invariably reveals that such behavior is not consistent. They are abnormally compliant and allow themselves to be manipulated, only to throw a violent temper tantrum at another time. Frequently aggression is turned toward self. Whereas some investigators (37) attribute self-inflicted injuries to pain "agnosia" or an inability to perceive appropriate warning through pain, others feel that the need for extremes of stimulation reflects masochistic gratification. Such aggression turned toward self is reminiscent of the behavior of monkeys reared in isolation (15).

It often happens that what seems to be a close mother-child relationship on casual observation is in reality infantile dependency or a desire to win approval. Thus, the impression of mother and child when first seen during an office visit may be misleading, especially since information of negativistic behavior—like tempers, fecal soiling, oppositional food refusal, garbage eating, and night wandering—are frequently withheld by the mother unless she is directly questioned about these signs.

A neurological sign: When lying supine, these deprived infants commonly adopt an infantile posture where the arms are abducted, externally rotated and supinated (28). Characteristically, this posture of tonic immobility is maintained for extended periods of time even while sitting upright or standing. It appears to be a manifestation of cerebral function at a subcortical level. The sign is nonspecific, since it has been described in severe organic brain disorders as well as in the maternal deprivation syndrome. Patients with PSD rarely adopt this posture spontaneously, probably because of the difference in age. However, we have demonstrated repeatedly in some patients that a sign can be provoked that may have similar significance. If an arm or leg is placed in a bizarre position, these patients will maintain the position for several minutes in catatonic-like fashion without being asked to do so.

Eating behavior is also characteristic. The majority of infants with the MDS (51) do not develop anorexia. When they are fed, they eat ravenously to the extent that there may be overflow vomiting. Mothers frequently use phrases like "He eats like a wolf," and "He eats more than I do," in describing their appetites (26, 51). Although it may be simply a sign of hunger, this phenomenon has been attributed to their inability to recognize satiety because of an impairment of body image and sense of self (45).

Eating behavior in PSD is more bizarre because these children scavenge through garbage cans, eat scraps of rotten food, and drink from toilet bowls or rain puddles. Like self-inflicted pain, these cravings may reflect a need for excessive stimulation or punishment. Although the majority eat repulsive matter with caloric value, some will eat, in addition, things like crayons and foam rubber. Like deprived infants, children with PSD require large volumes of food and drink. Although polyphagia suggests hunger, especially in a child who looks undernourished, polydipsia is evidently psychogenic because renal concentrating ability is normal.

ENDOCRINE FUNCTION AND METABOLISM

Endocrine abnormalities in patients with PSD were first described by Powell et al. in 1967 (43). The report stirred widespread interest because it seemed to document what heretofore had only been considered possible—a direct effect of the emotional state on neuroendocrine function and growth. Although similar GH deficits, as well as gonadal and adrenal dysfunctions, were known to occur in anorexia nervosa, it was possible that in anorexia nervosa endocrine dysfunctions were not due to psychologic factors, since patients were always severely emaciated and it had long been recognized that malnutrition affects pituitary function. By contrast, three of six patients with GH deficiency tested by Powell et al. had normal weights for height. Endocrine studies, which appeared after the original report, were recently reviewed in the psychiatric literature by Brown (6). Many questions concerning the cause of endocrine dysfunction and the pathogenesis of growth failure remain unsettled.

Growth hormone release after insulin-induced hypoglycemia was deficient in six of the eight cases with PSD studied by Powell et al. (43). The incidence of abnormality in cases studied subsequently was lower (5, 16-19, 27, 32, 44). GH release was defective also in response to other provocative stimuli, primarily arginine (5, 17, 18, 22, 44), but also exercise (32) and sleep (44). Baseline levels of circulating plasma GH were normal in PSD, whereas infants with the MDS—studied by Krieger and Mellinger (27)—had elevated plasma GH and responded further to provocative stimulation. They were similar in this regard to control infants with malnutrition due to organic disease who had comparable degrees of linear growth failure and a comparable weight for height (74 and 76 percent of normal, respectively).

Pimstone et al. demonstrated first in patients with kwashiorkor that elevated GH values drop within days of the institution of a protein diet (41). Subsequently, Krieger and Mellinger (27) tested random blood samples of three patients with PSD on the day of admission and found elevated GH,

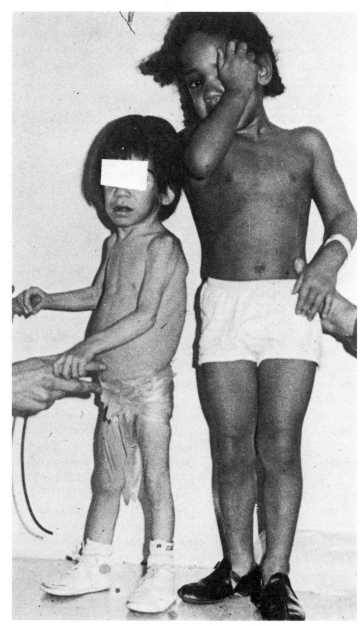

FIGURE 3. Thirty-seven-month-old girl with psychosocial dwarfism (weight 5.59 kg., height 75 cm), standing next to a normal age control.

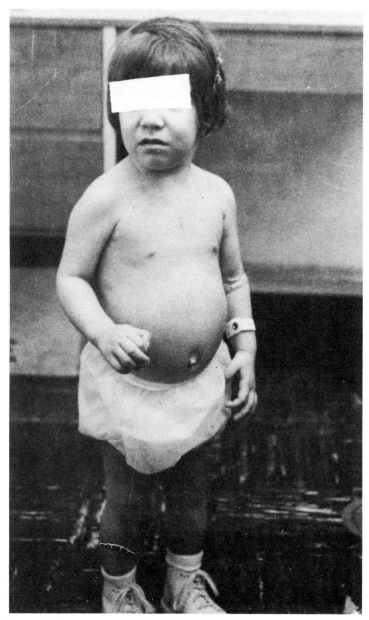

FIGURE 4. The same child after four weeks of hospitalization, during which time she gained 2.52 kg.

although, on later provocation, baseline levels were low and responses deficient. Their patients were different from the cases with PSD studied by Powell et al. (43) because they were younger and markedly underweight for height, as well as extremely short. Unresponsiveness to provocative stimuli seems to persist longer than elevation of baseline values, since abnormality was still present three weeks after the change in domicile. Moreover, one of three cases tested serially had regained normal height/weight proportions after six weeks, while the GH test remained persistently abnormal (27).

To evaluate the role that chronic malnutrition plays in the pathogenesis of GH dysfunction in PSD, it is necessary to study GH release in children of similar age and with equally severe degrees of linear growth retardation due to organic disease—but these are difficult to find. Greene (14) tested older children with cystic fibrosis who were underweight but not severely stunted and found elevated baseline levels and unresponsiveness to insulin-induced hypoglycemia. Similar observations have been reported for anorexia nervosa (33) and marasmic kwashiorkor (12). Unresponsiveness to provocation persisted in some malnourished infants (12) for at least one month after re-alimentation. High baseline GH levels with or without unresponsiveness to provocation are thus typical of malnutrition. Each abnormality has been seen in PSD, but the GH elevation may be difficult to detect because it may be as transient as in malnutrition, where it disappears after a few days of protein feeding.

It is not known whether a certain tissue level of GH throughout the day or the naturally occurring rise of circulating GH during slow wave sleep is necessary for growth. Wolff and Money (52) emphasized the importance of slow wave sleep for growth. They observed a relationship between periods of sleep disturbances and poor growth and suggest that one causes the other. However, changes in sleep and growth pattern were always associated with a corresponding change in domicile. A single observation by Powell et al. (44) is important because it disproves a direct link between sleep disturbances and growth. They observed a patient with PSD who had a normal sleep pattern, yet during slow wave sleep he showed repeatedly no rise in GH. Continuous measurements of circulating GH have apparently not been performed in the two deprivation syndromes.

Substitution therapy with GH should induce a growth spurt if nutrition is adequate and GH deficiency is, indeed, the cause of growth failure in PSD. This was tried in two published cases (10, 47) and this author has knowledge of two others who were treated with human GH prior to accurate diagnosis. Growth rate did not improve in the home environment.

Somatomedin levels are low in primary hypopituitarism, but also in malnutrition where GH is elevated, suggesting that somatomedin plays a role in feedback control. The finding of low somatomedin levels in PSD therefore is not proof that reversible hypopituitarism is the cause of growth failure in PSD (8, 49).

Neurotransmitter function studies promise to increase our understanding of the relations between growth and emotions, versus growth and nutrition. Dopamine and norepinephrine appear to play a central excitatory role in GH release, and drugs which increase hypothalamic serotonin content increase GH secretion but suppress ACTH (excluding 5-hydroxytryptophan, which stimulates adrenocortical secretion). Drugs which modulate these monoamine neurotransmitters can be used to investigate the pituitary hypothalamic axis. Imura et al. (18) gave propranolol to one patient with PSD and showed that the defective GH response to hypoglycemia can be reversed with this beta adrenergic blocking agent. Parra, who was working at the time with the John Hopkins group (38), also observed a better GH response to sequential arginine-insulin stimulation when infusing epinephrine and propranolol simultaneously with these provocative stimuli. The functional disorder of GH secretion in PSD thus appears to be caused by inhibition through beta adrenergic receptors.

Excretion of norepinephrine metabolites may be low during depressive states. In studying patients with affective disorders, Garver et al. (11) found that patients with low concentrations of urinary norepinephrine metabolites also had a low GH response to provocative stimuli. It is doubtful that similar data for PSD would be useful in evaluating the role of malnutrition because depressed patients are usually also anorexic.

Adrenocortical function and ACTH release have not been studied as extensively as GH, since only two centers report data and these are not in agreement. It is not known whether discrepancies are due to differences in technique or patient selection. The John Hopkins group (5, 43) measured ACTH reserve of patients with PSD with a natural stimulus for ACTH release, using metapirone, a drug which decreases circulating cortisol through blockage of 11-hydroxylase activity and thus increases negative feedback stimulation. They proved that the drug was absorbed, but since they used a dosage based on body weight, which is low relative to surface area, and since they gave the low dose for one day rather than the customary three, it is possible that cortisol production was not completely blocked. An unusually high percentage of their cases had an inadequate response, while the patients tested by the Detroit group (26, 27), who received the higher dose for three days, all had a normal response; a single patient of the Detroit group, who also received metapirone for only one day, had an inadequate response (27). Although the metapirone test was normal, four of their five patients with poor GH responsiveness also had an insufficient rise of plasma cortisol after insulin induced hypoglycemia (27), a phenomenon which need not be due to insufficient ACTH reserve. Patients with normal GH responsiveness to provocation (nine MDS; three PSD) showed a normal cortisol rise.

Patients with PSD tested by the Detroit group (27) also had in vivo tests of cortisol secretion rates (CSR), plasma cortisol, and ketogenic steroid (17-KGS) excretion (26). These tests corroborate the metapirone study in that they showed normal or excessive adrenocortical function. CSR was elevated in half of the patients tested (two or four PSD, and five of ten MDS). The elevation of CSR, which reflects cortisol production, emphasizes the need for an adequate metapirone dose to assure that plasma cortisol is effectively lowered. Urinary 17-KGS excretion did not reflect CSR, because 17-KSGs were only slightly elevated in five of seven cases with an elevated CSR. This was explained by difficulties in disposing of a cortisol load, which is typical of infants and anxious adults who consequently excrete metabolites other than 17-hydroxycorticosteroids. Mean plasma cortisol values were significantly higher on admission than before discharge, but admission values were more variable than discharge values, which suggests lack of a diurnal rhythm. Adrenocortical response to ACTH was normal.

Age controls with malnutrition due to organic disease were different because they had normal CSRs. Their 17-KGS excretion and adrenocortical reserve were normal; plasma cortisol values were on admission as variable and in the same range as values in MDS and PSD (26). These control data are in agreement with findings in children with marasmus from underdeveloped countries (2). Poor adrenocortical reserve in malnutrition has been cited (6) as evidence that MDS and PSD are different from malnutrition. However, the paper (3) referred to by the reviewer can be interpreted differently, which is also indicated by the published discussion of it; the data showed an adequate adrenocortical reserve if normalcy is judged by the response in multiples of the baseline values. There are, on the other hand, many reports in the literature of adrenocortical atrophy in patients dying of malnutrition, which indicates that the degree of malnutrition is an important consideration when making comparisons.

Since single plasma cortisol values are difficult to interpret when a diurnal rhythm is poorly established, and since an evaluation of adrenocortical function based on urinary metabolites may be misleading in certain conditions, 24-hour cortisol secretion rates appear to be the better test. These were measured in anorexia nervosa and normal values were obtained at a time when plasma cortisol was elevated due to a decreased turnover (4). This is similar to the abnormality in protein-caloric malnutrition, reported by Alleyne (2), who considers it a sign of relative overproduction because the pituitary does not respond to the elevation of plasma cortisol by decreasing ACTH release.

Gonadotropin and pubertal changes are currently being investigated by the John Hopkins group. They have physical observations on eight patients who were removed from their domicile after 12 and before 17 years of age and had onset of puberty either immediately (six) or within one to two years (two) (36). The prognosis for recovery may not always be as promising as suggested by these observations. I have followed one patient for ten years who was at the time of last contact 17 years old, but had no pubic and axillary hair, and had infantile penis and testes, with prepubertal values for plasma testosterone and 24-hour urinary 17-ketosteroid excretion. After removal from his mother's home at ten years of age, he had a remarkable catch-up growth, progressing from a height age of 20 months to one of five years within 18 months. However, since then his growth rate has remained normal for age, which has not been sufficient for further catch-up. He is an extreme example of delayed puberty, documented by endocrine data. It is not known whether he also represents an example of irreversible changes due to psychosocial deprivation, because it was not possible to monitor his new environment.

Thyro-metabolic function in PSD also has been studied, but only in two centers (5, 26, 27, 43). The incidence of low thyroxine and radioiodine uptake values was low among patients studied at John Hopkins (5, 43), who were older and less underweight than the patients studied in Detroit (22, 26, 27). In the latter group, mean thyroxine (by column) was low, similar to the mean of malnourished controls. These low levels were thought to reflect normal thyrometabolic function because basal metabolic rates (BMR) did not change much during recovery. The exceptions were one patient with PSD in each of two studies (26, 27) and a subsequent case (22) who showed clinical signs of acute starvation and skin and hair changes suggestive of hypothyroidism. The paradoxical finding of normal BMR's and low total thyroxine values in the majority of cases was attributed to normal free, viz. active thyroxine. However, this speculation was not confirmed in a subsequent study (29), which showed that free thyroxine may be low in patients with MDS or malnutrition when metabolic rates are normal for the patient's body composition. It remains to be shown whether this phenomenon is due to a relative increase in triiodothyronine. Low total thyroxine has been reported in marasmus and kwashiorkor, notably the study by Graham and

Blizzard from Peru (13), which provides appropriate control data. These investigators showed that free thyroxine may be high, normal, or low. High values were probably due to associated kwashiorkor, which is not likely a factor that influences thyroxine data in MDS and PSD.

The basal metabolic rate (BMR) has been measured by the Detroit group (22, 26, 27). The role of the basal energy expenditure is an important consideration in patients who are supposed to have a ravenous appetite *and* intake in the face of growth failure. The BMR in MDS is low for age, by and large normal for height age, i.e., body weight predicted from height, and elevated in relation to actual body weight. A high BMR per body weight is caused by a preponderance of metabolically active tissues, like brain and other parenchymal organs, over fat and muscle. As these tissues increase again during recovery, this BMR value decreases. By contrast, the BMR per weight predicted from height (i.e., height age) is stable during weight recovery (21). Exceptions are patients with clinical signs of severe malnutrition, evidenced by redundant skin folds, who have a low BMR for height age that rises within one or more weeks to a normal range, where it remains. This stable value, which is generally in the normal range for height age, thus seems to be the "normal" BMR for these patients.

Since adequacy of the caloric intake is customarily judged by norms that use body weight as reference standard, it becomes understandable why observers gain the impression that calorie requirements are abnormally high in MDS. Requirements are higher yet in PSD, because a majority has an elevated BMR for height age (22). Inefficiency of cellular metabolism is not the reason for the high BMR, because absolute values do not decrease during recovery.

A linear relationship between BMR and DNA content of parenchymal organs has been demonstrated in rats (30). Consequently, a typical eight-year-old patient with PSD, who has the height and skeletal proportions of a two-year-old but a higher BMR, appears to have more metabolically active cells than his normal two-year-old height control. In the absence of obesity or increased muscle mass, excess cellularity would have to be in internal organs. An increased cell density seems to develop over time as the height deficit develops, apparently because cell multiplication continues in parenchymal organs at a normal rate. This is suggested by the finding of a positive linear correlation between the deficit in height and the BMR elevation. Investigation of this hypothesis by histological or biochemical techniques would help to elucidate the role of GH deficiency in the growth failure, since it is unlikely that continued organ growth through cell multiplication would occur in patients with primary GH deficiency. Such patients do not have an elevated BMR for height age, suggesting that there is, indeed, a difference between PSD and hypopituitarism.

Studies of metabolic rate from underdeveloped countries are too numerous to quote and are difficult to interpret because of local differences in the type of malnutrition, including associated kwashiorkor. Moreover, the timing of the test in relation to realimentation or onset of weight gain, and the interval after a preceding meal are variable in different studies. Comparison of admission and recovery values suggests that the BMR is decreased (39) to a level lower than in the majority of cases with MDS and PSD from the USA. Marasmic patients from underdeveloped countries resemble in this regard those select patients with MDS or PSD who had clinical signs of severe malnutrition and low BMR's in a study that compared patients with and without redundant skin folds (29).

Energy balance and weight gain were studied in 16 of 24 infants with MDS (25) and it was found that the energy cost of weight gain is not different from that in controls with malnutrition due to organic causes, including congenital heart disease. However, these data cannot be extrapolated to PSD. Indeed, one home feeding experiment (22) showed that calorie intake was excessive during the second half of the observation period. The lesson to be learned from this experiment does not relate to energy efficiency, but rather to the demonstration that these patients *can* gain if *enough* food is given.

A negative energy balance may develop in the home environment of those patients with PSD who have histories of loose stools. Tests of absorptive and digestive function have not shown abnormality (5, 22, 46), although they were performed while the stools were still bulky and malodorous (22). It is possible that a mixed meal with natural roughage may be handled differently in this disorder than the single foodstuffs that are used in routine absorption tests. This was suggested by the finding of decreased nitrogen absorption in two of the three cases tested in one study (22). Malnutrition preceded the appearance of loose stools in the only two cases of this one study where the chronology of events could be documented (22). Recovery occurs in the hospital despite persistance of loose stools for several weeks, provided the patients are given as much food as they want.

These observations suggest that malabsorption is not the primary cause of growth failure, but intestinal losses may contribute in certain cases to the calorie deficit. The etiology of the loose stools remains unknown. Malnutrition, possibly complicated by gastrointestinal infection due to garbage eating, is one possibility; increased intestinal motility is another. The ravenous appetite that is typical of PSD and some cases of MDS is frequently attributed to malabsorption. Speculations concerning other causes for overeating include increased muscular energy expenditure due to tension or loss of sleep.

In evaluating energy balance, it is important to realize that overeating at the occasional meal described by parents does not indicate an adequate *average* intake over an extended period of time. Bearing in mind that a deficit of only five percent of the daily calorie requirement can cause growth failure, it should not be surprising that such a deficit can develop in a restrictive environment. This is the accepted view in infants with linear growth failure due to MDS who are underweight for height. Their intakes, like those of children with PSD, are often described as excessive (51), an account which is less believable in MDS than PSD, in view of the underweight and absence of loose stools.

Nitrogen balances of eight patients with MDS and one with PSD were included in a study of malnutrition (31) where patients were given, for three to 12 days, a diet which was insufficient for weight gain. Provision of more calories invariably caused a marked increase in nitrogen retention. The anabolic effect of GH on nitrogen balance is well recognized. Assuming, therefore, that reversal of the GH dysfunction, which occurs after the change in domicile, is necessary for resumption of growth and improved nitrogen retention, one would have to conclude that the emotional adjustment coincided in these patients always with the institution of a high caloric diet—an unlikely coincidence!

PATHOGENESIS

Developmental, affective, and behavioral abnormalities in MDS are a direct result of the infants' lack of sensory stimulation and social interaction. Abnormal social interaction—rather than the lack of it—seems to be the cause of the behavior abnormalities in PSD. On the other hand, incarceration has been documented in some cases (35), and the different treatment that these children receive, compared with siblings, has an isolating effect. The absence of significant intellectual deficit in half the cases of one study (22) also indicates that the insult may be different from that in MDS, although the later onset, mentioned above, may be responsible for this (24).

Growth failure in MDS is, according to most observers, the result of caloric undernutrition. That infants with MDS have not been offered enough food by the caretaker was demonstrated in one experiment (51) where understimulation was continued for a brief period, either in hospital isolation or in the home, but food was provided; weight gain occurred in all infants (11 of 13) who took enough calories. According to this study and accounts of the patients' eating behavior (26, 45, 51), anorexia is rare in MDS. The reasons that infants with good appetites are not fed and mothered adequately while cared for in the home are related to the mothers' psychological status (50). The majority have a personality disorder (9) and are unable to perceive and relate to the needs of others, including the child. The attitude of their infants facilitates underfeeding, since the infants frequently are or become undemanding. The conclusions that can be drawn from these observations about the pathogenesis of growth failure are supported by a primate study (20) which showed that monkeys reared in isolation eat well and grow normally, although the emotional insult was severe enough to cause fear, absence of social play, and autistic posturing.

The pathogenesis of the growth failure in PSD is more controversial because of the endocrine findings presented in the foregoing discussion, which are indicative of irregular GH release due to hypothalamic dysfunction. It is not known whether these GH abnormalities are sufficient to cause growth failure of the degree seen in PSD, whether they are the result of chronic and/or intermittent malnutrition, or whether a specific and purely emotional insult is operative in PSD which affects hypothalamic centers directly.

An analysis of 20 patients with a deprivation syndrome (24), who were at the time of diagnosis over three years old, suggested major differences in the environmental insult. These patients could be subdivided into two groups, based on characteristics of both mother and child, which seemed to reflect a difference in the maternal attitude toward the child. The smaller of two subgroups consisted of six patients whose mothers had a personality disorder like mothers of infants with MDS. Deprivation was readily suspected because mothers with personality disorders do not recognize their own shortcomings and therefore do not conceal the fact that they do not relate with, or care for the child. The incidence of deprivation of this variety decreased during the total period of observation, because no more cases were diagnosed after 1971. This was attributed to greater awareness of physicians and improved social service surveillance, leading to earlier diagnosis and treatment. Moreover, the possibility must be considered that growth failure can improve spontaneously, at least in this subgroup, because these mothers do not intentionally deprive or hang on to the child in need for a scapegoat. Since the child can therefore venture beyond the immediate sphere of influence by the mother with progressing maturity, it appears possible that many of these children will find food and nurturance from siblings, relatives and neighbors.

The majority of mothers (comprising the second subgroup) were different. Among their children no change in incidence of PSD was apparent over 14 years. Their demeanor and apparent affective relationship with the child made a good initial impression; they gave an informed history, had provided health care, and seemed to lead stable lives. However, hidden under the veneer of the "good mother" and neat homemaker were insecurity, paranoia, identity problems, and repression of conflict. The mother's attitude toward the child was restrictive, manipulative, and punitive. It was evident that the children were inconsistently handled, with demonstrative cuddling at one moment and severe punishment the next. Equally impressive was a difference in the behavior of these children, because garbage eating, violent tempers, intermittant oppositional food refusal, and self-inflicted injuries were seen only in this subgroup. Moreover, loose stools occurred exclusively among these children. By contrast, behavior abnormalities of the other six children consisted of rocking, fecal play and soiling. Patients in the larger subgroup appeared to be similar to cases described by other investigators and may represent an entity distinct from most cases of MDS.

These observations do not necessarily argue in favor of a specific emotional insult as a direct cause of growth failure in PSD, because food deprivation occurs in this environment through several mechanisms: food restriction as a form of abuse (22), oppositional food refusal by the child, anorexia during periods of depression, and iatrogenic food restriction imposed during treatment of the loose stools, which are frequently misdiagnosed as malabsorption syndrome. Indeed, home feeding experiments conducted in three patients with PDS (22, 33) had a similar outcome as the isolation experiments in MDS (51), and showed that patients with PSD can gain if they are given enough calories.

Because of unusual conditions in the environment of patients with PSD and mothers who cling to the child because they need a scapegoat, correct diagnosis is delayed. Chronic or intermittent malnutrition thus persists longer than may appear possible in a society where relatives, physicians, and social service agencies are expected to intervene. When the diagnosis is made, parents not infrequently leave town or fight temporary foster placement. Inability to admit failure in child rearing to themselves and their relatives distinguishes mothers in this larger subgroup of patients with PSD from mothers with character disorders who deprive small infants (MDS) but don't have similar ego needs. Although a specific emotional insult appears to be operative in PSD, which may have a direct effect on hypothalamic centers, the environment in most cases of PSD also contributes to prolongation of malnutrition that develops during infancy.

DIAGNOSIS

There is no symptom complex that establishes the diagnosis of MDS or

PSD, since all described findings—including malnutrition—can be the result of organic diseases that cause mental retardation or minimal organic brain dysfunction, disorders which are not infrequently associated with feeding problems. Neither can the diagnosis be definitely established by identification of psychosocial factors conducive to or consistent with deprivation. This is evidenced by the common finding of siblings who do not show overt evidence of grossly inadequate mothering. Diagnosis rests therefore on the demonstration that a growth spurt occurs and developmental and affective status changes upon a change in domicile.

Improvement is readily detected in infants because they start to gain weight immediately when they are underweight for height and not anorexic, and because the normal clustering of developmental milestones makes it easy to recognize an acceleration in the speed of maturation. The diagnosis is more difficult in PSD because weight gain cannot be expected if the patient is already proportionate in weight for height and recognition of linear catch-up growth requires several months. Endocrine abnormalities are not diagnostic.

Bias and overemphasis on adverse environmental conditions like illegitimacy, divorce, or alcoholism not uncommonly lead to a false diagnosis of MDS. Reliance on weight for age as an indicator of failure to thrive is misleading in cases where nonenvironmental causes for short stature exist, as in primordial dwarfism. This disorder is in many instances due to ill-defined prenatal insults, which may be suspected in cases with minor physical stigma or a low birth weight for length of gestation. The incidence of this disorder is highest among underpriviledged. Since MDS is prevalent in the same population group, misdiagnosis is frequent and can be prevented only by reliance on the therapeutic trial and demonstration of improved growth as an absolute prerequisite for diagnosis.

Failure of recognition, rather than overdiagnosis, is a problem is PSD, also because prejudice enters the diagnostic process all too often. The reasons are apparent, if one considers that a major subgroup of patients with PSD had the following characteristics: They were financially self-supporting, predominantly white (10 of 12) in an area where the majority of patients are black, and made a favorable impression on the initial interview (24).

CONCLUSION

The data reviewed in this presentation are compatible with the hypothesis that the two deprivation syndromes, MDS and PSD, which currently are distinguished only by age, represent a biological continuum, with partial recovery from malnutrition and persistence of linear growth failure in children with PSD. All observed endocrine and metabolic abnormalities have been described in malnutrition. Differences in endocrine function between the two syndromes can be attributed to changes that are known to occur during recovery from malnutrition.

The growth retarding environment has not been studied adequately. It is unlikely that the emotional insult is uniform, since two subgroups of patients with PSD can be recognized and similar division may be possible for infants with MDS. Although the possibility of a relation between endocrine dysfunction and a specific emotional insult deserves further study, malnutrition is a factor in the environment of patients with MDS and both subgroups of PSD. Malnutrition is aggravated by characteristics which develop in the patients, abnormal eating behavior, symptoms of malabsorption, and an increase in calorie requirements for size, caused by changes in body composition.

REFERENCES

1. AINSWORTH, M.D. 1962. The effects of maternal deprivation: A review of findings and controversy in the context of research strategy. Publication 14. World Health Organization Papers, p. 97.
2. ALLEYNE, G. A. O., and YOUNG, V. H. 1967. Adrenocortical function in children with severe protein-calorie malnutrition. *Clin. Sci.*, 33, 189.
3. BEAS, F., FERREIRA, E., and RIVAROLA, M. 1973. Adrenal cortical function in infants with malnutrition, as seen in Chile. In: L. I. Gardner and P. Amacher (Eds.) *Endocrine Aspects of Malnutrition, Marasmus, Kwashiorkor and Psychosocial Deprivation.* Santa Ynez, Ca: Kroc Foundation, p. 343.
4. BOYER, R. M., HELLMAN, L. D., ROFFWARG, H., KATZ, J., ZUMOFF, B., O'CONNOR, J., BRADLOW, L., and INKUSHIMA, D. K. 1977. Cortisol secretion and metabolism in anorexia nervosa. *N. Engl. J. Med.*, 298, 190.
5. BRASEL, J. A. 1973. Review of findings in patients with emotional deprivation. In: L. I. Gardner and P. Amacher (Eds.) *Endocrine Aspects of Malnutrition, Marasmus, Kwashiorkor and Psychosocial Deprivation.* Santa Ynez, Ca: Kroc Foundation, p. 115.
6. BROWN, G. M. 1976. Endocrine aspects of psychosocial dwarfism. In: E. J. Sachar (Ed.) *Hormones, Behavior, and Psychopathology.* New York: Raven Press, p. 253.
7. COLEMAN, R. W., and PROVENCE, S. 1957. Environmental retardation (hospitalism) in infants living in families. *Pediatrics* 19, 285.
8. D'ERCOLE, A. J., UNDERWOOD, L. E., and VANWYK, Y. Y. 1977. Serum Somatomedine—C in hypopituitarism and in other disorders of growth. *J. Ped.*, 90, 375.
9. FISCHHOFF, J., WHITTEN, C. F., and PETTIT, M. G. 1971. A psychiatric study of mothers of infants with growth failure secondary to maternal deprivation. *J. Pediatr.*, 79, 209.
10. FRASIER, S. D., and ROLLISON, M. L. 1972. Growth retardation and emotional deprivation; Relative resistance to treatment with human growth hormone. *J. Pediatr.*, 80, 603.
11. GARVER, D. L., PANDEY, G. N., DEKIRMENJIAN, H., and DAVIS, J. M. 1976. Growth hormone responsiveness to hypoglycemia and urinary MHPG in affective disease patients: Preliminary Observations. In E. J. Sachar (Ed.) *Hormones, Behavior, and Psychopathology.* New York: Raven Press, p. 233.
12. GODARD, C. 1973. Plasma growth hormone levels in severe infantile malnutrition in Bolivia. In L. I. Gardner and P. Amacher (Eds.) *Endocrine Aspects of Malnutrition, Marasmus,*

Kwashiorkor, and Psychosocial Deprivation. Santa Ynez, Ca.: Kroc Foundation, p. 19.

13. GRAHAM, G. G., and BLIZZARD, R. M. 1973. Thyroid hormonal studies in severely malnourished Peruvian infants and small children. In: L. I. Gardner and P. Amacher (Eds.) *Endocrine Aspects of Malnutrition, Marasmus, Kwashiorkor, and Psychosocial Deprivation.* Santa Ynez, Ca.: Kroc Foundation, p. 205.

14. GREEN, O. C., FEFFERMAN, R., and NAIR, S. 1967. Plasma growth hormone levels in children with cystic fibrosis and short stature. Unresponsiveness to hypoglycemia, *J. Clin. Endocr.*, 27, 1059.

15. HARLOW, H. F., ROWLAND, G. L. and GRIFFIN, G. A. 1964. The effect of total social deprivation on the development of monkey behavior. *Psychiat. Res. Rep.* 19, 116.

16. HELLMAN, D. A., and COLLE, E. 1969. Plasma growth hormone and insulin responses in short children. *Am. J. Dis. Child.*, 117, 636.

17. ILLIG, R. 1972. Wachstumshormon Untersuchungen bei 225 Kindern mit Minderwuchs. *Schweiz. Med. Wochenschr.*, 102, 760.

18. IMURA, H., YOSHIMI, T., and IKEKUBO, K. 1971. Growth hormone secretion in a patient with deprivation dwarfism. *Endocrinol.*, Jap., 18, 301.

19. KAPLAN, S. L., ABRAMS, C. L., BELL, J. J. CONTE, F. A., and GRUMBACH, M. M. 1968. Growth and growth hormone. *Pediatr. Res.*, 2, 43.

20. KEN, G. R., CHANROVE, A. S., and HARLOW, H. F. 1969. Environmental deprivation. Its effect on the growth of infant monkeys. *J. Pediat.*, 7, 833.

21. KRIEGER, I. 1966. The energy metabolism in infants with growth failure due to maternal deprivation, undernutrition, or causes unknown. I. Metabolic rate calculated from the insensible loss of weight. *Pediatrics*, 38, 63.

22. KRIEGER, I. 1973. Endocrines and nutrition in psychosocial deprivation in the USA: Comparison with growth failure due to malnutrition on an organic basis. In: L. I. Gardner and P. Amacher (Eds.) *Endocrine Aspects of Malnutrition, Marasmus, Kwashiorkor and Psychosocial Deprivation.* Santa Ynez, Cal.: Kroc Foundation, p. 129.

23. KRIEGER, I. 1974. Food restriction as a form of child abuse in ten cases of psychosocial deprivation dwarfism. *Clin. Pediatr.*, 13, 127.

24. KRIEGER, I. Deprivation syndrome in children three years and older. In preparation.

25. KRIEGER, I., and CHEN, Y. C. 1969. Calorie requirements for weight gain in infants with growth failure due to maternal deprivation, undernutrition, and congenital heart disease. A correlation analysis. *Pediatrics*, 44, 647.

26. KRIEGER, I., and GOOD, M. H. 1970. Adrenocortical and thyroid function in the deprivation syndrome: Comparison with growth failure due to undernutrition, congenital heart disease, or prenatal influences. *Am. J. Dis. Child.*, 120, 95.

27. KRIEGER, I., and MELLINGER, R. C. 1971. Pituitary function in the deprivation syndrome. *J. Pediatr.*, 79, 216.

28. KRIEGER, I., and SARGENT, D. S. 1967. A postural sign in the sensory deprivation syndrome. *J. Pediatr.*, 70, 332.

29. KRIEGER, I., and TAQI, Q. 1975. Free serum thyroxine level and basal metabolic rate. Aids to diagnosis in malnutrition and small-for-gestational-age dwarfism. *Am. J. Dis. Child.*, 130, 830.

30. KRIEGER, I., and TAQI, Q. 1977. Metabolic rate and body composition in rates nutritionally deprived before or after weaning. *Pediat. Res.*, 11, 796.

31. KRIEGER, I., and WHITTEN, C. F. 1969. Energy metabolism in infants with growth failure due to maternal deprivation, undernutrition, or causes unknown. Relationship between nitrogen balance, weight gain, and post-prandial excess heat production. 75, 374.

32. LACEY, K. A., HEWISON, A., and PARKIN, J. M. 1973. Exercise as a screening test for growth hormone deficiency in children. *Arch. Dis. Child.*, 48, 508.

33. LANDON, J., GREENWOOD, F. C., STAMP, C. B., and WYNN, V. 1966. The plasma sugar, free fatty acid, cortisol, and growth hormone response to insulin, and the comparison

of this procedure with other tests of pituitary and adrenal function. II. In patients with hypothalamic or pituitary dysfunction or anorexia nervosa, *J. Clin. Invest.*, 45, 437.

34. LEONNARD, M. F., RHYMES, J. P., and SOLNIT, A. J. 1966. Failure to thrive in infants. *Amer. J. Dis. Child.*, 111, 600.

35. MONEY, J. 1977. The syndrome of abuse dwarfism (Psychosocial dwarfism or reversible hyposomatotropism). *Am. J. Dis. Child.*, 131, 508.

36. MONEY, J., and WOLFF, G. 1974. Late puberty, retarded growth and reversible hyposomatotropinism (Psychosocial Dwarfism). *Adolescence*, 9 (33), 123.

37. MONEY, J., WOLFF, G., and ANNECILLO, C. 1972. Pain agnosia and self-injury in the syndrome of reversible somatotropin deficiency (psychosocial dwarfism). *J. Autism Child Schizo.*, 2, 127.

38. PARRA, A. 1973. Discussion. In: L. I. Gardner and P. Amacher (Eds.) *Endocrine Aspects of Malnutrition, Marasmus, Kwashiorkor and Psychosocial Deprivation*. Santa Ynez, Cal.: Kroc Foundation, p. 155.

39. PARRA, A., GARZA, Y., SARAVIA, J. L., HAZLEWOOD, C. F., and NICHOLS, B. L. 1973. Changes in growth hormone, insulin, and thyroxine values, and in energy metabolism of marasmic infants. *J. Pediatr.* 82, 133.

40. PATTON, R. G., and GARDNER, L. I. 1963. *Growth Failure in Maternal Deprivation.* Springfield, Ill.: Charles C Thomas Publishers.

41. PIMSTONE, B. L., WITTMAN, W., HANSEN, J. D. L., and MURRAY, P. 1966. Growth hormone and kwashiorkor. Role of protein in growth hormone homeostasis. *Lancet*, 2, 779.

42. POWELL, G. F., BRASEL, J. A., and BLIZZARD, R. F. 1967. Emotional deprivation and growth retardation simulating true idiopathic hypopituitarism. I. Clinical evaluation of the syndrome. *N. Engl. J. Med.*, 276, 1271.

43. POWELL, G. F., BRASEL, J. A., RAITI, S., BLIZZARD, R. M. 1967. Emotional deprivation and growth retardation simulating idiopathic hypopituitarism. II Endocrinologic evaluation of the syndrome. *N. Engl. J. Med.*, 276, 1279.

44. POWELL, G. F., HOPWOOD, M. J., and BARRATT, E. S. 1973. Growth hormone studies before and during catch-up growth in a child with emotional deprivation and short stature. *J. Clin. Endocrinol. Metab.*, 37, 674.

45. PROVENCE, S. A., and LIPTON, R. C. 1962. *Infants in Institutions.* New York: International University Press Inc., p. 147.

46. SILVER, J. K., FINKELSTEIN, M. 1967. Deprivation dwarfism. *J. Pediat.*, 70, 317.

47. TANNER, J. M. 1971. Isolated growth hormone deficiency; differential diagnosis. *Arch. Dis. Child.*, 46, 878.

48. THOMPSON, R. G., PARRA, A., SCHULTZ, R. B., and BLIZZARD, R. M. 1969. Endocrine evaluation in patients with psycho-social dwarfism. *Amer. Fed. Clin. Res.*, 17, 592. (Abst).

49. VAN DEN BRANDE, J. L., and DU CAJU, V. L. 1973. Plasma somatomedin activity in children with growth disturbances. In S. Raiti (Ed.) *Advances in Human Growth Hormone Research.* (Symposium) Baltimore, Md. p. 98.

50. WHITTEN, C. F., and KRIEGER, I. 1977. The maternal deprivation syndrome. In: *Problems Relating to Feeding in the First Two Years*. Columbus, Ohio: Ross Laboratories, p. 55.

51. WHITTEN, C. F., PETTIT, M. G., and FISCHHOFF, J. 1969. Evidence that growth failure from maternal deprivation is secondary to undereating. *JAMA*, 209, 1675.

52. WOLFF, G., and MONEY, J. 1973. Relationship between sleep and growth in patients with reversible somatotropin deficiency (psychosocial dwarfism). *Psychol. Med.*, 3, 18.

7

AN EXPERIENCE OF DEPRIVATION: A FOLLOW-UP STUDY

JARMILA KOLUCHOVÁ, PH.D.

Head of the Department of Psychology, Pedagogical Faculty, Palacký University, Olomouc, Czechoslovakia

INTRODUCTION

The diagnosis of psychic deprivation can be found in child psychiatry and clinical psychology only during the last 15 years. As this term is not used in the same manner by all authors, it is necessary to present our conception and definition. We define psychic deprivation, in accord with Langmeier and Matejcek (7), as a psychic state which occurs when a child is not given an opportunity to meet one or more basic psychic wants. We consider the following wants to be basic:

1) Establishment of permanent, positive emotional relationships with the mother (or mother substitute) and gradually with other close persons, allowing for the basic integration of personality and giving the child a feeling of security and self-worth.
2) A supply of objective, intellectual, emotional and social stimuli in adequate amount and variability.
3) Good basic conditions for learning, so that the surrounding world comes to make sense to the child and, gradually, more and more differentiated interactions between the child and its environment can be established.
4) Establishment of a feeling of identity and social value, as the child is accepted in the family and wider social groups.

At particular ages in the child's development, these wants are modified—their intensity being either increased or decreased. Also, in different historical periods the way and degree of meeting the wants are different, depending on social and cultural conditions. Nevertheless, under various circumstances, practical experiences, as well as research, indicate that the child's psychic wants are best met in an intact, well-functioning family.

It has been demonstrated that psychic deprivation is an important aetiopathogenetic factor for various difficulties and defects of psychic development. Consequently, from the point of view of clinical practice, it is particularly important that we identify psychic deprivation and formulate treatment plans.

SOME PROBLEMS IN DIAGNOSING PSYCHIC DEPRIVATION

Psychic deprivation is a gross damage of a child's development. Its clinical picture is rather diverse, conditioned by a number of factors, namely the age of the child and the length and severity of deprivational situation. In younger children psychic deprivation is manifested especially by retardation of psychomotor development and speech; in older ones it becomes evident by some eccentricities and fluctuations in their social behavior—e.g., emotional flatness is often seen in deprived children. We can often observe neurotic manifestations as well. Thus, severe deprivation can sometimes create an impression of psychotic disease. For example, we examined a two-year-old child who had been diagnosed as infantile Kanner's autism and a child who had been diagnosed at school age as reactive depression, although the correct diagnosis in both cases was severe deprivational damage, which was revealed after obtaining correct anamnestic data and after a detailed examination. Therefore, we do not consider it suitable to use the term "*deprivational syndrome*," because it cannot be explained as a fixed and explicitly defined set of symptoms.

The fact that deprivational damage can influence all spheres of psychic development and behavior makes the diagnosis of psychic deprivation both difficult and important. Sometimes we find that children who have suffered severe and prolonged deprivation, whether in inadequate families, often profoundly neglected and socially isolated, or living for a considerable period in an institutional environment, are misdiagnosed as oligophrenic. Distinguishing severe deprivation from oligophrenia is the most important differential diagnostic problem in this sphere. The clinical pictures of severe deprivation and oligophrenia are similar to some extent, which can lead to confusion of the two conditions, especially when tests are mechanically used and their results misinterpreted. The child may be diagnosed as imbecile, even if it is in fact grossly handicapped by deprivation. Especially in children up to the third year of age, socially isolated or living in an institutional environment without stimulation, we may see such profound retardation and developmental damage due to internal and external conditions of deprivation that it becomes very difficult to differentiate it from oligophrenia. As these children have no prospect of good development in their own family, it is sometimes necessary to intervene legally and take suitable therapeutic and educational measures.

If such a decision is to ensure the child's optimum development, a correct diagnosis is necessary. To this end, psychological findings should play a major role. Only psychological examination can reveal subtle differences between a severely deprived and an oligophrenic child. However, cursory outpatient examination will not serve. It is necessary to carry out repeated examinations aimed at the structure and dynamics of any developmental deficit. A skilled psychologist should not only assess the degree of retardation of the child, but also determine the outlook for further development. Such a psychological finding then makes a considerably greater contribution to the whole team of experts in determining treatment and placement than only the IQ expressed in numbers.

It is important to clarify the term "mental retardation," which is sometimes used interchangeably with mental deficiency and mental subnormality. We agree with Clarke (2) who says that this term "does not describe a clearly defined entity but rather a heterogenous group of conditions characterized by low or very low intelligence."

Clarke also points out that mental retardation encompasses both retardation caused by brain damage of varying etiology and retardation caused by extremely adverse sociocultural factors. We believe it is better to use the term mental retardation only as a general term for all forms of retardation or developmental damage where the main feature of the clinical picture is intellectual subnormality. Its use should be avoided in clinical practice where it is important to differentiate separate forms of mental retardation, especially on the basis of etiology and the quality of damage. It is only on the basis of such a clear description that it becomes possible to determine the degree of reparability.

POSSIBILITIES OF REVERSAL OF PSYCHIC DEPRIVATION

While stressing the importance of differential diagnosis between oligophrenia and severe deprivation, we must answer the question of the sense and purpose of this differentiation. There has been—even to the present day—a considerable therapeutic pessimism concerning severe deprivation, especially when it dates from an early age. There are some reports in the literature of accelerated development of children who had been severely deprived as a consequence of social isolation, but the cases are considered to be exceptional, and there is no detailed documentation or theoretical basis. Moreover, efforts have been directed chiefly to increasing IQ and far less at improvement in other areas. The major shortcoming of such reports has been the brief periods of follow-up.

The views on the irreparability of deprivational damage probably arose from the fact that severely deprived children, often abused, profoundly neglected or socially isolated in their family setting, remained permanently in a children's home after the withdrawal from the family. This may have brought about a certain increase in the intellectual level, but did not significantly develop the emotional and social components, nor the whole personality. As Clarke suggests, the pessimism, which had surrounded this problem led to passivity in looking for further possibilities to cure such children (1).

However, our longitudinal observation and investigation of severely deprived children have shown that deprivational damage is reparable to a much greater extent than was supposed. Many children, originally claimed to be permanently handicapped and even regarded as oligophrenic, are now at an average level and attend a regular school. We would stress again, however, that it is not enough to declare a child mentally retarded, determine its IQ and then observe whether it will increase. Nor is it acceptable to proclaim generally the reparability of mental retardation, as is frequently done. From the humane point of view, it is, of course, desirable to provide every mentally retarded child with maximum curative, educational and social care, but from the professional point of view it is necessary to realize that the degree of reparability and methods of reparation must be different for separate forms and stages of mental retardation. Accordingly, they must distinguish between deprived and oligophrenic children. An imbecile child will continue being such however well or badly it may be educated, while a deprived child, who only seemed to be at the imbecile level, can reach a high standard in specially favorable circumstances.

It has become evident that it is necessary to study real cases intensively and to observe deprived children longitudinally in their normal living conditions to be able to evaluate the possibilities of reparability of psychic deprivation and to find effective methods of reparation. Meanwhile, our research, which has always been based on this approach, has led us to the conclusion that we can be more optimistic than previously thought in predicting future outcome concerning deprived children. Our experience with the development of speech, too, contradicts the traditional view concerning the critical period for the development of speech. Successful development of speech was observed after passing to a stimulating environment as late as between the third and sixth year, and sometimes even later.

THE RESULTS OF THE RESEARCH

As noted above, our ability to answer complicated questions on psychic deprivation, especially where its differential diagnosis and reparability are concerned, must be based on a thorough, long-term study. Favorable prerequisites for such research arose in Czechoslovakia with the creation of new forms of substitute family care, the so-called "children's villages" and foster-family care for those children who are for various reasons not suitable for adoption. For a period of seven to ten years 70 children from such a children's village and 30 children from foster families have been observed by psychologists working with other experts.

The research, aimed at the general psychic and social development of the children, will go on until their maturity. The initial results of the research reported here proved to be positive and of great interest.

The children placed in foster families are those whose clinical picture is marked mainly by psychic deprivation of various kinds and degrees. They may be either children from children's homes without any prospect of returning to their original family or those taken away from their own inadequate families. However, slight deprivational damage in small children is not alone a sufficient indication for foster family care; if their psychic and somatic condition is otherwise good, they may be adopted. The children placed in foster families are usually severely deprived as a result of extended stay in children's homes or traumatized by frequent moves from one home to another. In addition, there are children with a small degree of oligophrenia, who must attend schools for the mentally retarded, as well as children with somatic and sensory afflictions, who are particularly sensitive to deprivation. Finally, there are also children who are placed in foster families because their parents are seriously ill—with schizophrenia, manic-depressive psychosis, heavy alcoholism, epilepsy, etc.

Understandably, the education of such children is rather demanding and therefore the foster parents must be very carefully selected; this could extend to a psychological examination. In children's villages, eight to 10 children of various ages and both sexes are brought up together by a foster mother; this family group lives in a family house. The "village" is socially linked up with the life of the real village surrounding it. The children attend school with the children of the regular village residents and thus they are in no way socially different or isolated from the normal life of the village.

In addition, there are also cases of foster parentage in natural families who may even have their own children. Usually, one or two children are placed in such families. These foster parents are also given a psychological examination to clarify the general structure of their personality, qualifications for bringing up children with educational difficulties, their motivation for foster parentage, and, finally, the stability of their married life and the whole environment of the family, especially as far as emotional and social relations are concerned.

Foster mothers for children's villages are specially trained for their work and foster parents are also thoroughly instructed in advance about the educational, social and other problems of their work and are given detailed information about the child entrusted to their care. They are also informed that there is a special advisory board at their disposal consisting of a social worker, a pediatrician and a psychologist. The foster parents know that the entire research project is connected with the activity of this advisory board and, therefore, they do not take them as unwelcome interference with the family, but as a help which they appreciate. At the same time this is also a kind of psychotherapy for them and an appreciation of their work.

The reaction of children coming to a foster family differed according to their age, their personality and their previous life experiences. Small children accommodated very quickly, although sometimes showing temporary reactions of anxiety. They clung to the close relationship with the members of the family, especially the foster mother; in various ways they demonstrated their fear of losing her and being sent back to the previous children's home environment. Older children kept on asking whether they would really stay there forever, whether somebody would not take them back, etc. Emotional relations between child and foster family were established very quickly; in families with their own children the position of the small adopted children was that of the youngest brother or sister overwhelmed with care and love. In very small children we could observe striking acceleration of their whole psychic development, especially of speech. The children quickly adapted socially, they were gay and contented, and the deprivational demonstrations (symptons) faded surprisingly quickly.

The development of intellectual ability of the children was most rapid during the first year of their stay in the foster family. The younger the children, the more remarkable was the progress.

Children up to the age of three added 15 to 20 points on the IQ scale. During the second and third years of the child's life in the foster family, the increase in IQ was slower, but during that time the remaining intellectual deficit caused by deprivational situation was usually made up. In classic studies dealing with psychic deprivation, the possibility of intellectual increase of deprived children during their school age is mostly not taken into account; their intellectual damage is considered to be persistent. However, we have found an increase in intellectual level even during school age—in some cases, a really notable increase, as will be noted below. While testing intelligence, we have also found that the deprivational situation afflicted mainly speech and the verbal component of intelligence; consequently, the progress in this area is slower and more difficult than in the performance component.

In school children we have also observed their school results and their general adjustment to school. We have recorded a conspicuous improvement; some children, who were behind in their school placement (because they had had to repeat a year or they had started attending school later than usual) could even skip one form with the help of the teacher and the family. This improvement of school performance is not determined only by the intellectual development, but more probably by the new emotional relationship to the foster mother and foster parents, and by their finding their place in the new family and the resulting feeling of security. All these factors motivate the child to perform at school and stimulate his ambition to achieve better school results and gain a good position in the class.

We have paid special attention to children, whose parents suffered from psychosis. The repair of deprivational damage in these cases was, on the whole, as good as in the others. There have not appeared any symptoms of their parents' disease, although some of the children are at the age of puberty.

Although it is impossible in this space to present all the data we have compiled in the course of several years, we think it useful to describe several cases at greater length. The children who have been observed fully for the longest period of time are monozygotic twin boys, whose development has already been described in detail in an effort to draw more general conclusions on the basis of this and some other observed cases (4, 5). Therefore, we will present here only a brief summary of their anamnestic data and psychic development, while concentrating in greater detail on their latest development, present state and prospects.

CASE HISTORY

The twins were born in 1960. Their mother died shortly after the delivery and the children lived in a home for infants until the age of 11 months.

Their development was adequate to their age. Then they lived for a short period of time with relatives and in a home for toddlers. When the boys were 18 months old, their father remarried and took the children to his new home. The children then lived in the family under most abnormal conditions until the age of seven. They were hated and cruelly beaten by their psychopathic stepmother; they were isolated from society, insufficiently fed, kept in a small, unheated closet, and often locked up in the cellar. When the matter came to light, the twins were treated at a hospital and then placed in a children's home. The somatic development at the age of seven was approximately equivalent to that of three-year-old children; they suffered from acute rickets and could barely walk and speak. The severe psychic deprivation, which seemed irreparable at that time (almost on the level of imbecility), started to improve in the children's home where they were placed. However, an outstanding improvement and acceleration of their psychic development, especially speech, occurred only after their coming to a foster family at the age of 9.

The manifestations of deprivation faded rather quickly in that family. There was extremely rapid intellectual development, as well as improvement in speech. One of the twins gained 17 points on the IQ scale between 9 and 10, which was the first year of their life with the family and their first year of school attendance. There was also the stimulating influence of the educational environment on their psychic development. The boys developed very close relations to their foster mother and to the whole family rather quickly, the relationship being of the same kind as in the natural family. This indicates that spontaneous adherence is possible even at a later age than usually admitted. In the development and forming of the personalities of the boys, no abnormalities or disorders appeared even at puberty. The boys' social development is very good: They are sociable and popular, with a very strong emotional bond to their family.

Since the time the children were removed from their original family, they have been continually observed. Besides the psychological examination by means of test and non-test methods, the observation of the boys in natural conditions was very thorough, especially in the family and in everyday group situations with their peers. Much more valuable information is obtained in these natural settings than in casual non-resident examination.

At present, the boys are just 17, their intelligence is slightly above the average, their IQs being between 105 and 110 and the structure and quality of both boys' intellectual functions being quite adequate. Thus, there has been a moderate increase in their intelligence and we can assume—in accordance with the general trend of their development—that IQ will develop somewhat further in the near future. The boys finished the basic 9-year school with average results. Earlier they had passed from the 4th class direct to the 6th. In accordance with their wish, they were admitted to an exacting vocational school of precision mechanics with a specialization in computers. A graduating examination will enable them to go on to a university. This kind of work corresponds with their intellectual level, technical talent, and interests; both are very fond of fine manual work.

The start of puberty of twins was delayed about one year in comparison with the average of our population. Even now their development, namely their interests and general expression, is on the level of children between 15 and 16, which corresponds with the level of their schoolmates at basic school rather than with that of students at the vocational school they will be going to. Now they are interested mainly in riding a bicycle, swimming, outdoor games; they play the piano well, they read a lot, and can play chess well.

As for their somatic condition, they are pubescently spindle-legged, both of them being rather slim and tall—almost six feet in spite of the fact that their parents were of medium height. Their height is surprising, also, because of the fact that at the time of their withdrawal from the deprivational environment there was deficit in the physical condition of both twins. The EEG record, made because of rather frequent headaches and previous serious injuries to the head evident from scars, is slightly abnormal; however, there are no attacks nor other neurological symptoms.

The general development and present state of the twins entirely contradict the original predictions of pediatricians and speech therapists that deprivational damage is irreparable, that the twins would be ineducable, that their speech would never develop, and that, as a result, they would be entirely excluded from the society of normal people. The reparation of gross deprivational damage occurred not only in the intellectual, but also in the emotional and social spheres, which we consider much more important.

CASE HISTORY

Following is a case that is of interest for evaluating the part played by genetic disposition and educational environment in the formation of personality. We present here a brief anamnesis of a girl born in 1965 and now living in the same family as the twins described above. This girl was withdrawn legally from her own family at the age of four as a consequence of almost total social isolation and cruel treatment by her psychopathic mother. The child had been tormented by hunger, she had been constantly kept alone in an unfurnished room, had slept on a straw mattress, and had not acquired the basic habits of body hygiene. This girl was placed in a children's home, where she displayed anxiety, agitation, and aggression. Her language ability was almost totally undeveloped and she was still incontinent. The teachers in the home considered her ineducable and it was decided that she should be placed in a mental institution.

The family in which the twins live happened to hear about this girl. Encouraged by the good development of the twins, they decided to adopt the girl into the family in spite of the fact that the prognosis for her development was rather pessimistic. Even though the child was difficult to care for in the family during the first weeks due to her agitation and anxiety, we were able to eliminate mental subnormality, although her retardation was considerable and deprivation symptoms conspicuous. The child started learning to speak rather quickly. She was bright and she began to attend a kindergarten.

However, this child has always presented a much greater educational problem than the twins. She attends a school for normal children and has an outstanding talent for music, but she has continued to have problems in her social relations. It is only with great difficulty that she joins in with other children or with her class group. Sometimes she is aggressive and intolerant with her contemporaries, although gentle and kind with younger children. Yet, sympathetic and consistent upbringing have produced some improvement which could not have been achieved in a children's home.

It is interesting to compare the girl with the twin boys. The deprivational history of the three children is rather similar and they now live in the same family and are given the same attention. Their different development in the social sphere could be explained by differing congenital dispositions but probably the chief factor is that the twins could relate to one another and so reduce their isolation. Moreover, the girl's mother is a severely psychopathic person with disorders in character and in social relations. There are no valid data about her father. On the other hand, the twins' mother was quite normal in intelligence and personality structure, while their father was characterised in the previous report (4) as passive and of below-average intellect. According to photographs and reliable reports, the twins seem to possess their mother's features, both physically and psychologically. But their better development in their social adjustment should be ascribed primarily to the fact that they could relate emotionally with one another and stimulate each other to some extent; thus, they did not experience the tormenting feeling of loneliness as destructively as would a totally isolated child.

THE FAMILY AS THE MAIN THERAPEUTIC FACTOR

The present findings, which are the result of a continuous and longitudinal observation, show convincingly that in the environment of a good foster family or in an artificially created family in a "children's village" even gross deprivational damage can be overcome, not only in the area of intellectual development, but in all aspects of the psyche. Such an environment influences in a positive way the forming of the children's personality and also helps in their social adaptation and in their finding a useful function or place in society.

All the children placed in substitute families are provided with all necessary medical care and the psychologist who observes their development also gives advisory and psychotherapeutic help to the foster parents and teachers. Although all these factors are important, it is necessary to stress that the environment of a family is an effective, integrating curative factor; foremost is the influence of the foster mother.

Our evidence concerning the possibility of remedying gross deprivational damage in a good substitute family has received considerable support (1, 3). However, it has also evoked disagreement, which we believe arises from a misunderstanding of our viewpoint (6). We do not underestimate the importance of either the mother-child relationship or the family environment for the forming of the child's personality, especially at an early age. We do not consider the child simply a passive recipient of stimuli from the family; rather, from an early age he is an active member of the family and contributes to the climate of the family. Deprivational damage must be considered a serious interference with and jeopardy of psychic development. Therefore, if a child is jeopardized by severe deprivation in its own family, if there is no prospect of reparation in spite of efforts on the part of society and various specialists, then it is necessary to withdraw him or her from the family and substitute for it the care of a children's home. But this environment, unless well selected, may also be dangerous in that it can add to deprivation. Further, any action in placing a child is dependent on the legal procedures in each country. Generally, a child's development and its mental health are better secured in the environment of a substitute family than in a children's home. This holds good despite the fact that considerable efforts are made to bring these homes as close to the life of the natural family as possible—by the design and furnishing of the setting, by the structure of the social life of the children, and by the whole regime of their daily life.

Since we consider the substitute family to be the most important therapeutic and rehabilitating factor, we obviously assign considerable importance to the mother-child relationship. We have been continually verifying that biological bonds—i.e. consanguineous parentage—are not absolutely essential. Adoptive or foster-mothers fulfill the functions of a mother far better than many a natural mother, even if they have not taken care of the child from birth, but only since the pre-school age, and even later, as has been confirmed by the foster-mother of the twins described above. Consequently, we summarize our research in the sphere of deprivation as follows:

1. We must rather carefully assess children whose anamnesis contains deprivation. It is important to know in a particular case whether there is oligophrenia or severe deprivation, or whether both factors cause the present state of the child.

2. Detailed psychological examinations and longitudinal observations are always necessary; their findings will help us to discover subtle differences between the similar clinical pictures of oligophrenia and deprivation and will enable us to predict development and explain suitable social and therapeutic arrangements.

3. Severe psychic deprivation, although originated at an early age, is to a great extent or totally reparable, on condition that the child receives psychological and medical care.

4. The main effective therapeutic factor, however, is a substitute family, the choice of which and its further supervising are shared by a team of professional workers. The environment of a family, stimulating and full of understanding, gives children a feeling of safety and secure relationships. The substitute family is a very successful therapeutic factor, according to our experience. Understandably, it is a very exacting and long-term therapy.

REFERENCES

1. CLARKE, A. D. B. 1972. Commentary on Koluchová's "Severe deprivation in twins: A case study." *J. Child Psychol. Psychiat.*, 13, 103.
2. CLARKE, A. D. B. and CLARKE, A. M. 1974. Mental retardation and behavioural change. *Br. Med. Bull.*, 2, 179.
3. CLARKE, A. M. and CLARKE, A. D. B. 1976. *Early Experience: Myth and Evidence*. London: Open Books.
4. KOLUCHOVÁ, J. 1972. Severe deprivation in twins: A case study. *J. Child Psychol. Psychiat.*, 13, 107.
5. KOLUCHOVÁ, J. 1976. The further development of twins after severe and prolonged deprivation: A second report. *J. Child Psychol. Psychiat.*, 17, 181.
6. KOLUCHOVÁ, J. 1976. Twins. *British Medical Journal*, 16 October, 897.
7. LANGMEIER, J. and MATEJCEK, Z. 1975. *Psychological Deprivation in Childhood*. Queensland University Press.

8

DISADVANTAGED INFANTS AS PARENTS

STEPHEN WOLKIND and FAE HALL

Family Research Unit
The London Hospital Medical College

INTRODUCTION

There can be little argument that a mother will significantly affect her baby during its infancy. Even if maternal love cannot be shown to be a mystical quality different from other factors which will impinge on the child, the impact of the mother must be overwhelming. Escalona (8) has pointed out that as a source of stimulation the human caregiver is more complex, more subtle and more variable than any other external stimulus to which the child will be exposed. In ideal circumstances, a mother's contacts with her baby are such that they will elicit from him the fullest range of responses possible in his repertoire of behaviour. In the absence of gross environmental and biological hazards, the infant's main need is to experience at least "good enough" mothering (29). A strong case can be made for "seeing a range of ill understood disorders of infancy, such as some sleeping and eating problems, avoidable illness and disturbances of growth and development as manifestations of mothering failure" (16, p. 289). In addition, the mother's influence during infancy will contribute, though not necessarily directly, to her child's ultimate intellectual and emotional state.

In some of the early child psychiatry research, a tendency developed to see all of a child's later difficulties as resulting directly from some charac-

The work reported in this chapter was supported by a generous grant from the Medical Research Council and a contract from the DHSS/SSRC Working Party on Transmitted Deprivation.

teristic of its mother—her overanxiousness, overprotectiveness, etc. In much of this work there is a total neglect of the infant's role in this relationship and of the effect of his behaviour on his mother. Perhaps partly as a reaction to the destructive manner in which some of these concepts entered clinical work through diagnoses such as "schizophrenogenic mothers," many workers began to concentrate on the infant side of the equation. From these studies it has become apparent that both the child and the mother have a part to play in determining the nature and possibly content of the interactions between them. Relatively simple infant characteristics such as its sex (14) have been shown to markedly affect the mother's behaviour. Paradoxically, we have probably reached a point where we now have more knowledge of how the baby affects its mother than of how her mothering ability is moulded by her own experiences, personality and expectations. In discussing in this chapter one of these latter areas, we are in no way seeing this as the sole or even most important determinant of the interaction or of the outcome for the child. Rather we are attempting to understand the antecedents of the contribution that one partner is bringing to a complex two-way relationship. In addition, we are crossing generations to ask whether the experiences which infants of disadvantaged mothers might receive in the early months and years will in turn determine how they will handle their own children.

VARIATIONS IN MATERNAL BEHAVIOUR

Clinical and social observation can leave no doubt about the presence of great variations in maternal behaviour. Even in a relatively homogeneous social group many differences can be seen; mothers may overprotect or neglect their child, while demonstrating a wide range of beliefs and child-rearing practices. In research, too, a striking feature of almost all studies is that no matter what sort of measure is used, whether a global term such as sensitivity (1) or more detailed observations (18), the same variation is seen.

It is less easy to understand the origins of these differences. With animal studies demonstrating the effects of hormones on mothering behaviour (26), a possibility could be biological variation. One attempt to examine this area in humans was that of Levy (12), who examined the relationship between "motherliness" and duration of menstrual flow. He found a direct and high correlation between the two, with "motherly" women having a longer flow. Interesting as this finding is, it clearly could be interpreted in a number of different ways.

Though biological factors are of undoubted importance, a far more promising field for enquiry would seem to be in socialization. In different societies very clear differences in mothering style have been described. Mead (13) has contrasted the Arapesh mother, who treats her baby as a soft vulnerable precious object needing to be protected and cherished with the Mundugumor mother, whom she describes as showing an active dislike of her child and discouraging intimate contact. Within our own society, social class differences in some aspects of handling have been described (2, 28); the most common finding is that there are lower levels of verbal interaction in working-class families. These studies all suggest that it is perhaps in each mother's own socialization, particularly during her childhood, that we might find the roots of her later behaviour. The mother's experience will reflect the values of the society in which she is brought up and the way in which these are interpreted on an individual level within her own family.

Support is given to this by the subjective feelings of mothers themselves, who, when questioned on the development of their child-rearing ideas, tend to recall their own family of origin. Stolz (25), from interviews with 78 women, found that 87 percent felt that their childhood experiences (either positive or negative) with their mothers had influenced the way they handled their own children. Forty-four percent also felt experiences with their fathers had been important. Psychoanalytic writers from their clinical experience with adult patients have also been impressed by this association: "The mother relationship in a woman is conditioned from the beginning by the various psychological influences of her own childhood development, upbringing and cultural environment" (7). In a more systematic enquiry on psychoanalytic lines, a similar conclusion was reached by Blake Cohen (3). In a study of 50 pregnant women, she found that those who were problem-free and were able to accept pregnancy and motherhood were particularly likely to have come from harmonious childhood homes and to have had a good relationship with their own mothers. From a clinical standpoint, the important issue clearly focuses on the converse of this finding. Do women from disadvantaged, disharmonious homes become those mothers who will have difficulties in coping both with their own problems and with their children?

THE DISADVANTAGED INFANT AS MOTHER

Harlow and his team have examined this question in the rhesus monkey. Females raised in infancy in total social isolation showed, in adulthood, gross abnormalities in mothering behaviour (24). They were either completely indifferent or violently abusive towards their infants. The degree of isolation and lack of parenting experienced by the females in their upbringing were, of course, far greater than would be found in any human situation, but the abnormalities of mothering found in Harlow's monkeys do suggest parallels with the behaviour of those human adults who are involved in the most serious form of parental failure: child abuse.

Rutter and Madge (21) have reviewed the literature on the families of origin of abusing parents. The parallel with the rhesus monkeys is heightened by their conclusion that, despite the lack of controls, "the findings are sufficiently striking for there to be little doubt that battering parents differ from the general population in the high proportion who experienced severely adverse parenting in their own childhood" (p. 235). In this same review these authors discuss the many difficulties involved in both defining and measuring disadvantage and poor parenting. There are problems in trying to assess psychological disadvantage which may have occurred many years previously. In particular, retrospective accounts of home atmosphere must be viewed with caution. One circumstance which can be enquired about, hopefully in a more objective fashion, is a child's early separation from its parents. For some time it was felt that all separation experiences were, in themselves, factors of major psychological importance, with inevitable long-term consequences. Even if the weight of evidence* now suggests that this is not so, it has become increasingly clear that certain sorts of separation can be recognized as highly sensitive indices of wider family problems and poor relationships. It is these problems which do, in fact, represent the most common type of psychological disadvantage to which a child can be exposed (19).

Frommer and O'Shea (9) have used these concepts to study the effects of childhood experience in a sample of primiparous women attending a pre-natal clinic. They enquired about any separations from her mother which the woman had experienced before the age of 11. As mothers themselves, those who reported separations were more likely to have difficulties in feeding their infants and would be more likely than the remainder to leave their two-month-old babies to feed from a propped bottle. Frommer and O'Shea went on to confirm that it was only a separation occurring in the context of a disturbed family relationship that was incriminated (10). In our study it is this limited but useful concept that we have used to define psychological disadvantage in childhood.

---

* See Howells, J. G. Separation and Deprivation. In Vol. 3 of this series, *Modern Perspectives in International Child Psychiatry*. Edinburgh: Oliver and Boyd, 1969.

THE FAMILY RESEARCH UNIT STUDY

Our work, a longitudinal investigation still in progress, can be regarded as being a three-stage study.

Stage 1—Over a one-year period all British-born primiparous women from an inner London Borough were given a brief screening interview when they first attended the obstetric clinics of the hospital serving the area. Five hundred thirty-four women, representing 95 percent of the total group, were successfully interviewed. The vast majority were Caucasian and of working-class origin.

Stage 2—From this group, three samples were selected for a more intensive interview study:

(a) A random sample of 105 married or cohabiting women.
(b) A random sample of 81 single women.
(c) A "risk" sample of 61 married women (14 of whom had already been selected for the random group) who, it was felt, on the basis of their replies to the screening interview, might be expected to have a greater than average chance of difficulties in mothering. The two main criteria which led to a woman's being included in the "risk" group were 1) a history of psychiatric illness and 2) her having as a child been separated from her parents for a reason suggesting ongoing family difficulties.

The selected women were interviewed with a semi-structured schedule when they were seven months pregnant and then at regular intervals after the birth of the child. All interviews were tape-recorded and an item was used for analysis only if in pilot studies there had been at least 90 percent inter-rater agreement for that item.

Stage 3—From the 233 women selected for stage 2, a subsample of 68 was randomly selected for an observational study at 20 weeks after the birth. Two weeks after each post-birth interview, detailed ethological observations were made of the mother and baby.

We can examine various aspects of the behaviour and attitudes of women who had disadvantaged childhoods from the data collected at each phase of the study. At the time of writing, it is possible to use information collected from the screening process, from the interview in late pregnancy and from the first interview and observation session after the birth of the baby when it was 20 weeks old.

Results

Stage 1—At this stage a disadvantaged childhood was defined as one 1) in which the woman had been separated for at least one month before the age of five or three months between the ages of six and 16 from one or both parents *and* 2) in which it appeared that this separation resulted from reasons suggesting chronic family disharmony or difficulties. These difficulties comprised family breakup through divorce or separation, prolonged parental illness, and admission of the child to a boarding school for social or psychological reasons. In addition, a separation for any reason was included if it resulted in the woman's having been admitted to local authority care. This was done because there is strong evidence that children admitted to "care" for any reason, no matter how apparently benign, tend to come from an unusual group of families (23), in particular ones characterized by a poor relationship between the parents (31).

Of the 534 women, 61 (11.4 percent) had experienced one of these separations. At this stage only relatively simple data were available. Shown in Table 1 are the proportions of women with and without a "disadvantaged" separation in childhood who were unmarried and in their teens at the time of their first pregnancy. In addition, for both groups, the mean score on the Malaise Inventory is shown. This instrument, a derivation of the Cornell Medical Index, gives a simple measure of neurotic ill health (20). The women were asked to complete the Malaise Inventory in a retrospective fashion describing their health as it had been before they became pregnant. The validity of this procedure and fuller details of the results of this stage have been described elsewhere (32).

The women in the disadvantaged group are clearly far more likely than the remainder to be unmarried and to be in their teens at the time of their first pregnancy. They have significantly higher scores on the Malaise Inventory.

Stage 2—Here it is possible to examine some aspects of the mothers' attitudes and health during pregnancy. For this analysis we have used only women from the two married samples. We have taken *all women with a disadvantaged background from the random and risk groups and have compared them with those women from the random group who come from a stable background*. At this stage a slight change in the definition of disadvantage was made. Examination of the screening data suggested that in our sample death of a parent in childhood was associated with a wide range of social and other difficulties throughout childhood and women with this experience were included in the disadvantaged group. In the random sample

TABLE 1

Stage 1 of study. Screening interview: Disadvantaged family of origin (i.e. childhood separation from "disrupted" family); age and marital status at first pregnancy, and pre-pregnancy "malaise" score.

	Disadvantaged N 61	Nondisadvantaged 473	
Unmarried	36(59.0%)	120(25.4%)	$X^2=29.57$ d of f= 1 p<.001
Teenagers	37(60.7%)	151(31.9%)	$X^2=19.55$ d of f= 1 p<.001
Malaise Score	6.04	3.72	t=5.31 var= 10.30 p<.001

of 105 women interviewed at seven months pregnancy, 24 percent had disadvantaged childhoods: This is a higher rate than was found in Stage 1. Only three of the women had experienced parental death; the rise mainly reflects the more intensive interviewing techniques used in the latter parts of the study. A similar effect has been described previously (10).

From the interview given in late pregnancy, it is possible to examine a wide range of variables. Only a sample is shown here, but it should be noted that a disadvantaged background was not associated with any excess of physical or psychiatric problems during pregnancy; nor was it associated with attitudes towards child-rearing, such as intention to breastfeed.

Table 2 shows, however, that on a number of variables marked differences *are* seen. The first three items can be seen as relating to the amount of support a woman is receiving during pregnancy. Those with the disadvantaged childhood are more likely to be having serious housing problems with either no home of their own or very inadequate accommodation. They are less likely to have their own mother available to support them or help with the baby after their return from the hospital. This difference is caused by a combination of their either having moved geographically away from their families, not having a mother alive, or of getting on badly with their mothers and not wanting their help. The measure of husband involvement was obtained by summating eight items based on the wife's account of her husband's attitude toward her and the baby-to-be and on her description of

TABLE 2

Pregnancy Interview (Stage 2). Social supports and attitudes of disadvantaged (separated) and nondisadvantaged (non-separated) groups.

N	Disadvantaged 43	Nondisadvantaged 72	
Major Housing Problems	17(39.5%)	12(16.7%)	X^2=6.11 d. of f=1 p<.05
Expecting Help from own Mother	16(38.1%)	42(58.3%)	X^2=6.06 d. of f=1 p<.05
Low Husband Involvement*	15(39.5%)	12(17.4%)	X^2=6.33 d. of f=1 p<.05
Planned pregnancy	20(46.5%)	52(72.2%)	X^2=6.90 d. of f=1 p<.01
Positive feelings on Learning of Pregnancy	24(55.8%)	54(75.0%)	X^2=4.96 d. of f=1 p<.05
Wanting Samed Sex Baby	27(62.7%)	25(34.7%)	X^2=7.47 d. of f=1 p<.01

*A full husband rating was available for only 38 of the disadvantaged and 69 of the nondisadvantaged group.

his help in actively preparing for the baby's arrival. Low husband involvement (defined as any husband whose score fell in the bottom quartile of the scores of the entire *random* sample) is more common in the disadvantaged group.

The next two questions look at the beginning of pregnancy. Mothers in the disadvantaged group were less likely to have planned their pregnancies and they were more likely to have had negative feelings when they first learned they were pregnant. The last question shows how the majority of women from a disadvantaged background experienced a definite desire for an infant of named sex. This was found far less frequently in the remainder, where the most common response was "either" or "I don't mind," almost invariably qualified with a remark such as "as long as it's healthy" or "I'll be pleased whatever it is."

Stage 3—Of the 68 women observed at home with their babies at 20 weeks, 20 came from families characterized by our definition of disadvantage. By a chance of sampling the disadvantaged mothers in this subgroup, as opposed to those in the larger samples in Stages 1 and 2, *did not differ from the remainder in age or marital status*. Full details of the observational technique and of the results at 20 weeks have been published elsewhere (33).

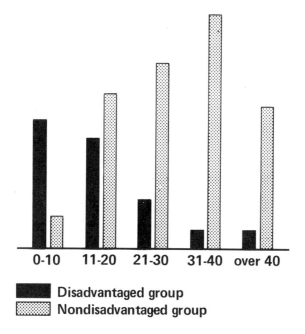

0-10   11-20   21-30   31-40   over 40

■ Disadvantaged group
▨ Nondisadvantaged group

Figure 1. Mothers from disadvantaged and stable
backgrounds. Number of non-caretaking touching
acts during observation period.

Basically, a variety of infant and mother behaviours were continuously recorded as they occurred during 100 15-second intervals of the baby's non-
feeding awake time. In addition to behaviour, the physical distance of the
mother from the baby was noted. The observations took place in the mother's
own home. No difference in the behaviour of the babies was noted between
the two groups. Very great differences, however, were found in the behaviour of the mothers. The disadvantaged mothers were far more likely to be
out of sight of the baby during the sessions. They were far less likely to look
at the baby, present it objects, vocalize to it or touch it in a non-caretaking
manner, i.e. caressing or kissing the baby or manipulating its limbs. The
very great differences between the groups in this latter activity are seen in
Figure 1. This is significant on a Mann-Whitney U test at $p < .001$.

Figure 2 shows a similar pattern for mother's vocalization to their babies.
This too is significant at $p < .001$. It was mentioned above that the disadvantaged mothers spent more time out of the sight of the babies. Even when
we control for this factor, the differences remain highly significant.

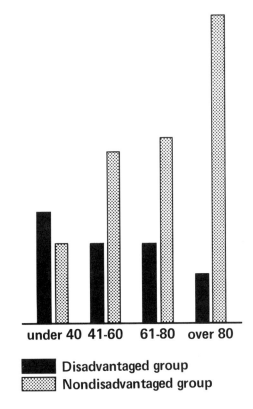

under 40 41-60   61-80   over 80

■ Disadvantaged group
▨ Nondisadvantaged group

Figure 2. Mothers from disadvantaged and stable backgrounds. Number of vocal acts during observation period.

DISCUSSION

Our measure of childhood disadvantage is clearly a very limited one. However, by basing it on a rigidly defined experience occurring in the woman's early life, it is most unlikely to be falsely selecting women without these experiences. Despite the fact that these circumstances were enquired about on two occasions, it remains possible that some subjects with disadvantaged childhoods were not identified. Even if our measure is taken not as absolute fact, but rather as a woman's *adult perception of childhood disadvantage*, it is striking how it has selected a group of women who differ from the remainder on a variety of measures. As a first step, it is necessary to determine whether the characteristics of this group are in themselves causes for concern; are they likely to suggest an adverse outcome for these women's children?

The Screening Data (Stage 1)

The three factors associated with the disadvantaged group are high rates of unwed mothers and teenage mothers, and a higher mean score on the pre-pregnancy malaise score. Illegitimate children have been shown to have higher rates of behavioural and learning difficulties than do other children. Convincing evidence has been produced to suggest that this is more related to accompanying social difficulties than to any defects in the mothers (6), but certainly higher rates are found. There is considerable overlap between marital status and low maternal age. Nationally, 50 percent of births to teenagers are illegitimate, compared with eight percent for older women. Having a mother in her teens at the time of birth also seems to be a definite risk factor for a child. In addition to the high rate of illegitimacy in this group, teenagers are more likely to have a second baby after only a brief interval; also, for teenagers who are married the divorce rate is twice as high as for older women.

Oppel and Royston (17) attempted to disentangle the effects of age from the associated variables. They compared younger mothers (17 and under) with an older group (18 to mid-twenties) matched for marital status and social disadvantage. The younger mothers were less involved emotionally with their children and had less desire to control them. Their children had more behavioural problems and were of lower intelligence than those of the older women. These findings are hardly surprising; although a mother, the teenager is still an adolescent. Adolescence in our society is a time when a young person is having to come to terms with new feelings and emotions and is adapting to new social roles. To have in addition to cope with the demands of a baby whose dependency *and* autonomy must be accepted is perhaps too great a burden. An interesting feature of the malaise scores is that the higher scores of the disadvantaged group are almost identical to the scores of mothers of disturbed children in the Isle of Wight study (20). Though this last point is very indirect, taken with the other two factors, it suggests that a disadvantaged childhood is associated later not just with differences, but with difficulties.

Stage 2

The association of disadvantaged maternal childhood with later difficulties is reinforced by the findings from the second stage of the study. Some of the features associated with the disadvantaged group suggest a poor outlook. An unplanned pregnancy may not be a disaster for a couple. Though unexpected, it may immediately become welcomed, but a significantly higher proportion of the disadvantaged group started their pregnancy with negative feelings. The picture is made gloomier by the lack of support available for the women. They are more likely to have poor housing and have less possibility of direct help from both husbands and mothers. The low involvement of the husbands, in particular, seems a cause for concern. Brown and his colleagues (4) have demonstrated how a distant relationship with husbands left mothers looking after preschool children more vulnerable to depression.

The desire for a child of named sex is a small but perhaps important finding. It does seem to suggest a rather unreal attitude towards the baby-to-be—a desire to possess an object for self-gratification rather than the acceptance of a new individual in its own right. This links with a finding we have reported elsewhere that the disadvantaged mother is less likely than others to see her four-month-old baby as "a person" (11).

Stage 3

These points seem to lead directly to the differences found at the third stage of the study. Perhaps if the baby is not seen as an autonomous being, the mother feels little need to attempt interaction. Tulkin and Kagan (28) have attempted to explain the low level of verbal stimulation by working-class mothers as reflecting their feeling that a baby is unable to experience adult emotions and so there is little point in talking to it. They found, however, equally high levels of physical contact in all social groups. In our disadvantaged sample there are low levels of both forms of interaction—physical and verbal.

Though this finding may be highly suggestive of a poor outcome for the infant, it must, in fact, be treated with caution, since there is not a great deal of hard evidence linking low levels of stimulation to later outcome. Yarrow and co-workers (34) found that in boys, but not in girls, higher maternal physical contact in infancy was related to higher IQ at age 10, and that mothers' communication with their infants was related to later social competence. Murphy (15) reported on 31 mothers of "above average competence in handling their babies." She found that both low and high extremes of attention, body contact and talking to the baby were related to less good coping capacities in the child. Certainly these papers would suggest that the findings from stage 3 of our study tend to point to the same conclusion as do those from the earlier two stages. It is with this type of data, however, that one can see how crucial the infant's own characteristics and reactions to the low stimulation may be in determining the final outcome.

THE MECHANISM OF THE ASSOCIATION

We are focusing on the relationship between disadvantage in childhood and later maternal behavior both to find out how the disadvantaged childhood affected the mothers in our study *and* to speculate on whether their behavior will have long-term effects on their children.

The first model to be considered is one which proposes a "critical period" in an individual's infancy. This would hypothesize that if during this fixed time span the child were to be handled insensitively, it would in adulthood never be able to itself handle a baby sensitively. More baldly, this would state that the unloved child will grow up unable to love. An analysis of our stage 1 screening data examining the age at which the family breakdown occurred showed that the effect was independent of whether the separation occurred before or after the age of five (32). Breaks starting before the age of five were no more likely to be associated with difficulties than those occurring after that age. This conforms both to general experience—parents *are* seen who, though severely deprived in early childhood, cope well and effectively with their own children—and with the mass of data which shows that, excluding special experiences such as multiple hospital admissions, early events, such as separation, do not *in themselves* seem to leave lasting effects (5).

One type of early experience has, however, been shown to relate later to a difficulty, perhaps rather akin to the marital and parenting patterns described above. Children admitted before the age of three to children's homes continue to show a quality of "disinhibition" or lack of awareness of appropriate social boundaries (30). Though it has been felt on clinical grounds that this was inevitably associated with an inability ever to maintain a one-to-one relationship, recent work on adopted children has shown that even this is not necessarily so. Tizard (27) has demonstrated how children with this characteristic can be successfully adopted. They may remain over-friendly to strangers but certainly are able to relate to their adoptive parents.

Results such as these clearly indicate the need for an alternative model. It could be argued that a woman's early family experiences do not, in fact, relate directly to her mothering behaviour. Perhaps it is the poor housing, the low involvement of the women's husbands or the unplanned pregnancies which are really the causal factors. If this is so, this, of course, only pushes the question one step back: Why are disadvantaged women more likely to marry uninvolved husbands, etc.? This could evolve into a continued series of questions and answers which, in all probability, would eventually take us back to the disadvantaged childhood itself. Perhaps it is this theoretical exercise that in practice does occur. If a "critical period" theory is likened to a journey on a non-stop express train, this alternative process can be compared to being on a behind-time local train. It will make many stops at which it will be possible to get off, but, as the stops are very brief and the train is getting increasingly crowded, leaving, though possible, is not easy and becomes progressively more difficult as more stops are passed. It can, however, be done; Blake Cohen (3) has described in her study how some women with very adverse childhoods had married very supporting and caring husbands. These women coped excellently with both pregnancy and motherhood. Change can occur even in adulthood. Stolz (25), in addition to finding that most women looked upon their families of origin as influencing their mothering, found that an equal number had recently adopted or rejected practices observed in other parents. Though the difficulties in changing an individual's circumstances should not be underestimated, this model does offer more ground for hope than one based on a biological critical period. Tizard's adopted group did well because they made a total break with an earlier life. Should these speculations prove correct, the task for future intervention research may be to seek in a woman's life points where far less drastic changes can be effective.

FATHERS

Although the title of this chapter speaks of disadvantaged *parents*, we have, in fact, spoken only of mothers. We will end with at least an apology of an attempt to deal with fathers. A very high proportion of infants show an attachment to their fathers and in some cases this appears to be the babies' most important relationship (22). In Murphy's study (15), she noted that in some families a mother's low level of interaction with a baby was compensated for by a very high level of stimulation by the father. Clearly the role of the father can be crucial for a child's development.* If our knowledge of the origins of maternal variation is limited, that of paternal variation is virtually nonexistent. Biller (2) suggests there is strong evidence

---

* See Howells, J. G. Fathering. In *Modern Perspectives in International Child Psychiatry*, Edinburgh: Oliver and Boyd, 1969.

that a male's adjustment to marriage is related both to his relationship with his father and his parents' marital relationship. So little is known, however, of the different patterns of fathering that we cannot say if these same factors are implicated in this too. There is an urgent need to examine fathering in more detail; in child development work it often seems far too easy to forget that it takes two to make a baby!

REFERENCES

1. AINSWORTH, M. D., BELL, S. M. V. and STAYTON, D. J. 1971. Individual differences in strange-situation behaviour of one-year olds. In: H. R. Schaffer (Ed.) *The Origins of Human Social Relations*. London: Academic Press.
2. BILLER, H. B. 1974. Paternal Deprivation. Lexington, Mass.: Lexington Books.
3. BLAKE COHEN, M. 1966. Personal identity and sexual identity. *Psychiatry 29*, 1.
4. BROWN, G. W., BHROLCHAIN, M. N. and HARRIS, T. 1975. Social class and psychiatric disturbance among women in an urban population. *Sociology, 9*, 225.
5. CLARKE, A. M. and CLARKE, A. D. B. 1976. *Early Experience, Myth and Evidence*. London: Open Books.
6. CRELLIN, E., PRINGLE, M. L. K. and WEST, P. 1971. Born Illegitimate: Social and educational implications. National Foundation for Educational Research.
7. DEUTSCH, H. 1945. *The Psychology of Women, Vol II*. New York: Grune and Stratton.
8. ESCALONA, S. K. 1969. *The Roots of Individuality*. London: Tavistock.
9. FROMMER, E. A., and O'SHEA, G. 1973. Antenatal identification of women liable to have problems in managing their infants. *Brit. J. Psychiat., 123*, 149.
10. FROMMER, E.A., and O'SHEA, G. 1973. The importance of childhood experience in relation to problems of marriage and family building. *Brit. J. Psychiat. 123*, 157.
11. HALL, F., PAWLBY, S. J. and WOLKIND, S. N. In Press. Early life experiences and later mothering behaviour: A study of mothers and their 20-week old babies. In: D. Shaffer and J. F. Dunn (Eds.) *The First Year of Life*. London: Wiley.
12. LEVY, D. M. 1942. Psychosomatic studies of some aspects of maternal behaviour. *Psychosom. Med. 4*, 223.
13. MEAD, M. 1962. *Male and Female*. Harmondsworth: Penguin.
14. MOSS, H. A. 1967. Sex, age and state as determinants of mother-infant interaction. *Merrill-Palmer Q. 13*, 19.
15. MURPHY, L. B. 1974. Later outcomes of early infant and mother relationship. In: L. J. Stone, H. T. Smith and L. B. Murphy (Eds.) *The Competent Infant*. London: Tavistock.
16. OPPE, T. E. 1975. Speculations on the relevance of developmental psychology to paediatrics. In: Parent-Infant Interaction. Ciba Foundation Symposium 33 (new series). Amsterdam. Associated Scientific Publishing.
17. OPPEL, W. C. and ROYSTON, A. B. 1971. Teenage births: Some social, psychological and physical sequelae. *Amer. J. Publ. Hlth. 61*, 751.
18. RICHARDS, M. P. M. and BERNAL, J. F. 1972. An observational study of mother-infant interaction. In: N. Blurton-Jones (Ed.) *Ethological Studies of Child Behaviour*. Cambridge: Cambridge University Press.
19. RUTTER, M. L. 1972. *Maternal Deprivation Reassessed*. Harmondsworth: Penguin.
20. RUTTER, M. L., TIZARD, J. and WHITMORE, K. 1970. *Education, Health and Behaviour*. London: Longman.
21. RUTTER, M. L. and MADGE, N. 1976. *Cycles of Disadvantage*. London: Heinemann.
22. SCHAFFER, H. R. and EMERSON, P. E. 1964. The development of social attachments in infancy. *Monogr. of Soc. Res. in Child Develop., 29*. No. 2.

23. SCHAFFER, H. R. and SCHAFFER, E. B. 1968. *Child Care and the Family*. London: Bell.
24. SEAY, B., ALEXANDER, B. K. and HARLOW, H. F. 1964. Maternal behaviour of socially deprived monkeys. *J. Abn. Soc. Psychol.*, *69*, 345.
25. STOLZ, L. M. 1967. *Influences on Parent Behaviour*. London: Tavistock.
26. TERKEL, J. and ROSENBLATT, J. S. 1968. Maternal behaviour induced by maternal blood plasma injected into virgin rats. *J. Comp. Physiol. Psychol.*, *65*, 479.
27. TIZARD, B. 1977. *The Adoption of Children from Institutions after Infancy in Child Adoption*. London: Association of British Adoption and Fostering Agencies.
28. TULKIN, S. R. and KAGAN, J. 1972. Mother-child interaction in the first year of life. *Child Dev.*, *43*, 31.
29. WINNICOTT, D. W. 1971. *Play and Reality*. London: Tavistock.
30. WOLKIND, S. N. 1974. The components of "affectionless psychopathy" in institutionalized children. *J. Child Psychol. Psychiat.*, *15*, 215.
31. WOLKIND, S. N. and RUTTER, M. 1973. Children who have been "in care": An epidemiological study. *J. Child Psychol. Psychiat.*, *14*, 95.
32. WOLKIND, S. N., KRUK, S. and CHAVES, L. 1976. Childhood separation experiences and psychosocial status in primiparous women: Preliminary findings. *Brit. J. Psychiat.*, *128*, 391.
33. WOLKIND, S. N., HALL, F. and PAWLBY, S. J. In Press. Individual differences in mothering behaviour: A combined epidemilogical and observational approach. In: P. Graham (Ed.) *Epidemiological Approaches in Child Psychiatry*. London: Academic Press.
34. YARROW, L. J., GOODWIN, M. S., MANHEIMER, H. and MILOWE, I. D. 1974. Infancy experiences and personality development at ten years. In: L. J. Stone, H. T. Smith and L. B. Murphy (Eds.) *The Competent Infant*. London: Tavistock.

9

THE ESSENCE OF MOTHERING CHILDREN UNDER FIVE

GEORGE L. LIPTON, M.B.B.S., F.R.A.N.Z.C.P.,
M.R.C. PSYCH., F.R.A.C.P.

Director of Mental Health Authority and
Austin Hospital Child Psychiatry Training Programme;
Director of Child and Adolescent Psychiatric Services,
Austin Hospital, Melbourne;
Senior Associate, Department of Psychiatry
Melbourne University, Australia

and

BRUCE J. TONGE, M.B.B.S., M.R.A.N.Z.C.P.,
M.R.C. PSYCH., D.P.M.

Lecturer, Department of Psychiatry,
Melbourne University;
Consultant Child Psychiatrist,
Austin Hospital, Melbourne, Australia

INTRODUCTION

In this chapter a distillation and examination of the maternal contribution to mother-child relationships will be undertaken in an attempt to define the essence of mothering and whether there are any necessary features and components of a mother's interaction with her child which facilitate and promote his gradual but certain attainment of maturity.

A review of the literature concerning mother-child interaction does not provide an adequate and comprehensive model of the essential basic features of mothering behavior(5). Many models of maternal function are based on psychoanalytic theory(6, 62). These models often concentrate on specific aspects of mothering, such as breastfeeding. The emphasis has been on the effects of these aspects of mothering on the development of the child's inner world, particularly in relationship to emotional disorder and personality development. These contributions have highlighted the importance of empathy between mother and child(56), the role of the mother as revealed by studies of the effects of disruption and lack of continuity in the provision of maternal care(6, 45), the effects on the child's development of the mother's attitudes and feelings towards her child(44), and the importance for the development of the child's conscience and impulse control of the manner in which a mother gratifies her child's needs(21). These models and concepts of mothering based on psychoanalytic theory are difficult to test empirically by experiment and observation(18).

Others have tackled the problem of providing a model of maternal function by developing observational scales and measures of maternal behavior(8, 14, 51, 52). Inferences are drawn by the experimenter concerning the meaning of certain observed behaviours in the complex sequence of mother-child interactions. Important aspects of the mother's contribution to the interaction, such as attentional cycling(9), reciprocity(30), and maternal affectional contact(14), have been described, but the question of what are the basic and essential features of mothering remains.

The term *mothering* includes a wide range of activities, but in particular "love, the development of enduring bonds (attachment), a stable but not necessarily unbroken relationship, and a 'stimulating' interaction are all necessary qualities, but there are many more"(47, p. 28).

If there are any essential and basic qualities of mothering, it must be demonstrated that these mothering interactions remain constant in form, although they may vary in content and style. A model of mothering which remains constant in form throughout the developmental process will be presented. In particular, the analysis and consequences of this model as it applies to mothering behaviour towards children under five years of age will be examined. The mother-child relationship comprises at least three components: 1) the contribution of the child, 2) the contribution of the mother, and 3) the nature of their mutuality, reciprocity and interplay of activity. For the purposes of this chapter attention will be focused predominantly on the maternal component of the mother-child interaction. The contribution of the child's endowment and other factors in his development will be dealt with elsewhere in this book. It is recognised that parents must adapt to the developmental changes in their child and that children have the ability to modify and alter parental action.

Before defining the essence of mothering we must consider mothering by whom, for whom and for what purpose.

Mothering by Whom

Mothering is initially the role of motherhood and is therefore a normal function of a mother who is able to remain in a relationship with her child. Later, others, like fathers or teachers, may assume and express some of the aspects of mothering, provided they have a psychological tie to, and some responsibility for the nurturing of, the child. Therefore, mothering is performed by any adult who becomes the female psychological parent of the child. "Whether any adult becomes the psychological parent of a child is based on day-to-day interaction, companionship, and shared experience. The role can be fulfilled either by a biological parent or by an adoptive parent or by any other caring adult—but never by an absent inactive adult, whatever his biological or legal relationship to the child might be" (24, p. 19).

Mothering for Whom

Mothering is for children. We shall look at the nature of mothering for children up to the commencement of their primary school education at about the age of five years.

Mothering for What Purpose

The purpose of mothering is to facilitate and promote a child's development from a state of symbiosis and total dependence through to maturity and independence. Maturity is a complex concept implying the attainment of a variety of personal qualities and social skills. The mature individual is able to appropriately differentiate between his own subjective inner world and the external world and to test reality. He has a developed sense of self which includes a secure gender identity, a sense of autonomy and self-esteem, an awareness of his own capacities and limits, and an ability to control impulses and delay the immediate gratification of needs through the expectation and hope of eventual gratification. In particular, maturity implies the ability to tolerate anxiety, to be able to cope with the unavoidable experiences of separation and loss that occur in life, to have the capacity to be alone, and to cope with repressive experiences without ego disintegration.

A great deal of mother's behaviour is a reflection of her relationship with, and nurture of, an individual who has emerged from a unique unity with her and who now has the task of separating from her to become an individual with an identity in his own right. Mahler's description of the psychological birth of the human infant is organised around the principle of the emergence of the infant as an individual from a pre-individual phase of psychic symbiotic unity with his mother(36).

The hallmark of maturity is, therefore, to be seen in the individual's capacity to relate effectively with others and to be capable of intimacy(37), empathy, and mutuality in relationships.

The psychobiological and social aspects of maturation occur in the setting of adequate cognitive and physical development. The mature adult therefore has the capacity not only to reproduce biologically but to act as a psychological parent and to have empathy for her child. Thus, a measure of the success of mothering is for the child in turn, when grown up, to be able to mother. Psychobiological and social survival of the species is thereby assured(28).

THE PLACE OF MATERNAL EMPATHY

Maternal empathy, or the concept of a mother's feeling herself into her infant's place(59), is central to appropriate maternal behaviour and is implied in every element of the model of maternal behaviour proposed in this chapter. Empathy is difficult to define and yet is intuitively understood by most people. It has been defined as the capacity of a person "instinctively and intuitively to feel as another does"(38, p. 113). The mother temporarily gives up her ego for that of the child and the latter in sensing the empathiser's response may take the initiative of communicating more of his experience and feeling thus providing the stimulus for what may become a mutual empathic response(39). This definition of empathy is different from what may be called "intellectual empathy"(4), in which persons identify with each other in terms of their verbalised thoughts only. It also differentiates empathy from sympathy, where expressed feelings for the child are derived from a projection onto the child of the feelings of the mother. Sympathy has little concern for the child's actual feelings and is not synonymous with maternal understanding.

Empathy is a direct instinctual or intuitive reaction to the child's needs. Empathic understanding is arrived at by a process of self-reflection that leads the parent to an understanding of the motivations of both her own reactions and the child's behaviour. Only an empathic understanding of the ongoing process between herself and the child can guide a mother's interaction with the child to a successful outcome(3). It is this capacity for empathic understanding that allows a mother to take action that is compatible with the child's inner reality, her own inner reality and external reality. Such a capacity will allow the mother to recognise her child's anxiety and whether or not it is within his coping means.

Empathic mothering facilitates a child's development from a state of symbiosis to maturity and is the psychic correlate of what is observed in successful mothering behaviour.

MODEL PATTERN OF MOTHERING BEHAVIOUR

There is a model pattern of mother-child interactions in which the mother's contributions are specific. This model contains within it the essence of mothering. The essential formula of this behavioral pattern may be characterised in the sequence of events discussed below.

There are two essential states in which the mother-child relationship exists and in each of the states there are specific maternal functions. There are also specific maternal functions in the interface or transitional areas between the two states of being.

The State of Togetherness

The mother and child are in a state of togetherness, the quality of which may range, according to the child's phase of development, from initial symbiosis(34) to subsequent mutually empathic communion(38).

The major maternal functions in this state of togetherness are *holding*(60, 62) and refuelling.(36). It is in this state of togetherness, in the mutuality of the mother-child relationship, that the child recovers from the emotional results of his foray into separateness. After a period of togetherness, mother again pushes out, the timing and style of her actions depending on her sensitivity to and empathic awareness of her child's inner state and developmental needs.

The Function of Pushing Out

The mother allows or encourages activity which interferes with the state of togetherness and leads to a state of separateness. The mother encourages her child to be separate, actively pushing him into the environment and providing, or ensuring the availability of, environmental stimulation. We define this as the pushing out function of the mother.

The State of Separateness

Challenged thus by the maternal behaviour of pushing out into a stimulating situation, the child is provoked to respond. The response may be immediate distress. He may attempt to master the situation with either success and gratification or failure and eventual frustration leading to distress. Alternatively, he may become progressively overwhelmed with excitement.

The major maternal function during this state is to carefully provide *a dosing of experience and stimulation* for the child and to titrate his experience against his internal state through her empathic awareness of his inner experience and needs.

The Function of Reunion

Sooner or later the child becomes distressed or overexcited with his independent activity. The mother responds to this by actions which reunite the child to her in a state of togetherness. The timing and style of her actions depend on her sensitivity to and empathic awareness of her child's inner state of need, regardless of his overt behaviour. Reunion thus acts to return the child to a state in which mother acts as an auxiliary ego when the child's immature ego is threatened or overwhelmed(22, 29).

While it is recognised that this model as stated does not represent the entire subtle and infinite ranges of behaviour which are evident in mothering, we believe that this functional breakdown of mothering serves to delineate those aspects of mothering behaviour which can generally be identified. It is recognised throughout this chapter that a mother's behaviour occurs in concert with the behaviour and development of her child(8, 30, 48). The focus will be on those aspects of mother which influence the pattern of behaviour. A mother's own response to her child is an amalgam of her own background and experience, together with the stimuli provided by the child and the environment, both in actuality and as perceived by her. A response by a mother which is seen as appropriate and empathic to one child may be quite unempathic and inappropriate to another. Even the same child may experience his mother's response in different ways at different times according to his feeling state. It is, therefore, important in examining mothering behaviour to constantly view it against the background of the changing state and needs of the child and to constantly view the *congruity* of her total response to her child's needs. The mother, therefore, may be in or out of tune with her child.

The model proposed shares concepts with other models of maternal behaviour(3, 8, 29, 36, 45, 47, 60, 62) and has the advantage of being particularly relevant clinically. It allows for a fine discrimination in the clinical examination of mothering behaviour within the context of mother guidance, and it also alerts the clinician to elements of mothering patterns which may be specifically distorted.

Togetherness

The paradigm of the state of togetherness is to be found in the relationship between mother and child early in the child's life when mother is in the state of Primary Maternal Preoccupation. Winnicott's concept of Primary Maternal Occupation describes the state within which most mothers meet the needs of their infants in the first few weeks after birth:

> Only if a mother is sensitised in the way I am describing can she feel herself into her infant's place, and so meet the infant's needs. These are at first body needs and they gradually become ego needs out of the imaginative elaboration of physical experience.
> There comes into existence an ego-relatedness between mother and baby from which mother recovers, and out of which the infant may eventually build the idea of a person in the mother. From this angle the recognition of the mother as a person comes in a positive way, normally, and not out of the experience of mother as the symbol of frustration. The mother's failure to adapt in the earliest phase does not produce anything but the annihilation of the infant's self. . . .
> In the language of these considerations the early building up of the ego is therefore silent. The first ego organisation comes from the experience of threats of annihilation which do not lead to annihilation and from which repeatedly, there is recovery. Out of such experiences confidence in recovery begins to be something which leads to an ego and to an ego capacity for coping with frustration(59, p. 304).

Togetherness begins, therefore, as the physical reality of a mother responding to her infant's immediate needs, refuelling him (literally with milk, for example), and not allowing him to experience annihilatory stress. These physical beginnings of togetherness and refuelling provide the foundations for the later psychic experience of being refuelled through mutuality with a reliable mother. Further, it establishes the basis for the empathic mutuality, "feeling herself into her infant's place"(59), which will become an important basis for mother's continuing judgements about the child's state and about whether to expose him to being "pushed out" or "reunited."

The state of mutuality which represents togetherness has different forms in accordance with the child's developmental level. Initially, in the state of Primary Maternal Preoccupation during the first few weeks, mother is most likely to preempt or respond to the child's distress and needs with the minimum delay, thus refuelling him and, so far as possible, minimising his overt distress. The relationship is one of fusion, with the mother responding to bodily needs.

Subsequently, as maternal preoccupation subsides, there develops the more mutual but heavily infant-centred state of psychic symbiosis where togetherness appears to be experienced as a state wherein mother and child feel themselves to be as one(34, 36).

With increasing individuation, as the child develops from this pre-individuated symbiotic state, the state of togetherness loses its initial fused quality and is seen more and more as a state of empathic communion between mother and child. Although this meeting of minds and feelings with its intense mutuality may be enhanced by physical contact and nurturing, it is not, at later stages, dependent on these. Its essential nature is psychological. It is grounded in the many experiences of separating and then reuniting with a reliable mother. These experiences allow for increasing individuation of each from the other when the possibility of return with close intimacy is securely predictable. *It is in her capacity to let the child individuate as well as to allow him to return to empathic mutuality when necessary that a mother's love and concern for her child best expresses itself.* From this a child can develop the capacity to love, without togetherness threatening either his development of autonomy or his capacity for meaningful intimacy.

In this state of togetherness mother acts as a protective shield(29) and at the same time provides the child with the model of care, integration and coping experiences which Sandler has called the qualitative organising component of maternal functioning(50). The incorporation of this component into the developing infantile ego may subsequently guide it in its synthesising function.

The model presented is cyclic. It is predetermined, however, by the mother's capacity for empathic mutuality, which must precede the vicissitudes of separation and individuation if the child is to be ideally protected from the ego-disintegrative effects of his early ventures into separateness and of his own inner processes.

Pushing Out

A child's need for experience and stimulation at all ages and in accord with his developmental level and tolerance has been stressed by many authors(5, 11, 28, 36, 42, 47, 48). It is necessary for a child to experience reality, both in the form of frustration and in terms of his capacity to achieve mastery. To most appropriately achieve these stepping stones there must be a very sensitive and empathic rapport between mother and child in which the mother exposes the child to experiences in careful doses(23). Mother's role will depend on the constitution and sensitivities of her child, the circumstances in which they find themselves and the moment-to-moment reactions which the child displays. Clearly, there are some children who have a great curiosity and proclivity for moving away and exploring or attempting other activity, whereas other children may be more passive and have a tendency to remain satisfied in continued mutuality with mother. The term pushing out refers to both the active process of mother's encouragement of her child to undertake some experience, and the apparently opposite activity of restraining the child who wishes to undertake a form of activity which is not in his best interests or is beyond his capacity. The value in the concept of pushing is that, whatever be the child's internal state and wishes for activity, it is in the final analysis the responsibility of the mother to push the child into a graduated series of experiences. This responsibility should be seen as an *active*, rather than restrictive or passive, component of mothering.

The degree of activity will depend on the developmental level of the child. In the earliest phase of mothering the place for pushing out is minimal because the child's capacity for independent action and toleration of frustration is minimal and his response to being exposed to this may be catastrophic. Later on, early in the first year of life, the child will have been exposed to sufficient experiences of recovery from experiential anxiety to enable him to confidently deal with some degree of frustration and to seek independence within narrow limits. He becomes more able to deal with internal and external psychic events. It is now that mother must increasingly assume that component of behaviour which we have described as pushing. Her child can now tolerate a gap of time between her pushing and his regression to catastrophic experience if her behaviour places him under stress. As the child's intellectual and emotional growth continues and his capacity to deal with his world increases, she will push him more and more into activities of independence, encouraging his own cognitive development and social functioning. By the time he is five he will be able to tolerate, and should indeed enjoy the challenge of, being pushed into preschool and other social situations in which he is without his mother for significant periods of time.

In applying the model pattern of mothering to the care of children under five, it is important to recognise that, while the pattern pertains throughout, there is nevertheless a major difference between the mothering of the preindividuating child (first few weeks of life) and the individuating child. With the former, mother's responses are directed predominantly to the biological needs of the child and her pushing out functioning is minimal. With the individuating child, she will increasingly respond to his psychological and developmental needs. Her pushing functioning will be more prominent as a natural aspect of the mother-child relationship.

It is tempting to imagine on theoretical grounds that the primary maternal preoccupation of the first few days or weeks after birth might represent in itself the reunion and refuelling functions of maternal behaviour after the very significant pushing out which is represented by the birth process.

The empathic understanding, which allows mother to take action that is compatible with the child's inner reality, her own inner reality and external reality, demands that she take responsibility for the environment into which he is pushed. This refers not only to the physical and material facilities but also to the social facilities and the people with whom the child may interact. At younger ages, apart from the mother herself, these facilities tend to be simple toys, familiar domestic items and restricted, carefully monitored social contacts. As the child grows, the facilities required increase in complexity. By age five the child is meeting a wide range of people and requires a wide variety of opportunities for play, socialisation, adventure and learning.

In order to be able to push out and to encourage separation and individuation, mother may face conflicts within herself. Every independent step the child takes increases the psychological distance between himself and his mother. Mother, also, must face the loss inherent in the developing separation. Her usual responses to separation and loss are therefore aroused. If her anxieties in this area have not been resolved, they may subtly present themselves as a variety of distortions of the pushing out process. It requires a mature empathy and capacity for dealing with separation and aggression in order to respond realistically to the child's ego, which is often silent, rather than to his id, whose frustrations make themselves known so forcibly. The mother must fail the id but never the ego of the child(60).

Separateness

As a result of mother's pushing behaviour, the child now finds himself in a situation where he is, for a variable period of time and to a variable degree, independent, doing activities as he wishes, responsible for his actions and, to a greater or lesser degree, alone. The mother's behaviour will considerably determine whether this state is pleasurable, rewarding and pro-

ductive, or frightening, inhibiting and counterproductive. The essence of
the maternal attributes in this situation is her empathic awareness of the
state of the child's experience as it feels to him at the time of its occurrence.
She must have a capacity to be meaningfully in tune with his levels of
interest, excitement and frustration and to respond accordingly.

In the state of separateness: 1) The child shows interest or motivation, or
is induced to do so by a sensitive mother, and moves towards a situation or
activity. 2) The child finds pleasure or challenge in the situation and pursues
it seeking to continue and master the experience. In mastering a variety of
experiences the child has an opportunity to develop attitudes, capacities
and skills. 3) After a period of interest or challenge with more or less gratification, the child will experience negative internal states such as fatigue,
frustration, overexcitement or a loss of interest. While it is often possible
to divert a child to other interests, or for the child himself to become attracted to other activity, sooner or later a state of distress supervenes. He
may make overt communication or it may become apparent through his
behaviour that his capacity to function is becoming interfered with. At such
a time and without support, a child may become acutely or gradually more
insecure and more regressed in behaviour. Finally, if allowed to continue,
this regression becomes a severe experiential crisis with deteriorating function and a fearful state of aloneness, helplessness and passivity. It is a
critical aspect of maternal functioning that she reliably intervenes to prevent
this ultimate regressive state of annihilatory terror being experienced by her
child.

In the state of separateness the mother's role can most readily be understood in terms of *dosing* her child with experience, titrating his experience
against his internal state. She uses her own self both to help him contain his
distress and regressive responses and to reward his progress. In pushing a
child out into activity and allowing him to pursue it mother provides doses
of life situations in accordance with a variety of factors (23). Some of these
are: 1) congenital activity type and constitutional sensitivity of child(17); 2)
the physical status of the child(10); 3) his mental capacity; 4) his age; 5) the
type of life experience he is undergoing; 6) the effects desired by the mother
as a result of those experiences; and 7) The society's attitudes towards the
child(43). All these factors, if taken into account, will lead to the gradual
pushing out of the child into increasingly complex life situations. Graduated
doses of experience, with reliable support and prevention of overwhelming
anxiety or frustration, stimulate further learning and mastery. The more an
infant has seen and heard the more he wants to see and hear(41).

When pushed into new life situations, the child has the opportunity to learn the content of that situation, as well as his own physical and emotional limits. However, in order for the child to discover these limits, he must be given the opportunity of experiencing them, which means that he should be allowed to continue the experience to the point at which anxiety is experienced. A mother must therefore not only be in touch with her child's state of feeling, but must also be able herself to tolerate some degree of his distress, in order to accurately dose him, not only with life experience, but also with the frustration that such experience may engender.

Overdosing the child with experience to the point of helplessness and terrified regression may lead to a child's becoming fearful of any potentially anxiety-provoking situation which is perceived as leading to intolerable anxiety. On the other hand, underdosing a child, that is, providing only stimulations which present little challenge, may equally interfere with progressive realistic and structured individuation. The child, overprotected from anxiety, and prevented from learning to experience and tolerate normal frustrations, may view any anxiety as overwhelming.

At all times good enough mothering will involve a complex interplay with the child to help contain his anxiety or other disruptive feelings related to his experience and yet enable him to continue towards mastery in whatever way is available to him.

> ". . . we found that an infant classified as having a smooth relationship, when placed on the floor, usually turns away from the mother immediately in order to explore and play; from time to time he will drift back on his own initiative to make brief contact with the mother. She, on her part, tends not to interfere with the play until the baby is seeking some sort of interaction with her. If, for instance, the baby attracts her attention from across the room to show a toy the mother at once responds. If the baby comes to her and seems to want to be picked up she picks him up; she does not, however, pick him up if that involves interrupting his play. So the shift from exploration to proximity seeking proceeds quite readily on the initiative of the baby the mother being responsive to his initiative. . . .
>
> . . . some of these mothers were really extraordinary in the extent to which they respected the babies' activities. And if they had to interrupt him for purposes of feeding or changing they would not just grab the baby—they would time their intervention carefully and then first talk or play with him to get him into the right mood before going on to the next activity(1, pp. 281-2).

Her increasing and decreasing involvement and the style in which she becomes involved will constantly and sensitively vary. At one time the involvement may be verbal, at another, a cuddle, and at yet another, direct help with a task. Yet at all times she will expect the child to individually act, enjoy and master to the extent of his capacities, and increasingly become responsible for his own behaviour. For example, a two-year-old playing with flour and making a mess might be expected to symbolically help his mother clean up, a four-year-old might be expected to clean up but mother will have to follow to complete the job, while an eight-year-old might be expected to fairly efficiently complete the task.

The mother must be prepared to move in, bringing to an end the state of separateness, when her empathic understanding of her child suggests to her that he has reached the limits of his tolerance and before he decompensates too severely. This requires fine timing and judgement, since such an intervention should be neither too premature nor unduly delayed.

Reliability and consistency of mothering are recognised as essential for healthy child development(63). There is a wide range of distress which may be experienced by any child. Reliable mothering exists for that child if he can reasonably expect her to intervene whenever his anxiety reaches predictable levels of tolerance.

Predictability of intervention is the foundation stone of consistent mothering. If mother has an inflexible way of dealing with situations irrespective of the child's internal state, she may, in fact, be unreliable from his point of view. A mother who times the feeding of her baby in response to her empathic awareness of his need is more likely to be experienced as a reliable mother than one who is reliable to a schedule which may bear no relationship to her child's needs. This concept of reliability, in relation to needs and internal states of the child, is of critical importance in development, since it allows him to experience increasing degrees of anxiety or fear with the confident expectation of eventual resolution. Increasing exploration of the inner and outer world is facilitated. Confidence, increasing personal integration, and decreasing fear of personal annihilation follow. Thus, through mother's reliability, as subjectively perceived by the child, the child may constantly benefit from "threats of annihilation which do not lead to annihilation and from which there is recovery"(59, p. 304).

Reunion

Empathic reunion is the way in which mother reliably brings to an end the state of separateness, when the child's inner state of negative feeling approaches intolerable limits and the child requires holding and refuelling. Where a mother is reliable in her approach, active in its implementation where necessary, and the reunion is regularly followed by a refuelling empathic intimacy, a child's self-esteem is confirmed. His self-esteem arises from the internalisation of the maternal attitudes, which place him as being of preemptive importance when he is distressed. His recurrent return to a regressed togetherness with mother, in the form of their empathic communion, allows him to view intimacy as gratifying.

Reunion is a rescuing and relieving phenomenon. It is not antithetical or threatening to subsequent further autonomy. Reunion is a function of mother at the interface of separateness to togetherness, just as pushing out is a function of mother at the interface of togetherness to separateness. The child may often initiate these interface activities, but both are to be seen as active maternal functions and are the responsibility of the mother, depending on her empathic knowledge of the child's inner needs, which may at times be at variance with his apparent overt communication. For example, a mother may actively bring the child to herself, against his protest, when she is aware of his gradual loss of control over his feelings and his need to be soothed and refuelled within a protective togetherness.

CONSEQUENCES OF DISTORTIONS IN THE PATTERN OF MOTHERING BEHAVIOUR

In the preceding discussion, mothering behaviour has been considered in an idealised way. Even the most empathic and relatively non-neurotic mother will fluctuate in the quality of mothering she provides at different times and in different situations. Despite such variations, it is the expectable norm of her behaviour which constitutes the essence of her mothering.

Distortions and deviations of mothering behaviour and its consequences may also be examined within this framework. Psychological problems arising out of her past life experience may interfere with a mother's capacity to attach, to love, or to be empathic in a meaningful way. These mothers are at risk of being unreliable even though, with considerable motivation, they struggle to develop intellectual understanding of the task(61). The resultant inappropriate interplay in the mother-child interaction may be reflected in the child's developing personality and behaviour, either at the time or subsequently.

Mothering failure may occur in one or more combinations of the elements of maternal functioning described. Distortions of mothering style may occur in the following ways:

1) Consistent mothering style *but*:
   (a) excessive mothering function;
   (b) insufficient mothering function.
2) Inconsistent mothering style and function.

The specific consequences that follow from distorted mothering will be outlined for each component of mothering function.

It is obvious that distortions of mothering functions in any one aspect of the mother-child relationship will necessarily influence the other aspects of the relationship. For example, anything that interferes with togetherness will also be reflected in the state of separateness.

Nevertheless, there is clinical value in considering distortions of mothering in terms of the specific mothering functions, namely holding and refuelling, pushing out, dosing of stimuli, and reuniting. These functions will be considered within the context of the state within which each occurs.

Distortions of Mothering Function in the State of Togetherness

In togetherness, mother acts as a protective shield(29), holding the child(60, 62), and refuelling him emotionally(36). Through this experience of mutuality, the child is able to sustain a sense of well-being and safety. The major developmental and personality derivatives to be gained by the child from the mutuality of empathic togetherness are the ability to trust and the development of self-esteem(15). Distortions of mothering functions in this state are consistent but excessive holding; consistent but insufficient holding or refuelling; and inconsistent holding and refuelling.

Consistent but excessive holding is seen in its most extreme form in those cases where a mother is unable to allow her child to individuate and a symbiotic psychotic relationship evolves. In such a case, where the child remains a narcissistic component of mother, either psychosis or severe cognitive developmental deviation may occur in the child(33, 35, 57, 58). These extreme distortions of mothering function usually occur in the context of maternal psychosis or severe personality disorder. When there is a lesser degree of distortion, many childhood difficulties relating to intolerance of the anxiety of separation may result. This will be further discussed within the consideration of the problems manifest in the stage of separateness.

When there is consistent but insufficient holding or refuelling, the holding may be appropriate in manner but does not fully meet the child's real needs. This may occur when the mother is anxious, guilty or depressed. These maternal states of distress interfere with empathic functioning. In such situations the child is held and allowed to regress but is pushed out before his anxiety is mastered and his needs met. Refuelling is inadequate. If repeated, the child may become overstimulated without adequate opportunity for recovery. This may lead to so-called precocious development and pseudomaturity in the child. This has been linked with subsequent adolescent identity confusion and crisis(16, 29).

In its extreme form, insufficient holding is manifest in the absence or loss of the mothering person. The short-term consequences of such a loss are well-known as the syndrome of distress, manifest in the child by protest, despair and then detachment(7, 44, 47, 53, 54). The long-term effects are less certain. It is likely that untoward long-term effects of such loss are minimised when a child has had adequate experience of empathic mothering prior to the loss and effective mothering care is resumed subsequently, even if by a different mothering figure. On the other hand, if the child has not experienced adequate empathic mothering prior to loss, then there is a significant chance that the child will develop behavioural problems and eventual psychiatric disorder in adult life(46).

When there is inconsistent holding and refuelling, the child is unable to experience the "average expectable environment"(25). The inconsistency may derive from within the mother, as a result of her own personality or emotional state, or it may derive from the child, when he makes demands that even the mature effective mother cannot meet(29). Such demands may be made by a child as a result of his own constitutional sensitivities(17), or because of physical handicap(10, 49).

Recurrent unpredictable failure of the mother to hold her child and to act as an auxiliary ego in support of his immature ego can be seen to act as cumulative trauma(29) and "the consequences of (this) will become manifest at some future date"(20, p. 106).

The child who experiences inconsistent management and variable affectional relationships is at risk of developing deviant behaviour, usually of an antisocial nature(7, 12, 46, 55).

Children who have not experienced effective togetherness with their own mother may subsequently themselves have difficulties as parents, the origins of their own mothering deficits being derived from their inadequate childhood experiences. They tend to use projection onto the child as an important defense against closeness, perceiving their child as persecuting or unloving just as they had experienced their own parents(4, 32).

From the foregoing it can be seen that repeated failure in the ability of the mother to provide adequate togetherness for her child, to hold and refuel him consistently and empathically with due regard to his level of anxiety and regression, can lead to serious developmental consequences, particularly in the area of personality development.

Distortions of the Pushing Out Function

The good enough mother is able to push her child out into a phase and age appropriate state of separateness. As described, this pushing out will arouse within the mother her usual response to separation and loss. If her anxieties in this area have not been resolved, they may subtly present themselves in the form of her being unable to effectively push her child out into an appropriate experience or separateness. An excessive experience of mutuality is thereby encouraged.

If she has difficulty with her own aggressive impulses, she may perceive the pushing out process and the consequent anxiety of her child as an unacceptably hostile act on her part and be unprepared to provide this active form of mothering.

Alternatively, the mother may attempt to cope with these problems by overcompensation, pushing the child out beyond his endurance.

Distortions of Mothering Functions in the State of Separateness

Phase and age appropriate separateness provides for the child sufficient doses of social, physical, cognitive and linguistic stimulation. From this aspect of mothering, in time, the mature attributes of mastery, autonomy, social skills, the ability to work and play, and the capacity to cope with anxiety and conflict are formed. Distortions of mothering functions in this state are consistent but excessive pushing out; consistent but insufficient pushing out; and inconsistency in the child's experience of separateness.

Consistent but excessive pushing out includes those behaviours of mother which lead to the child being in a state of separateness beyond his tolerance and implies a concomitant decrease in togetherness. The child must sink or swim with relative lack of support. The nature of the experience for the child depends on the environment, which may be either relatively stimulating or impoverished. The dose of stimulation in the environment provided by the mother varies independently of the extent of her pushing out.

When there is excessive separateness in a stimulating environment, the child pushed out beyond his capacity will experience the anxiety of overstimulation. Repeated provocative overstimulation(31) leads to mounting anxiety in the child, which, if unrelieved, may lead to the experience of helplessness. As discussed under the heading of "insufficient holding," repeated overstimulation for the child may result in pseudomaturity and precociousness. If the stimulation is completely overwhelming, then the child may withdraw from activity. The mother providing this overstimulation is usually preoccupied with her own emotional problems. This is one way in which maternal neurosis, depression, anxiety or guilt may impinge upon the child. He, given tasks beyond his phase, may have his immature defenses overwhelmed and may retreat to neurotic decompensation.

When there is excessive separateness with an impoverished environment, the child experiences excessive pushing out as a deprivation. The empty room or cot with an absent mother are extreme examples of this type of inappropriate separateness. The deprivation the child experiences is loss of maternal care in both its holding and stimulating aspects. This is not necessarily equivalent to loss of the mother figure(26). Developmental retardation and deviation are the well-documented consequences of privation of stimulation(13, 47) in a child who has been excessively pushed out. For example, a child excessively pushed out into an environment which lacks vocal and auditory stimulation will have developmental delay and distortion in his speech and conversational abilities. Speech is learned and refined in the reciprocal and stimulating nature of conversation(2, 19, 27).

Consistent but insufficient pushing out includes those behaviours of mother which prevent a child from experiencing an adequate state of separateness and are therefore associated with an increase of inappropriate togetherness. The child does not have adequate opportunity to experience and test his capacities. Overprotected from normal anxiety, the child is unable to learn to tolerate normal frustrations and may experience any anxiety as overwhelming. The mother fails to provide sufficient doses of stimulation. A subtle problem in dosing may appear in the "good mother" who is so sensitive to her child's needs that she responds even before he becomes anxious or can assert himself in any way. "The child is left with two alternatives: either to be in a state of permanent regression merged with the mother or else to stage a total rejection of the seemingly good mother(60, p. 593).

When there is inconsistency in the child's experience of separateness, the child will have difficulty in establishing effective defenses against anxiety, since his support from mother comes haphazardly in relationship to his state of anxiety. This situation frequently occurs when a family or personal crisis prevents effective mothering because the mother is preoccupied with her own concerns. If this distortion is short-term, then the child exhibits a reactive disorder in his behaviour. If the pattern of unpredictability continues, then more significant personality distortions may emerge. The child may be prevented from developing a sense of mastery and autonomy, this being expressed in adult life as impaired abilities to work and relate effectively with others.

Distortions of the Reuniting Function

From the reliable mother's active reuniting function the child develops a sense of worth and the trust that surrender of the self to another in a relationship is gratifying and will not lead to a loss of self. Failure of mother to provide effective reunion and holding for the child may set the scene for difficulty in adult interpersonal relationships, particularly in those intimate relationships in which regression may occur. Distortions and problems in marital and sexual relationships may emanate from this.

CONCLUSION—THE ESSENCE OF MOTHERING

Mothering is for children but is also a very gratifying, challenging, and developmental experience for the mother herself. It provides her with an opportunity to re-experience the unique mutuality which exists between mother and child, this time approaching the situation with her maturity, adult intellect, feeling, and experience. In allowing her to experience a profound and loving intimacy, mothering also reaffirms for her her own individuality and the fact that love and intimacy with a person are entirely compatible with separateness and psychological distance, without either experience destroying the sense of self of either partner or threatening the continuity of the relationship.

Mothering of children under five, in particular, provides the experience of being in or out of a state of togetherness and yet at all times having a responsibility for the care and protection of the child's developing faculties.

While all aspects of mothering, insofar as possible, are in response to cues provided by the child or the environment around him, mother, as a protective shield, is required at all times to be active rather than passive in her attitudes. The described functions of holding and refuelling, pushing out, dosing and titrating the child's experience, and finally reuniting with him to rescue him or to refresh him are constantly at play in her relationship with the child and take many forms according to necessity and appropriateness.

The good enough mother functions in these complex ways with little awareness that she is doing so. Many of her responses are spontaneous, based on an inner awareness of what her child's needs are at any moment.

The psychic function which facilitates and allows for the smoothness of her caring for her child is that of empathic awareness and understanding of her child. This depends on her ability to achieve genuine psychic mutuality with another. This faculty depends to a considerable extent on her own experiences of having been mothered, understood, protected, and yet allowed to develop a capacity for autonomy and intimacy.

The essence of mothering the young child, therefore, must lie within the sensitive functioning of the mother in relation to the child's moves towards and away from her. The essential features of her attitudes and performance are her empathic, although perhaps unconscious, understanding of his needs and moves, and her ability to actively respond to her own mothering intuitions.

REFERENCES

1. AINSWORTH, M.D.S. 1971. Mother infant interaction: Characteristic and dynamics (Discussion) In: H.R. Schaffer (Ed.) *The Origins of Human Social Relations.* London: Academic Press.
2. ANDERSON, B.J. 1977. The emergence of conversational behaviour. *J. Communication,* 27:85.
3. BENEDEK, T.B. 1970. Motherhood and nurturing. In: E.J. Anthony and T. Benedek (Eds.) *Parenthood, Its Psychology and Psychopathology.* Edinburgh and London: Churchill Livingstone.
4. BISHOP, F.I. 1975. Perception, memory and pathological identification as precipitating factors in parental attacks on children. *Med. J. Aust.,* 21:243.
5. BLANK, M. 1976. The mother's role in infant development. In: E.N. Rexford, L.W. Sander, and T. Shapiro. (Eds.) *Infant Psychiatry, A New Synthesis.* New Haven and London: Yale University Press.
6. BOWLBY, J. 1953. *Child Care and the Growth of Love.* Harmondsworth: Penguin Books.
7. BOWLBY, J. 1969. *Attachment and Loss.* Vols. 1 & 2. New York: Basic Books.
8. BRAZELTON, B. F., KOSLWOSKI, B., MAIN, M. 1974. The origins of reciprocity: The early mother infant interaction. In: M. Lewis and L.A. Rosenblum (Eds.) *The Effect of the Infant on its Caregiver.* New York: Wiley-Interscience.
9. BRAZELTON, B.T., TRONICK, E., ADAMSON, L., ALLS, H., and WISE, S. 1975. Early mother infant reciprocity. In: *Parent-Infant Interaction: Ciba Foundation Symposium 33.* (New Series) Associated Scientific Publishers.
10. BURLINGHAM, D. 1961. Some notes on the development of the blind. *Psychanal. Study of Child,* 16:121.
11. CALL, J.D., and MARSCHAK, M. 1966. Styles and games in infancy. *J. Am. Acad. Child Psychiat.,* 5:193.
12. CRAIG, M.M. and GLICK, S.J. 1965. *A Manual of Procedures for Application for the Glueck Prediction Table.* London: Univ. London Press.
13. DENNIS, W. 1960. Causes of retardation amongst institutional children. *Iran. J. Genet. Psychol.,* 96:47.
14. DUNN, J.F. 1975. Consistency and changes in styles of mothering. In: *Parent-Infant Interaction: Ciba Foundation Symposium 33* (New Series). Associated Scientific Publishers.
15. ERIKSON, E. H. 1965. *Childhood and Society* (Rev. Ed.) London: Hogarth Press.
16. ERIKSON, E.H. 1968. *Identity, Youth and Crisis.* New York: W.W. Norton.
17. ESCALONA, S.K. 1953. Emotional development in the first year of life. In: M.J.E. Senn, (Ed.) *Problems of Infancy and Childhood.* New York: Josiah Macy Jr. Foundation.
18. ESCALONA, S.K. 1958. The impact of psychoanalysis upon psychology. *J. Nerv. Ment. Dis.,* 126:429.
19. FREEMAN, M., and TONGE, B.J. 1977. A case study of emotional and cognitive growth: A joint treatment approach. *Aust. J. of Human Comm. Dis.,* 5:61.
20. FREUD, A. 1958. Child observation and prediction of development. *Psychoanal. Study Child.,* 13:92.
21. FREUD, A. 1966. *Normality and Pathology in Childhood.* Harmondsworth: Penguin Books.
22. FREUD, A. 1970. A discussion with Rene Spitz In: *The Writing of Anna Freud.* Vol. VII. New York: International Universities Press.

23. FRIES, M.E. 1946. The child's ego development and the training of adults in his environment. *Psychoanal. Study Child*, 2:85.
24. GOLDSTEIN, J., FREUD, A., and SOLNIT, A.J. 1973. *Beyond the Best Interests of the Child*. New York: The Free Press.
25. HARTMANN, H. 1939. *Ego Psychology and the Problem of Adaptation*. New York: International Universities Press.
26. HOWELLS, J.G. 1970. Fallacies in child care: 1. That "separation" is synonymous with "deprivation." *Acta Paedo. Psychiat.*, 37:3.
27. JAFFE, J., and FELDSTEIN, S. 1970. *Rhythms of Dialogue*. New York: Academic Press.
28. KAUFMAN, I.C. 1970. Biological considerations of parenthood. In: E.J. Anthony, and T. Benedek, (Eds.). *Parenthood, Its Psychology and Psychopathology*. Edinburgh: Churchill Livingstone.
29. KAHN, M.R. 1963. The concept of Cumulative Trauma. *Psychoanal. Study Child*, 18:286.
30. KLAUS, M.H., TRAUSE, M.A., and KENNEL, J.H. 1975. Does human maternal behaviour after delivery show a characteristic pattern? In: *Parent-Infant Interaction: Ciba Foundation Symposium 33* (New Series) Associated Scientific Publishers.
31. KRIS, E. 1962. Decline and recovery in the life of a three year old; data in psychoanalytic perspective on the mother child relationship. *Psychoanal. Study Child*, 17:175.
32. LIPTON, G.L. and TONGE, B.J. 1977. Bring Mum in too—The inpatient management of crises in mother-infant relationships. Presented at 1977 Annual Congress of R.A.N.Z.C.P. Australia.
33. MAHLER, S.M. 1952. On child psychosis and schizophrenia. *Psychoanal. Study Child*, 17:286.
34. MAHLER, M.S., and GOSLINER, B. 1955. On symbiotic child psychosis. *Psychoanal. Study Child*, 10:195.
35. MAHLER, M.S. 1965. On early infantile psychosis. *J.Am. Acad. Child Psychiat.*, 4:554.
36. MAHLER, S.M., PINE, F., and BERGMAN, A. 1975. *The Psychological Birth of the Human Infant*. New York: Basic Books.
37. MEARES, R. 1977. *The Pursuit of Intimacy*. Melbourne: Nelson.
38. OLDEN, C. 1953. On adult empathy with children. *Psychoanal. Study Child*, 8:111.
39. OLDEN, C. 1958. Notes on the Development of empathy. *Psychoanal. Study Child*, 13:505.
40. PAUL, N.L. 1970. Parental empathy. In: E.J. Anthony, and T. Benedek (Eds.). *Parenthood, Its Psychology and Psychopathology*. Edinburgh: Churchill Livingstone.
41. PIAGET, J. 1950. *The Psychology of Intelligence*. London: Routledge.
42. PRINGLE M.K. 1975. *The Needs of Children*. London: Hutchinson Educational.
43. RICHARDS, M.P.M. 1971. A comment on the social context of mother infant interaction. In: H.R. Schaffer, (Ed.) *The Origins of Human Social Relations*. London: Academic Press.
44. ROBERTSON, J. 1958. *Young Children in Hospital*. London: Tavistock Publications.
45. ROBERTSON, J. 1962. Mothering as an influence on early development. A study of well-baby clinic records. *Psychoanal. Study Child*, 17:245.
46. RUTTER, M. 1971. Parent child separation: Psychological effects on the children. *J. Child Psychol. Psychiat.*, 12:233.
47. RUTTER, M. 1972. Maternal Deprivation re-assessed. Harmondsworth: Penguin Education.
48. SANDER, L.W. 1962. Issues in early mother child interaction. *J. Am. Acad. Child Psychiat.*, 1:141
49. SANDLER, A.M 1963. Aspects of passivity and ego development in the blind child. *Psychoanal. Study Child*, 18:343.
50. SANDLER, J. 1960. The background of safety. *Int. J. Psychoanal.*, XLI.
51. SCHAEFER, E.S. 1959. A circumplex model for maternal behaviour. *J. Abnorm. Psychol.*, 59:226.
52. SCHAEFER, E.S., BELL, R. Q. and BAILEY, N. 1959. Development of a maternal behaviour research instrument. *J. Genet. Psychol.*, 95:83.
53. SPITZ, R. 1945. Hospitalism. *Psychoanal. Study Child*, 1:53.

54. SPITZ, R. 1946. Hospitalism—a follow-up report. *Psychoanal. Study Child*, 2:113.
55. WEST, D.J. 1969. *Present Conduct and Future Delinquency*. London: Heinemann.
56. WINNICOTT, D.W. 1949. *The Ordinary Devoted Mother and Her Baby*. London: Tavistock Publications.
57. WINNICOTT, D.W. 1949. Mind and its relation to psyche-soma. In: *Collected Papers*. New York: Basic Books.
58. WINNICOTT, D.W. 1952. Psychoses and child care. *Collected Papers*. New York: Basic Books.
59. WINNICOTT, D.W. 1958. Primary maternal preoccupation. In: *Collected Papers: Through Paediatrics to Psychoanalysis*. London: Tavistock Publications.
60. WINNICOTT, D.W. 1960 The theory of the parent infant relationship. *Int. J. Psychoanal.*, 41:585.
61. WINNICOTT, D.W. 1962 Providing for the child in health and in crisis. In: *The Maturational Processes and the Facilitating Environment*. New York. International Universities Press.
62. WINNICOTT, D.W. 1965. *The Family and Individual Development*. London: Tavistock Publications.
63. WINNICOTT, D.W. 1970 The mother infant experience of mutuality. In: E.J. Anthony, and T. Benedek (Eds).) *Parenthood, Its Psychology and Psychopathology*. Edinburgh: Churchill Livingstone.

10

THE FATHER-INFANT RELATIONSHIP

FELTON EARLS, M.D.

Assistant Professor in Psychiatry,
Children's Hospital Medical Center;
Associate in Medicine,
Children's Hospital Medical Center;
Instructor in Pediatrics,
Harvard Medical School,
Boston, Mass.

and

MICHAEL YOGMAN, M.D.

Associate in Medicine,
Children's Hospital Medical Center;
Instructor in Pediatrics,
Harvard Medical School,
Boston, Mass.

INTRODUCTION

Not surprisingly, children may be as prone to hold a stereotypical view of the father's role as adults are. Statements such as a father is "the ruler of the household and telivision [sic]set" or "a person hoo[sic] coaches your baseball team when he's not the coach" (21, 60) present contrasting roles of fathers as disciplinarian and as teacher. The stereotype restricts the various roles that fathers may have to older children and adolescents. Babies and young children are thought to need a different kind of nurturance which is the exclusive domain of mothering.

This chapter challenges the stereotype by acknowledging that fathers can and do form a significant relationship with infants and young children, one that is qualitatively different from the mother-child relationship. Sections of this chapter will discuss recent studies on the nature and quality of the father-infant relationship, as well as disturbances in the relationship. Medical and behavioral conditions in the infant which require knowledge of variability in the father-infant relationship are examined in regard to clinical management and social policy.

HISTORICAL BACKGROUND

References describing the father-child relationship in the literature of child psychiatry, pediatrics, and psychology were quite rare until about five years ago. Clinical practice began changing 10 or 15 years ago when maternity units in various hospitals in the United States started permitting fathers to view the birth process. Over the past 10 years, popular interest in revising routine labor and delivery practices in the United States has evolved from a rather intellectual, middle-class movement, with roots in the women's movement, to a broadly based and widely practiced social phenomenon. The revisions have been many: relaxation techniques, "natural" childbirth, the Lamaze methods, and home-based delivery. Fundamental to all of them is the arrival of the father as a participant-observer in the childbirth process.

What has produced such changes in this country and why are they now occurring? Are the changes witnessed in this country applicable to other societies that differ in social, cultural and economic structure? Indeed, why are we writing a paper on the father-infant relationship now, given its relative absence from the literature in our professions for centuries?

Writings about the history of fathers' role in ancient cultures describe overall family structure but provide little information on the father-infant relationship. For example, though we know that the ancient Hebrews practiced polygamy while Greeks and Romans practiced monogamy and that male adults were dominant over women, comments about infants are limited to reports of infanticide (81). In ancient China and in Arab countries we know that Confucian and Islamic ideas both stressed reverence and love for the father as a function of his age and sex (53, 30). While it seems clear that patriarchy or male dominance represented a common theme of major religious and philosophical traditions, we know little about whether this implies that fathers were cold, distant and uninvolved with their infants in all of these cultures, or whether they tended to be more involved in some than in others.

According to Stone's (102) social history of the family in England, the nuclear family as we now know it was formed by 1500. Family life at that time was characterized by a rigidly patriarchal structure, high rates of infant and maternal mortality, and harsh discipline of children. Infant care practices consisted of wet nursing, swaddling of infants, and what would be considered in our present society as indifferent attitudes towards children. Marriage was a bargaining process, an event negotiated to secure title or property rights. By 1750 shifts occurred in the philosophical thinking about the importance of the individual and early experience, and Stone argues that there began to be more evidence of deeper personal relationships within marriages and in parent-child relationships. This shift has steadily influenced the evolution of the contemporary Western nuclear family. To what extent economic, demographic and political forces have contributed to changing the character of relationships within families is open to question, but it is certain that industrial and technological developments of the past 200 years have gone far in stabilizing our current pattern.

By 1950 a new phase of family and social relationships appears to have begun, perhaps in response to reaching the limits of industrialized growth in Western Europe and the U.S. This phase is characterized by demographic changes, the availability and efficacy of new forms of contraception, and changes in social values, placing increasing amounts of significance on individual fulfillment, emotional involvement, and sexual equality. It is in the context of this third epoch in the modern history of Western Europe and the United States that revised definitions of men's roles (80) and fathers' roles, in particular, are emerging.

PHYLOGENETIC AND ANTHROPOLOGICAL BACKGROUND

Attempts to review phylogenetic evidence of the role of fathers in order to better understand the uniquely human aspects of fathering uncover no simple evolutionary trend (63, 83, 93). While in most species mothers care for infants, in others caretaking is shared by both males and females (herring gull, fox, penguin), and in some, male caretaking predominates (stickleback, midwife toad, seahorse) (93). The range of activities for highly involved males includes defending territory, nest-building, keeping a vigil over the eggs and keeping the brood together in the stickleback (105), to the predigestion and regurgitation of food for the infant in the wolf, to protection, play and transport in the coyote and fox.(93). Within primates, the range is also wide. The marmoset, a new world monkey, assists during birth, premasticates food during the first week and carries the infant at all times except during nursing during the first three months (33). The barbary macaque engages in social chatter with infants from birth, and encourages the beginning locomotion which functions to orient the infant towards interaction with other troop members (16). However, male primates are by no means universally nurturant. Male tree shrews, bush babies and langurs are known to be hostile towards infants of their species, while male feral chimps show little interest in and have little contact with their infants.

Variability in male caretaking exists not only between species, but among individuals within species. Both in the wild and in captive groups, rhesus males are either aggressive or indifferent to young. However, under laboratory conditions, when the female rhesus is removed from the group, males increase their caretaking behavior and engage in more intense and reciprocal play with infants (84). Even males reared in social isolation are capable of forming affective social relationships (29), although males reared in strict social isolation are still less nurturant toward their young than females raised under comparable circumstances (19).

Attempts have been made to suggest what environmental or ecological factors favor male caretaking across species. Trivers (108) used the concept of "parental investment" to describe the influence of natural selection on parent-infant behavior as an evolutionary mechanism which increases survival of the offspring. Variables said to be associated with higher male parental investment include: monogamous social organization with prolonged pair bonding, the defense of territory, familiarity with mother, close kinship ties, permissive mother-infant interaction, and relative isolation from other conspecifics (63, 83, 110).

Anthropological data provide further insights into the way social and cultural variables influence the level of paternal care of infants. In cultures such as the Arapesh, fathers play an active and joint role with mothers throughout pregnancy, as well as in caring for infants after birth (37). More commonly, in non-industrialized cultures fathers play only a minor role with infants compared to mothers (6). However, analyses of social organization in different cultures (110, 111) suggest that males have a closer relationship with their infants when families are monogomous, when both parents live together in isolated nuclear families, when women contribute to subsistence by working, and when men are not required to be warriors.

Taboos and rituals both restrict and enhance the father's role in many cultures. The couvade ritual has been most widely discussed. In its classic form (107), the father takes to bed during the mother's pregnancy, labor and delivery as a means of sharing in the experience. Rivere (89) has reviewed anthropological evidence on the couvade and presented a novel interpretation which assigns the father the responsibility for creating the spiritual part of the infant, while the mother carries the responsibility for physical creation.

In summary, phylogenetic and anthropological data underscore the diversity in male-infant caretaking roles. The limited data suggest that ecological factors may be more powerful determinants of male parenting than biological factors.

NORMAL ADAPTATION IN THE FATHER-INFANT RELATIONSHIP

Empirical studies of the father-infant relationship can be seen as part of a broader attempt to understand a social world of infancy that includes not only fathers, but grandparents, friends, siblings, peers and strangers. Previous conceptualizations of infant social development focused almost exclusively on the mother-infant relationship, whether the importance of the mother was tied to her gratification of instinctual drives in psychoanalytic theory or to her association with the feeding experience in social learning theory. While attachment theory conceptualized the infant as active rather than passive in seeking the caregiving and love necessary for survival, this theory also argues for the uniqueness and exclusiveness of the mother-infant relationship(9). No theory acknowledged a meaningful direct role for fathers until the child entered the Oedipal period and began to identify with the father (27) or until the father could play a clear instrumental role in the family such as teaching his child to throw a ball(73).

Several shifts have occurred in the last ten years which have legitimized the study of the father-infant relationship. Many of these studies have been reviewed recently (68,50,58,37,24). First, secular changes in infant care documented by Bronfenbrenner (14) have resulted in fathers playing a more active role. These secular changes include families in which both parents work and caretaking is shared (38) and an increase in single-parent families in which father is primary caretaker (67), as well as a shift in the father's role in the family from a more authoritarian one to a more individualized and flexible one in which the father is permitted a more direct interaction with his infant.

Secondly, our understanding of the mother-infant relationship has been modified by findings that the feeding experience is not as critical as once thought (34), that social responsiveness and stimulation are the key dimensions contributing to psychological development (87), and that infants could be attached to fathers who were not primary caretakers (96). It has been suggested that studies of maternal deprivation were, more accurately, studies of parental deprivation.

Interest in the father-infant relationship has come at a time when the field of infancy research has taken on vigorous new studies in characterizing a wide range of perceptual, cognitive and social competencies innately possessed or acquired quite early in development by infants (42, 101). In the first minutes after birth, the newborn cannot only see, but will visually track and respond positively to presentation of a human face (10). He cannot only hear, but prefers speech sound to pure tones (25) and a female vocal pitch over any other. Not only will the newborn turn to the human voice repeatedly, but his body will move in perfect synchrony with the articulated structure of adult speech (23). By six days of age, the newborn has learned to prefer the smell of his own nursing mother's breast pad to that of any other nursing mother's breast pad (59). Many of these competencies represent biological preadaptations which influence caregivers to insure the infant's survival.

These processes of mutual recognition and regulation by both infant and parent (43) demand a major revision in our thinking about infants as capable of influencing caregivers (55). Any theory of the father-infant relationship consequently must account for bi-directional influences of the infant on the father and the father on the infant. A theory of the father-infant relationship must also recognize that these reciprocal influences can be direct as well as indirect, mediated through the mother or another family member so that the family is often the meaningful unit of analysis. We suggest that the father-infant relationship is similar to the mother-infant relationship in that infants can elicit competent, loving care from both male and female adults.

To simplify the review process, we will consider what is known about the father-infant relationship by separately examining five developmental periods: preconceptual, prenatal, neonatal, one to six months, and six to 24 months. Since much of the data presented is based on studies done in the United States over the last five years, caution should be exercised in generalizing the findings beyond contemporary United States society.

Preconceptual and Prenatal Periods

The availability of contraception means that prospective mothers and fathers can not only choose whether or not to have children, but when to have them. While demographic data in the U.S. document a shift toward postponing the age of having a first child in many families, what factors influence that decision and what consequences derive from delaying the age of childbearing have not been investigated. It is likely, however, that the decision to have children is viewed by increasing numbers of men and women as a major transition in adult development. Whether or not males actively make a choice is probably influenced by such variables as prior sex education, early experiences as a child, available role models of fathering, and current marital experiences. An example of how intricate this decision can be for a male is given by Gurwitt (32), who described the psychodynamic responses of a young man whose wife became pregnant and delivered a baby girl while he was undergoing psychoanalysis. As this man approached the decision to have a baby, the internal turmoil and change that accompany a reworking of past and current relationships with mother, father, siblings and wife are described. The father's drivenness at moving and settling into a new home had the symbolic quality evidenced in his associations of preparing a nest. Similarly, the intensity with which he completed and defended his doctoral dissertation represented his attempt to complete his own creation prior to embarking on the shared creation of a baby.

While the classic studies of Bibring (7) have given us detailed insights into the mother's prenatal experiences, no comparable studies exist for fathers. Gurwitt (32) in his case report discusses two aspects of the prenatal experience: first, the man's reactions to changes in his wife's physical and psychological status throughout the pregnancy and second, a reworking of significant relationships and events early in his life. As was true in Bibring's studies, Gurwitt finds it "remarkable" that by the time of the birth of the child the preceding turmoil had been covered by an "amnesic blanket." As part of a larger study of family psychological adaptations to first pregnancies, Liebenberg's study (56), in which 64 normal, expectant fathers were interviewed on several occasions during pregnancy, is of interest. Initially, most of the fathers were pleased about the pregnancy, but worried about the accompanying increased emotional and financial responsibilities. Many of them identified with their wives and expressed envy at her ability to have a baby. Sixty-five percent of the fathers in her study developed complaints similar to those of pregnant women: fatigue, nausea, backache, headaches, and vomiting; a few transiently gained 10-20 pounds, and several stopped smoking and switched from drinking coffee to milk. This finding is similar to that of Trethowan (107), who described psychosomatic symptoms in expectant fathers.

While studies of men becoming fathers are few, the limited data suggest that the period prior to the birth of the baby may be similar, as well as different, for fathers and mothers. It appears similar in that it is a time requiring readjustment for both as the roles of spouse and parent become integrated. This process for the father is different in the degree of biologic freedom afforded males during the parturition process. This may require a father to search for alternative vehicles for creation, i.e., through work or through being a protector or provider for his wife and subsequent child. The emotional "crisis" for the prospective father is to balance his desires to be emotionally available to his spouse with his desires to be creative and to provide security for his family through work.

Birth and the Newborn Period

Fathers are now increasingly encouraged by obstetric services to accompany their wives during labor and delivery. This practice is finding support in research work. For example, Anderson and Standley (3) have shown that husband support during this time lessens the degree of maternal distress. Another study has looked more directly at the experience of fathers during the immediate postnatal period. Thirty fathers of healthy firstborns were given a questionnaire 48-72 hours after birth to examine their emotional responses toward their babies. Half the fathers had been present in the delivery chamber and half had not. The questionnaire documented the powerful impact on the father of seeing and holding the newborn. The data suggested a nonsignificant trend that fathers present at the birth were better able to recognize their own newborns, were more certain that the baby was really theirs, and felt more comfortable holding them(31). The study suggests that immediate physical contact between father and the newborn may be a more crucial variable in the developing relationship than the father's viewing the birth process. A sub-sample of the fathers were also interviewed in conjunction with the questionnaire presentation. These fathers emphasized their desire to touch, pick up, move, hold and play with their newborn and were particularly impressed by the liveliness, reflex activity and movements of the baby: "When she starts moving I go and pick her up and she starts moving in your hands and your arms and you can feel her moving up against you. It's like a magnet (31, p. 525)." While these descriptions may be more characteristic of fathers, other reports appear characteristic of either parent: feelings of extreme elation, relief that the baby is healthy, feelings of pride and increased self-esteem and feelings of closeness when the baby opens its eyes(90). Fathers' descriptions of their newborns have also been reported to be more sex-typed than mothers', as evidenced by postpartum interviews on day one in which fathers rated sons as firmer, more alert, stronger and hardier, and daughters as softer, finer featured and more delicate(91).

While debate goes on about the existence of a sensitive period for maternal contact with newborns(43), no comparable studies exist for fathers. However, in one study of a small sample of five fathers, the sequence in which fathers touch their newborn over the first three days of life has been shown to be the same as with mothers: first with fingertips and then with full palms, and first on the extremities and later on the trunk(44), although the fathers took longer before they displayed this progression. Whether this sequence is specific to parents or characteristic of human adults, generally, is yet to be determined.

Studies of father-newborn interaction in the postpartum period suggest that fathers and mothers are equally active and sensitive to newborn cues during the postpartum period. In general, the conclusions hold for middle-class and lower-class families, and in both dyadic (father-infant) and triadic (mother-father-infant) situations(69-71). These studies also suggest differences between father-newborn interactions and mother-newborn interactions: Fathers held, rocked and provided more auditory and physical stimulation to their infants. Using questionnaires, these studies found that fathers of newborns believe that their babies need more stimulation and affection and are more perceptually competent than mothers do(72). Pedersen (74), studying four-week-old babies, has shown that fathers have an indirect influence on their babies as well, mediated through support of mother, that resulted in a more effective mother-infant relationship. While these studies describe how fathers and mothers interact with their newborn babies, little is known about the baby's contributions in the newborn period. It is reasonable to assume that a father's sleep rhythms are modified by a new baby's entrance into a home. Considering Sander's studies (94) on the entrainment of biorhythms for mothers and infants, one wonders about similarities and differences in this process for fathers and infants as organization takes place in the larger system of the family.

The First Six Months

Infants as young as two weeks of age have been studied during face-to-face interaction with their fathers in a laboratory setting, as part of a longitudinal study over the first six months. Microanalyses of videotape data enabled Yogman, Dixon and their colleagues (112, 113) to show that infants by two months of age could display different expressive patterns during interaction with fathers, as compared with mothers or strangers. Significant differences in individual behaviors, such as infant frown, smile and remaining still (absence of limb movement), were found with fathers as compared with mothers and strangers (see Figure 1) and suggest that infants can differentiate fathers, at least in the context of an interactive setting. Adults in these studies also differed in their behavior with infants, as evidenced by differences in vocalization and touching patterns. Over the six months, mothers vocalized with soft, repetitive, imitative burst-pause talking (47.0 percent of time) more often than fathers (20 percent) and strangers (11.9 percent), while fathers touched their infants with rhythmic tapping patterns (43.9 percent of time) more often than mothers (27.7 percent) or strangers (29.1 percent).

While these behavioral descriptions of father-infant interaction capture some of the communicative content of these interactions, analyses of the structural and regulatory aspects of these exchanges are likely to be more useful in understanding the developing father-infant relationship. Using methods for analyzing the structural characteristics of social interaction developed by Brazelton et al. (11) and Tronick (109), Yogman, Dixon and Tronick (115) found both similarities and differences during father-infant and mother-infant interaction by three months of age. Using data such as the level of affective involvement, the timing of transitions and the amount of meshing between partners, they suggest that the interaction of young infants with fathers, as well as with mothers, is a reciprocal and jointly regulated process in which both partners modify their actions in response to the feedback provided by their partner(12). While the transitions are simultaneous with both parents, they differ in sequence and quality: With fathers transitions are accentuated from peaks of maximal attention to valleys of minimal attention, while with mothers attentional shifts are more gradual and modulated. They also found differences in "interactive games" (100), in keeping with the differences in adult behavior: Mothers and infants played more verbal games, while fathers and infants played more tapping games with a quality and temporal structure more likely to be associated with an increase in the infant's attention and arousal. They characterized interactions with fathers as heightened and playful and interactions with mothers as smoothly modulated and contained.

While these studies document the social capacities of fathers and young infants, we know very little about the actual experiences of fathers and infants at home during these first few months, a period of transition and adaptation to the new baby. Pedersen (75), who has done home observations with infants aged five months, finds that the father's behavior with his infant is closely related to the quality of his relationship with his wife. Given his earlier findings that the baby's alertness and motor maturity at four weeks of age are associated with the husband's support of his wife (74), it appears that the baby's behavior may have a continuing influence at five months. The importance of father-infant interaction at this time is suggested by the report that, at least for males, a high degree of father involvement based on home observation is associated with greater social responsiveness during a Bayley test at five months of age(77).

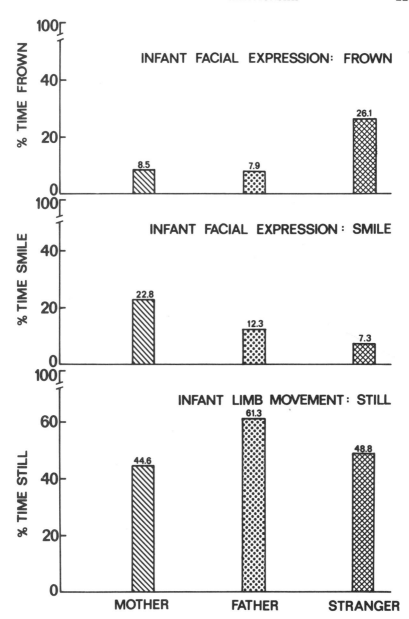

FIGURE 1. Infant (0-2 months) expressive displays. Percent of time infants under two months frown, smile or are still with mother, father and stranger.

Attachment and the Second Year

The study of the father-infant relationship with infants between six and 24 months focuses almost exclusively on the development of attachment, as defined by Bowlby(9) and Ainsworth(2), or on some revision of this definition. They ask such questions as: Do infants greet, seek proximity with and protest on separation from fathers as well as mothers? These studies give rather conclusive support to the existence of father-infant attachment. By seven to eight months of age, in environments considered to have relatively low degrees of psychosocial stress, infants are attached to both mothers and fathers, and prefer either parent over a stranger(50). During the second year, most studies also show attachment to both mother and father (48, 21, 52), although, in the more stressful setting of a laboratory, some studies have shown that infants prefer mothers between 12 and 18 months (5, 22, 51). The issue of preference for mother or father depends on what measure is used, but independent estimates by Kotelchuk (46) and Schaffer and Emerson (96) produce similar results. Both demonstrate that between 12 and 21 months 51 to 55 percent of infants show maternal preferences, 19 to 25 percent show paternal preferences and 16 to 20 percent show joint preferences.

Clinically important and yet not well studied are the influences on father-infant attachment. Pedersen and Robson (76) report that father's investment in caretaking, as well as the level of stimulation and play he provides, is positively associated with the greeting behaviors in eight-to-nine-month-old babies. Infants whose fathers participate highly in caregiving show less separation protest and cry less with a stranger than infants whose fathers are less involved(47).

Given that infants are attached to both mothers and fathers, how are their relationships different? First, mothers and fathers interact differently: Fathers engage in more play than caretaking activities with six-month-olds (85) and more often pick up their infants (eight months) to play physical, idiosyncratic games, while mothers are involved in more caregiving, play with toys, and conventional games such as peek-a-boo(50). In the second year, fathers were better able to engage their children in a play situation. Their play was more likely to be physical, arousing, and briefer in duration, and they reportedly enjoyed the bouts of play more than mothers(21). Infants at eight months responded more positively to play with fathers than mothers (50) and in the second year not only preferred to play with fathers but were judged to be more involved and excited with them(21). It is fascinating to note that fathers' physical play with their infants correlates most highly with mothers' verbal stimulation (.89) and toy play (.96) (21). These are maternal behaviors found in other studies to be part of a pattern of "optimal maternal care" (20).

All of these studies have been based on the assumption that the quality of the father-infant relationship is more important than the quantity, given some as yet to be defined lower limit. Reports of father involvement vary widely, from a mean of eight hours/week spent playing and 26 hours/week available at home with nine-month-old babies(76), to 30 minutes/day spent alone with the infant (one-twelfth that of mother)(78). When one looks at specific activities (feeding, cleaning, play), fathers spend much less time than mothers, although a greater proportion of fathers' time with the baby is spent in play than mothers' (37.5 percent vs. 25.8 percent)(47). Even though fathers do not spend as much time with their babies as mothers, at least one-quarter to one-half of fathers are involved in some caretaking responsibilities and almost 90 percent often play with their infants(47,65,88).

The influence of the father-infant relationship on later cognitive, social and emotional development has not been well studied. Concurrent predictions of infant Bayley scores at 16 and 22 months were related to father's ability to engage the child in play and to anticipate independence on the part of the child(21). Most attempts to assess the impact of the father-infant relationship on later development have looked at father-absent families and the relationship to sex-role identification. Father-absence, particularly prior to age five(62), has been shown to influence masculine sex-role adoption and cognitive style among boys (8,36,17) and heterosexual roles among girls(40). Since these studies have been criticized for confounding both the underlying reason for the father's absence and its effect on the mother, the focus has shifted to understanding the differential relationship of fathers with sons and daughters during infancy. Studies show that not only do fathers vocalize and play more with sons than daughters, but this is especially true for firstborn sons(70,71). Studies of infant preferences show that male infants prefer fathers at least by a year of age(5,99).

In summary, studies of the father-infant relationship suggest that the pregnancy experience is a time of developmental transition for fathers as well as mothers, that both the father and the infant are ready for meaningful social interaction from birth, and that an attachment bond exists between them by the end of the first year.

NONADAPTIVE MODES IN THE FATHER-INFANT RELATIONSHIP

The preceding section has adequately demonstrated that once the father's sperm successfully impregnates the ovum, his biologic and social commitment to the pregnancy and the first years of his infant's life has just begun. We now proceed to discuss how the event of becoming a father may be perceived as a psychologic stress and result in poor adaptation to the role of father. Recognition of fathering as a psychologic stress capable of producing major psychiatric disorder is intricately bound to the psychodynamic model of etiology. The most provocative paper to appear in this literature is that of Zilboorg(117), who explored stressful adaptations to the role of parent as a rationale to explain the dynamics of depressive illnesses in men and women. The existence of a variety of unconscious barriers to parenthood were examined, such as the hatred of one's own father serving as a barrier to the wish to become a father. An example typical of the cases presented in the paper is that of a man who lost his own father when six years old who became suicidally depressed during his wife's pregnancy. The development of depressive disorders in the 37 intensively studied cases was viewed by the author as an extreme attempt to resolve an incestuous drive rooted in the Oedipal condition. The use of psychodynamic explanations to describe the unconscious roots of major psychopathology in men who are fathers or expectant fathers in other studies has followed in the tradition of Zilboorg. Feelings of hostility and dependency directed toward the infant overtly or covertly pervade the clinical picture of acute depressive and psychotic illnesses in men, usually in their fourth decade of life. This clinical presentation is not limited to fathers having their first experience with pregnancy.

What we find most important in the Zilboorg paper is the attention given the interaction between psychodynamic and sociocultural factors. Having explained depression as an attempted resolution of unconscious forces, the author goes on to compare the clinical appearance of this illness in men with postpartum depressions and psychoses in women. His conclusions require one to reexamine the boundaries and limitations of sex-roles in Western society. First, he found that paranoia was an unusually common symptom in disorders in males, but quite uncommon in women. Further, he found that men appeared to be more often psychotic or extremely regressed in their morbid behaviors than women. It appeared that depressive symptoms alone were not sufficient to resolve emotional conflict in the men. The chief reason for this given by Zilboorg was the social stigma attached to depression or depressive symptoms in males. Society instructs men to view symptoms such as passivity, impotence and crying as a threat to their self-images. Men had few adaptive alternatives to resolve the psychologic stress associated with fathering. Zilboorg carefully documents each maladaptive alternative: murder, pathological projection (claiming that the child is not his), rivalry with the infant, passivity or femininity (it is here that Zilboorg discusses the couvade phenomenon), and sadism towards the child (harsh punishment).

We have concentrated on Zilboorg's paper because of its originality in describing major psychopathology associated with fathering. Several case studies already reviewed by Lacoursiere (49) and by Earls (24) extend Zilboorg's findings and interpretations to other clinical samples. The case material leaves much to be desired in determining how necessary and sufficient such explanations really are to the development of psychiatric illness. Zilboorg was offended by Kraepelinian psychiatrists who were content to stop at the level of phenomenology in describing psychopathological reactions, and missed the meaning of life experiences in the onset of depressions. Although current developments in the biochemical basis of depression represent progress in explaining vulnerability of certain persons to become depressed, the danger of sterile associations in psychiatric research persist. Perhaps methods such as those used by Brown (15) to describe life events in the etiology of depression will eventually lend credence to psychodynamic interpretations such as those so eloquently described by Zilboorg.

It is fortunate that the incidence of major psychiatric illness related to fatherhood is low. Rettersol (86) has estimated that the incidence of father-precipitated psychosis is no greater than two percent of all psychoses in men based on hospital admission statistics. There is little known about lesser degrees of psychopathology associated with fatherhood. For example, Trethowan (106) estimated that approximately 11 percent of a normal population of men experienced some psychosomatic symptoms associated with expectant fatherhood, and a paper by Hartman and Nicolay (35) suggests that antisocial behavior may accompany the event of becoming a father. The few studies that do exist require replication before much credence can be given to their findings(104). It is also unfortunate that none of the studies has prospectively followed a group of fathers experiencing a psychiatric illness or psychiatric symptoms during pregnancy to see what consequences these might have for the father-infant relationship.

In light of these comments on the association between the perceived stress of becoming a father and psychopathology, it is worthwhile considering to what extent father absence as a social maladaptation may be associated with symptoms of anxiety or depression. On clinical grounds we have been impressed with how often the timing of a father's exit from the home environment coincides with the last trimester of pregnancy and the first few postnatal months. We know of no research data to support this impression, but it remains an interesting clinical question.

CLINICAL MANAGEMENT

It is beyond the scope of this chapter to develop a full thesis on how transformations occurring in Western societies are affecting family life. Two recent reports from the United States have already characterized these changes as profound(41, 64). Changing definitions of men's and women's roles in society, the changing forms of marriage, increasing rates of separation and divorce, and postponement of childbearing to later ages are only a few indicators of the direction that these transformations are taking. These social changes require adaptations in the helping professions. Our final concern in this chapter is to provide a clinical framework for medical practitioners—nurses, pediatricians, child psychiatrists, family physicians, and social workers—working with fathers and infants. Having given a perspective on adaptive and unadaptive modes of fathering, we would like to consider clinical situations in which an evaluation of the father's role and his active participation in the management process is necessary.

To put in perspective the current needs and dilemmas confronting modern families, it is necessary to begin with a brief historical digression. Over the past 200 years, families have become less self-sufficient in passing on the essential skills of life and work to children. As these functions have eroded, various agencies or agents of society have taken their place—the school, physicians, nutritionists, and others—leaving parents with a diminished sense of authority and control over the rearing of their own children. In this sense, the "experts" have taken the place of a more natural social support system, leaving parents in the role of what one report has termed the "weakened executive" (41). Up to now, doctors and social workers have regarded fathers as voluntary parents; no harm is done by their presence and investment in child-rearing as auxiliaries to the mother, but no critical deprivation results from their lack of emotional investment either. So deeply ingrained is the idea of the critical exclusivity of the mother-child relationship in health services that we still refer to such services as "maternal-child" clinics or departments. It is essential to revise this bit of clinical ideology to include fathers on an equal basis with mothers.

To encourage clinical thinking on when to involve fathers in the management of developmental problems of infants, we provide several examples from our own clinical experience. The examples give only a preliminary account of an ideal state of affairs in which fathers as well as mothers would be routinely involved in clinical work with infants.

1) *A suspicion exists that psychopathology exists in the father.* As indicated in a previous section of this chapter, the stress of expectant parent-

hood may in itself be sufficient cause to produce a psychopathological reaction. The particular form that the reaction takes may depend on a genetic predisposition, the past experience of the father, or both at some level or interaction.

2) *A father may be experiencing high degrees of psychosocial stress without manifest psychopathology*, for instance, as in employment-related difficulties. We have been impressed with the degree to which such paternally related stresses appear to influence the clinical presentation of developmental and behavioral problems in the infant. This influence is often masked by the mother's chief complaint or by other circumstances in the family. The clinician must proceed in unraveling the problem with a high index of suspicion, sensitivity, and skill.

3) *There is an indication or an implication of marital tension.* It strikes us that clinicians quite commonly fail to interview the father when the mother indicates the marriage is a problem. By failing to do so, the clinician takes the risk of entering into a collusion with the mother to isolate the father and minimize his significance to the infant.

4) *It is not uncommon for the father to serve as a protective factor in a family undergoing a stressful situation.* This may be most evident when the mother has a physical or a mental disorder. Failure to recognize the father's role in such a case is a serious clinical error. More commonly, in families in which both parents are employed, each parent serves as a psychological buffer for the periodic absences and stresses of the other.

5) *Child abuse is either evident or suspected.* It has been reported that fathers are less commonly the perpetrators of violence towards children than mothers(82). However, the issue is far from settled and clinical work is confronted with at least two problems in deciding what specific contributions fathers have made to cases of child abuse. The first is knowing to what extent other acts of domestic violence are prevalent. In this connection fathers may be facilitators or accessories to acts of violence towards children which are carried out by another family member. The second problem relates to the need to distinguish biologic from substitute or social fathers (the latter are, in most cases, the mother's paramours). There is some evidence that substitute fathers are more commonly the perpetrators of violence towards children conceived from a prior relationship of the mother than biologic fathers are towards their own children(82).

Controversy exists over to what extent an abusive parent is likely to have a psychiatric disorder. The studies of Smith et al. (97) and Baldwin and Oliver (4) both indicate high degrees of personal and social deviance in families which contain a seriously abused child. A sobering and bleak account of abuse in several generations of a single family pedigree is reported by Oliver and Taylor(66). They found over 40 seriously neglected or abused children in the pedigree. Several family members were retarded, psychotic or had a profound personality disorder. The index child's father and his side of the family contributed as greatly to the overall picture of family maladaptation as the mother and her side of the family. This single report may not be atypical of many cases of serious abuse, as argued by Baldwin and Oliver in their community-wide study. In less extreme cases of abuse, parental psychopathology does not appear to be relevant and often only single children are abused. Nevertheless, the clinician is still faced with the responsibility of assessing the psychologic and social status of the parents.

6) *Intervention programs for "high-risk" infants typically fail to separate maternal and paternal reactions, roles and responsibilities.* A content analysis of several programs indicates, once again, the emphasis on mothers, with the expectation that they will carry the major responsibility as agents of change. When fathers are included they appear to be less efficient in carrying out specific program tasks than mothers. For instance, in a program described by Bricker (13), fathers were more dependent on the constant direction and encouragement of trainers than mothers. Mothers eventually achieved independence from the trainers and were able to embellish the intervention procedures in ways that fathers were not. When fathers remained involved in the program, they seemed to play the primary role of emotional supporters to their wives, rather than of change agents with their infants. It would be important to know what part the staff of this program had in generating high or lowered levels of expectation towards fathers, but this is not reported.

Two reports of studies that directly attempted to modify father-infant interaction are relevant to increasing the efficacy of father involvement in the management of high-risk infants, although the infants included in the program were not defined as high-risk. Zelazo et al.(116), working with a group of fathers of 12-month-old sons characterized by relatively low degrees of father-infant interaction, instructed one-half of the group to play with their sons for 30 minutes a day. At follow-up, one month later, infants in the intervention group showed greater degrees of proximity-seeking to their fathers in a free play context than infants in the non-intervention group.

In another Swedish report, Johannesson (39) gave instructions to fathers on various aspects of infant care (bathing and feeding) during the lying-in period. Fathers in the experimental group were found to have higher degrees of infant caretaking activity than those in a matched control group on the bases of a maternal questionnaire given six weeks following discharge. Yogman et al. (114) reported a longitudinal study of face-to-face father-infant interaction in a family where the infant was temperamentally irritable at birth. A sequence of interactive difficulties with frequent infant gaze aversion was followed by more reciprocal interactions and eventual adaptation. Extension of this study to larger numbers of temperamentally difficult children may prove to be an effective technique in the primary prevention of behavior problems in older children.

There are, at least, two issues at stake in the evaluation of the father's role in the care of a "high-risk" infant. (In this case, we restrict use of the term "high-risk" to infants who are born with some recognized physical or mental abnormality, e.g. cerebral palsy, Down's syndrome, prematurity. The term has also been used to define infants who are born to mothers who are considered to be at high-risk for defective parenting. We know of no instances in which the term has been applied to infants born to fathers who are considered to be at high-risk of defective parenting.) The first is to assess the father's reaction to the presentation of an abnormal infant. Grief reactions are common and their effect on the health and psychological status of fathers has not been well described(98). It is also important to assess the effect of the abnormal child's presence on family relationships, particularly the parents' marriage. There is conflicting evidence on the degree to which the presence of an abnormal child in a family contributes to marital separation and divorce. Kolin's study (45) in New York state of children born with a meningomyelocoele found that 46 percent of the parents were divorced by the time the children were of school age. This finding is contradicted by other studies which report that separation and divorce are no commoner in such families than in the general population. Further, there is the suggestion by Martin (61) that divorce only occurs in situations in which there has been marital strain prior to the birth of the child.

Gath's case-control study (28) of families experiencing the birth of an infant with Down's syndrome is of particular interest. In nearly a third of the families with an abnormal infant, the marriage was characterized by severe degrees of tension or separation during the 18 months following birth, compared to a total absence of this degree of marital strain in the control group. Nevertheless, half the marriages were reported to have high degrees of warmth and positive regard. Other studies have suggested that the presence of an abnormal infant might serve as a positive catalyst to a marriage, but none has reported it as convincingly as Gath's study. Exactly what role fathers have in determining the direction of the effect is not clear. Gath found that the source of marital tension commonly was sexual dissatisfaction. This may have been a reflection of the father's grief and mourning after having produced a defective offspring. However, in those cases of increased marital satisfaction, it was noted that many of these same parents continued to grieve throughout the two-year study period. It will be important in subsequent clinical research to isolate the individual contribution of both the parents to marital stability or disruption.

7) *In some of the situations listed above adolescent fathers are likely to be a prevalent age group in clinical samples* (e.g., child abuse). Yet, specially designed preventive and intervention programs for adolescent girls rarely involve fathers. A substantial body of literature exists on adolescent mothers suggesting that early sexual activity and subsequent pregnancy are manifestations of emotional disturbance(1), although this position has been recently disputed by Schaffer et al. (95). Very little is known about the emotional status or the motives for reproduction in adolescent males. Correcting this clinical situation and increasing our knowledge of adolescent fatherhood will contribute to improved services and may direct the way towards effective intervention in the high rates of unwanted pregnancy in this age group. However, aggressive efforts are necessary to involve young males in obstetrical services designed for mothers. Lorenzi et al. (57) report that, when the adolescent mother finds a permanent relationship with the putative father, a second pregnancy occurs within 18 months of the first, and that this pregnancy carries a higher biologic risk for the infant than did the first. While impermanence of relationships between adolescent parents is certainly common, it is rather surprising to find how often they desire a permanent relationship. Several studies have documented that 40 to 50 percent of clinic samples of adolescent mothers have maintained a relationship with a single male, the putative father, for a period of more than two years following the first pregnancy(26,79). This suggests that increased vigilance by health practitioners is necessary to involve young men in family planning, obstetrical services, and pediatric programs serving adolescent populations. It is clear, however, that in addition to vigilance, a good deal of creativity and flexibility will be required to make interventions successful.

CONCLUSION

In the absence of more knowledge about the variety of emotional and social meanings attached to fatherhood, we must speculate that there is a kind of social "plasticity" associated with the phenomenon. At least the options open to a man as to what role he will take as a father seem to be more varied than those available to a woman who becomes a mother, perhaps only because the biologic component of parenting is weaker in men and more easily shaped by social influences. It follows from the clinical literature that in societies that permit men to take a variety of alternative psychologic and social roles, psychopathology should be more limited than in a society that offers narrow and constricted choices to men. Even more fascinating is the possibility that generational effects may accrue from having men become more deeply invested in pregnancy as a shared experience and develop stronger emotional bonds with infants. Is it possible, for instance, that the concept of Oedipal rivalry between fathers and sons is a sociocultural byproduct of a cultural tradition in which fathers are relatively detached from the day-to-day caretaking routines of their infants and young children? The question that intrigues us, standing at the threshhold of what appears to be a certain revolution of sexual roles and relationships in our society, is how the continued and deepening investment of men in pregnancy and early child care will alter the way their sons respond to their subsequent fatherhoods.

Social policy changes are also having a profound effect on stabilizing the direction of influences in the father-child relationship. For a sample of some of the ways these social policies are taking effect, consider the following examples. A recent study from the U.S. reports that, in 38 percent of contested custody cases, fathers were granted custody. In fact, laws in several American states are changing to make it easier for fathers to obtain custody. Levine(54) has interviewed fathers who are the sole or primary caretakers of children and discusses this as a social phenomenon of great importance to the welfare of children. Sweden has recently offered men the option of taking paternity leave to care for their babies. Others have suggested that men be allowed greater access to their babies in hospital nurseries and that they be allowed routinely to have extended contact with their babies on the first day of life. Beyond the lying-in period, the need for flexible work schedules and part-time employment, as well as improved sex and parent education in high school for adolescent males, has been emphasized. Given our limited knowledge, any attempt at revising social policies should increase the options available to fathers and their families rather than promote specific alternative prescriptions.

Even when social policy and clinical management in pediatrics and child psychiatry satisfactorily reflect appreciation and greater knowledge of the father-infant relationship, men will still have to make personal choices regarding fatherhood. High paternal investment may require a reduction or compromise in competitive urges. On the other hand, low paternal investment, especially in families in which both parents work, can carry the risk of marital strain and family tension. Pursuit of an optimal balance between home and work may prove to be a vanishing ideal for some. But for many men the emotional rewards of parenthood may give rise to the sense of renewal, creativity and fulfillment. Such were the surprises of Bertrand Russell as captured in this passage from his autobiography:

> When my first child was born, in November 1921, I felt an immense release of pent-up emotion, and during the next ten years my main purposes were parental. Parental feeling, as I have experienced it, is very complex. There is, first and foremost, sheer animal affection, and delight in watching what is charming in the ways of the young. Next, there is the sense of inescapable responsibility, providing a purpose for daily activities which skepticism does not easily question. Then there is an egoistic element, which is very dangerous; the hope that one's children may succeed when one has failed, that they may carry on one's work when death or senility puts an end to one's own efforts, and, in any case, that they will supply a biological escape from death, making one's own life part of the whole stream, and not a mere stagnant puddle without any overflow into the future. All this I experienced, and for some years it filled my life with happiness and peace (92, p. 150).

REFERENCES

1. ABERNETHY, V. 1974. Illegitimate conception among teenagers. *Amer. J. Public Health*, 64:662.
2. AINSWORTH, M.D.S. 1973. The development of infant-mother attachment. In: B. Caldwell and H. Ricciuti (Eds.), *Review of Child Development Research* Vol. 3. Chicago: University of Chicago Press.
3. ANDERSON, B.J. and STANDLEY, K 1976. A methodology for observation of the childbirth environment. Paper presented to the American Psychological Association, Washington, D.C.
4. BALDWIN, J.A. and OLIVER, J.E. 1975. Epidemiology and family characteristics of severely-abused children. *Brit. J. Preventive and Social Medicine*, 29:205.
5. BAN, P.L. and LEWIS, M. 1974. Mothers and fathers, girls and boys: Attachment behavior in the one-year-old. *Merrill-Palmer Quarterly*, 20:195.
6. BARRY, H. and PAXSON, L.M. 1971. Infancy and early childhood: Cross-cultural codes. *Ethnology*, 10:467.
7. BIBRING, G. 1959. Some considerations of the psychological processes in pregnancy. *Psychoanalytic Study of the Child*, 14:113.
8. BILLER, H. 1970. Father absence and the personality development of the male child. *Developmental Psychology*, 2:181.
9. BOWLBY, J. 1969. *Attachment and Loss* (Vol. 1), New York: Basic Books.
10. BRAZELTON, T.B. 1973. *Neonatal Behavioral Assessment Scale*. Clinics in Developmental Medicine, No. 50. London:S.I.M.P. with Heinemann Medical; Philadelphia: Lippincott.
11. BRAZELTON, T.B., TRONICK, E., ADAMSON, L. ALS, H. and WISE, S. 1975. Early mother-infant reciprocity. In: R. Hinde (Ed.), *Parent-Infant Interaction*. Amsterdam: Elsevier.

12. BRAZELTON, T.B., YOGMAN, M.W., ALS, H. and TRONICK, E. 1979. The infant as a focus for family reciprocity. In: M. Lewis and L. Rosenblum (Eds.), *The Social Network of the Developing Infant*. New York: Plenum.

13. BRICKER, W.A. and BRICKER, D.A. 1976. The infant, toddler, and preschool research and intervention project. In T.D. Tjossem (Ed.) *Intervention Strategies for High Risk Infants and Young Children*. Baltimore: University Park Press, p. 545.

14. BRONFENBRENNER, U. 1961. The changing American child: a speculative analysis, *Journal of Social Issues*, 17:6.

15. BROWN, G. 1974. Meaning, measurement and stress of life events. In B.S. Dohrenwend and B.P. Dohrenwend (Eds.) *Stressful Life Events: Their Nature and Effects*. New York: Wiley, p. 217.

16. BURTON, F.D. 1972. The integration of biology and behavior in the socialization of Macaca Sylvana of Gibraltar. In: F. Poirier (Ed.) *Primate Socialization*. New York: Random House.

17. CARLSMITH, L. 1964. Effects of early father absence in scholastic aptitude. *Harvard Education Review*, 34:3.

18. CASSELL, T. and SANDER, L. 1975. Neonatal recognition processes and attachment: the masking experiment. Paper presented to Society for Research in Child Development, Denver.

19. CHAMOVE, A., HARLOW, H.F., and MITCHELL, G.D. 1967. Sex differences in the infant-directed behavior of preadolescent rhesus monkeys. *Child Development*, 38:329.

20. CLARKE-STEWART, K.A. 1973. Interactions between mothers and their young children. *Monographs of the Society for Research in Child Development*, 38: (6-7, Serial No. 153).

21. CLARKE-STEWART, K.A. 1977. The father's impact on mother and child. Paper presented to Society for Research in Child Development, New Orleans.

22. COHEN, L.J. and CAMPOS, J.J. 1974. Father, mother, and stranger as elicitors of attachment behaviors in infancy, *Developmental Psychology*, 10:146.

23. CONDON, W. and SANDER, L. 1974. Neonate movement is synchronized with adult speech. *Science*, 183:99.

24. EARLS, F. 1976. The fathers (not the mothers): Their importance and influence with infants and young children. *Psychiatry*, 39:209.

25. EISENBERG, R.B. 1976. *Auditory Competence in Early Life: The Roots of Communicative Behavior*. Baltimore: University Park Press.

26. EWER, P. and GIBBS, J. 1975. Relationship with putative father and use of contraception in a population of Black ghetto adolescent mothers. *Pub. Health Rep.*, 90:417.

27. FREUD, S. 1923. *New Introductory Lectures on Psychoanalysis*. New York: Norton.

28. GATH, A. 1974. The impact of an abnormal child upon the parents. *Brit. J. Psychiat.*, 125:568.

29. GOMBER, J. and MITCHELL, G. 1974. Preliminary report on adult male isolation-reared Rhesus monkeys caged with infants. *Developmental Psychology*, 10:298.

30. GOODE, W.J. 1963. *World Revolution and Family Patterns*. Glencoe: Free Press.

31. GREENBERG, M. and MORRIS, N. 1974. Engrossment: The newborn's impact upon the father. *American Journal of Orthopsychiatry*, 44:520.

32. GURWITT, A. 1976. Aspects of prospective fatherhood. *Psychoanalytic Study of the Child*, 31:237.

33. HAMPTON, J.K. and HAMPTON, S.H. 1966. Observations on a successful breeding colony of the marmoset. *Folia Primatologica*, 4:265.

34. HARLOW, H.F. 1958. The nature of love. *American Psychologist*, 13:673.

35. HARTMAN, A. and NICOLAY, R. 1966. Sexually deviant behavior in expectant fathers. *J. Abn. Psychol.*, 71:232.

36. HETHERINGTON, E.M. 1966. Effects of paternal absence on sex-typed behaviors in negro and white preadolescent males. *Journal of Personality and Social Psychology*, 4:87.

37. HOWELLS, J.G. 1969. Fathering. In: J.G. Howells (Ed.) *Modern Perspectives in International Child Psychiatry.* Edinburgh: Oliver and Boyd.
38. HOWELLS, M. 1973. Employed mothers and their families. *Pediatrics, 52*:252.
39. JOHANNESSON, P.W. 1969. Instruction in child care for fathers. Dissertation at University of Stockholm.
40. JOHNSON, M.M. 1963. Sex role learning in the nuclear family. *Child Development, 34*:315.
41. KENISTON, K. (Ed.) 1977. *All Our Children.* New York: Harcourt, Brace, and Jovanovich.
42. KESSEN, W. 1970. Human infancy. In: P. Mussen, (Ed.) *Carmichael's Manual of Child Psychology.* New York: Wiley.
43. KLAUS, M. and KENNELL, J. 1976. *Maternal-Infant Bonding.* St. Louis: Mosby.
44. KLAUS, M. KENNELL, J., PLUMB, N., and ZUEHLE, S. 1970. Human maternal behavior at the first contact with her young. *Pediatrics, 46*:187.
45. KOLIN, I. SCHERZER, A. NEW, B., and GARFIELD M. 1971. Studies of school-age children with meningomyelocoele: social and emotional adaptation. *J. Pediatrics, 78*:1013.
46. KOTELCHUK, M. 1973. The nature of the infant's tie to his father. Paper presented to the Society for Research in Child Development, Philadelphia.
47. KOTELCHUK, M. 1975. Father-caretaking characteristics and their influence on infant-father interaction. Paper presented to American Psychological Association, Chicago.
48. KOTELCHUK, M. 1976. The infant's relationship to the father: experimental evidence. In: M. Lamb, (Ed.) *The Role of the Father in Child Development.* New York: Wiley.
49. LACOURSIERE, R. 1972. Fatherhood and mental illness: a review and new material. *Psychiatric Quart., 46*:109.
50. LAMB, M. 1975. Fathers: forgotten contributors to child development. *Human Development, 18*:245.
51. LAMB, M.E. 1976. Effects of stress and cohort on mother-and father-infant interaction. *Development Psychology, 12*:435.
52. LAMB, M.E. 1977. The development of mother-infant and father-infant attachments in the second year of life. *Developmental Psychology, 13*:637.
53. LANG, O. 1946. *Chinese Family and Society.* New Haven: Yale University Press.
54. LEVINE, J.A. 1976. *Who Will Raise the Children? New Options for Fathers.* Philadelphia; J.P. Lippincott.
55. LEWIS, M. and ROSENBLUM, L. 1974. *The Effect of the Infant on its Caregiver.* New York: Wiley.
56. LIEBENBERG, B. 1973. Expectant fathers. In: Shereshefsky, P. and Yarrow, L. (Eds). *Psychological Aspects of a First Pregnancy and Early Postnatal Adaptation.* New York: Raven Press.
57. LORENZI, M.E., KLERMAN, L.V. and JEKEL, J.F. 1977. School-age parents: How permanent a relationship? *Adolescence, 12*:13.
58. LYNN, D. 1974. *The Father: His Role in Child Development.* Monterey, Ca.: Brooks/Cole.
59. MACFARLANE, A. 1975. Olfaction in the development of social preferences in the human neonate. In: R. Hinde, (Ed.) *Parent-Infant Interaction* (Ciba Foundation Symposium, No. 33), Amsterdam: Elsevier.
60. McGRATH, L. and SCOBEY, J. 1969. *What is a Father?* New York: Simon and Schuster.
61. MARTIN, P. 1975. Marital breakdown in families with spina bifida cystica. *Dev. Med. Child Neurol., 17*:757.
62. MISCHEL W. 1976. Sex typing and socialization. In: P. Mussen, (Ed.) *Carmichael's Manual of Child Psychology.* New York: Wiley.
63. MITCHELL, G.D. 1969. Paternalistic behavior in primates. *Psychological Bulletin, 71*(6):399.
64. NATIONAL ACADEMY OF SCIENCES 1976. Toward a National Policy for Children and Families. Washington, D.C.
65. NEWSON, J. and NEWSON, E. 1963. *Patterns of Infant Care in an Urban Community.* New York: Penguin.

66. OLIVER, J.E. and TAYLOR, A. 1971. Five generations of ill-treated children in one family pedigree. *Brit. J. Psychiat.*, *119*:473.
67. ORTHNER, D., BROWN, T. and FERGUSON, D. 1976. Single-parent fatherhood: An emerging life style. *Family Coordinator*, *25*:429.
68. PARKE, R. 1979. Perspectives on father-infant interaction. In: J.D. Osofsky (Ed.) *Handbook of Infancy*. New York: Wiley.
69. PARKE, R.D., O'LEARY, S.E. and WEST, S. 1976. Mother-father-newborn interaction: effects of maternal medication, labor, and sex of infant. *Proceedings of the American Psychological Association*, p. 85.
70. PARKE, R.D. and O'LEARY, S. 1976. Father-mother-infant interaction in the newborn period. In: K. Riegel and J. Meacham (Eds) *The Developing Individual in a Changing World* (Vol. 2). The Hague: Mouton.
71. PARKE, R. and SAWIN, D. 1975. Infant characteristics and behavior as elicitors of maternal and paternal responsibility in the newborn period. Paper presented to Society for Research in Child Development, Denver.
72. PARKE, R. and SAWIN D. 1977. The family in early infancy: Social interactional and attitudinal analyses. Paper presented to Society for Research in Child Development, New Orleans.
73. PARSONS, T. and BALES, R. 1954. *Family, Socialization and Interaction Process*. Glencoe: Free Press.
74. PEDERSEN, F.A. 1975. Mother, father, and infant as an interactive system. Paper presented at American Psychological Association, Chicago.
75. PEDERSEN, F.A., ANDERSON, B.J. and CAIN, R.Z. 1977. An approach to understanding linkages between the parent-infant and spouse relationships. Paper presented at the Biennial meeting of the Society for Research in Child Development, New Orleans.
76. PEDERSEN, F.A. and ROBSON, K.S. 1969. Father participation in infancy. *American Journal of Orthopsychiatry*, *39*:466.
77. PEDERSEN, F., RUBINSTEIN, J. and YARROW, L. 1978. Infant development in father-absent families. *Journal of Genetic Psychology*.
78. PEDERSEN, F., YARROW, L., ANDERSON, B. and CAIN, R. L. 1979. Conceptualization of father influences in the infancy period. In: M. Lewis and L. Rosenblum (Eds.) *Social Network of the Developing Child*. New York: Plenum.
79. PLATTS, K. 1968. A public agency's approach to the natural father. *Child Welfare*, *47*:530.
80. PLECK, J. and SAWYER, J. (Eds.) 1974. *Men and Masculinity*. Englewood Cliffs, N.J.: Prentice-Hall.
81. QUEEN, S.A. and ADAMS, J.B. 1952. *The Family in Various Cultures*. Chicago: J.B. Lippincott.
82. RIGLER, D. and SPINETTA, J. 1972. The child-abusing parent: A psychological review. *Psychological Bulletin*, *77*:296.
83. REDICAN, W.K. 1976. Adult male-infant interactions in nonhuman primates. In: M.E. Lamb, (Ed.) *The Role of the Father in Child Development*. New York: Wiley.
84. REDICAN, W.K. and MITCHELL, G. 1973. A longitudinal study of paternal behavior in adult male Rhesus monkeys: 1. Observations on the first dyad. *Developmental Psychology*, *8*(1):135.
85. RENDINA, I. and DICKERSCHIED, J.D. 1976. Father involvement with firstborn infants. *Family Coordinator*, *25*:373.
86. RETTERSOL, N. 1968. Paranoid psychosis associated with impending or newly established fatherhood. *Acta Psychiat. Scand.*, *44*:51.
87. RHEINGOLD, H. 1956. The modification of social responsiveness in institutional babies. *Monographs of the Society for Research in Child Development*, 21, No. 63.
88. RICHARDS, M.P.M., DUNN, J.F. and ANTONIS, B. 1977. Caretaking in the first year of

life: the role of fathers, and mothers' social isolation. *Child Care, Health and Development*, 3:23.

89. RIVIERE, P.G. 1976. The couvade: a problem reborn. *Man*,9:423.
90. ROBSON, K. and MOSS, H. 1970. Patterns and determinants of maternal attachment. *Journal of Pediatrics*, 77:976.
91. RUBIN, J.Z., PROVENZANO, F.J. and LURIA, Z. 1974. The eye of the beholder: Parents' views on sex of newborns. *American Journal of Orthopsychiatry*, 44:512.
92. RUSSELL, B. 1958. *The Autobiography of Bertrand Russell* (2 Vols.) London: Allen and Unwin.
93. RYPMA, C.B. 1976. The biological bases of the paternal responses. *Family Coordinator*, 25:335.
94. SANDER, L.W., JULIA, H., STECHLER, G., BURNS, P. and GOULD, J. 1975. Some determinants of temporal organization in the ecological niche of the newborn. Paper presented at I.S.S.B.D., Guildford, England.
95. SCHAFFER, D., PETTIGREW, A., WOLKIND, S. and ZAJICEK, E. 1978. Psychiatric aspects of pregnancy in schoolgirls: a review. *Psychological Medicine*, 8:119.
96. SCHAFFER, H.R. and EMERSON, P.E. 1964. The development of social attachments in infancy. *Monograph of the Society for Research in Child Development*, 29, No. 94.
97. SMITH, S., HANSON, R. and NOBLE, S. 1974. Social aspects of the battered baby syndrome. *Brit. J. Psychiat.*, 125:568.
98. SOLNIT, A. and STARK, M. 1961. Mourning and the birth of a defective child. *Psychoanal. Study of Child*, 16:523.
99. SPELKE, E., ZELAZO, P., KAGAN, J., and KOTELCHUCK, M. 1973. Father interaction and separation protest. *Developmental Psychology*, 9:83.
100. STERN, D. 1974. The goal and structure of mother-infant play. *Journal of American Academy of Child Psychiatry*, 13:402.
101. STONE, L.J., SMITH, H. and MURPHY, L.B. 1973. *The Competent Infant*. New York: Basic Books.
102. STONE, L. 1977. *The Family, Sex and Marriage in England 1500-1800*. New York: Harper and Row.
103. TEW, W., LAURENCE, T., PAYNE, S. and RAWNSLEY, K. 1977. Marital stability following the birth of a child with spina bifida. *Brit. J. Psychiat.*, 131:79.
104. TOWNE, R. and AFTERMAN, J. 1955. Psychosis in males related to parenthood. *Bull. Meninger Clinic*, 19:19.
105. TINBERGEN, N. 1952. The curious behavior of the stickleback. *Scientific American*
106. TRETHOWAN, W. 1965. The couvade syndrome. *Brit. J. Psychiat.*, 111:57.
107. TRETHOWAN, W.H. 1972. The couvade syndrome. In: Howells, J. (Ed.) *Modern Perspectives in Psychoobstetrics*. Edingurgh: Oliver and Boyd
108. TRIVERS, R.L. 1972. Parental investment and sexual selection. In: Campbell, B. (Ed.) *Sexual Selection and the Descent of Man 1875-1971*. Chicago: Aldine.
109. TRONICK, E. 1977. The ontogenetic structure of face to face interaction and its developmental functions. Paper presented to Biennial Meeting, Society for Research in Child Development, New Orleans.
110. WEST, M.M. and KONNER, M.J. 1976. The role of the father: an anthropological perspective. In: M. Lamb (Ed.) *The Role of the Father in Child Development*. New York: Wiley.
111. WHITING, B. and WHITING, J. 1975. *Children of Six Cultures*. Cambridge: Harvard University Press.
112. YOGMAN, M.W. DIXON, S., TRONICK, E., ADAMSON, L., ALS, H., and BRAZELTON, T.B. 1976. Development of social interaction of infants with fathers. Paper presented at Eastern Psychological Association, New York.
113. YOGMAN, M., DIXON, S., TRONICK, E., ADAMSON, L., ALS, H., and BRAZELTON, T.B., 1976. Father-infant interaction. *Pediatric Res.*, 10:309.

114. YOGMAN, M. DIXON, S., TRONICK, E., ALS, H., and BRAZELTON, T.B. 1976. Parent-infant interaction under stress: the study of a temperamentally difficult infant. Paper presented to American Academy of Child Psychiatry, Toronto.
115. YOGMAN, M., DIXON, S., and TRONICK, E. 1977. The goals and structure of face-to-face interaction between infants and fathers. Paper presented to Society for Research in Child Development, New Orlenas.
116. ZELAZO, P.R., KOTELCHUCK, M., BARBER, L., and DAVID, J. 1977. Fathers and sons: an experimental facilitation of attachment behaviors. Paper presented at the Biennial Meeting of the Society for Research in Child Development, New Orleans.
117. ZILBOORG, G. 1931. Depressive reactions to parenthood. Amer. J. Psychiat., 10:927.

11

NEWBORN ORIENTATED PATERNAL BEHAVIOR: IMPLICATIONS FOR CONCEPTS OF PARENTING

Joyce Sullivan, Ph.D.

Head, Department of Home and Family Life,
Florida State University, Tallahassee

and

Darrell McDonald, M.S.

Director, The Family Development Birth Center
Los Angeles, California

FATHERING—MYTH OR REALITY?

The importance of the paternal role in the development of the child is one of the least understood concepts in human development. Empirical research in the field of parent-child relationships has largely been derived from data collected from maternal-child observations and interviews with mothers (25). The use and abuse of the term parenting have generated widespread myths and inaccurate assumptions inherent in commonly held concepts basic to parent-child relationships. The term parenting *per se* has been equated and confused with the concept of mothering to the extent that the paternal role has been almost totally ignored. The imbalance of concern for the maternal role at the expense of the paternal role has caused a distortion of interpretation of research in parent-child relations. Only in recent years have attempts been made to delineate distinctive paternal roles in relation to the infant and young child.

The somewhat limited amount of research which is available on the father's role frequently reflects negative connotations. Several researchers have reported that fathers are depicted in the literature as being relatively weak and inferior at parenting when compared with mothers (8a, 39). Children frequently view their fathers as hardworking, serious individuals who are extremely limited in the expression of joy and love (13). The call of occupation, whereby the majority of children are left to maternal care or maternal concern for that care, has, in general, caused fathers to all but abdicate their parenting roles. Brenton (9) suggests the concept of fathering is missing in contemporary culture. Young girls play with dolls, fuss over babies and actively practice caregiving skills. The fact that little girls will someday become parents is almost implicit in their cultural upbringing. This is not true with young boys.

In addition, wives generally view the appropriate role of the husband/father primarily as the provider, rather than the parent. In a study of 600 women in the Chicago area, 87 percent of the respondents selected the provider role as the most important function for their spouse over the roles of father and husband (26). Thus, in very subtle ways, mothers reinforce the expectation that parenting for men is not a primary or necessarily significant role.

Illustrations of females as the significant caregivers for young children in the child development texts perpetuate the notion that men do not belong in careers which involve care and concern for young children. The standard operational procedures of many traditional hospital maternity wards often regard the father as an afterthought or, perhaps, as a symbolic fringe benefit afforded the mother in consideration for her efforts in labor and delivery. The cultural warping of fathering roles in contemporary society could lead one to marvel that today's father accepts any nurturant parenting roles.

The significance of paternal role in the development of young children is extremely difficult to assess within the multiplicity of influences which act or react as contributing forces on human development. Numerous studies of children in fatherless homes have attempted to ascertain the effect of paternal deprivation on children. In a review of over 400 varied and somewhat fragmentary studies of children reared in fatherless homes, no conclusive significant evidence was found to substantiate the fact that children in fatherless homes were deficient in any aspect of development (17).

The inability to identify the effects of specific paternal roles with any degree of certainty has led researchers to examine the quality and quantity of father interaction with infants and young children. Several studies have quantified the amount of time fathers spend with young children. Findings range from an average of 37 seconds per day (34) to an average of eight hours per week (33) of father interaction time with infants under one year of age.

Some credit has been attributed to fathers in the dimension of sex-role development (1a, 3). However, little or no significant influence has been associated with the paternal role concerning processes of cognitive development or social learning. Lamb (22, 23) has extensively reviewed the literary accounts of maternal influence in these realms of child development, noting the lack of reference to paternal influence.

The critical importance of the maternal relationship with the child has been thoroughly documented for more than a quarter of a century (12). The literature includes numerous and detailed investigations substantiating that separation and/or maternal deprivation may result in pathogenic behavior in the child (4a, 6).

Only recently, however, have investigators examined the effects of paternal deprivation on child development (1a, 1b). The effects of optimal fathering on the development of young children has virtually been ignored by researchers. Unwed fathers, single fathers, divorced fathers and widowed fathers have received extremely limited attention in research.

If theorists are right regarding the tremendous amount of human intellectual, social and emotional potential available for development in the early years of life (4, 18), it is difficult to imagine why more attention has not been given to the role of the father in the early developmental years of the child—especially in societies where occupational patterns of husbands and wives are beginning to parallel. Assuming that it is advantageous for infants and young children to be involved with more than one significant person during early development, it is important to understand the full potential of fathers as full-fledged parents. If this perspective has validity, it behooves researchers to closely examine the processes of fathering as well as mothering. Variables which enhance and optimize the potential of fathering might be critical for both the child and the father.

MATERNAL AND PATERNAL BEHAVIORS WITH THE NEONATE

Pregnancy and lactation ascribed to the female have no doubt, been instrumental in the lack of concern for the paternal role during pregnancy, birth and early infant development. Since the mother carries the fetus en utero and lactates, she naturally develops an unique relationship with the infant. Recent studies on maternal-newborn bonding indicate evidence of powerful mechanisms available in the dynamics of the mother-infant relationship immediately postpartum, which if acted out, might help assure the performance of continual nurturant behavioral patterns during early infancy (20).

Maternal species-specific behavior following birth has received extensive attention in the ethological studies. Numerous investigations report predictable species-characteristic behavior of females directed toward their offspring (37). The initial characteristic maternal-neonate behaviors of most mammalian species are critically important to the survival of the young and to the continued willingness of the female to nurture her offspring. These characteristic behaviors may be dramatically altered if the mother and newborn are separated following birth.

There are few studies describing nonhuman male behavior patterns during the immediate postpartum period. The available literature suggests a marked uniformity of male-neonate behavior among noncaptive primates of monogamous social groups (35). These behaviors include inspecting, touching, carrying, cleaning, grooming and protecting infants.

Recent research has focused upon the phenomena of predictable and sequentially ordered newborn-oriented human maternal characteristic behavior that appears functionally related to the quality of the maternal-to-infant bond. Several studies have investigated initial newborn contacts and note remarkably uniform maternal behavior directed toward the newborn. Rubin (38, p. 829) reports that mothers move gradually from very small areas of physical contact to more extensive contacts. The maternal sample studied exhibited "a definite progression and an orderly sequence in the nature and amount of contact" during first encounters with their new infants. Initially, only fingertips were used to touch, then the lengths of the fingers and palms; still later, the arms were employed to touch and hold the infant. The direction of contact area was from the periphery of the mother's body inward, centripetally. The multipara progressed through these stages just as the primipara, although the progression appeared to be more rapid with the more experienced mother. Rubin (38) elaborates: "The initial contact made by the mother with her child are exploratory in nature; fingertips are used predominately. . . . The mother will usually run one finger up and over the baby's hair, rather than her hand. . . . She will trace his profile and contours with her fingertips. If she turns his head . . . she uses her fingertips; if she has to support his head . . . she uses the index finger and thumb (no palm); if she has to turn him over, she contacts him with her fingertips" (p. 830).

More recently, Lang (24) reported strikingly similar behaviors exhibited by most mothers experiencing home births. Prior to initial nursing, almost all of the mothers (N=52) began touching and stroking their newborn with the tips of the fingers. Mothers frequently initiated physical contact with their newborn by tracing the contours of the infant's head or other extremities. While holding their infants, most mothers assumed the *en face* posture and vocalized to them in an unusually high-pitched voice.

To objectively quantify human behavior at first encounters with the neonate, Klaus et al. (21) recorded the behavior of 12 mothers by taking pictures every second using remote controlled apparatus. Each fifth frame of the first nine minutes was then examined for stability and uniformity of newborn-oriented maternal behaviors. Detailed quantifications noted maternal fingertip touching, palming and progressive contact with specific areas of the infant's body. Results indicated strikingly uniform and stable newborn-oriented maternal behaviors. An identical sequencing of contact behaviors was observed in all mothers. Contacts began with fingertip touching of the infant's extremities, proceeding to encompassing palm contact with the infant's trunk or head.

The simultaneous increase of maternal interest in the infant's face and eyes also appears to be consistent from case to case. Klaus et al. (21) measured this interest by the amount of time spent in the *en face* position and the verbalized interest expressed concerning the infant's eyes.

It should be noted that these data were derived from behaviors exhibited in a highly structured parturient environment. All the mothers were in the same supine position when presented with their newborn, and all the infants were placed on the bed in the same position relative to the mother. No third person was present. Also, mothers had been separated from their infants prior to initial contact for a period ranging from 30 minutes to 13½ hours (average 5.3 hours).

From these studies, fragmentary evidence emerges that intial human maternal-newborn behavior appears to be stable and may be predictable within a specifically defined and controlled environment. Due to the impact that the environmental milieu may impose on species-characteristic behavior (31), investigations should present criteria of the parturient environment. Since mass hospital birthing is a relatively recent cultural development, it is suggested that this environment may not be uncritically conceptualized as a "natural" environment for human parturition (10).

Only a limited number of studies have focused on paternal behaviors during first encounters with their newborn. Researchers investigating father participation in early experimentation involving hospital rooming-in units suggest the neonate has a pronounced effect on paternal behavior (19, 27,

30). More recently, obstetricians have also reported that fathers exhibit an intense behavioral preoccupation with their neonates during early interactions (7, 29, 41).

A study at Charing Cross Hospital, London, investigated 15 fathers who were present at birth and 15 fathers who had initial contact with their newborn immediately subsequent to the birth (15). Results of this study suggest that neonates have a marked impact on initial paternal behavior. The investigators proposed the term "engrossment" to characterize the intense psychological involvement of fathers with newborns.

The researchers reported that one characteristic of paternal engrossment was an acute visual awareness of the neonate. This finding was consistent for both fathers present and fathers not present at the delivery of their offspring. One father elaborated, "When you wave yourself at her, wave your hand, she seems to try to follow you with her eyes . . . and once she looks at you, I don't know if she sees or not, but once she looks at you, and she's got really blue eyes, really dark and beautiful, really beautiful" (15, p. 526).

Another paternal behavior reported by Greenberg and Morris (15) was tactile awareness of the newborn; they stated, "There is a desire for and pleasure in the father's tactile contact with the newborn. . . . The fathers have the desire to touch, pick up, move, hold, and play with the newborn and they find it extremely pleasurable to carry this out" (p. 523).

Parke O'Leary and West (31a) compared the behavior of 19 fathers and mothers when first interacting with their newborn at University Hospital, Madison, Wisconsin. Observations made 48 hours after birth of middle-class, well-educated, caucasion subjects indicated that, behaviorally, fathers were very involved participants with their newborns and interacted with them as readily as did mothers. The data revealed that fathers spent an inordinate amount of time looking at and touching their newborn. Repeating the investigation with a large sample of lower-class, racially heterogeneous fathers in the Cincinnati, Ohio area resulted in similar findings.

PATERNAL BEHAVIOR AT INITIAL NEWBORN
CONTACT IMMEDIATELY FOLLOWING BIRTH

An investigation recently completed (28) was designed to systematically examine initial newborn-oriented paternal behaviors to determine if these behaviors might be stable and uniform. The following discussion reports the results of this investigation and the implications for new insights in the concept of parenting.

Selection of the Birth Environment

The birth environment selected is located in the Medical Arts Center, Kingston, Pennsylvania, under the supervision of William Hazlett, M.D. and Eleanor Mullen, R.N. In this birth environment the mother and father are prepared to effect the process of birth without direct intervention of the attending physician and nurse. The decor of the birth room is home-like in terms of furnishings, color, draperies and wall hangings. A noninstitutional single bed is used during birthing. Mothers may assume any position during birth which they find comfortable. Almost total privacy is maintained during labor and following delivery. During this period the mother and baby are unobtrusively monitored by the nurse. A fully equipped obstetrical unit is located adjacent to the Medical Arts Building in the Nesbitt Memorial Hospital.

The birth environment selected was based on criteria established to assure total spontaneity of the paternal behaviors under investigation. Seven newborn-oriented behaviors were delineated and examined for stability and uniformity to determine if these behaviors might be validly conceptualized as characteristic of human fathers (1).

Following the identification of the birth environment, a series of observations of father-assisted births in the noninterventive birth environment were conducted. Slides taken during these observations and a collection of slides of previous births in this environment were analytically reviewed. The initial observations and subsequent examination of the slides indicated that a more extensive investigation was warranted. Permission to videotape a consecutive sample of father assisted births was granted and subsequently two small video cameras were mounted on the walls of the birth room. Coax cables were installed connecting the cameras to a video recorder and a video monitor in a room directly across a hallway from the birth environment. From this monitor room, the birth and the immediate postpartum period were observed. This arrangement permitted most paternal behaviors to be observed on the video monitor and simultaneously recorded on videotape cassettes.

Paternal Behavior Identified and Defined

The initial pilot studies and the consecutive sample of videotaped recordings provided reference sources used to identify seven newborn-oriented

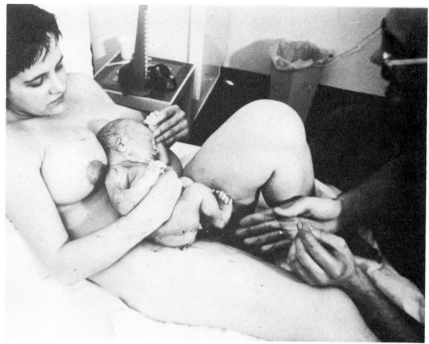

FIGURE 1. Paternal Shooting Behavior (Photo by E. Mullen)

behaviors, which were repetitiously exhibited by the fathers experiencing birth in the defined environment. These behaviors, illustrated in Figures 1 through 6, were defined* as follows:

> Shooting Behavior—The arms are extended from a vertical position at the shoulder and/or elbow toward the neonate. Fingers may or may not be extended and one or two arms or hands may be presented in the shooting posture.
> *Fingertip contact behavior*—Discernibly distinct motions of the fingers and/or thumbs, including up and down poking motions (21), stroking motions (24), or circular motions.
> *Palm contact behavior*—Paternal contacts the newborn with the entire surface of one or both palms including lengths of the fingers (38).
> *Hovering behavior*—A posture is assumed beside the bed in a standing, kneeling, sitting, or squatting posture or on the bed in a sitting or kneeling posture as the torso bends at the waist extending the head

*A detailed description of these behaviors may be found in the original research (28).

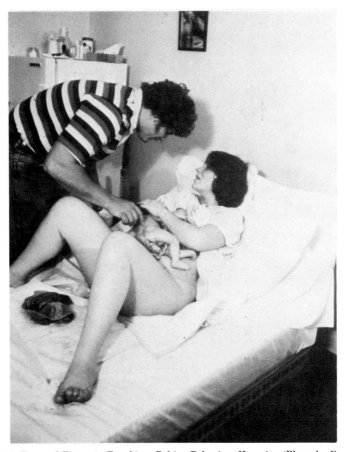

FIGURE 2. Paternal Fingertip Touching, Poking Behavior, Hovering (Photo by E. Mullen)

and shoulders toward and/or over the newborn. This posture results
in presenting the paternal face frontally toward the neonate.

Visual behavior—The father's face is presented toward the newborn
and his chin is elevated to an angle which intersects with the infant.

Prolonged gazing behavior—The father assumes a visual contact posture and exhibits this behavior continuously for an uninterrupted interval of ten seconds or more.

Face-to-face presentation behavior—Discernible posturing behavior
which results in presenting the face frontally in proximity to the neonate's face and aligned as fully as possible on the same vertical plane
of rotation elevation (26a, 36).

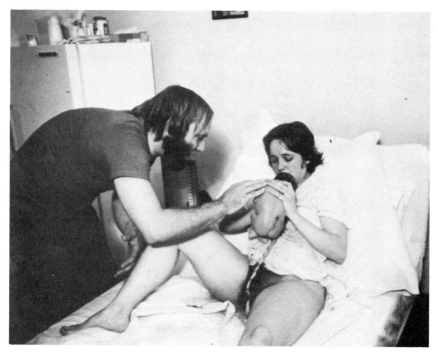

FIGURE 3. Paternal Fingertip Contact Behavior, Progressing to Palming Behavior (Photo by
E. Mullen)

Sample

Early in 1977, seven consecutive parturient couples who elected to birth
in the noninterventive environment and in father-assisted deliveries were
requested to participate in the study. The paternal sample was heterogeneous on several demographic variables, including socioeconomic background, ethnicity, educational level, age, geographical origin, parity and
occupation. It was a first birth for three of the couples. One father had
been present during one prior birth and had experienced noninterventive
access to the neonate immediately postpartum. Two of the fathers had been
present at a previous sibling birth but did not have access to the neonate
immediately postpartum. Thus, for all fathers except one, active involvement during birth and immediate and noninterventive access to the neonate
was a novel experience.

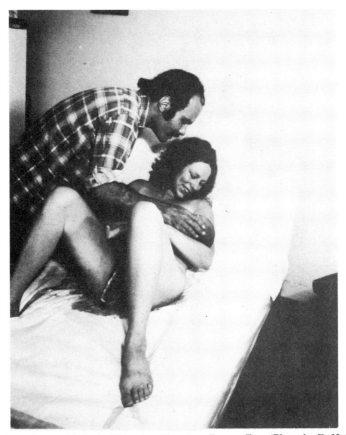

FIGURE 4. Paternal Palming Behavior, Hovering, Face-to-Face (Photo by E. Mullen)

Procedure

Between May and September 1977, the birth and the immediate postpartal period of seven cases were recorded on a Sanyo VTC7100 one-half-inch video recorder. Similar to the procedure in the Klaus et al. (21) investigation of maternal behaviors, the initial nine minutes immediately following birth were extracted from each of the seven videotaped cases. The initial nine-minute period of each case was then divided into three intervals, each of three minutes duration. These intervals were played at four-to-one slow motion on the VTC7100 and simultaneously transferred to soundless, three-quarter-inch videotape cassettes.

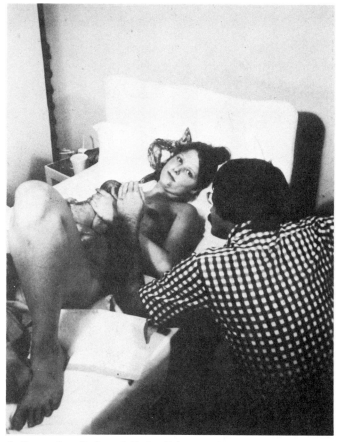

FIGURE 5. Face-to-face Prolonged Gazing Behaviors. Note Father Shields the Eye of the Neonate to Facilitate Gazing eye-to-eye (Photo By E. Mullen)

A secluded room was provided with a series of four video monitors wired to permit four observers to simultaneously, yet independently, view the slow-motion videotapes. The viewing carrels were isolated to assure the behaviors were independently scored. The observers were trained to discern the behaviors under study and attained significant reliability prior to scoring the sample cases (p = .01). Inter-observer reliability measures computed from the scoring of the behaviors indicated significant agreement was maintained during the quantification sessions (p = .01).

The technique used to quantify the behaviors required the observer to

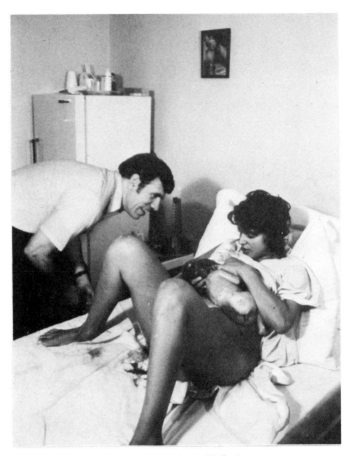

FIGURE 6. Paternal Hovering Behavior (Photo by E. Mullen)

depress a hand-held button as each of the selected paternal behaviors was exhibited and to release the button as the behavior ceased. Wires were routed from each observer button to an Easterline Angus Operation Recorder which provided graphic records of each observer's responses. The graphic recording charts were printed with time/date grids which made it possible to divide each three-minute observation interval into 288 units. Since it required 12 minutes to view each three-minute interval at four-to-one slow motion, each grid unit was equated to a time frame of two and one-half seconds. Frequency counts of the number of grid units on the charts divided by 288 (the total number of possible units) yielded interval proportion scores for each behavior exhibited during each three-minute observation interval (actual time). Observers identified and quantified one behavior at a time, resulting in each observer viewing each three-minute interval of each case seven times (once for each behavior under investigation). Thus a four by three by seven repeated measures paradigm may be conceptualized, whith an N of 84 and a sample size of seven.

Design and Statistical Treatment

Multiple Linear Regression (MLR) analysis and F-tests were used to calculate significant linear relationships between the paternal behaviors and the observation intervals under investigation; significance was established at alpha = .01. The Sign test was employed to test the directionality of the emergence of contact behaviors. The data were normalized and corrections for multiple comparisons and upward biased variance estimates were computed. The independent (predictor) variables included in the study were the three intervals, the subjects, the observers and neonate gender. The dependent (criterion) variables included the seven paternal behaviors under investigation.

Major Findings

Criterion variance accountability. To determine the criterion variance that can be uniquely attributed to the observation intervals, the three sampling periods were tested for accountability of criterion variance while the remaining predictor variables were covaried. The computations revealed the differences among the three intervals accounted for a significant amount of the criterion variance over and above the criterion variance accounted for by the covariates (p = .01).

The stability of initial paternal behaviors. Before the paternal behaviors were considered significantly stable, criteria was established requiring that each behavior be exhibited at least one-third of the first observation interval, as measured by the mean proportion score of each behavior. This criteria was based on the incidence of initial maternal-newborn behavior (21). Six of the seven behaviors studied complied with the established criteria. Palming behavior was exhibited only 11 percent of the time during the first interval and was, therefore, not considered stable. The statistical comparisons are presented in Figure 7.

The singularity of initial paternal behaviors. To determine if the initially stable behaviors might be significantly unique, the proportion scores (amount of time spent) of each initial interval behavior were compared with the

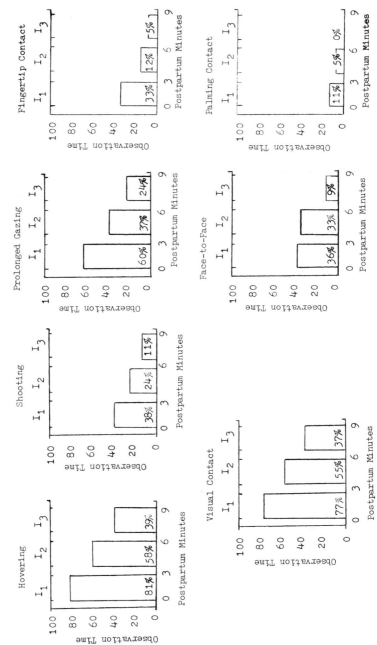

FIGURE 7. Interval (I) Proportion Scores of Seven Newborn-Oriented Paternal Behaviors Exhibited During the First Nine Postpartal Minutes

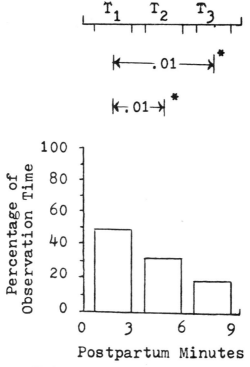

FIGURE 8. The Initial Three Minutes of Seven Neonate-Oriented
Paternal Behaviors Compared With the Same Behaviors Exhibited During Two Consecutive Three Minute Observation Intervals Of the Immediate Postpartum Period

* Two behaviors did not attain the .01 level of significance when the initial interval
was compared with the second interval: Face-to-face behavior (p = .075) and palming behavior (p = .205). Palming behavior did not attain the .01 level of significance
when the initial interval was compared with the third interval (p = .076). Eleven of
the fourteen one-tailed tests were significant at the .01 level. Multiple Linear Regression techniques were employed to compare each behavior between the intervals. I
= interval

interval proportion scores of the same behaviors exhibited during the subsequent intervals. Statistical analysis indicated that five of the six initially
stable (first interval) behaviors maintained stability during the second interval. Similar computations comparing each initial interval behavior with
the same behaviors exhibited during the third interval revealed all the initially stable behaviors were significantly diminished. These data strongly
indicate that stable and characteristic newborn-oriented paternal behaviors

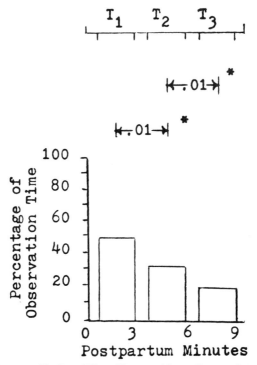

FIGURE 9. The Initial Three Minutes of Seven Neonate-Oriented Paternal Behaviors Compared With the Same Behaviors Exhibited During the Second Three Minute Interval and the Second Three Minute Interval Behaviors Compared With the Third Interval Behaviors

* Two behaviors did not attain the .01 level of significance when the initial interval was compared with the second interval: Face-to-face behavior (p = .075) and palming behavior (p = .205). Fingertip contact did not attain the .01 level of signigicance when the second interval was compared with the third (p = .122). Eleven of the fourteen one-tailed tests were significant at the .01 level. Multiple Linear Regression techniques were employed to compare each behavior between the intervals. I = interval

exhibited during the first three minutes of neonatal life are significantly more intense than these same behaviors when examined three and six minutes later. The significance of these comparisons are illustrated in Figure 8.

Once it was determined that the initial interval behaviors were characteristically stable and significantly more intense during initial encounters with the newborn, the behaviors were then examined to determine if they might emerge in uniform and predictable fashion across the three observation intervals. The first interval behavior was compared with the same behavior exhibited during the second interval; the second interval behaviors were then compared with the same behaviors exhibited in the third interval. F-tests were computed comparing the proportion of observation time these behaviors were exhibited between these intervals. These computations indicated the initial newborn-oriented paternal behavioral repertoire underwent uniform changes during the observation period that were significantly directional (one-tailed tests were computed). The significance of these comparisons are illustrated in Figure 9.

Sequencing of paternal contact behaviors. The ethological and human maternal research findings indicate characteristic newborn-oriented physical contact behaviors emerge sequentially. Thus, for this investigation, criteria were established which required paternal-newborn contact behaviors to also emerge in a sequentially uniform fashion if they were to be considered stable. Each of the fathers sampled made first contact with their newborn using the tips of their fingers, later proceeding to palming contact. This singular ordering of behavior was remarkably characteristic among the subjects studied (p = .001 as measured by the Sign test). The paternal sample examined initiated first contacts with their newborns in much the same centripetally ordered pattern reported to be characteristic of mothers.

Examination of the data indicated that the fathers exhibited markedly stable behavior upon initially encountering their newborn. Further, the intensity of these initially stable behaviors was significantly diminished when compared with subsequent samplings of the same behaviors; also, the initially stable behavioral repertoire emerged in a predictably uniform manner.

DISCUSSION

Results of the McDonald (28) investigation raises questions about parental-infant bonding and contemporary institutionalized birthing practices. The findings are not unlike results demonstrated in recent research examining maternal-newborn characteristic behaviors. The "burst" of stable and uniformly characteristic paternal behaviors oriented toward the newborn during the initial three minutes postpartum appear to be strikingly similar to initial newborn-oriented characteristic maternal behaviors which have been identified and discussed by Rubin (38), Klaus et al. (21) and Lang (24). These studies suggest further research is needed to determine if, in fact, there may be universally present behavior which is species-characteristic of human fathers and mothers at initial encounters with their newborn.

The following discussion centers on the complementary relationship between the stable, yet spontaneous, paternal behaviors delineated in the McDonald (28) investigation and stable, yet spontaneous, newborn behaviors and preferences documented in other investigations. The complementary quality of the interfacing of these behavioral repertoires appears to be functional in optimizing the quality of the father-to-newborn affectual bond.

Paternal hovering behavior results in the father's face being in proximity to the neonate and frontally presented. This posture locates the father's face in an area relative to the neonate which facilitates the newborn coming into visual contact with the paternal face. It has been demonstrated that the undrugged and untraumatized newborn, in the first minutes of life, will exhibit a preference for the human face and scan the environment to seek out this particular stimuli (14). Once a face is located, newborns will "lock-on" to it and spend prolonged periods engaged in eye-to-eye contact. These spontaneously exhibited visual interactions appear to release paternal engrossment and facilitate the formation of the paternal bond to the newborn. Paternal hovering behavior, then, by resulting in the father's face being presented in proximity to and directed toward the neonate, facilitates visual interactions with the newborn by presenting differentially preferred stimuli. Neonatal responses, in turn, facilitate paternal engrossment with the newborn and the formation of the paternal-newborn bond (15).

Paternal visual contact behavior was also pervasive during the initial observation interval. The available data indicate that fathers become visually encaptured by the newborn. Findings in the McDonald (28) study revealed most visual contact (60 percent) occurred during episodes of prolonged gazing (exceeding ten continuous uninterrupted seconds). This marked visual preoccupation with the newborn is harmonious with newborn preferences for looking at the closely presented human face.

Newborn-oriented paternal face-to-face presentation posturing also appears to be harmoniously interfaced with newborn behaviors and preferences. When face-to-face presentation behavior occurred, the fathers exhibited discernible behavior which resulted in presenting their face frontally to the infant's face and aligning their face as closely as possible to the same vertical rotational plane of elevation as the infant's face. This spontaneous yet stable paternal behavior appears to be particularly efficacious in precipitating neonate responses, since it has been demonstrated that infants respond differentially when the face is presented in the 0° presentation (i.e. *en face*) as opposed to the 90° or 180° facial presentation (43).

Thus, neonates exhibit visual preferences for the human face, and for the face to be presented on the same vertical rotational plane of elevation as their own face. Within the face, neonates find the configuration around the eyes particularly interesting (11,16,36,40). This neonate preference is synchronous with parental face-to-face presentation behavior. The complementary quality of stable newborn behaviors and stable paternal behaviors results in prolonged periods of paternal-newborn eye-to-eye gazing and appears to enhance father-to-newborn bonding (36).

The most interesting evidence indicated by the McDonald (28) investigation reveals that paternal behaviors directed toward the newborn immediately postpartum (in a noninterventive environment) closely parallel maternal behaviors which have been identified at first encounters with her newborn. Thus, both maternal and paternal newborn-oriented behaviors appear to be stable and uniform. Since the literature suggests that characteristic maternal-newborn behaviors may be functional in establishing the mother-to-newborn psychological bond, is it not unreasonable to theorize that stable and characteristic newborn-oriented parental behaviors may be functional in establishing the father-to-newborn bond?

A complementary relationship between stable paternal behaviors and stable newborn behaviors has been postulated. Further, the harmonious interfacing of these behavioral repertoires is suggested to be functional in establishing the paternal-to-newborn bond. These implications raise important questions concerning sibling-newborn interactions and the dynamics of family bonding.

Initial research investigating the processes of father-to-newborn bonding indicates that fathers may effect this psychological bond via behaviors similar to those exhibited by mothers at initial newborn encounters. Paternal bonding suggests powerful and meaningful implications for the nature of paternal-child interaction and for the process in which this interaction is not only allowed but encouraged.

Maternal and paternal roles need to be regarded as separate phenomena. The fact that maternal influences on the development of children are critically important does not suggest that paternal influences on the development of the child are unimportant. Parenting should be referred to as two distinct and complex systems of offspring-oriented behaviors. The unique and complementary nature of the maternal and paternal behaviors, both individually and collectively, needs to be addressed in the process of human development.

REFERENCES

1. BARNETT, S. 1973. Animals to man: The epigenetics of behavior. *Ethology and Development* (Clinics in Developmental Medicine No. 47, Spastics International Medical Publications). Philadelphia: J. B. Lippincott.

1a. BILLER, H.B., 1971. Father, child, and sex roles. *Paternal-determinants of personality development*. Lexington, Mass.: Heath-Lexington Books.

1b. BILLER, H.B. 1974. *Father power*. New York: David McKay.
2. BILLER, H.B. 1975. *Father, Child and Sex Role Paternal Determinants of Personality Development, 18*, 245-266.
3. BILLER, H.B. 1976. The father-child relationship: Some crucial issues. In: C. Vaughan and T. Brazelton (Eds.), *The Family—Can It be Saved?* Chicago: Year Book Medical Publishers.
4. BLOOM, B. 1964. *Stability and Change in Human Characteristics*. New York: Wiley.
4a. BOWLBY, J. 1951. *Maternal care and mental health*. (WHO, Geneva).
5. BOWLBY, J. 1958. The nature of the child's tie to his mother. *International Journal of Psycho-Analysis*.
6. BOWLBY, J. 1969. *Attachment and Loss* (Vol. 1). London: Hogarth Press and Institute of Psycho-Analysis.
7. BRADLEY, R. 1962. Father's presence in delivery rooms. *Psychosomatics, 3*(6), 474-479.
8. BRAZELTON, T. 1973. The effect of the maternal expectations on early infant behavior. *Early Child Developmental Care, 2*, 259-273.
8a. BRENTON, M. 1966. *The American Male*. New York: Coward-McCann & Geoghegan.
9. BRENTON, MYRON. 1972. The paradox of the American father. In: L. Howe, (Ed.), *The future of the family*. New York: Simon and Schuster.
10. BUREAU OF THE CENSUS. 1975. Historical Statistics of the United States; The Department of Commerce (Series A 57-72, p. 11). Washington, D.C.; The United States Government Printing Office.
11. FANTZ, R. L. 1965. Visual perception from birth as shown by pattern selectivity. *Annals of the New York Academy of Sciences, 118*, 793-814.
12. FREUD. S. 1940. *An Outline of Psychoanalysis*. New York: Norton.
13. FUCH, L. 1973. *Random Matters*. New York: Random House.
14. GOREN, C. C. 1975. Visual following and pattern discrimination of face-like stimuli by newborn infants. *Pediatrics, 56*(4).
15. GREENBERG, M., and MORRIS, N. 1974. Engrossment: The newborn's impact upon the father. *American Journal of Orthospychiatry, 44*(4).
16. HAITH, M. M., KESSEN, W. and COLLINS, D. 1969. Response of the human infant to level of complexity of intermittent visual movement. *Journal of Child Psychology, 7*,52.
17. HERZOG, E., and SUDIA, C. 1968. Fatherless homes: A review of research. *Children, 15*, 177-182.
18. HUNT, J. 1961. *Intelligence and Experience*. New York: Ronald Press.
19. JACKSON, E. 1948. A hospital rooming-in unit for newborn infants and their mothers. *Pediatrics, 1*, 28-43.
20. KLAUS, M. and KENNELL, J. 1976. *Maternal-Infant Bonding*. St. Louis: C. V. Mosby Co.
21. KLAUS, M., KENNELL, J., PLUMB, N., and ZUEHLKE, S. 1970. Human maternal behavior at first contact with her young. *Pediatrics, 46*, 187-192.
22. LAMB, M. 1975. Fathers: Forgotten contributors to child development. *Human Development, 18*, 245-266.
23. LAMB, M. E. 1976. *The Role of the Father in Child Development*. New York: Wiley.
24. LANG, R. 1972. *Birth Book*. Palo Alto, Ca.: Genesis Press.
25. LeMASTERS, E. 1977. *Parents in Modern America*. Homewood, Ill.: Dorsey.
26. LOPATA, H. 1965. The secondary feature of a primary relationship. *Human Organization*, Summer, *15*, 177-182.
26a. LUDINGTON, H. 1977. Postpartum development of maternicity. *The American Journal of Nursing*, July.
27. McBRYDE, A. 1971. Compulsory rooming-in in the ward and private newborn service at Duke Hospital. *The Journal of the American Medical Association, 145*, 625-628.
28. McDONALD, D. 1978. Paternal behavior at initial newborn contact immediately following birth. Unpublished thesis. University of Akron, Akron, Ohio.
29. MILLER, J. 1964. Fathers in the delivery room. *Child and Family, 3*, 3-11.

30. MONTGOMERY, J. 1952. Rooming-in of mother and baby in the hospital. *Illinois Medical Journal, 102,* 191-196.

31. NEWTON, N. 1977. Effect of fear and disturbances on labor. In: Steward and Stewart (Eds.), *21st Century Obstetrics Now!* (Vol. 1) NAPSAC, Chapel Hill, N.C.: NAPSAC.

31a. PARKE, R. D., O'LEARY, S. and WEST, S. 1972. Mother-father-newborn interaction; effects of maternal medication, labor, and sex of infant. *American Psychological Association Proceedings.*

32. PARKE, R. D., and O'LEARY, S. E. 1976. Father-mother-infant interaction in the newborn period: Some findings, some observations and some unresolved issues. In: K. Riegel, and J. Meacham (Eds.), *The Developing Individual in a Changing World, Volume II, Social and Environmental Issues.* Mouton: The Hague.

33. PEDERSON, F., and ROBSON, K. 1969. Father participation in infancy. *American Journal of Orthopsychiatry, 39,* 466-472.

34. REBELSKY, F., and HANKS, C. 1971. Fathers' verbal interaction with infants in the first three months of life. *Child Development, 42,* 63-83.

36. REDICAN, W. 1976. Adult male-infant interactions in nonhuman primates. In: M. Lamb (Ed.), *The Role of the Father in Child Development.* New York: Wiley.

36. ROBSON, K. 1967. The role of eye-to-eye contact in maternal-infant attachment. *The Journal of Child Psychology and Psychiatry, 8*(13).

37. ROSENBLATT, J. 1975. Prepartum and postpartum regulation of maternal behavior in the rat. *Parent-infant interaction* (Ciba Foundation Symposium 33). New York: Scientific Publishers.

38. RUBIN, R. 1963. Maternal touch. *Nursing Outlook, 11,* 828-831.

39. RUITENBECK, W. 1967. *The Male Myth.* New York: Dell.

40. STECHLER, G., and LANTZ, E. 1966. Some observations on attention and arousal in the human infant. *Journal of the American Academy of Child Psychiatry, 5*(517).

41. STENDER, F. 1968. *Fathers in the Delivery Room.* Bellevue, Washington: The International Childbirth Education Association.

42. VAUGHAN, V. 1976. Perspectives from ethology. *The Family—Can It Be Saved?* Chicago: Year Book Medical Publishers.

43. WATSON, J. S. 1973. Smiling, cooing, and "the game." *Merrill-Palmer Quarterly, 18*(323-339).

12

THE YOUNG CHILD AND
HIS SIBLINGS

Dora Black, M.B., F.R.C. Psych., D.P.M.

Consultant Child Psychiatrist, Edgware General Hospital, Edgware, and Honorary Consultant, The Hospital for Sick Children, London,

and

Claire Sturge, M.B.B.S., D.C.H., M.R.C. Psych., M. Phil.

Consultant Child Psychiatrist, Northwick Park Hospital, Harrow and Kingsbury Child and Family Centre, London

INTRODUCTION

Most children have siblings. Of a sample of children born in 1964 (26) five out of six children had at least one sibling by age 11. In the Ipswich Thousand Family Survey (50) 84.5 percent of families contained more than one child. In this study it was shown that at all ages a child spends more time relating to siblings than to father and by age ten is spending as much time relating to a sibling as to mother. Although common sense dictates that siblings must have a profound effect on each other, this subject has received scant attention.

The effects on the child of one or more siblings could be:

    (a) loss or deprivation of parental attention;
    (b) changes in the family configuration with consequent changes in the interactions between parents and child;
    (c) direct experience of interaction with the sibling(s).

For many young children the birth of a brother or sister provides their first experience of separation from their mother, as well as their first experience of sharing. Yet sibling relationships, both normal and abnormal, have received comparatively little attention from psychologists and psychiatrists. The recent interest in the origins of social behaviours and in the nature of attachment has tended to focus attention on parent-child relationships and peer relationships to the exclusion of the sibling relationships. Clinicians, too, have interested themselves little in the subject. A recent textbook of psychiatry (92) has only two references to siblings in the index. The psychoanalytic literature contains many references to sibling rivalry in case studies but there has been little attempt to examine in a systematic way the impact on a young child of the birth of a sibling or the effects of illness, handicap or death. Indeed, the majority of studies which purport to examine the effect on families of the presence of an ill or handicapped child ignore the siblings or mention them only in passing. With the development of family therapy there has been an increasing acknowledgement of the importance of sibling-sibling interaction (e.g. 82, 27). This may stimulate more systematic research, for at present there are no longtitudinal studies which examine the development of normal sibling relationships.

In this chapter, we review the four main areas of interest and research to date on the effects on children of siblings:

1) the reactions of young children to the birth of a sibling;
2) some personality traits, including intelligence, which seem to be related to ordinal position, sex differences and age gap between siblings;
3) factors associated with size and type of sibship; and
4) effects on young children of chronic illness, handicap, either physical or mental, and death of a brother or sister.

Some pathological sibling relationships are also considered.

REACTIONS OF YOUNG CHILDREN TO THE BIRTH OF A SIBLING

There is a dearth of research on the reactions of young children to the birth of a sibling, although many authors, for example Winnicott (122), Thomas et al., (111) and Moore (78), refer to the experience of a young child of having a new brother or sister as a major traumatic event and use such terms as displacement and dethronement. Even in the 19th century, the importance of this event was recognised in clinical practice; Descuret in 1841 (25) described a case of a seven-year-old wasting away after the birth of a sibling and a "radical cure" effected by putting the seven-year-old to the mother's breast. There is, however, no good study examining the reactions of young children to this event at the time. Legg et al. (66) studied children in 21 families through the arrival of a further sibling. There was no attempt to control for ordinal position, age gap or many intervening events, e.g., change of house. They showed that most of the children showed regressive reactions, many exhibited aggression towards the new baby and one developed an imaginary companion—a reaction also referred to by Nagera (79).

Thomas et al. (111) confirm these findings. Of the 18 families in which a younger sibling was born during the course of a study on temperament, over half the children showed moderate to marked disturbance. This disturbance took the form of either regression or aggression expressed towards the baby. Similarly, Powers (83) studied children three months before and after the birth of a sibling and showed adjustment difficulties and various problems in the control of anxiety in most of the children.

Taylor and Kogan (109), who observed mother-child interactions in eight dyads before and after the birth of a sibling, showed that both mother and children exhibited less warmth towards each other after the arrival. In a study currently being undertaken by one of the authors looking at the reactions of firstborn children to a new arrival, all children under four showed some negative reactions. As well as regression and aggression expressed towards the baby, some children showed aggression towards the mother, some to others, e.g., peers or pets; and some children exhibited a depressive type of reaction. In spite of the many opinions on the subject, there is insufficient research material to allow analysis either of the type of reaction shown at different ages or the "optimal age gap" in the sense of the age of children at which they show least disturbance when the next sibling is born.

Looking at the animal literature, Rosenblum (89) has shown that certain primates show reaction to the birth of a sibling. Pig-tail monkey infants showed a marked disturbance with the prominent onset of self-sucking behaviour and decrease in play and general activity. Chimpanzees, although affectionate to younger siblings, also push them off their mother's breast.

PERSONALITY DIFFERENCE ACCORDING TO ORDINAL POSITION, SEX AND AGE GAP BETWEEN SIBLINGS

On the personality traits (including intelligence) of siblings, particularly as related to ordinal position, there is an abundance of research, literally thousands of papers. This may be largely because ordinal position is such a simple variable for which to control. Most studies are on college students, usually by questionnaire, relating their ordinal position to such factors as intelligence, achievement, affiliation. In fact, there are enormous methodological problems in this type of research. Completed family size and social class have both been shown to be much stronger determinants of intelligence, achievement and some other personality traits than sibling position (40,88). Of course, social class and family size are not independent variables. For example, the significance of the finding that first children are overrepresented among eminent people depends mainly on whether family size, social class, and population trends are adequately controlled for. In addition, age gap and sex differences between siblings and, again, social class and family size have been shown to be as important as actual ordinal position (123).

In the following sections we will summarize the more consistent findings.

Intelligence and Eminence

The evidence for a birth order effect on intelligence is contradictory. Early writers, e.g. Francis Galton (33) and Havelock Ellis (28), produced evidence for the firstborn's being more intelligent than later born children, but methodologically their work is unsound. Terman (110) and Altus (2) argue that there is an overrepresentation, but not a general tendency, of firstborns among the highly intelligent. In large studies, Douglas (26) and Eysenck (29) found no evidence for the firstborn, being generally more intelligent than others. But this is contradicted by the largest study ever to date, on nearly 400,000 19-year-olds in the Netherlands (7), which is methodologically impeccable. They showed that within each family size, intelligence (tested on the Raven Matrices) declines with birth order and that the lastborn shows the greatest intellectual differential drop, i.e., greater than is accounted for by their ordinal position. They showed, as others (80) that intelligence declines with family size. Only children score relatively low, at about the level of the first child in a four-child family. On the basis of these figures, Zajonc and Markus (123) develop a fascinating model—the confluence model. According to this model, the intellectual growth of the child depends on his intellectual environment and this environment is diluted by having other siblings, particularly if younger. However, intellectual development is enhanced by having a younger sibling, near in age, to teach. This last explains the handicap to last and only children. The model also takes age gaps into account as an important variable.

If firstborn children are more intelligent than others, this might explain the general finding that they attain eminence more often than later born children. This view has been adhered to over a long period from Galton (33) and Cattell (19), through Altus (2) to Sutton-Smith and Rosenberg (108). But much doubt can be thrown even on this finding because of methodological weaknesses (cf. 100).

Psychiatric Disturbance

By far the most research has been done on sibling position and schizophrenia, with varying results, but these studies are not relevent here. Suffice it to say that the arguments of Hare and Price (40) throw doubt on all the findings to date.

In childhood most associations between disturbance and birth order are negative or contradictory. Thus there appears to be no relationship in autism or anorexia nervosa. Tuckman and Regan (117) and Shrader and Leventhal (104) found that firstborns were more often referred for child guidance help than lastborn children. Douglas (26), on the other hand, in a population study, found an excess of lastborn children with problems of bedwetting and maladjustment. This perhaps fits in with the developmental study of McFarlane (74) indicating that later born children have earlier externalised problems whereas firstborn children have later internalised problems. The explanation of these contradictory results may be that parents are more anxious about firstborns and so they are referred more often. Both Hersov (43) and Smith (106) found an overrepresentation of youngest children amongst school-refusers. Their control for family size current in the population was inadequate, but Berg et al. (8) confirmed this finding among adolescent school-refusers from three- or four-child families with good population controls.

Personality Traits

Most of the vast amount of research looking for associations between personality and sibling status is only relevant to the present chapter through inference. Findings regarding firstborn or lastborn children, or children with a particular sexed sibling, or with a particular age gap between them and their sibling(s) suggest that the existence of that sibling or siblings has had a marked and specific effect on the child. For this reason we briefly review the topic in spite of the lack of research actually examining the effect of the siblings on each other, directly or indirectly.

In this type of research, in addition to the methodological problems in dealing with sibling status mentioned, there are the problems of the reliability and validity of the tests for measuring personality traits. Also, many of the studies are with adults and their relevance to childhood is not clear.

The main areas of research interest have been: (a) ordinal position; b) age and sex differences between siblings; c) parental determinants of differences between siblings.

There are studies on almost every sibling constellation (see Sutton-Smith and Rosenberg's book, *The Sibling*, which tries to bring all these findings together(108)). The most consistent findings are of personality differences between firstborns and children in any other sibling position and, to a lesser extent, between lastborns as well as only children and children in other positions. Firstborn children, of either sex, are more dependent (affiliative), achieving and conforming (97, 119, 102, 85) and serious and sensitive (72). Only children (of course, also firstborns) are similar in their dependence and achieving, but Rosenberg's (108) work shows that first children with siblings have greater drives for achievement than those without. Only children apparently have greater self-esteem than first children with siblings and do not suffer any particular disadvantages. Youngest children resemble only children in these respects more than they resemble any other sibling position.

Not all studies are in agreement in these findings but the above represents the majority view (108). One of the reasons for the disagreement probably is the failure in many studies to control for sex and for the age gap between adjacent siblings. By far the most comprehensive studies taking these variables into account are those of Helen Koch (56-59). In large studies of five- and six-year-old children from two-child families, children did better on tests of mental ability if they had a brother within four years of age. Boys with "not-much-older" sisters were "sissy" on various scales as compared with boys with brothers.

Cornoldi and Fattori (21), in a study of college students, showed that firstborns with siblings less than three years younger showed greater affiliation needs than those with wider spacing.

These few findings extracted from the enormous literature (there is a listing of 1000 references (101)) illustrate the complexity of the subject. It is clear that sibling status, including ordinal position, family size, sex and age gaps, is important for the developing personality of the child. How these variables interact and how they are affected by the child's innate temperament and total life situation remain largely a mystery—and a very complex one.

Research on parents' behaviour with their children is more useful, particularly since at its base is a desire to understand how sibling differences are caused. Several studies have shown differences in parental, usually maternal, behaviour towards first- as opposed to secondborn children. This has been shown in infant-feeding (112), which is more efficient with second children, and in other behaviours: mothers are less warm and more restrictive, interfering and inconsistent with firstborns (23, 45, 64, 65), but also give them more attention (51, 65, 90). Cushna (23) showed mothers' expectations of firstborns far exceeded those for their other children; there were also differences in their expectations according to sex. Hilton (45) has used her results to formulate a hypothesis as to why firstborns develop such high dependence needs. She showed in a study of mother-child interaction that mothers were more interfering, extreme and inconsistent with their firstborn than with later-born children. She suggests that this undermines the first-born's attempts to develop reference points for self-evaluation and therefore results, in a broad sense, in marked dependence on the parents for this evaluation. All these studies on parents' behaviour show much more consistent results than those for birth order effects and are mainly based on observed differences in behaviour.

There seem to be no studies on sibling interaction as such which throw light on how the presence of siblings affects a child's development. The presence of siblings protects against some of the adverse effects of maternal separation (41). In Koluchová's study (61) of severe and prolonged deprivation, the twins, although severely deprived, made a full recovery, unlike another lone child; this suggests the presence of the other twin had a protective effect during the depriving experience (see chapters on twins in Sutton-Smith and Rosenberg (108) who discuss how these interactions could theoretically affect development).

SOME PARTICULAR SIBLING CONSTELLATIONS

The Only Child

In spite of early assumptions that only children were "spoiled brats" studies have shown that they have no specific disadvantages (18,48). Certain personality traits in only children are different from those in children with siblings (see above). There is a tendency for many children to display marked characteristics of the opposite sex (39). This appears to result from a particularly strong identification with the opposite sexed parent in one-child families. Belmont and Marolla's work (7) suggests, unlike that of Davis (24), that only children have no intellectual advantage.

Twins

There is extensive work on twins regarding their morbidity, their development, their concordance rates for personality, illness and deviance. Here we are concerned with the way in which having a twin affects the other twin. In this area there are a few direct observational studies. Of special interest is the finding of Costello (22), based on extensive observational work, that mothers are limited in their capacity to mother and that twins therefore each receive little more than 50 percent of the attention that a singleton receives. This may largely explain the finding that twins lag in development, especially linguistically (24), and is borne out by the finding that where a twin has died early in life, the level of intellectual functioning of the surviving twin is much nearer that of a singleton child (86). In Burlingham's classic study (12) of three identical twin pairs, she showed the dynamic interaction between the twins with their roles, in terms of dominance and passivity, interchanging, their similarity being continually reinforced both by their twin and by others. Helen Koch also studied twin relations (60). She found that same-sexed non-identical twins showed more problems than monozygotic twins. They were more aggressive and competitive and she postulated this was because they suffered the same comparison as monozygotic twins but without the twinship support between them. Opposite-sexed twins also had more problems than monozygotes.

The Large Family

There have been no findings suggesting any advantages to children in large sibships. There are studies showing membership of a large family to be associated with lower intelligence and poorer linguistic skills (80), antisocial behaviour (93), and pathology in adult life, e.g., alcoholism (105). Large family size is, of course, also related to low socioeconomic status, but the associations mentioned above hold even when social class is controlled for.

Sibling Interactions

A few general comments regarding sibling interactions are in order though one hesitates to state the obvious, especially in the absence of research confirmation.

The arrival of a new sibling is most likely met with resentment, whatever the age of the child. The resentment arises from the child's displacement within the family and is probably most difficult for the first child, who has no experience of sharing parental attention. An unexpected last child may present particular problems for the penultimate because he or she is displaced from the favoured last child position. Sibling rivalry occurs as a result of competition for parental favours. Regressive behaviours may be an attempt to receive that very close care and attention from which the new baby seems to be benefitting. If the new sibling is of the same sex as the child, rivalry may be heightened; if it is of the opposite sex, castration anxieties may result.

But there are also many positive aspects to this experience (27). Some children become rapidly more mature. A new baby brings out gentle maternal feelings, even in boys. The helplessness of the new baby may give the older child a feeling of superiority and mastery. The opportunity to teach can benefit both the younger and older child. Children learn to share and to cope with relationship problems. The younger child has someone to model, if even in a "reactive" sense of making opposite-sexed siblings behave more determinedly according to their sex (as suggested by some of Koch's work). Female siblings tend to make boys more masculine but not vice-versa. Balint (5) suggests that the occupation of a role by an older sibling may exclude a younger sibling from it, e.g., a girl with a very feminine older sister may take the role of her male counterpart. This would agree with the idea in many theories of family functioning of role assignment to each member of the family.

Sibling relationships are, of course, dynamic and continually changing. Many variables come in to this in addition to size and type of sibship, age gaps and birth order. The marital relationship, family patterns, new siblings, temperament of the individual and external factors all play a part. Sibling experience also plays a part in the success of marriages (54).

PATHOLOGICAL SIBLING RELATIONSHIPS

Sibling Incest

This is probably relatively common, though the incidence is obviously difficult to assess. Approximately 15 percent of the total of all types of incest are between siblings (70). The reason it is thought to be so rarely encountered in practice is that in many cases it apparently has no ill effects. Certainly, compared with other sorts of incest (70, 120), the perpetrators and their families are less abnormal and show many fewer signs of aftereffects.

Sibling Murder

Again, it is difficult to establish the frequency of sibling murder. Although the victim is classified as murdered, the murderer, if under 10, is not classified as such because he is below the age of criminal responsibility in England and Wales. In addition, some murders of this type are no doubt classified as accidental—where, for example, a child is drowned but, in fact, the family knows a sibling pushed him into deep water. In the period 1972-76, in England and Wales, children known to the police to have been murdered by a sibling have varied between three and seven per year. There are several single case histories of fratricide (1). The suggestion is that, in addition to the jealous feelings about the sibling (always younger), the child who murders has also been a witness or a victim of marked violence in his own life.

GENERAL EFFECTS OF ILLNESS AND HANDICAP ON FAMILY LIFE

Effects on Siblings

The majority of sibling reactions to illness and handicap are non-specific and common to siblings of children suffering from a wide range of conditions. The specific effects are considered below. Most parents report that the siblings of ill and handicapped children are affected to some extent, although in many cases the effects may be beneficial, such as the development of desirable character traits—tenderness, compassion, generosity, and protectiveness (6,13,63). Younger siblings are more likely to be adversely affected, especially if the ill child takes up an undue proportion of the mother's time (13) or there are many disruptions in family life due to hospital stays or financial hardship. Among older siblings, girls seem most vulnerable (30,36), probably because of excessive demands made on them to act as substitute mothers and mother's helpers. Most studies have not attempted to distinguish factors which modify the effect of the illness or handicap on the siblings but it is likely that the following factors will be ameliorating—mildness of the handicap (55), a large age gap between the affected child and his sibling (34,35,44,55), moderate family size(36,55), good marital relations(55), financial and housing security, and good professional and community support (37,38,55,98).

Psychiatric Disorder

Psychiatric symptomatology in siblings of ill or handicapped children, when it occurs (various authors report an incidence of from 0-50 percent), is non-specific; there is no characteristic disorder in the siblings of ill and handicapped children. Diseases which are known to be familial (e.g., muscular dystrophy, certain degenerative brain diseases, haemophilia, cystic fibrosis) and those which are life-threatening appear to affect siblings to a greater degree than chronic but non-fatal or non-familial conditions such as mental retardation or most physical handicaps.

Symptoms commonly reported among siblings are attention-seeking behaviour (55), jealousy (75,44), rivalry, (102) and aggression, which may be displaced from the handicapped child onto other children. The well sibling, if given an opportunity, will express many fears arising from his identification with the handicapped child (55), such as fear of physical attack, shame and embarrassment (20). Older children may have anxieties about their future—their marriage prospects and their chances of bearing an affected child (20).

Size of Family

Certain handicapping conditions may even affect the size of the family itself and thus determine whether there will be any younger siblings at all (47, 113, 114). Holt (47) has calculated that 34 fewer than predicted children were born in 160 families, where further pregnancies were possible, following the birth of a subnormal child. The reasons given for limitation of family size are the fear of another subnormal child and the attention needed by the child. A few families deliberately embark on pregnancy to prove that they are normal(6). Salk et al. (94) found that about half of their haemophilic families limited further pregnancies. Mothers of children with terminal illnesses may embark on another pregnancy; Friedman (32) found that 20 percent of his sample of mothers of terminally ill children were pregnant.

It seems that accurate genetic advice and counselling about contraception, amniocentesis and abortion should be available and *offered* to all affected families. It may be that Fraser and Latour's (31) finding that there was *no* reduction in fertility in the families of mongols they studied was the result of the availability of such counselling.

Effects on Family Life

All chronic illness and handicap has an impact on family life. Fewer outings are possible for the family or the married couple—especially as babysitters who are willing to undertake or can be trusted with the care of an ill or handicapped child are rare (81). The need of the child for special care may make it impossible for the mother to return to work (44) or for the father to accept a promotion if it means longer hours of work or moving away from a specialized centre (13,99). Thus financial hardships may be added to the other stresses of living with illness or handicap.

The parents' marriage is put under strain by the presence of an ill or handicapped child. In some cases the relationship will be strengthened, but often the additional care required by the child will lead to tension and possibly breakup. This, of course, will affect not only the handicapped child, but his siblings.

Most illness in children is acute and self-limiting or recovers swiftly with treatment. More children are now treated at home as we have come to realize the traumatic effects of separation and hospitalization. There are many studies which concentrate on the psychosocial effects of illness on the affected child and his parents. Unfortunately, in none of the studies reviewed below were the siblings interviewed and few of the studies compare their findings with a normal control sample. The criticisms of Kelman (53) about the design of studies on brain-injured children's families are relevant to all these studies.

The chronic physical illnesses which have been best studied are cystic fibrosis (13, 118), chronic renal failure (49,62,95), leukaemia (7,67,73), and congenital heart disease (3,68,71). With the exception of the latter, which consists of a heterogenous group of disorders, with widely differing prognoses, all these chronic illnesses are life-shortening and life-threatening and require an enormous investment of time and energy by parents for their treatment. The findings of various studies are very similar. Between one-third and one-half of the siblings are reported by their parents to have troubling signs and symptoms of disturbance. An important finding is the improvement in siblings following an improvement in the health of the child, for example, when stabilized on renal dialysis (49) or renal transplant (62), or in the less seriously ill children with heart disease (68).

The only controlled study (68) found that siblings did not differ significantly from well-baby controls on measures of general adjustment and personality variables. Those siblings who received more maternal "pampering" were better adjusted, although patients with high scores on "pampering" fared worse. This measure appeared to reflect different attitudes in the two groups—maternal pampering being the opposite of neglect in the sibling group, while it was a measure of overprotectiveness, as opposed to normal rearing, in the patient group. This confirms Kew's (55) finding that well children in families with a handicapped member are more likely to be neglected and to show attention-seeking behaviour. The only other controlled study in this area (44) also found no significant differences between siblings and controls.

Other Illnesses

Although asthma and eczema are the commonest chronic physical disorders in childhood, there appear to have been few systematic studies on the impact on family life of these diseases. Reddihough et al. (87) found that 40 percent of siblings were observed by both the parents and the asthmatic to ignore the asthma attacks. An equal number were helpful. Parents thought that 12 percent of siblings were frightened by the attack, but the asthmatic children themselves thought only 2 percent of their siblings were scared. In these and other chronic diseases, the extent of handicap is likely to determine the degree of disturbance in the child and his family. The epidemiological studies of Rutter and his colleagues (93) showed that in these two disorders and in epilepsy the vast majority of children were either not handicapped by their disease or only mildly handicapped. By contrast, handicap of a moderate, severe or extreme degree was common in brain disorders such as cerebral palsy, hydrocephalus, etc. and present in all severely subnormal children. Chronic degenerative familial brain disorders, while rare, have a particularly tragic impact on siblings who watch the dementia and death of their brother or sister, only to then become aware of the same symptoms in themselves. Atkin (4) describes these families as "doomed" and has pertinent and helpful suggestions about meeting their needs. Travis (116), like Atkin a social worker specializing in helping the families of chronically ill children, looks at the special problems posed by most common chronic illnesses and their impact on parents and siblings.

Physical Handicap

Physical handicap is usually non-progressive and may be very varied in its degree of severity. In two studies, Hewett et al.'s (44) of cerebral palsied children, and McMichael's (75) of children attending a special school because of severe handicap, about one-third of the siblings were jealous or otherwise disturbed. The former study was controlled and the findings were not significantly different from siblings in ordinary families. Minde et al.'s study (76) of a group of physically handicapped children in special schools attempts to correlate parental behaviour with outcome. The finding that parents who strive to make their handicapped child feel "like anyone else" undoubtedly took care away from well siblings accords with Kew's (55) suggestion that the presence of a handicapped child is "a social event capable of disrupting the balance of forces in an entire family group." His study, the only one in this area to focus on the siblings, uses the clinical material from 538 families to elaborate theories of family functioning—of which the concept of role allocation in the family seems most fruitful. The presence of a handicapped child may distort role allocation so that the well sibling may be overvalued or may have to achieve *all* the parental expectations.

Mental Handicap

Studies of the siblings of the mentally handicapped have been more satisfactory than those we have described above. At least two controlled studies are reported (34,36,37) and teenage siblings of the mentally handicapped have been interviewed (17,38).

Holt (46) studied 201 families containing a severely retarded child. Of the 432 siblings, 24 (mainly younger sibs) were reported as being very fearful because of repeated physical attacks by the retarded child, and 19 (mainly older siblings) were felt to be tired and doing poorly at school because of having to help unduly in the house. A further 20 were attention-seeking or withdrawn and 10 experienced severe shame and embarrassment which seemed related to the parents' attitudes towards mental handicap.

Tizard and Grad (114), comparing the families of mentally handicapped children living at home and families of those in institutions, found that twice as many of the institutionalized group had a sibling who was maladjusted or mentally backward (26 percent compared with 12 percent). It was likely that the presence of two handicapped or difficult children in the home was the main reason for the parents' seeking institutional care and the authors did not find evidence that keeping the retarded child in the family was a potent source of stress to the siblings. However, the families with a handicapped child at home were significantly more likely to have limited social contacts, compared with the institutionalized group.

Gath (34) compared the school-age siblings of 22 children with Down's syndrome (mongolism) living at home with children with surgically treated cleft lip/palate using the Rutter behavioural questionaires. No differences were found between either index group and the population norms.

In another, larger study (35), Gath compared randomly selected classroom controls with each sibling of 108 mongol children living at home. Significantly more of the female siblings than of the controls, had antisocial disorders. This was more marked if the mother was over 40 at the birth of the handicapped child, if the family contained more than five children and if they belonged to social class IV and V. The most common symptoms were poor peer relationships (75 percent), restlessness (64 percent), disobedience (55 percent), misery (53 percent), and tempers and irritability (53 percent).

Gath's first study (34) controlled more carefully for family size and ordinal position and it is possible that the greater incidence of antisocial disorder in the index group is a reflection of the lower social class and larger family size of that group compared with the controls; these are factors which are known to influence deviancy. In order to study this, Gath (36) compared the female with the male siblings of the mongol children studied in the previous paper (35). Eighteen percent of the brothers of mongols and 14 percent of the sisters were rated on the Rutter teachers' scale as deviant. Compared with the control population used by Rutter (93) significantly more female siblings were disturbed, whereas the incidence of disturbance in the males was similar to the controls. The vulnerable girls were mainly firstborn and were usually more than three years older than the handicapped child. Gath considered that the girls were at risk because of their greater responsibility for domestic work and child care in the family compared with their non-handicapped brothers and points out that girls, while more resistant to developing antisocial disorder than boys, can succumb if the stress is great enough.

A prospective controlled study by the same author (37) compared the amount of time mothers of normal babies and mothers of mongols spent with the older sibling before the baby's birth and between one and two years' afterwards. The older siblings of mongols had more of mother's time than the older siblings of normal babies. All the mongols were only two years old at the end of the study but it is possible that differences between this study and the previous ones reflect the improvements in counselling and support available for the families of the handicapped in the last few years. However, it may also be due to the fact that the mongol child is less mobile and therefore less of a nuisance when small, although this is not the case when he is older.

Caldwell and Guze (17) studied 32 retarded children and examined one of their siblings (10-16 years) for intelligence and manifest anxiety by means of Standford Binet tests and a structured clinic interview. They were comparing the siblings of retarded children at home and in institutions. There were no significant differences between the home and institution based groups. Graliker et al. (38) interviewed 21 teenage siblings of mentally retarded children under six years of age living at home. These siblings accepted the handicapped child and were free from significant problems in those families where the parents shared a common attitude towards the handicap. The good mental health of these siblings may have been a function of the fact that all the families were being counselled. There was no control group.

San Martino and Newman (96) present four case studies of the siblings of retarded children seen at a child guidance clinic and suggest that there is important work to be done by intervening early to prevent morbidity in the families of handicapped children. They suggest that parental guilt for having produced a handicapped child is projected onto the normal sibling, who is then held responsible for the trouble. Parental anger towards the well sibling is really displaced from the handicapped one and the normal child identifies with his sibling to ward off anxiety and to increase parental acceptance. Studying the family myths may lead to a useful treatment plan. A similar mechanism is proposed by Kaplan (52) in her single case study, as a result of which she suggests that group discussions with the siblings of the retarded may prevent morbidity.

The Death of a Sibling

Childhood bereavement as a specific stress which may affect personality development and mental health has been given considerable attention (10,11,91). However, most studies have been concerned with the death of a parent; there have been few studies of the effect of sibling loss.

Cain, Fast and Erickson's (16) paper, the only comprehensive survey of the reactions of children to sibling death, is based on a retrospective case note study of psychiatric patients. It is by no means a systematic study and lacks scientific method, but it is rich in case material and attempts to classify the disturbed reactions under a number of headings, including guilt reactions, distorted concepts of death, disturbed attitudes, phobias, cognitive disturbances, etc. They emphasize the need to include all the family members in plans made for helping bereaved families and the importance of paying particular attention to the effect of the death on family dynamics. They draw attention again to the concept of developmental level of the child in trying to understand his or her reactions and they recognize the extensive and varied reactions to the death and the possibility of later as well as immediate reactions. These reactions are as much a result of the behaviour of those around them as of the child's own internal responses (15).

Lindsay and MacCarthy (69), in reviewing the sparse literature on the siblings of dying children, draw attention to the conflict between the needs of the parents to withdraw and mourn and the needs of the other children for warmth and care. The stress of a death of a child or impending death is severe and parental reactions are likely to be crucial in determining the coping capacity of the siblings, especially the younger ones.

The impact of stillbirth and miscarriage on siblings has received even less attention. Cain et al. (14) have published a clinical study of psychiatric patients of all ages where a miscarriage appeared to have a disruptive psychological effect on the children. We know of no systematic studies in this area.

Summary

Interactions between well siblings and the ill, dying and handicapped and how they affect behaviour, development, and personality appear to have attracted little research attention. Most studies find about one-third of siblings affected and it is likely that the stresses on parents resulting from having an ill or handicapped child affect the quantity and quality of their interactions with their other children. Where early support and intervention services exist, siblings cope better. It is probable that most sibling problems arising from the presence of an ill or handicapped child could be prevented or mitigated if such services were extended and improved. The need for research into coping strategies and modifying factors is obvious.

CONCLUSIONS

In this chapter we have attempted to review what is a confused and uneven research literature. It might be helpful to summarise and bring together the more important findings.

A child's position in a sibship is reflected in certain personality traits and his liability to develop childhood psychiatric disorders. The evidence is that this is a result of the interactions between parental attitudes, the child's temperament and his relations with his siblings. But there is little research trying to tease out these relationships in spite of the generally observed major upheaval in a child's life when a sibling is born. In psychosocial research not only the birth of a sibling but also the leaving home, hospitalisation or death of a sibling are considered major life events and contribute significantly to acute and chronic physical and mental diseases of children (42).

The quality and quantity of research into the effects on children of illness, handicap and death of a sibling are generally poor, with the notable exception of the work of Gath and Hewett (34,35,36,37,44). Life experiences of these kinds are likely to have their impact modified by temperamental variables and the child and parental attitudes as mentioned above.

The most fruitful approach, though not based on research, to understanding the complex interactions between family members lies in the theory of family systems. Systems theory views the family as a unit as greater than the mere sum of the attributes of the individual members. It consists of various subsystems which are dynamic in themselves and interact with each other, for example, the spouse and sibling subsystems. Minuchin (77) sees the sibling subsystem as "the first social laboratory in which children can experiment with peer relationships. Within this context children support, isolate, scapegoat and learn from each other. In the sibling world, children learn how to negotiate, cooperate and compete. They learn how to make friends and allies, how to save face while submitting, and how to achieve recognition of their skills. They may take different positions in their jockeying with one another and those positions, taken early in the sibling subgroup, can be significant in the subsequent course of their lives'' (p. 59).

Attempts are being made to understand role assignment within families (115) and this could lead to a reformulation of the adjustments necessary in the family dynamics where there is a new arrival or loss of a family member. Siblings obviously have a great impact on each other. We see their learning to cope, with the help of parents, with change, envy, sharing, competitiveness and rivalry as constructive since it gives the opportunity to develop essential social skills. In childhood the advantages and disadvantages of having siblings perhaps balance out; there is very little handicap in being an only child. However, the advantage of the sibling experience is perhaps shown in adult life in that only children appear to make less successful marriages (121).

The clinical implications of the few available findings are that it is important to develop a body of knowledge of the effect on children of various life events, in order that parents can be counselled in dealing with these. In addition, knowledge of the common patterns of sibling interaction and how these can be modified by the factors we have been considering would be of enormous value to parents and clinicians alike.

REFERENCES

1. ADELSON, L. 1972. The battering child. *J. Amer. Med. Assn.*, 222, p. 159.
2. ALTUS, W.D. 1966 Birth order and its sequence. *Science*, 151, p. 44.
3. APLEY, J., BARBOUR, R.F., and WESTMACOTT, I. 1967 Impact of Congenital Heart Disease on the Family: Preliminary Report. *Br.Med.J. I*, 103.
4. ATKIN, M. 1974 The 'doomed family.' In: L. Burton (Ed.), *Care of the Child Facing Death*. London: Routledge & Kegan Paul.
5. BALINT, M. 1963 The younger sister and prince charming. *The International Journal of Psychoanalysis*, Vol. 44, p.226-227.
6. BARSCH, R.H. 1968 *The Parents of the Handicapped Child. The Study of Child Rearing Practices*. Springfield, Ill.: Thomas.
7. BELMONT, L. and MAROLLA, F.A. 1973 Birth order, family size and intelligence. *Science*, 182, p.1096.
8. BERG, I., BUTLER, A., and McGUIRE, R., 1972. Birth order and family size of school phobic adolescents. *Br.J.Psych.*, 121, 509.
9. BINGER, C.M., ABLIN, A.R., FEUERSTEIN, R.C. KUSHNER, J.H., ZOGER, S., and MIKKELSEN, C., 1969 Childhood leukemia, emotional impact on patient and family. *New Eng.J.Med.*, 280:8, 414.

10. BLACK, D. 1978 The Bereaved child. *J.Child Psychol.Psychiat.,19:287-292.*
11. BOWLBY, J. 1961 Childhood mourning and its implications for psychiatry. *Amer.J.Psychiat.,* 118:481.
12. BURLINGHAM, D 1952. *Twins—A Study of Three Pairs of Identical Twins.* London: Imago.
13. BURTON, L. 1975 *The Family Life of Sick Children.* London: Routledge & Kegan Paul.
14. CAIN, A.C., ERIKSON, M.E., FAST, I., and VAUGHAN, R. 1964 Children's Disturbed reactions to their mothers' miscarriage. *Psychosomatic Med.,* 26:1, 58.
15. CAIN, A.C., and CAIN, B.S. 1964 On replacing a child. *J.Amer.Acad. Child Psychiat., 3,* 443.
16. CAIN, A.C., FAST, I., ERICKSON, M.E. 1964 Childrens disturbed reactions to the death of a sibling. *Amer.J.Orthopsychiat., 36,* 741.
17. CALDWELL, B.M. and GUZE, S.B. 1960 A study of the adjustment of parents and siblings of institutionalized and non-institutionalized retarded children. *Amer.J.Mental Def., 64,* 845.
18. CAMPBELL, A.A. 1933 A study of personality adjustments of only and intermediate children. *J.of Genet.Psychol., 33,* 197.
19. CATTELL, J.M. 1917 American men of science. *Science Monthly,* 5, p. 371.
20. COLEMAN, R.F. 1967 Groupwork with brain-injured children and their siblings. Report of the 4th Annual Conference of the Association for Children with Learning Disabilities. New York.
21. CORNOLDI, C. and FATTORI, L.C. 1976 Age-spacing in first-borns and symbiotic dependence. *J.Personality. Soc.Psychol.,* 33 4, 431.
22. COSTELLO, A. 1974 Are mothers stimulating? *New Scient.,* May 9.
23. CUSHNA, B. 1966 Agency and birth order differences in very early childhood. Paper presented at the meeting of the American Psychological Association in September, New York.
24. DAVIS, E.A. 1937 *Development of Linguistic Skills in Twins.* Univ. Minnesota Press.
25. DESCURET, J.B. 1841 Jalousie dans un enfant de sept ans. in "La Medicine des passions". Transl. by A.B. Hooton (1971) *Bull.Hist.Med.* 45, 380.
26. DOUGLAS J.W.B. 1944 *The Home and the School: A Study of Ability and Attainment in the Primary School.* London: MacGibbon & Kee.
27. EINSTEIN, G. and MOSS, M.S. 1967 some thoughts on sibling relationships. *Soc.Case Work,* 48, 9
28. ELLIS, HAVELOCK 1926 *A Study of British Genius.* Boston: Houghton, Miffton.
29. EYSENCK, H.J. and COOKSON, D. 1970 Personality in primary school children. 3 - Family Background. *Brit.J.Educ.Psychol.,* 40, p.117.
30. FARBER, B. 1959 Effects of severely mentally retarded children on family integration. *Monographs of the Society for Research in Child Development, 24,* 2.
31. FRASER, F.C. and LATOUR, A. 1968 Birth rates in families following birth of a child with mongolism. *Amer.J.Mental Def., 72,* 883.
32. FRIEDMAN, S.B., CHODOFF, M.D., MASON, J.W. and HAMBURG, D.A. 1963. Behavioural observations on parents anticipating the death of a child. *Pediatr., 32,*610.
33. GALTON, F. 1883 *Enquiries into Human Faculty* (170). London: Eugenics Society.
34. GATH, A. 1972 The mental health of siblings of congenitally abnormal children. *J.Child Psychol.Psychiat., 13:3,* 211.
35. GATH, A. 1973 The school-age siblings of mongol children. *Brit.J. Psychiat., 123:573.* 161.
36. GATH, A. 1974 Sibling reactions to mental handicap: A comparison of the brothers and sisters of Mongol children. *J.Child Psychol.Psychiat., 15:3,* 187.
37. GATH, A. 1978 *Downs Syndrome and the Family.* London.: Academic Press.
38. GRALIKER, B., FISHLER, K. and KOCH, R. 1962 Teenage reaction to a mentally retarded sibling. *Amer.J.Mental Deficiency, 66,*838.
39. GUNDLACH, R.H. and RIESS, B.F. 1967 Birth order and sex of siblings in a sample of

lesbians and non-lesbians. *Psychol. Reports*, 20,61.

40. HARE, E. H. and PRICE,J.S. 1970 birth rank and schizophrenia with a consideration of the bias due to changes in birth rate. *Brit.J.Psychiat.*, 116, 409.

41. HEINICKE, C. and WESTHEIMER, I.J. 1965 *Brief Separations*, London: Longmans.

42. HEISEL, J.S., REAM, S., RAITZ, B.S., RAPPAPORT. M. and CODDINGTON, R.D. 1973 The significance of life events as contributing factors in the disease of children. III A study of pediatric patients. *J.Pediatr.*, 83 (i) 119.

43. HERSOV, L.A. 1960 Persistent non-attendance at school. *J. of Child Psychol. Psychiat.*, 1 (2), 130.

44. HEWETT, S, NEWSOM, J. and NEWSOM, E. 1970 *The Family and the Handicapped Child.* London: George Allen & Unwin.

45. HILTON, I. 1967 Differences in the behaviour of mothers towards first and later-born children. *J.of Personality & Soc.Psychol.*, 7, 282.

46. HOLT, K.S. 1958 The home care of severely retarded children. *Pediatrics*, 22:4 744.

47. HOLT, K.S. 1958b The influence of a retarded child upon family limitation. *J.Mental Def. Res.*, 2,28.

48. HOOKER, H.F. 1931 The study of the only child at school. *J.of Genet.Psychol.*, 39, 122.

49. HOWARTH, R. 1976 "The psychosocial impact of renal dialysis of children at home." Paper presented at Conference of the European Working Party on Children with Chronic Renal Disease, Heidelberg.

50. HOWELLS, J.G. 1976 *Principles of Family Psychiatry*. London: Pitman Publishing Ltd.

51. JACOBS, B.S. and MOSS, H.A. 1974 Birth order and sex of sibling as determinants of mother-infant interaction. Paper presented to Amer. Psycho. Ass.

52. KAPLAN, F. 1969 Siblings of the retarded, In: S.B. Sarason and J.L. Doris (Eds.), *Psychological Problems in Mental Deficiency* New York: Harper & Row.

53. KELMAN, H.R. 1964 The effect of a brain-damaged child on the family. In: H.G. Birch, (Ed.), *Brain Damage in Children*. New York: Williams & Wilkins.

54. KEMPER, T.D. 1966 Mate selection and marital satisfaction according to sibling type of husband and wife. *J.Marr.Fam.Living.*, 28, 346.

55. KEW. S. 1975 *Handicap & Family Crisis—A Study of the Siblings of Handicapped Children*. London: Pitman Publishing.

56. KOCH, H.L. 1954 The relations of "primary mental abilities" in five and six year olds to sex of child and characteristics of his sibling. *Child Develop.*, 25, 209.

57. KOCH, H.L. 1955a. The relation of certain family constellation characteristics and the attitudes of children towards adults. *Child Develop.*, 26, 13.

58. KOCH, H.L. 1955b. Some personality correlates of sex, sibling position & sex of sibling among five and six year old children. *Genet.Psychol.Monog.*, 52, 3.

59. KOCH, H.L. 1956 Children's work attitudes and sibling characteristics. *Child Develop.*, 27, 289.

60. KOCH, H.L. 1966 *Twins and Twin Relations*. Chicago:University of Chicago Press.

61. KOLUCHOVÁ, J. 1976 The further development of twins after severe and prolonged deprivation. A second report, *J.Child Psychol.Psychiat.*, 17 (3) 181.

62. KORSCH, B.M., NEGRETE, V.F., GARDNER, J.E., WEINSTOCK, C.L., MERCER, A.S., GRUSHKIN, C.M. and FINE, R.N. 1973. Kidney transplantation in children: Psychosocial follow-up study on child and family. *J. Pediatr.*, 83:3, 399.

63. KRAMM, E.R. 1963 Families of Mongoloid Children. Childrens Bureau Publication No. 401. Washington, D.C.: U.S. Government Printing Office.

64. LASKO, J.K. 1954 Parent behaviour toward first and second children. *Genet.Psychol.Monogr.*, 49, 96.

65. LAWSON, A. and INGLEBY, D.J. 1974 Daily routines of pre-school children, effects of age, birth order, sex, social class and developmental correlates. *Psychol.Med.*, 4, 399.

66. LEGG, C., SHERICK, I. and WADLAND, W. 1971 Reaction of pre-school children to birth of a sibling. *Child Psychol. & Human Develop.*, 5 (1) 3.

67. LEWIS, I.C. 1967 Leukemia in childhood: Its effects on the family. *Aust.Paediat.J.*, *3*, 244.
68. LINDE, L.M., RASO, F.B., DUNN, O.J. and RABB, E. 1966 Attitudinal factors in congenital heart disease. *Pediatrics*, *38*,92.
69. LINDSAY, M. and MACCARTHY, D. 1974 Caring for the brothers and sisters of a dying child. In: L. Burton (Ed.), *Care of the Child Facing Death*. London: Routledge & Kegan Paul.
70. LUKIANOWICZ, N. 1972 Incest. *Brit.J.Psychiat.*, 120,301.
71. MAXWELL, G.M. and GANE, S. 1962 The impact of congenital heart disease upon the family. *Am.Heart J.*, *64*,449.
72. MCARTHUR C. 1956 Personalities of first and second children. *Psychiatry*, 19, 47.
73. MCCARTHY, M. 1975 Social aspects of treatment in childhood leukemia. *Soc.Sci. & Med.*, 9:263.
74. MCFARLANE, J.W., ALLEN, L. and HONZIK, M.P. 1954 A developmental study of the behaviour problems of normal children between twenty-one months and fourteen years. Univ. of California Publications in Child Develop. 2.
75. MCMICHAEL, J.K. 1971 *Handicap—A Study of Physically Handicapped Children and Their Families*. London: Staples Press.
76. MINDE, K., HACKETT, J.D., KILLOU, D. and SILVER, S. 1972 How they grow up. 41 Physically Handicapped Children and their Families. *Amer.J.Psychiat.*, *128*, 1554.
77. MINUCHIN, S. 1974 *Families and Family Therapy*. London: Tavistock.
78. MOORE, T. 1975 Stress in normal childhood. Society Stress and Disease. Vol. 2 In: Levi. (Ed.), *Childhood and Adolescence*. Oxford University Press.
79. NAGERA, H. 1969 The imaginary companion. Its significance for ego development and conflict solution. *Psychoanal. Study Child*, 24. 185.
80. NISBET, J.D. 1958 Intelligence and family size. 1949-1954. *Eugen. Rev.*, 49, 201.
81. P.E.P. 1966 *Mental Subnormality in London: A Survey of Community Care*. London: P.E.P.
82. POLLAK, O. (1960) A family diagnosis model, *Social Serv. Rev. 34*, 19.
83. POWERS, E.A. 1969 Children's adjustment to a sibling birth and its relations to ego functions. *Dissert.Abst.Int.*, 30, 5B, 2406.
84. POZNANSKI, E. 1969 Psychiatric difficulties in siblings of handicapped children. *Clinical Paediatrics*, 8:4.
85. PRICE, J. (1969) Personality difference within families: Comparison of adult brothers and sisters. *J.of Biosoc.Sci.*, 1, 177.
86. RECORD, R., MCKEOWN, T. and EDWARDS, J.H. 1969 An investigation of the difference in measured intelligence between twins and singletons. *Ann. Hum.Genet.*, 34,11.
87. REDDIHOUGH, D.S., LANDAU, L., JONES, H.J. and RICKARDS, W.S. 1977 Family anxieties in childhood asthma. *Aust.Paediatr.J.*, 13, 295.
88. ROSEN, B.C. 1961 Family structure and achievement motivation. *Amer.Sociol.Rev.*, 26, 574.
89. ROSENBLUM, L.A. 1971 Infant Attachment in Monkeys. In: H.R. Schaffer (Ed.) *The Origins of Human Social Relations*. London: Academic Press.
90. RUBENSTEIN, J. 1967 Maternal attentiveness and subsequent exploratory behaviour in the infant. *Child Develop.*, 38, 1089.
91. RUTTER, M. 1966 *Children of Sick Parents*, London: Oxford University Press.
92. RUTTER, M. and HERSOV, L. 1976 *Child Psychiatry: Modern Approaches*. London: Blackwell.
93. RUTTER, M., TIZARD, J., and WHITMORE, K. 1970 *Education, Health and Behaviour*. London: Longman.
94. SALK, L., HILGARTNER, M. and GRANICH, B. 1972 The psychosocial impact of haemophilia on the patient and his family. *Soc.Sci.& Med.*, *6*, 491.
95. SAMPSON, T.F. 1975 The child in renal failure. *J.Amer.Acad.Child Psychiat. 14*:3, 462.

96. SAN MARTINO, M. and NEWMAN, M.B. 1974 Siblings of retarded children: A population at risk. *Child Psychiatry & Human Development*. 4 (3), 168.
97. SCHACHTER, S. 1959 *The Psychology of Affiliation*. Stamford, California: Stanford Univ. Press.
98. SCHONELL, F.J. and WATTS, B.H. 1957 A first survey on the effects of a subnormal child on the family unit. *Amer.J.Mental Deficiency, 61*,210.
99. SCHONELL, F.J. and RORKE, M. 1960 A second survey on the effects of a subnormal child on the family unit. *Amer.J.Mental Deficiency, 64*.862.
100. SCHOOLER, C. 1972 Birth order effects: Not here, not now. *Psychol. Bull.* 78, 161.
101. SCHUBERT, D.S., WAGNER, M.E. and SCHUBERT, H.J. 1976 One thousand references on sibling constellation variables. Ordinal position, sibship size, sibling age-spacing and sex of sibling. *Cat.Sel.Docum.Psychol.*, 7, 70.
102. SEARS, R.R., MACOBY, E. and LEWIS, H. 1957 *Patterns of child rearing*. Illinois: Row, Peterson, Evanston.
103. SHERE, M 1956 Socio-emotional factors in the family of twins with Cerebral Palsy. *Exceptional Children*, 22:196.
104. SHRADER, W.K. and LEVENTHAL, T. 1968 Birth order of children and parental problems. *Child Develop.*, 39 (4) 1165.
105. SMART, R.G. 1963 Alcoholism, birth order and family size. *J.Abn.Soc.Psychol.*, 66, 17.
106. SMITH, S.L. 1970 School refusal with anxiety: A review of sixty-three cases. *Brit.J.Psychiat.*, 15, 257.
107. STONE, N.D. 1968 Familial factors related to placement of mongoloid children. American Foundation for the Blind. *Research Bull.*, 15, 163.
108. SUTTON-SMITH, B. and ROSENBERG, B.G. 1970 *The Sibling*. New York: Holt Rinehart.
109. TAYLOR, H.K., and KOGAN, K.L. 1973 Effects of birth of a sibling on mother-child interaction. *Child.Psychiat.&Hum.Develop.*, 4, 53.
110. TERMAN, L.M. 1925 The Mental and Physical Traits of a Thousand Gifted Children. Genetic Studies of Genius Vol. 1.
111. THOMAS, A., BIRCH, H.G., CHESS, S. and ROBBINS, L.C. 1961 Individuality in response of children to similar environmental situations. *Amer.J.Psychiat.*, 117, 798.
112. THOMAS, E.B., TURNER, A.M., LIEDERMAN, P.H. and BARNETT, C.R. 1970 Neonate-mother interaction: effects of parity on feeding situations. *Amer.J.Psychiat.*,117, 798.
113. TIPS, R.L., SMITH, G.S., PERKINS, A.L., BERGMAN, E., and MYERS, D.L. 1963 Genetic counselling problems associated with trisomy 21, Down's disease. *Amer.J.Mental Def.*, 68, 334.
114. TIZARD, J. and GRAD, J.C. 1961 *The Mentally Handicapped and Their Families*. London: Maudsley Monograph 7. O.U.P.
115. TOMAN, W. 1961 *Family Constellation: Theory and Practice of a Psychological Game*. Springer Publishing Co.
116. TRAVIS, G. 1976 *Chronic Illness in Children*, Stanford, Calif.: Stanford University Press.
117. TUCKMAN, J. and REGAN, R.A. 1967 Ordinal position and behaviour problems in children. *J.Health Soc.Behav.*, 8, 32.
118. TURK, J. 1964 Impact of cystic fibrosis on family functioning. *Pediatrics, 34*, 67.
119. WARREN, J.R. 1966 Birth order and social behaviour. *Psychol.Bull.*,65(i) 38.
120. Weinberg, S.R. 1955 *Incest Behaviour*. New York: Citadel.
121. WELLER, L., NATAN, O. and HAZIN, O: 1974 Birth order and marital bliss in Israel. *J.Marr. and the Fam.*, 36, 794.
122. WINNICOTT, D.W. 1964 *The Child, the Family and the Outside World*. London: Penguin Books.
123. ZAJONC, R.B. and MARKUS, G.B. 1975 Birth order and intellectual development. *Psychol.Rev.*, 82(i) 74.

13

IMPRINTING AND THE YOUNG CHILD

W. Sluckin, B.Sc.(Eng.), B.Sc., Ph.D., F.B.Ps.S.

Professor of Psychology,
University of Leicester, England

THE IMPRINTING PHENOMENON

It has been known for a long time that newly hatched birds of the so-called nidifugous species, such as ducklings, goslings, domestic-fowl chicks, quail chicks and the like, tend to form attachments to conspicuous moving figures. Under natural conditions the young bird is usually attracted to its own mother. Experimental studies have shown that the developing attachment is not primarily due to life-supporting physiological rewards of food, water or heat, though these strengthen the bond, but to the mere exposure to the mother-figure. Both in nature and in the laboratory, the initial approach and following responses of very young nidifugous birds develop into preferences for, or attachments to, the figures so approached. This phenomenon was given by Konrad Lorenz the name of imprinting. He originally thought that it took place very rapidly, that it occurred only during a critical period early in the animal's life, and that, once imprinting had been established, it was irreversible(14).

Since those early days many experimental studies have demonstrated that imprinting is a gradual process; that is to say, the longer the exposure to a given figure, the firmer the imprinting will be. Nor is imprinting confined to as narrowly restricted a sensitive period as originally believed. Most importantly, filial imprinting, which shows itself in a short-term preference for the familiar object, is not irreversible(20). Sexual imprinting, that is, directing courtship at figures which had become familiar to the individual in infancy, is another matter. Sexual imprinting in certain bird species (such as estrildine finches) has been found to be largely unalterable(12), although it is non-existent in other species, such as the cuckoo and the American cowbird.

The tendency to approach salient figures and to follow them if they recede is inborn and inherited. The tendency to imprint, that is, to form attachments without conventional reinforcements, is likewise innate. However, the process of imprinting, of becoming attached to a *specific* type of figure, is a learning process. Thus, it is now universally agreed that imprinting is a form of learning, although there is no universal agreement about precisely how it is related to other types of learning(26).

Perhaps it needs to be re-emphasized that a distinguishing feature of imprinting is that it takes place even when the approach and following responses of the hatchling remain unrewarded by heat (newly hatched birds do not require water or food until several hours later). In the laboratory a chick may readily acquire a preference for, say, a moving box; it thus forms a "tie" to the box as a result of visual exposure to it. In nature, mother hen would normally provide her chicks with shelter and warmth and would lead them to water and food. There is evidence that such rewards speed up and strengthen the developing attachment, but they are not a *sine qua non* of imprinting. Thus, as a training procedure or a learning process, imprinting is different from both classical and operant conditioning. Whether it is ultimately explicable in terms of conditioning is an issue with which learning theorists are grappling(28). It may be said, however, that it is an issue which is somewhat esoteric. And it may be added that, like imprinting, many other learning processes refuse to fit neatly into global learning theories; examples are imitation, song learning in birds, language learning in young children, the development of specific hungers and the acquisition of certain food aversions.

When it is said that the young precocial bird (one that has fully developed vision and hearing and is capable of locomotion, soon after hatching) imprints to the first conspicuous figure it encounters, it should not be assumed that all stimulus figures are potentially equally attractive to it. On the contrary, some stimuli are intrinsically more attractive to a given species than others and, therefore, more likely to become objects of attachment. Intermittent stimuli, such as flickering lights or jerkily moving objects, are by far the best for imprinting purposes. The size of the figure matters; if it is very small, it will be pecked, and if it is very large, it will be snuggled against. Its colour matters, too; however, studies of colour preference have proved much more difficult than expected, because these preferences not only vary a great deal among different species but also depend on such environmental factors as temperature(5).

There is one last point that must be made in outlining the basic features of the imprinting phenomenon, or classical imprinting, as it is sometimes called. This concerns the relationship between imprinting and fear. Early research workers formed the impression that very young birds were relatively fearless. At that stage they were thought to be imprintable. As fear developed through maturation, the imprintability of the young bird was thought to wane and eventually cease. Later, it became clear that the very process of imprinting entailed the development of fearfulness. What happens is that exposure to a given figure results in a gradual imprinting to that figure. This, in turn, means that the young animal recognizes a strange figure as such when it sees it. It is attracted to the familiar and it draws away from the unfamiliar; thus, it shows fear of the unfamiliar just because it is now capable of recognizing it. Therefore, the development of fear is not independent of imprinting; rather, it is in a large measure a consequence of it(19). This is an important conclusion, which may have implications for the understanding of the growth of attachments and fears in the human infant.

CRITERIA OF IMPRINTING

In order to consider the role of imprinting in the psychological development of the child we must be clear about the characteristics of imprinting and the criteria by which to judge whether our observations point to imprinting or otherwise. We have already outlined the most important features of imprinting, but before turning to the problem of criteria we may draw the reader's attention to a common source of confusion about imprinting, namely the variations in the usage of the word itself. Most workers in the area apply the term imprinting to the particular type of early learning, as described in the last section. This usage embraces both filial and sexual imprinting, but excludes what is known as associative learning. Some writers, however, go further and apply the term, rather loosely, to a variety of forms of early and later learning which do not obviously fit the paradigm of conventional conditioning(27). Perhaps it is fairly harmless to use the term imprinting in a variety of ways, as long as the theoretical status of imprinting within the field of learning remains somewhat undetermined. In this chapter we are not insisting on the narrowest possible definition of imprinting; at the same time we shall see how some very broad interpretations of what is imprinting are quite misleading.

We may now ask how we can properly determine whether a duckling or a chick is actually imprinted. In the first place we must use a training procedure which excludes the possibility of attachment through conditioning. In other words, we must ensure that learning is by exposure and not through associated reinforcement. Outside the laboratory we can never be quite sure that an observed attachment has come about solely by imprinting. Assuming that the training has been as specified, how do we *test* the young bird for imprinting? The answer is less simple than may seem, owing to the safeguards that must be taken to ensure that such inferences as we make from our observations are fully justified.

The most commonly used test of imprinting is the so-called choice test. Suppose that we wish to find out whether our animals can imprint under certain conditions and duration of exposure to figure A. Animals are first individually trained and then individually tested for discrimination between the familiar figure A and a strange figure B. However, we cannot infer that imprinting has taken place if our animals prefer A to B because the chosen figure may be inherently more attractive to them than the other one. Therefore we need to satisfy ourselves also that control animals familiarised with B and called upon to choose between A and B do choose B. Only then can we conclude that our experimental animals have developed an imprinted preference for the familiar figure.

There are, of course, also other indicators of imprinting. Imprinted animals separated from the imprinting figure give characteristic "distress" calls, whereas control animals make no such vocalisations. Again, exposure-trained animals, separated from the figure and reunited with it after the sensitive period, will readily approach it or recognise it as familiar; control animals, however, without the prior experience of the figure, will approach it, if at all, much more warily. Imprinted young birds allowed to stay in the proximity of the mother-figure do not follow the figure slavishly. After a while such animals appear to take no notice of the figure and busy themselves otherwise. However, when disturbed, they run back to the figure and stay close to it, while control animals without prior exposure learning will not pass this "run-to-mother" test(25).

More interestingly, perhaps, imprinted animals will work (for example, by pecking the key in a suitably constructed apparatus—a form of the Skinner Box) to gain access to, or merely to see, a familiar figure; control animals that had not been so imprinted, and are past their sensitive period, are not disposed to do any work to gain sight of such a figure(11). Last but not least, a stringent criterion of imprinting is one of direction of sexuality. In certain circumstances, early filial imprinting will manifest itself at maturity as sexual imprinting, that is, as courtship directed at familiar-type figures, even if such are not the natural mates of the imprinted animal. Whether such sexual imprinting in birds has any implications for the human species is a matter for speculation. Before we look, however, at any possible imprinting in the human species, we must consider what is known about imprinting in mammalian species in general.

IMPRINTING IN MAMMALS

There is no doubt that newborn precocial mammals show approach and following responses to a marked degree. Lambs, kids, calves and foals can be commonly seen following their mothers. Among rodents, infant guinea-pigs are born with full powers of vision and hearing and are capable of locomotion soon after birth. Like hooved animals, infant guinea-pigs will soon after being born follow moving objects, which under natural conditions would be their mothers. Whether such following responses lead in precocial mammals, as they do in nidifugous birds, to imprinting had for a long time been a matter of doubt. Experimental studies had been lacking until the late 1960s. The first to be investigated was the guinea-pig, a classic and conve- nient laboratory animal. Using procedures similar to those customarily used in the studies of imprinting of chicks, ducklings and the like, it was possible to establish that exposure-trained guinea-pigs display preferences or attach- ments to familiar figures(10,24).

Whether imprinting may be said to occur in altricial mammals whose young are born in an immature state, often blind, and always incapable of independent locomotion, is a much more controversial question. The be- haviour of puppies has been studied extensively(22). It has been reported that early in the life of a puppy, during the so-called period of primary socialisation, the puppy develops an attachment to human beings. That is the time when the true taming of the animal occurs; it is said that this taming, though reinforced by feeding, depends essentially on exposure to human beings. For this reason the period of primary socialisation has been equated by some writers with imprinting. Nevertheless, it is extremely dif- ficult in altricial animals such as rats, cats and dogs to separate out exper- imentally early in life the various factors that are implicated in the formation of attachments by such animals. In other words, it is somewhat uncertain whether in altricial animals attachment of the young to parent-figures is or is not rooted in imprinting.

The behaviour of infant rhesus monkeys has been studied even more extensively than that of puppies. The well-known experiments concerning the relationship of infants to "wire mothers" and "cloth mothers" conducted by H.F.Harlow and co-workers(8) have succeeded in separating the roles of feeding experience and feeling experience. Although the "wire mother" is a source of milk and the "cloth mother" is not, the infant monkey invariably develops an attachment to the latter rather than the former, apparently as a result of what has been called contact comfort. However, the formation of such attachments by infant monkeys involves *associative* learning, and this is procedurally different from classical imprinting. In the case of laboratory-trained chicks or ducklings, visual experience alone leads to the development of attachment. In the case of Harlow's monkeys, both visual and tactile experiences play a part. It is the feel of the toweling material, the contact comfort, that makes for attachment. However, the monkey learns at the same time to *associate* the appearance of the "cloth mother" with the comforting feeling. Later, it recognises the "cloth mother" at a distance by sight. It will not go to a "monster" that has the same pleasant feel. The learning process, then, is not precisely the same as in classical imprinting. Therefore, there is some doubt as to whether it is justified to regard attachments so formed by infant monkeys as imprinting.

THE PATHOLOGY OF IMPRINTING

Imprinting investigated under laboratory conditions may be thought of as pathological in that the young animals form attachments to "unnatural" objects, such as flickering lights, moving boxes and other conspicuous figures, rather than to their own parents. Similar "unnatural" imprinting sometimes occurs also in the farmyard, when, for example, ducklings are hatched under a domestic-fowl hen; such ducklings can be seen to follow the mother hen around, and there is no doubt that they are firmly imprinted to her. Among mammals, dogs, for example, become devoted to their human masters. And one may wonder whether there is an element of imprinting in the strong attachments that children are capable of developing for animals. Sexual, no less than filial, imprinting can become misdirected in animals. But perhaps it is too far fetched to ascribe human sexual deviance to misimprinting.

Another form of pathology—or psychopathology, for we are dealing with pathology of behaviour—occurs when imprinting is being experimentally delayed or hindered. If a highly attractive figure is not available, a less attractive one will become the object of imprinting. In addition to being imprinted to the mother, the young become imprinted to one another. When reared singly, they become imprinted to the more salient features of their environment and show fear when placed in unfamiliar surroundings.

When normal imprinting is prevented, behavioural development becomes abnormal. Animals lacking a suitable mother-figure are less exploratory and consequently learn less or learn more slowly. Not surprisingly, their social development suffers. Above all, lack of suitable objects of attachment has been found to lead to abnormal sexuality in the males of such diverse species as the jungle-fowl(13) and the rhesus macaque monkey(23). Whether such findings have any relevance for the explanation of human behaviour remains uncertain. Extrapolations from animal studies to human psychopathology are notoriously fraught with risks.

IMPRINTING AND THE HUMAN SPECIES

Although the human infant is born in a fairly mature state compared with many mammalian species (e.g., its eyes are open and functional), it is far from capable of locomotion. How could imprinting in babies be contemplated in the absence of approach and following responses? No thoughts were apparently expressed before the late 1950s that imprinting might be a component of human early learning. Then, a suggestion was made that the smiling response in babies could parallel in some ways the approach and following of young precocial birds(7). Imprinting—it was further speculated—might result if this smiling were directed always at the same person. Maternal deprivation was viewed as constituting an absence of imprinting. Therefore, the long-term effects of maternal deprivation in children might be similar in their pathology to the long-term consequences of the lack of an adequate imprinting figure in precocial birds and mammals.

Suggestions of this nature, although not implausible, are devoid of support of empirical evidence. Yet, similar suggestions continue to be made. Thus, it has been said more recently that the very young human infant, while unable actually to follow a moving figure, does nonetheless follow the figure with its eyes—and such visual following could be the basis of human imprinting(4). A much more far-fetched speculation has been that imprinting could sometimes occur in the intrauterine environment before birth. Subsequently such infants—it was said(15)—would not be drawn to any external figures and, therefore, would exhibit symptoms of infantile autism. Speculations of this kind are purely conjectural, and it is impossible to see how they could be put to any empirical test.

Observational and experimental evidence of imprinting in human infants which might be properly scrutinised was first adduced in the early 1960s(18). It was reported that newborn infants exposed experimentally to the sound of 72 paired beats per minute (a heartbeat-like sound) for four days gained more weight and cried less than infants in the control group. The explanation of this finding was in terms of intrauterine auditory imprinting to the mother's heartbeat. It was argued that after birth the experimental infants thrived because of the presence of the familiar sound, whereas their control counterparts were miserable because the familiar sound was absent; under natural conditions young infants are frequently held by the mother close to her body, and are thus not consistently deprived of the sound of the beating heart. Let us examine step by step this claim of auditory imprinting to the mother's heartbeat which has been repeated on later occasions(16).

First of all, the question arises as to whether the original experiment was sufficiently rigorously conducted to warrant confidence in the findings themselves. In other words, would attempts at replication, using strict experimental controls, yield similar results? Secondly, could auditory imprinting occur in the womb? Thirdly, assuming the findings, i.e., increase in weight and decrease in crying, to be valid, could they be ascribed to prior imprinting in the womb?

Attempts to substantiate the original findings have been unsuccessful, even though extensive and thorough investigations were made(3,29). The most that was found was that sounds of many kinds could have a soothing effect on babies; this would surprise no one. Further, the question of auditory imprinting in general is an interesting one. There is no special reason why young animals should not, as a result of exposure, form attachments to sounds, much as they do to visual stimuli. Certain bird species, like the chaffinch, have an innate ability to produce a rudimentary song, but they learn the full song in the first year of their life from the adult members of the species. Although this type of learning has been compared to imprinting, it is clearly not classical imprinting; there is no element of preference or attachment here. In fact, it is well attested that, so far as is known, auditory imprinting—as opposed to visual imprinting—does not occur in birds(6). There is no evidence of it in mammals either, although it is not, of course, impossible that it exists in some species and is as yet undiscovered.

Lastly, the explanation as to why sounds, including heartbeat, may have a soothing effect on human babies presents a challenging problem; but to explain this effect in terms of imprinting *in utero* is unparsimonious and highly conjectural. In any case, to establish imprinting two groups of subjects are needed, one exposure-trained with a given type of stimulation and one untrained. Only if the trained subjects show signs of attachment and the untrained do not can prior imprinting be inferred. And it is not possible to have control individuals *in utero* unexposed to the heartbeat sound!

THE DEVELOPMENT OF THE CHILD'S ATTACHMENTS

In spite of everything that has been said so far, the concept of imprinting does appear to be applicable to human development. There is no doubt that the human infant normally develops an emotional tie to its mother and/or other adults and children. How do these attachments come about? What kind of learning is involved? One possibility is that the infant's attachment to its mother develops in accordance with the rules of Pavlovian conditioning. Mother becomes a conditioned stimulus, a signal, for food and other creature comforts. Thus the infant responds to the mother-figure much as it does to the unconditioned stimuli themselves. Another possibility is that the child's repertoire of activities is channeled through intermittent reinforcement into attachment behaviour, according to the laws of operant conditioning. In other (simpler) words, the child's initial signs of affection for the mother are repeatedly rewarded by the care and love that the child receives, and the child's attachment, because it pays, is continually stamped in. Yet another possibility is that the mother, being the most familiar figure in the child's life, becomes the object of attachment through exposure learning, or imprinting. It could be that attachment to mother and father and siblings and others around develops as a result of *all* these learning processes at once, and other factors besides. Much behaviour and many feelings acquired through experience cannot in the present state of knowledge be readily ascribed to one or another learning mechanism. Attachment is no exception to this.

In the late 1950s, Bowlby(1) rejected the prevalent view shared by psychoanalysis and learning theory that attachment was rooted in the feeding experience and the infant's dependency on its mother. He and others saw the beginnings of attachment in the infant's proximity-seeking, which focused progressively on the mother(21). What was emphasized, but not to the total exclusion of other factors, was that exposure to the mother and contact with her were in themselves a crucial feature in the growth of attachment. This is a process akin to imprinting, if not exactly equivalent to classical imprinting. In a broadened sense of the term, imprinting could be regarded as the key factor in the development of the child's attachments and preferences(2). To be sure, imprinting could not be unequivocally demonstrated in the human infant, but much circumstantial evidence makes it likely that imprinting-like learning is an important element in the development of social attachments in early childhood.

A powerful case has been made by Bowlby(2) for regarding attachment behaviour of the human infant as continuous, in terms of evolutionary development, with attachments displayed by the young of infrahuman species.

If this is accepted, then the study of abnormalities of behaviour resulting from deprivation or disruption of early social bonds is probably relevant to human psychopathology. We should be straying too far from the topic of imprinting if we attempted to give a comprehensive review of the long-term effects of bond disruption in animals. We may mention, however, that prevention of proper attachment formation in infancy and its long-term consequences have been fairly extensively investigated in several species of infrahuman primates. The most severe effects include, in males, inability to mate, and, in females, failure to exercise normal maternal care(9). There is much observational data to show that the development of "sense of security" in animals is associated with the formation of normal attachments. What is uncertain, and where much more research is needed, is how effective in animals the recovery from disturbances in bond formation can be.

As for human beings, the literature claiming long-term damage consequent upon distortions of early attachment relationships is voluminous. The validity of the more sanguine claims has been severely questioned. However, conclusions that cannot be seriously doubted include a higher incidence of delinquency among children from broken homes and some tendency in those who have experienced many early separations towards psychopathic character traits(17). Whether such conclusions indicate inadequate imprinting in the individuals in question during their early childhood is a moot point.

REFERENCES

1. BOWLBY, J. 1958. The nature of the child's tie to its mother. *Int.J.Psychoanal.*, *39*, 1.
2. BOWLBY, J. 1969. *Attachment and Loss.* Vol. 1. London: Hogarth Press.
3. BRACKBILL, V., ADAMS, G., CROWELL, D. H. and GRAY, M.L. 1966. Arousal level in neonates and preschool children under continuous auditory stimulation. *J. exp. Child Psychol.*, *4*, 178.
4. BRODY, S. and AXELROD, S. 1971. Maternal stimulation and the social responsiveness of infants. In: H. R. Schaffer (Ed.), *The Origins of Human Social Relations.* London: Academic Press.
5. DAVIS, S. J. and FISCHER, G.J. 1978. Chick colour approach preferences are altered by cold stress: colour pecking and approach preferences are the same. *Anim. Behav.*, *26*, 259.
6. GOTTLIEB, G. 1971. *Development of Species Identification in Birds.* Chicago: University of Chicago Press.
7. GRAY, P. H. 1958. Theory and evidence of imprinting in human infants. *J. Psychol.*, *46*, 155.
8. HARLOW, H. F. 1960. Primary affectional patterns in primates. *Amer. J. Orthopsychiat.*, *30*, 676.
9. HARLOW, H. F. and HARLOW, M. K. 1966. Learning to love. *Sci., Amer.*, *54*, **244**.
10. HARPER, L. V. 1970. Role of contact and sound in eliciting filial responses and development of social attachments in domestic guinea pigs. *J. comp. physiol. Psychol*, *73*, 427.
11. HOFFMAN, H. S., SEARLE, J. L., TOFFEY, S. and KOZMA, F. 1966. Behavioral control by an imprinted stimulus. *J. exp. Anal. Behav.*, *9*, 177.

12. IMMELMANN, K. 1972. Sexual and other long-term aspects of imprinting in birds and other species. In: D. S. Lehrman, R. A. Hinde, and E. Shaw (Eds.), *Advances in the Study of Behavior, Vol. 4*. New York: Academic Press.
13. KRUIJT, J. P. 1962. Imprinting in relation to drive interactions in Burmese Red Junglefowl. *Symp. zoo. Soc. Lond., No. 8*, 219.
14. LORENZ, K. 1937. The companion in the bird's world. *Auk, 54*, 245.
15. MOORE, D. J. and SHIEK, D. A. 1971. Toward a theory of early infantile autism. *Psychol. Rev., 78*, 451.
16. MORRIS, D. 1967. *The Naked Ape*. London: Cape.
17. RUTTER, M. 1972. *Maternal Deprivation Reassessed*. Harmondsworth: Penguin Books.
18. SALK, L. 1962. Mothers' heartbeat as an imprinting stimulus. *Trans. N. Y. Acad. Sci., 24*, 735.
19. SALZEN, E. A. 1962. Imprinting and fear. *Symp. zoo. Soc. Lond., 8*, 199.
20. SALZEN, E. A. and MEYER, C. C. 1967. Imprinting: reversal of a preference established during a critical period. *Nature, 215*, 785.
21. SCHAFFER, H. R. and EMERSON, P. E. 1964. The development of social attachments in infancy. *Monogr. Soc. Res. Child Dev., 29*, No. 3, 1.
22. SCOTT, J.P. 1958. Critical periods in the development of social behavior in puppies. *Psychosom. Med., 20*, 42.
23. SEAY, B., ALEXANDER, B.K. and HARLOW, H.F. 1964. Maternal behavior of socially deprived rhesus monkeys. *J. abn. soc. Psychol., 69*, 345.
24. SLUCKIN, W. 1968. Imprinting in guinea-pigs. *Nature, 220*, 1148.
25. SLUCKIN, W. 1970. *Early Learning in Man and Animal*. London: Allen & Unwin.
26. SLUCKIN, W. 1972. *Imprinting and Early Learning*. London: Methuen.
27. SLUCKIN, W. 1974. Imprinting reconsidered. *Bull. Br. psychol. Soc., 27*, 447.
28. SLUCKIN, W. 1975. Towards an explanation of imprinting. *Rev. Latinoamer. Psicol., 7*, 299.
29. TULLOCH, J.O., BROWN, B. C., JACOBS, H. L., PRUGH, D. G. and GREEN, W. A. 1964. Normal heartbeat sound and the behavior of newborn infants: a replication study. *Psychosom. Med., 26*, 661.

14

CROSS-CULTURAL APPROACH TO CHILD PSYCHIATRY AS APPLIED TO THE INFANT AND YOUNG CHILD

Klaus Minde, M.D., F.R.C.P. (C)

Professor of Psychiatry, University of Toronto;
Director, Psychiatric Research Unit, The Hospital for
Sick Children, Toronto, Canada

and

Nancy J. Cohen, Ph.D.

Assistant Professor of Psychiatry, University of Toronto;
Senior Research Associate, Psychiatric Research Unit,
The Hospital for Sick Children, Toronto, Canada

INTRODUCTION

Although psychiatrists have pursued an interest in questions concerning culture and human behaviour over the past 50 years, the actual application of cross-cultural findings to issues of illness, treatment, and prevention is quite new (28,50). As in other aspects of medicine and psychiatry, study and treatment of children, especially very young children, have lagged behind even further.

In the present chapter we will examine some of the possible influences of culture on child development in the first few years of life and consider the application of cross-cultural findings to the care of young children in developing countries. In societies where mental health care for children is in its early stages, recognition of the role of cultural beliefs, practices and explanations of behaviour should play an important role in dictating mental

295

health care and the training of practitioners. Consideration of the effects of culture in the early years is especially important, since at this time the child is thought to be both particularly receptive and particularly vulnerable to environmental influences. Also, by comparing development across cultures we have an opportunity not only to learn more about the cultures themselves but also to examine assumptions about the universality of significant dimensions of child development.

Our task potentially could cover many behavioural and biological disciplines and, within these, numerous phenomena. For our purposes here, we will focus primarily on selected biological, social, and psychological aspects of normal and abnormal development we feel are most relevant to understanding psychiatric disabilities and modes of adaptation in the first few years of life. We have chosen to emphasize developmental theory and research findings and discuss methodology only cursorily since excellent reviews of the latter are presented elsewhere (58,61).

HISTORICAL ASPECTS OF THE STUDY OF CHILD DEVELOPMENT AND CULTURE

The study of the growth and development of children in Western countries has a different history from the study of these phenomena in non-Western cultures. In the Western world, it began in response to various external pressures to better the health and education of children, in contrast to many other traditional scientific disciplines which developed within the academic structure. Throughout the 19th century, both educators and physicians increasingly came to realize that the development of children was the responsibility of society at large (1). By the end of the century, improvements in the expertise in these professional areas led to expansion of educational and health facilities for children. Later, in the late 1890s and first two decades of the 20th century, significant advances in techniques of experimentation and measurement in psychological and biological disciplines led physicians, educators and psychologists to begin carrying out relevant research. For example, it was recognized that there were scientific norms for growth in height and weight and mental abilities against which children's health and intelligence could be measured (43, 100). It was not until the 1920s that academic psychologists began to play an active role in expanding the field of developmental research. Thus, at the beginning of the century first clinicians and then researchers concerned with child development began to accumulate data, refine methodology, and build theories appropriate for their respective problems and applications.

The study of child development in non-Western cultures, in contrast, grew out of the western academic tradition in anthropology, a discipline more concerned with understanding existent social and cultural institutions than in creating pressures for change. When psychiatrists came to be interested in cross-cultural comparisons in the 1920s it was for theoretical reasons aimed primarily at proving or disproving various aspects of psychoanalytic theory (46, 59, 67). Subsequently, the research interests of cross-cultural psychiatrists shifted to describing and comparing belief systems across cultures with regard to cause and cure of mental illness (47, 115) and to determining the epidemiology of psychiatric disorders among non-Western societies (18, 34, 77). As mentioned earlier, the actual application of cross-cultural knowledge to clinical psychiatry has come about only recently.

In order to put into perspective the current state of knowledge concerning culture and infant development, we first will briefly trace the major theoretical trends that provided the bases for early research on the influence of culture on development: maturational theory, psychoanalytic theory, learning theory and ethological theory. For the most part, each has dealt with the question of the relative importance of hereditary and environmental influences on child development and thus says something about the malleability of the developmental process.

Maturational theory, as popularized by Gesell (35), held that development occurred because of a prearranged scheme or plan within the body. Through detailed observation of infants and young children, Gesell documented that the order of attainment of developmental tasks remained fairly constant in children and called this phenomenon "biological programming." For Gesell this held true in all the four major fields of ontogenetic organization, i.e., motor, adaptive, language, and personal-social behaviour. Although he realized that each organism would go through developmental or "seesaw" fluctuations (36), with a progressive movement toward stability, he never conceded that these fluctuations might be due to environmental facilitation or retardation of development.

Another theoretical trend came about as the work of Freud and his followers created an awareness of dynamic conceptions of mental processes. Like the maturationalists, Freud was convinced that the basic structure of human development—and especially of human personality—was genetically determined and that people mature psychologically according to principles that apply universally. However, he also believed that the functional aspects of each individual's personality are shaped by experience in a social context. His greatest influence on developmental theorizing was his insistence on the importance of early experience for laying down patterns that would endure through the life span. This added both motivational and emotional variables to the study of child development and provided the clinician with a theoretical framework of child development for the understanding of personality development.

The third trend in psychological theorizing was learning theory, which was derived from Pavlov's work on the conditioned reflex in animals. Watson and his followers (108, 109) began to apply Pavlov's principles to children, claiming that the course of development could be shaped in a particular direction by controlling environmental input. Dissatisfied with the simplistic notions of learning espoused by Watson, a number of researchers introduced what came to be known as social learning theory; this combined learning theory and psychoanalysis to achieve a better understanding of the role of motivation in the learning process (44, 75, 94). Subsequently, other brands of social learning theories became influential in stressing the effects of various child-rearing practices (95) and in creating an awareness that children learn by imitation, a process that can take place without external control by rewards and punishments (6).

At this juncture it is interesting to see how these views affected the study of children in non-Western societies. Early field research in anthropology took place at a time when anthropologists considered the role of genetic factors alone to be relevant. To a large extent this was due to an unfortunate association of early theories of genetic differences with notions of racial supremacy that were popular among 19th century explorers and missionaries (71).

Margaret Mead, whose work marked the beginning of detailed anthropological work with young children in other cultures, initially suggested using children from different cultures to provide a "crucial experiment" for the testing of developmental theories (71). The first contribution in this area was made by Malinowski (66) in response to Freud's view that, although experience influences how the Oedipal conflict is represented, the existence of the conflict itself is genetically determined and thus inevitably universal in the development of a boy reared in a nuclear family. To disprove Freud, Malinowski went to a matrilineal society in the Trobriand Islands to perform the crucial experiment. In this society the roles of mother's lover and son's father were played by two different male adults; the former was played by the child's biological father and the latter by the mother's brother. Observations of the father-son relationships showed that the Oedipal conflict as known in Western patrilineal society did not appear. Mead supported Malinowski's conclusions with her studies of adolescent girls in Samoa (69) and New Guinea (70) by showing that adolescent turmoil associated with puberty in American society was a function of cultural factors, i.e., the homogeneous and relatively isolated nuclear household's lack of a strong peer culture.

Subsequently, Mead came to realize that it was too simplistic to assume that cultures could be compared according to some single theoretically relevant variable (74). One solution to this problem was provided in the period after World War II when John Whiting and his colleagues (5, 6, 111, 114) introduced a combined psychological and anthropological approach to the study of child development and culture which became the model for a considerable amount of research on social and personality development in childhood over the next two decades. Whiting's contribution was an important one because it introduced quantitative and deductively-oriented methods to the field of anthropology which up until that time had relied primarily on descriptive information for its data base. Influenced by both psychoanalytic and social learning theories, much of the work done by Whiting and his colleagues focused on relating various child-rearing practices to societal structure and cultural beliefs and to specific adult behaviours and personality traits. For example, Whiting and Child (111), using an ethnographic atlas, coded information from 70 cultures in relation to child-rearing practices for five systems of behaviour judged to be salient in all cultures: feeding, toilet training, sex training, handling of aggression, and handling of dependency. The most prominent finding was that, in general, severe or punitive child-rearing practices tended to be related cross-culturally to anxious preoccupation with the particular motivational system under consideration, e.g., dependency, whereas relative indulgence tended to be unrelated to cultural beliefs and personality. These results were interpreted as raising questions about the psychoanalytic concept of fixation as being due to either excessive frustration or excessive indulgence at a given psychosexual stage.

The cornerstone of the above theories and research was that early experience invariably influences later behaviour. While the concept of the predictability of later behaviour through the study of child-rearing appeared to be logical, psychologists and anthropologists came to see that their approach was still too simplistic and that a linear early input-later output model of development had severe limitations. The limitations became apparent through studies using data obtained from naturalistic observation of children which showed that children are rarely passive recipients of experience but must be seen as active agents in their intellectual and social development (8, 11, 64). Furthermore, the well-established findings regarding neonatal individuality (101) and the longitudinal studies tracing variations in the course of development as infants with different temperaments interact with their environments (102) obviously challenged a linear model of development which explained behaviour as a result of either genetic or experiential factors.

The impetus for this shift came about from two theoretical approaches that gained influence in the 1960s. One was Piaget's (86) theory concerning the adaptive nature of cognitive development and the second was ethological theory as applied to the study of human social behaviour (3, 11, 12, 53). In particular, the ethologists re-introduced factors generally overlooked in the years during which social learning theory held sway, namely factors related to genetic "programming" of both infants and mothers which are seen as an outcome of processes oriented toward adaptation. Although the under-pinnings of this process are biological, for modern ethologists (12, 53) such programming is not simply an unfolding of fixed, stereotyped responses. The behaviours of the infant, and even more so of the mother, are to some extent modifiable by experience, while at the same time being considered instinctive. The ethological orientation allows one to go beyond the mere demonstration of differences between children to examine how behaviour develops and is influenced by experience.

In practice, to understand this complex interactive process would mean taking into account, simultaneously, multiple measures of biological and behavioural characteristics of the mother and child and the context in which the child develops, including both the immediate environment and the beliefs and attitudes of the particular culture. Obviously, to accomplish this is a monumental task and one which researchers only recently have been willing to tackle (58). However, it also is a task which lends itself to the study of infants since child-rearing practices are more amenable to systematic observation during infancy than during later periods of childhood. In the next sections we will consider recent progress which has been made in attempting to understand within different cultural contexts the effects these multiple influences have on two aspects of normal development of critical importance in infancy—cognitive development and the development of social relationships.

CULTURE AND NORMAL DEVELOPMENT

Cognitive Development

Because of the infant's limited behavioural repertoire, there are more items on infant tests of cognitive development related to sensorimotor abilities rather than to mental abilities. Although these infant test scores do not necessarily predict later intellectual level, they do give some indication of the current level of development of central nervous system functioning. The study of infant sensorimotor development is especially appealing to cross-cultural researchers, since there are a number of relatively culture-free, standardized tests available for ordering milestones (61).

While it has long been accepted that sensorimotor development can be retarded by early unfavourable experiences (25, 116), the belief that it can be accelerated is relatively new. Since the work of Faladé (27) in Senegal and Géber (31) in Uganda, it has been widely held that African infants are precocious in their psychological development. For example, using the Gesell Scale, Géber examined 252 Ugandan infants during their first year of life (31, 33), finding the greatest acceleration in locomotor development, although other aspects of development such as language, prehension, manipulation, adaptivity, and personal-social behaviour were also precocious. Working in the same culture, Ainsworth (3) reported similar findings using the Griffiths Scale. Since, in Géber's study, 37 of the Ugandan infants were found to show precocity within the first 24 hours after birth, the author initially felt the differences were due to genetic factors. However, her later comparison of Westernized and traditional village families (32) suggested that infant care practices were largely responsible for the differences in rate of development.

In a recent comprehensive review of the literature on infant precocity, Werner (110) reported the results of 50 studies, all of which showed infants reared in traditional pre-industrial communities in Africa, Asia, North, Central and South America, Europe, the Near East and the Pacific Islands to be accelerated on various measures of psychomotor development. The African sample showed the greatest acceleration, followed closely by Central American infants and those from various parts of the Indian subcontinent. The acceleration was most conspicuous after birth and during the first six months of life. Although some of the reviewed studies suggest the possibility that these neonatal differences are genetically influenced, the continuing precocity in the first year of life typically has been attributed to commonalities in child-rearing practices in the pre-industrial societies (3, 32, 110). For example, in most of these cultures infants receive almost constant sensory, kinesthetic and tactile stimulation while they are carried on their mother's back or hip during her daily routines. In addition, they are breastfed frequently and handled by various members of the extended family.

More recently, investigators have de-emphasized the issue of general precocity and have examined the relationships between specific cultural practices and their influence on motor development. For instance, Super (99) tested 20 Kipsigis Kenyan infants in their first year and found a distinct pattern of development rather than overall precocity. Advancement was found in skills that were either specifically trained or encouraged by child care practices in that culture, i.e., sitting, upright progression toward walking, head control, grasping, and strength and coordination of the legs. Skills which the Kipsigis infant got little or no opportunity to practice, i.e., rolling from back to stomach, did not show precocity. Among the Baganda of Uganda, Kilbride and Kilbride (48) also found that sitting and smiling behaviour could be accelerated through training and reinforcement. Similar patterns have been found in studies of Zambian infants (37, 38) who, possibly because of their mothers' habit of carrying them on their back supported by a body sling and the infant's consequent need to shift position, showed stepping, crawling and grasping motions early on.

A contrast in developmental pattern has been observed among an isolated group of Indians in Southern Mexico, the Zinacantecos (13, 15). Among the Zinacantecos infants, soon after birth, are clothed in a long heavy skirt that extends beyond their feet and then are wrapped in additional layers of blankets. According to the Indians' belief, these layers keep the children from "losing parts of their souls." It is also a practice that severely restricts most activity. Also, during the first three months infants' faces are kept covered to protect them from the "evil eye," a practice which necessarily restricts visual stimulation.

Neonatal testing and observation showed that, although Zinacantecan infants were small at birth compared to American infants, nevertheless, they were better coordinated, able to maintain quiet, alert states for long periods and made a smooth transition from one state to another. Developmental testing during the first year also showed that the Zinacantecan infants consistently lagged one month behind North American children in mental and motor development. This developmental lag may be accounted for, to some extent, by the limited social and visual stimulation these children experienced as a result of the above cultural beliefs and practices. Yet Brazelton et al. (15) found the quiet, inactive Zinacantecan children to be well adapted to their culture, which strongly emphasizes conformity. These investigators also stressed the interactional significance of this behaviour, saying that these babies, who were quiet at least partly due to early treatment, may have influenced their own parents who were generally quiet and alert. This last suggestion is supported by Greenfield (40), who has noted that in both the Zambian and Zinacantecan cultures, the type of infant, the way adults interact with him, and the values of the culture all fit together to form a harmoniously functioning system; thus a change in any one part of the system obviously would have repercussions in the rest, making it meaningless to try to distinguish cause and effect.

The transactional relation between the infant's needs and child-rearing practices is particularly striking when our knowledge includes traditions associated with the birth of an infant. For example, the Zinacantecan infant starts life physically inactive, is then tightly swaddled and carried horizontally on his mother's back in a way that restricts movement. As noted above, this swaddling also is a successful adaptation to the environment; the child is kept warm in the cold mountain climate and protected somewhat from exposure to infection. Moreover, a quiet baby is less likely to explore and get into dangerous situations.

In a Guatemalan Indian culture studied by Kagan and Klein (45), infants also were isolated in infancy and spent the first 10 to 12 months in a darkened hut with little social stimulation or opportunity for manipulating objects. When tested periodically during their first year the Guatemalan infants, compared to American infants, were passive and unalert and were retarded three to four months on various indicators of cognitive development, i.e., attentiveness, object permanence and language. Nevertheless, in the same culture, by age 11, the children's performance on tests of perceptual analysis, inference, recall, recognition and memory was comparable to American norms. These findings suggest that infant retardation may be reversible. If this is so, cognitive development in the early years is more resilient than was thought to be the case.

The acceleration of some non-Western infants on standardized tests, when it does occur, usually is relatively short-lived. In fact, between the first and second year test scores begin to fall so that after the age of two these infants generally score below infants in Western cultures (31, 37, 110). There are two possible explanations for this. One is that this break in development is a result of discontinuity between what might be considered to be nearly optimal child-rearing conditions and ones that are traumatic or depriving. Around the age of two there often is a change in diet, especially in areas where adequate nutrition is not available. Also, breastfeeding often stops because the mother has given birth to another child and thus the attention and level of stimulation given to the older child may be reduced abruptly; in some cultures the older child actually moves to another house (4).

Support for the hypothesis that precocity disappears as a result of discontinuity in caretaking practices comes from studies in which a drastic change in infant handling is *not* in evidence. For instance, Brazelton et al. (15) showed that Zinacantecan infants did not show a change in test scores but lagged consistently one month behind North American infants in motor and mental development throughout the first year. Similarly, the Guatemalan infants who spent the first year in a darkened hut subsequently appeared to be passive and unalert (45). Thus, these quiet children initially got little stimulation from parents or others and with little change in their level of stimulation tended to continue to be quiet and calm.

Further support for the discontinuity hypothesis comes from studies of "Westernized" upper-middle-class urban infants from the same African and Indian ethnic groups. The Westernized African infants were not initially as accelerated as traditionally reared rural infants, although they were superior to Western infants in motor development in the first year. During the second year of life, however, in contrast to the traditionally reared infants, they continued at an accelerated level when compared to Western infants of similar socioeconomic status.

A second explanation is that the break in development has something to do with the nature of the tests used and the situation in which the child is tested (84). With increased age the test items become less sensorimotor and more mental, at which point the fact that the test norms are established in the West rather than in the infant's own culture may become more important. Also, the older infant may be more uneasy with the strange tester and the demands of the test situation.

At this point it is important to consider the significance of these early developmental data for later growth and development. Brazelton (13, 14) noted that a passive, alert infant contributes to the viability of the isolated culture of the Zinacantecans. He suggested that interplay between the quiet, nonmotoric infants, who were unusually sensitive to auditory and visual stimuli, and the reinforcement for passive behavior from the environment produced the quiet, imitative, suspicious adults in the culture. Their capacity to work for monotonously long periods without relief contributed to their viability under the stringent environmental forces around them.

In many developing countries, the child-rearing practices suited ideally for pre-industrial living are likely to have to change during a cultural transition period. In this case one might ask whether early cultural practice may impede the development of cognitive competence necessary to master a changed environment. While a final answer to the question is not possible, the results of Kagan and Klein (45) suggest we can be optimistic about the malleability of human behaviour. Their work implied that children have a genetic potential for various types of mental competence which can be activated by environmental demands at various times. Thus, in a population in which disease is endemic and infant mortality rates are high, a mother is concerned with immediate survival issues and might justifiably ignore suggestions to stimulate her infant's behavioural and cognitive development so that he can perform well in school some years hence. She also may perceive encouraging the child to explore his environment and to become independent as increasing the chances for mortality through predation, infection or accident. Thus, it may be presumed that, if active exploration and experimentation, rather than obedience and imitation, had been the goal of cultural adaptation, the teaching procedures among Zambians and Zinacantecans would be quite different.

In summary, we can see that cognitive development of infants in various cultures appears to differ with the needs and requirements of the local culture. Despite such differences, however, there is evidence that the general malleability of human experience is present for a good number of years and that changes which may be necessitated by cultural demands can be met.

Development of Social Relationships

Before looking at how and why social relationships might vary across cultures, we will outline some universal phenomena in the process of developing social relations which, in addition, have special relevance for infants. The primary and most important early social relationship is an affective bond or attachment which develops and persists over time between the infant the the adult who is his primary social caretaker, usually the mother. In the West, this process goes through various stages. In the first months of life, the infant begins to be able to discriminate between his mother and others and is more responsive to his mother. In the second half of the first year, this process takes a particular turn and the infant may express distress when the mother leaves his sight (separation anxiety). Attachment is reflected in other behaviours as well, e.g., greeting the mother after an absence, clinging, and following. All of these behaviours serve to keep the infant near his caretaker and signal to the caretaker that the infant is in need of protection.

Comparative studies have indicated that the sequence of stages in the attachment process is universal, although timing may vary from culture to culture (3, 37). A good example of such a study is the one done by Mary Ainsworth (3) among the Ganda of Uganda in East Africa. Ainsworth went to the homes of infants ranging from two to 11 weeks of age and observed them there on alternate weeks for a period of approximately six months. She showed that attachment behaviour, as indicated by separation anxiety, developed in Ganda infants about four months earlier than in American infants. She also showed that the quality of an infant's attachment to his mother might be quite different from the quality of his attachment to the person who cared for and fed him. Other investigators have confirmed the early appearance of separation anxiety in traditional societies in Zambia

(37), the Kalahari Desert (52), and rural Guatemala (60). This early close attachment is probably best explained by the fact that in all of these cultures at all times the infant remains very close to the primary caretaker during the first months of life and his cries are immediately responded to, often by breastfeeding. In contrast, in Western cultures infants tend to be more physically isolated, particularly at night, and consequently may be attended to less promptly. These cultural differences have suggested to some workers that proximity and sensitivity to the infant's signals are crucial elements in the formation of strong attachment (3, 11, 52).

However, it is important at this point to stress that development is not a uniform concept but proceeds only through the interplay of biological, psychological and cognitive forces. Both the psychological precocity and the early attachment of Ugandan infants appear to be a consequence of special patterns of interaction. The two may be related in that one causes the other. For instance, some investigators (60, 93) have suggested that an infant must have a mental representation of his mother to perceive her departure; thus, the more rapid cognitive development of traditionally reared infants may be at least partially responsible for the observation of early attachment in these infants. It must be recognized, however, that the relationship may go in the other direction or that precocious cognitive development and early attachment are not causally related at all.

The practice of keeping an infant close and responding to him rapidly most likely reflects an adaptive response to particular environmental conditions. The most accepted hypothesis about why the human species solved the problem of how to protect itself through reciprocal infant-mother attachment behaviours is the ethological view. This view holds that it evolved from primates who depended on hunting and gathering to sustain themselves (4, 11, 53). While out on expeditions it was necessary for an infant to be carried or to be trusted to stay near his/her caretaker. In addition, the infant was equipped with the curiosity to explore, which helped in learning characteristics of the environment and in gaining adaptive skills.

Particular environmental conditions, however, may influence the degree to which proximity seeking and exploration are shown (62). For instance, as we mentioned earlier, in cultures in which disease and high infant mortality are endemic, isolation from contact with other people and restriction of exploration may be important for survival (15, 45). Another environmental influence may be related to economic aspects of the culture. Berry (9) and Konner (52) observed that early independence training seems to be encouraged among peoples who hunt and gather, whereas obedience and responsibility tend to be favoured traits in societies that accumulate wealth, i.e., by farming or cattle raising (5, 83), or in which a mother's workload necessitates the training of older children to take on domestic chores (57, 113). An obedient child who can babysit and contribute to food and craft production, thus freeing the parents to do productive labour in such situations, is an obvious asset.

Finally, the frequent practice in traditional societies of breastfeeding infants on demand and weaning late, i.e., often not until the child is two to three years of age, is important in areas in which malnutrition is common. In southern Nigeria, LeVine (62) observed that mothers adjusted the age of weaning to the size of the child. Since height and weight often are used as crude indicators of health status in malnourished populations, this adjustment of weaning age would appear to be a medically sound practice.

A final issue in child-rearing which has frequently been addressed in cross-cultural comparisons is the question of whether multiple caretakers produce effects which are detrimental to the establishment of secure affectional bonds. Some 50 years ago, Mead (69) suggested that Samoan adults tend to have "shallow" emotional relationships because the large number of caretakers in an extended family prevented the formation of adequate emotional capacities. Yet today, studies in both Western and non-Western societies clearly indicate that many infants form primary attachments with more than one person (3, 52, 57). Ainsworth also provided evidence to suggest that the quality of the infant's attachment to his mother was related to the number of people in a Bagandan household. This finding is born out by Konner (52) who studied the !Kung of the Kalahari Desert. He noted that over the first year the !Kung children showed decreasing contact with their mothers, but that this was made up for to some extent by the infant's interacting with older children. In support of this he cited observational data of two to five year olds in London and of the !Kung, showing that English children were more likely to be face-to-face with the mother than were the !Kung but less likely to be face-to-face with other children. This suggests that, despite early intensive contact between !Kung mothers and infants, the infants may form a qualitatively different kind of attachment to their mothers, possibly because of the availability of the company of groups of children of various ages.

As mentioned earlier, one aspect of the theoretical shift that has occurred in the last two decades came about with the understanding that individual differences in infants, as well as in caretakers, must be recognized to understand the developmental process. Thomas and Chess (102) have shown the significance of temperamental traits, e.g., activity level and adaptability, as they interact with the environment. To date, the relationship between temperamental individuality and socialization has been mentioned only in passing in comparative studies, e.g., Brazelton et al. (13, 14). Thus, more systematic research in this area is clearly warranted.

In summary, as was the case with cognitive development, it appears that idiosyncratic child-rearing strategies for adaptation and survival have evolved and become the norm in particular cultures. Thus, while certain aspects of social development are universal, e.g., attachment, variations in development also occur which can be directly related to cultural needs and requirements.

PRESENT CONCEPTS OF DEVELOPMENT

In the preceding sections we have tried to give a brief historical review of some of the main themes of theory and research relating culture and human development. These deliberations have made it clear that child development is a complex process. They also have shown that there are many ways to conceptualize and explain general laws that govern the development of children. While some of these themes have become less important as our knowledge has increased, others have retained or regained their credibility over the years. Although the following principles may not be accepted by every expert in child development, they do represent a consensus of a good many contemporary scientists.

1) *No single concept of development does justice to all the phenomena which we observe in the developing organism.* There appears to be a lower age limit for the appearance of developmental phenomena, which is primarily determined by the maturation of the central nervous system. However, it is presently not known whether there are upper prime bounds for the acquisition of a given ability, such that if the appropriate stimulus conditions are not provided within a given interval the ability will never appear. Also, we do not know how far optimal conditions can accelerate the development of particular abilities.

2) *The child is an important shaper of his environment.* Children do not merely react to their environment; the environment reacts to them as well. Parents have their own needs and whether or not their particular infant meets these needs will affect the parents' response and therefore the environment in which a child grows. An active, exploring child may prove a delight to parents who value such qualities, but may arouse frustration and anxiety in parents who would have preferred or need a more passive and non-challenging child to fit into the cultural context. This means that the

feelings and responses of the basic caretakers will be influenced by the degree to which the child meets their preexisting needs. The more they are satisfied, the more they will be able to value the child and hence provide him with an environment for optimal growth.

This principles also implies that a specific developmental level can be reached by different routes. Since new developmental levels may allow for extensive re-organization of behaviour, past problems may not persist in present psychological functioning. Thus a newborn infant who is difficult to care for and causes frustrations in his mother may, through maturationally preprogrammed appearance of the social smile at six to eight weeks, change his caretaker's attitude completely and contribute to a mutually much more satisfying developmental process. It is clear that such phenomena also make it difficult to predict accurately the final outcome of the child's emotional development, because each new developmental stage can provide chances to revise earlier adaptations to life. For example, an initially clumsy child may later on succeed in school and thereby gain the confidence he needs for success in his society.

3) *Development is not a phenomenon which affects only one particular sphere of life, such as emotions or intelligence, but is the sum total of various interlocking forces and embraces changes in biological, intellectual, emotional and social behaviour.* These forces constantly interact and influence their mutual progression. Hence, development in all areas should be examined in any assessment of possible cognitive or emotional deviations in children.

CULTURE AND ABNORMAL DEVELOPMENT

There is an extensive literature on causes and factors thought to adversely influence the psychosocial development of children. As we consider some of these, the following general points should be kept in mind.

(a) Adverse factors may be equally important in many cultures or may be quite culture-specific.
(b) Factors which are statistically associated with a particular psychosocial abnormality may not cause this abnormality. For example, poor school achievement may be associated with delinquency, but both problems may be caused by specific cultural expectations within the family.
(c) Factors which cause a psychological disorder may be different from those which perpetuate it. For example, a mother may beat and injure her infant because of her own unresolved needs, while the child's later behavioural abnormality may be due to the inflicted cerebral damage.

Biological Factors

Temperament

Individual differences in temperament among children can be observed and measured within a few weeks after birth (7, 10). The constellation of these "temperamental traits," which describes the way in which a child habitually interacts with the world around him, has been shown to predict some later behavioural difficulties in middle-class children in developed countries (39, 103). While critics initially questioned the usefulness of the concepts of temperament for children other than physically healthy middle-class children, Chess and her colleagues have found an almost identical distribution of temperamental characteristics among mentally retarded children (19), lower class children (42, 104), and a group of children whose mothers had prenatally been infected with rubella (20). Furthermore, they confirmed the increased incidence of disturbed children who showed particular temperamental clusters in all these groups.

To date only one study employing non-Western samples has been cited (102). DeVries and Sameroff found that infants of three East African tribes (Kikuyu, Digo and Maasai) could be classified by their mothers according to the Chess and Thomas temperamental criteria. It is of interest, however, that the distribution of the various temperamental traits was quite different from those of Western samples. For example, the African children were generally less adaptable, less approaching, and showed a poorer mood than their Western peers. In addition, they were more distractible and more persistent. There were also differences between the three tribal groups: Maasai infants were most active, Kikuyu least adaptive and approaching, and the Digo infants less rhythmic. It is presently not clear how much of this difference is related to the cultural inappropriateness of the questionnaire and how much reflects basic genetic or child-rearing differences. These differences also may reflect perception of the infant with respect to some cultural expectations for certain desirable infant characteristics. As yet, there are no studies which have investigated any possible association between early temperament and later behavioural abnormalties in these African children.

Brain disorder

Brain injury or cerebral dysfunction as indicated by cerebral palsy or epilepsy has been found to increase the risk of mental health problems in all societies in which it has been studied (92, 96). A number of factors appear to contribute to the development of mental disturbance, including psychosocial stress, intellectual impairment and temperamental changes which may be associated with damage to the brain, and changes in the coping abilities of the brain-injured child. Brain injury is especially important in developing countries where the majority of young children brought to mental health clinics suffer from the behavioural and intellectual sequelae of post-natally acquired brain damage (76, 79). Public health measures which will help in the eradication of illnesses which lead to brain damage (especially malaria in sub-Saharan Africa) will thus have a very major impact on the mental health of African children.

Malnutrition

A significant number of children born in non-technological societies experience serious protein-calorie malnutrition during the early years. Such malnutrition is thought to be responsible for more deaths among these young children than all other causes combined (68). When malnourished infants do survive, they typically are smaller, more vulnerable to infection and more limited intellectually than well-nourished children (10). In a review of studies on malnutrition, Birch (10) concluded that the effects of malnutrition vary with the stage of development at which it is experienced. Thus, some investigators have shown that if severe protein-calorie malnutrition occurs in the first year and continues for an extended period without remediation, impairment of intellectual and motor performance is quite profound. However, if nutritional rehabilitation occurs within the first five to six months, reduction of intellectual functioning below normal levels is less likely (23, 117). When malnutrition occurs later, i.e., at two to three years or after, the behavioural effects are less severe and more amenable to treatment (23). The above conclusions are drawn from studies of children suffering from severe malnutrition. The sequelae of mild to moderate malnutrition found in many socially disadvantaged populations are less clear, although it generally is believed that they are slight and relatively reversible (49). It should be noted that even when malnutrition is successfully rehabilitated in infancy it is not certain whether there are long-term effects on behaviour which can be neither detected nor treated early in life.

It is imperative to realize that studies which deal with the consequences of inadequate nutrition are usually dealing with children who live socially disadvantaged lives. The exact degree to which nutritional and environmental disadvantages interact is presently not known. However, the work of Cravioto and De Licardie (22) suggests that the intellectual deficit in undernourished preschool children is only regained when, in addition to adequate nutrition, there is an adequate environment for the child.

Physical handicaps and illness

In developed countries it has been found that chronic physical illnesses and handicaps are associated with an increased rate of mental health problems (81, 87, 98). Parents may become oversolicitous toward their ill or handicapped child; the child may suffer from the consequences of frequent separations and hospitalizations; siblings may be neglected.

Less is known about the impact of physical disorders on the psychological functioning of children in developing countries. Clinical experience certainly indicates that many children seen in mental health clinics also suffer from a physical illness or handicap (78). On the one hand, this may reflect a high incidence of physical conditions in the general population. On the other hand, it may be related to local customs which do not tolerate illness over a long period and which may interpret physical malfunctioning as an indication of hostile outside forces (85).

Cognitive Factors

It previously has been documented that emotional problems are more common among mentally retarded children in all cultures. In addition, it is known that children in the developed countries who have specific disorders involving learning and language development present with a greater number of psychosocial problems than children without such disorders (24, 29, 89). The degree to which similar correlations exist in developing countries is not clear. We have previously reviewed a number of recent studies which have shown a close correlation between the type of caretaker stimulation an infant receives during his first year of life and his performance on standardized cognitive and motor tests. For example, Super (99) reported that Kipsigis infants were advanced relative to Americans in sitting, standing, and walking, but not in crawling and rolling over. The former activities were actively encouraged by their caretakers; the latter were not. Similar data were reported by Konner (52) on the precocious development of sitting and posturing among !Kung infants of the Kalahari desert. It could well be postulated that the failure of the infant to perform cognitively well in the areas of culturally determined importance (such as posturing among !Kung infants) could lead to adverse consequences for his mental health.

Social Factors

Family discord

Another social factor which has consistently been shown to be associated with behavioural disturbances in the West is family discord (90). Some evidence for the validity of this finding in less technological societies comes from the work of Minde (76, 78) in Uganda. Minde found that there were signs of severe family discord in a high percentage of 100 children attending a mental health clinic. Forty-four percent had lost one or both parents through separation and 22 percent had been sent away to relatives for more than six months because of an acute family crisis. In this particular sample, 10 percent of all patients were between one and three years of age at the time of referral. While most of these children presented with symptoms related to some type of cerebral damage, the incidence of family discord among the very young children was nearly identical to that of an older, behaviourally disturbed group.

A similar incidence of social disorganization was found among 48 children in three rural African communities who were identified by their primary school teachers as "generally difficult and badly behaved" and who scored within the abnormal range on a behaviour questionnaire (80). Here, 39 percent came from broken homes and 41 percent had been placed away from their families. In this study a matched control sample of well-behaved children was available. Among these children, only 14 percent came from broken homes and 12 percent had been sent away from their original families. Since these data came out of a general survey of the rural areas, they have the advantage of reflecting the unmet psychiatric needs of rural African communities.

Socioeconomic class

In the West, research on the relationship between social class and psychological disturbance in children has yielded inconsistent results (90), although there is evidence to show that psychological problems are more common in children of the inner cities than in those living in rural areas (91). Rutter (90) has suggested that it is not social class per se which is at the root of disturbance but factors, such as family discord, overcrowding, low intelligence, and perinatal complications leading to brain damage, which are often associated with low socioeconomic class. We already have shown in the above discussion that many of these variables are potentially important in other cultures as well.

Associations between social class and psychological problems also have been attributed to class differences in mother-infant interaction patterns. At one time it was believed that lower-class mothers were less warm and caring, and stimulated their infants less; in turn it was assumed that this led to a "deficit" in attachment and cognitive development (21). In fact, when class differences do occur—and not all studies show that they do (7, 63)—they disconfirm the notion that lower-class infants necessarily are deprived. For instance, Tulkin (106) observed mother-infant interactions in middle- and lower-class dyads in the first year of life. In his sample, middle-class mothers talked to their infants more and provided them with a greater variety of stimulation than did working-class mothers. Yet, lower-class mothers spent just as much time in close proximity to their infants, held them as much and responded to their infants' interactional invitations as positively as did middle-class mothers. However, while holding among middle-class mothers appeared to be the primary vehicle for face-to-face encounters between the mother and her infant and served as a preparatory step for verbal interactions, in lower-class mothers the same activity was followed by silent comforting behaviour. This suggests that identical behaviours, i.e., holding, may have different meanings for various groups of mothers.

Somewhat different findings were reported by Lewis and Wilson (65), who found that the main differences between social class levels occurred in the frequency of touching, holding, and smiling at the baby. The higher the class, the lower the frequency of behaviour. In turn, holding and touching were positively related to a measure of cognitive development in infancy. Although the exact nature of the relation between social class and maternal-infant interaction variables is not yet clear, these data undoubtedly have led to a shift in thinking about the nature and importance of class differences.

Our previous consideration of cognitive development in traditionally reared non-Western infants yielded results in line with those of Lewis and Wilson with lower-class mothers. At least in the first year of life, both of these groups of infants were at an advantage in terms of cognitive development, probably because of the high levels of tactile, kinesthetic and visual stimulation they received. In this context it is interesting to note that in recent years middle-class North American upbringing has shifted in the direction of encouraging these types of stimulation with the increased use of body and back carriers for infants.

In the one non-Western study specifically concerned with social class, Leiderman and Leiderman (57) observed infants and their caretakers in a rural East African community. They found significant differences in the behaviour among families who had different economic resources; families who had more wealth (determined by cash income, land owned, number of cattle and chicken owned, source of water supply) provided their children with alternate caretakers more frequently than did less wealthy families. These secondary caretakers, in turn, were significantly older (mean age =

20.2 years) in the families of high than in those of a low economic level (mean age = 13.9 years). The older alternate caretakers showed a higher rate of interaction with their charges. The infants of the higher economic group scored significantly superior on both mental and motor tests. This suggests that economic advantage either through a combination of genetic selection, better nutrition and maternal health or through differential post-natal experiences is related to early infant behaviour.

In summary, it appears that membership in a low socioeconomic class does not necessarily lead to deficits in development or to poor mental health. However, in both Western and non-Western societies, low socioeconomic class frequently is associated with biological and social factors which place the child at risk, e.g., family discord, poor nutrition.

Psychological Factors

It has been well demonstrated that variations in the psychosocial development of children are strongly associated with particular qualities in the parent-child interaction. For example, prolonged early parent-child separation often has been linked with later psychological disturbance (2, 12, 105). More importantly, Rutter and his group (88, 116), in a detailed study of the families of psychiatric patients, found that children who had been separated from both parents came from more disturbed families than children who had never been separated. This suggests that the parental interaction prior to the separation was already disturbed and that, at least in Rutter's study, the later antisocial behaviour of the children arose less from the separation than from the associated marital discord preceding the separation. This association is supported by studies which have shown that a separation experience caused by the death of one or both parents is not associated with an increase in later psychopathology of children (41).

While no precise parallel studies from the developing countries exist, there is some evidence that Western findings may apply to African children as well. Thus Mugyenyi, Farrant, and Minde (82) assessed the effects of institutionalization on 20 Ugandan infants aged five to 27 months. They paired ten infants who had been in the institution for less than 4.7 months with ten whose average stay was ten months and compared them on a number of cognitive and emotional developmental variables. Both groups of children scored equally well on all psychological and behavioural measures, indicating that institutionalization per se does not necessarily retard the emotional and cognitive development of young children in developing countries.

Further support for Rutter's findings comes from the studies of Minde in

Uganda. In one study (80), broken homes but not the death of one parent distinguished disturbed from control children. Minde (77, 79) also reported that children from polymatric families (families in which there were two or more mother figures) were overrepresented among both his clinic attenders and children who were identified as disturbed by both their teachers and parents, as well as by a psychiatric examination in the community survey. For example, 31 percent of all the disturbed children versus only 14 percent of the controls came from polymatric homes. While the underlying reason for this association is not clear at present, it seems that this was not an outcome of the quality of the children's attachment(s) but a result of children with more than one mother playing off their various caretakers against each other. This in turn led to inconsistent disciplining and, possibly, to psychiatric symptomatology.

In summary, then, it appears that many of the variables which are associated with retarded or deviant development of either a cognitive or emotional nature are similar among different cultures. What differs are the motives underlying a pathogenic environmental influence, e.g., father leaving a rural area to find work in the city, and the channels through which it reaches the organism, e.g., being sent to a relative when a sibling is born.

TREATMENT AND PREVENTION

In developed countries psychiatric treatment related to infants is itself in the infancy stage. In developing countries it is virtually nonexistent. This relative lack of concern with the mental health of this age group is probably related to:

(a) the unwillingness or hesitation of parents to refer their very young children to a mental health specialist because "parents *should* know themselves" how to handle young children;

(b) the reluctance of many psychiatrists to take seriously the complaints of mothers or fathers of young children, which in turn may be based on the concept that "things will work themselves out" with a young child;

(c) the low community disturbance value of young children and the consequent lack of government funding for specific remedial programmes;

(d) the frequent relative lack of knowledge about early child development among both medical and non-medical professionals dealing with children;

(e) the unavailability of specific intervention programmes for young children which have been scientifically evaluated;

(f) the view often encountered in developing countries that as long as hunger and disease are so very common, treatment of mental health problems must be seen as a luxury.

All the above points appear reasonable at first glance; yet they go against our present knowledge that normal development depends on the relatively smooth coordination of biological, cognitive, emotional and social influences on an intrinsically active organism. Thus, early intervention, while it may not directly influence the final outcome of a specific condition, will at least enable us to provide a child with the building blocks he/she needs to reach the presently obtainable developmental equilibrium. Such early intervention obviously must include the whole child, that is, it cannot separate the physical aspects from the emotional aspects of his development. This premise appears intrinsically logical and has been borne out by evidence from controlled investigations. For example, Lechtig, Delgado, Lasky, Klein, Engle, Yarbrough and Habicht (56) demonstrated that impaired psychosocial functioning in Guatemalan families predicted childhood malnutrition. Malnutrition and poor health, in turn, caused significant physical and neurological disorders which secondarily increased psychiatric disability.

From the previous considerations we can state a number of principles that are important for prevention and treatment of mental illness:

(a) Good general health measures are of utmost importance for the improvement of mental health of young children. Specifically, emphasis must be given to adequate prenatal maternal nutrition, proper prenatal and perinatal obstetrical care and the general immunization of young children.

While these general health measures have been documented to be of practical value, there are less adequate data regarding the impact on child development of social welfare measures. Nevertheless, the following points typically are generally agreed to be important.

(b) Unstable and discontinuous patterns of parenting are unfavourable for child development. Specifically, this means that, whenever possible, we should offer early guidance and education for parents of infants. It also means that short-term care outside the family, such as in day care centres, should provide relief for stressed parents and a consistent caretaker for the young child. Failing these measures, we must recognize the need for an early decision to be made with respect to foster or adoptive care for young children whose parents seem unlikely to be able to look after them.

(c) There is also clear evidence, at least in the Western literature (26), to indicate that hospitalizations for children under the age of five should be avoided as much possible. When they are medically necessary, they should be kept as brief as possible and free parental visiting privileges should be mandatory for all children.

(d) Our data unequivocally suggest that high priority must be given to the task of rearing children and meeting their developmental needs. This can best be done through the training of physicians, educators, nurses and other paramedical personnel to better understand and meet the psychosocial needs of children. In practice this will mean giving these professionals an awareness of differences in individual children's needs and the recognition that children are influenced by the emotional climate that surrounds them. Professionals from various disciplines must also learn to work together and help each other, since children have needs which traverse the competencies of any one specialty. This abdication of narrowly defined professional roles is especially important in developing countries where the trust and belief in mental health principles and the education of parents about child development can be greatly enhanced through a continuing relationship between a parent and another modelling adult. Once such a link is securely established, we can begin to undertake the necessary studies which would allow us to evaluate and monitor urgently needed programmes to provide specific assistance to the young child.

(e) The application of anthropological knowledge to medical care is a relatively recent development. In the past there was a moralistic tendency among both anthropologists and psychiatrists which interfered with the application of their knowledge in an objective manner (72). Often they denounced traditional beliefs and practices as damaging to the children's needs. Currently, in a number of settings, traditional concepts of mental illness and its treatment are being incorporated into modern health care practice for adults (54). This type of innovation for children should be heartily encouraged.

(f) Finally, economic and social life in developing countries is changing rapidly. As in all societies that have experienced a technological revolution, family and community structures, as well as child-rearing and educational practices, are undergoing changes. In our earlier discussion, it was suggested that child-rearing practices in traditional societies appeared to be adapted to strategies for survival, thus creating a smooth "fit" between infant care practice and cultural needs and values. Parents who have been reared in a traditional way and subsequently adopt a Westernized way of life often reject the folk wisdom of their ancestors; at the same time, they may not yet feel comfortable with what has replaced this. Although we presented data to suggest that young children are malleable enough to meet changing environmental demands (45), during a cultural transition period the pattern of parent-child relationships often is neither traditional nor Western. A period of confusion and conflict may ensue which increases the risk for emotional ill health in both the infant and his/her parents (55, 112). The shift toward Westernized life-styles also means that the extended family system once available to absorb and cater to abnormal infants and young children is disappearing. Given these social changes, there is a need for accumulating knowledge about psychological and social concomitants of cultural transition in developing nations and for development of educational and treatment services to help individuals arrive at a new fit between child care practices and cultural values.

It is obvious that future clinical and research work in the area of children's mental health must be planned and executed by indigenous scientists, since only then can medical, social, psychological, and anthropological data be productively integrated to serve children and families in individual countries. Such a process undoubtedly will create a wealth of new knowledge and understanding about the interplay of cultural and other forces on development and surely will assist us "Westerners" in our attempts to cope with our own ever-changing cultural structures.

REFERENCES

1. ABBOTT, G. 1938. *The Child and the State.* Chicago: University of Chicago Press.
2. AINSWORTH, M.D. 1962. The effects of maternal deprivation: A review of findings and controversy in the context of research strategy. In: *Deprivation of Maternal Care: A Reassessment of its Effects.* Public Health Papers No 14. Geneva: World Health Organization.
3. AINSWORTH, M.D. 1967. *Infancy in Uganda.* Baltimore: John Hopkins University Press.
4. AINSWORTH, M.D. 1977. Infant development and mother-infant interaction among Ganda and American families. In: P. H. Leiderman, S.R. Tulkin and A. Rosenfeld (Eds). *Culture and Infancy.* New York: Academic Press.
5. BACON, M., BARRY, H., AND CHILD, I. 1959. Relation of child training to subsistence economy. *Amer. Anthropologist,* 61:51.
6. BANDURA, A., AND WALTERS, R.H. 1963. *Social Learning and Personality Development.* New York: Holt.
7. BECKWITH, L. 1972. Relationship between infants' social behavior and their mothers' behavior. *Child Develop.,* 43:397.
8. BELL, R... 1974. Contributions of human infants to caregiving and social interactions. In: M. Lewis and L. A. Rosenblum (Eds). *The Effects of the Infant on its Caregiver.* London: Wiley.
9. BERRY, J.W. 1966. Temne and Eskimo perceptual skills. *Int. J. Psychol.,* 1:207.
10. BIRCH, H.G. 1972. Malnutrition, learning, and intelligence. *Amer. J. Public Hlth.,* 62:773.
11. BOWLBY, J. 1957. Ethological approach to research in child development. *Brit. J. Med. Psychol.,* Pt. 4:230.
12. BOWLBY, J. 1975. *Attachment and Loss. Vol. II: Separation, Anxiety and Anger.* Harmondsworth: Penguin.

13. BRAZELTON, T.B. 1972. Implications of infant development among the Mayan Indians of Mexico. *Human Develop.*, 15:90.
14. BRAZELTON, T.B. 1977. Implications of infant development among the Mayan Indians of Mexico. In: P.H. Leiderman, S.R. Tulkin and A. Rosenfeld (Eds.). *Culture and Infancy.* New York: Academic Press.
15. BRAZELTON, T.B., ROBEY, J.S., AND COLLIERS, G.A. 1969. Infant development in the Zinacanteco Indians of southern Mexico, *Pediatrics*, 44:274.
16. BURTON, R.V. AND WHITING, J.W.M. 1961. The absent father and cross-sex identity. *Merrill-Palmer Quart.*, 7:85.
17. CAREY, W.B. 1970. A simplified method for measuring infant temperament. *J. Pediat.*, 77:188.
18. CEDERBLAD, M. 1968. A child psychiatric study on Sudanese Arab children. *Acta Psychiat. Scand.*, Suppl. 200.
19. CHESS, S., AND KORN, S. 1970. Temperament and behavior disorders in mentally retarded children. *Arch. Gen. Psychiat.*, 23:122.
20. CHESS, S., KORN, S., AND FERNANDES, P. 1971. *Psychiatric Disorders of Children with Rubella.* New York: Brunner/Mazel.
21. COLE, M., AND BRUNER, J. 1971. Cultural differences and inferences about psychological processes. *Amer. Psychol.*, 26:867.
22. CRAVIOTO, J., AND DE LICARDIE, E.R. 1968. Intersensory development in school age children. In: N. S. Scrimshaw and J. E. Gordon (Eds). *Malnutrition, Learning and Behavior.* Massachusetts: MIT Press. p. 252.
23. CRAVIOTO, J., AND ROBLES, B. 1965. Evolution of adaptive and motor behavior during rehabilitation from kwashiorkor. *Amer. J. Orthopsychiat.*, 35:449.
24. DAVIE, R., BUTLER, N., GOLDSTEIN, H. 1972. *From Birth to Seven: A Report of the National Child Development Study.* London: Longman.
25. DENNIS, W. 1960. Causes of retardation among institutional children. *J. Genet. Psychol.*, 96:47.
26. DOUGLAS, J.W.B. 1975. Early hospital admissions and later disturbances of behavior and learning. *Dev. Med. Child Neurol.*, 17:456.
27. FALADÉ, S. 1955. Le Developpement Psycho-moteur du Jeune Africain Originaire du Senegal au Cours de sa Premiere Annee. Paris: Foulon.
28. FAVAZZA. A.R. AND OMAN, M.1978. Overview: Foundations of cultural psychiatry. *Am. J. Psychiat.*, 139:293.
29. FOLSTEIN, S. AND RUTTER, M. 1977. Infantile autism: Genetic study of 21 twin pairs. *J. Child Psychol. Psychiat.*, 18:277.
30. FRANK, L.K. 1939. Cultural coercion and individual distortion. *Psychiatry*, 2:11.
31. GÉBER, M. 1956. Developpement psycho-moteur de l'enfant Africain. *Courrier*, 6:17.
32. GÉBER, M. 1960. Problemes poses par le developpement du jeune enfant Africain en fonction de son milieu social. *Le Travail Humain.*, 23:99.
33. GÉBER, M. AND DEAN, R.F.A. 1957. Gesell tests on African children. *Pediatrics*, 30:1055.
34. GERMAN, J.A. 1972. Aspects of clinical psychiatry in sub-Saharan Africa. *Brit. Psychiat.*, 121:461.
35. GESELL, A. 1928. *Infancy and Human Growth.* New York: Macmillan.
36. GESELL, A. 1954. The autogenesis of infant behavior. In: L. Carmichael (Ed.) *Manual of Child Psychology* New York: Wiley.
37. GOLDBERG, S. 1972. Infant care and growth in urban Zambia. *Human Develop.*, 15:77.
38. GOLDBERG, S. 1977. Infant development and mother-infant interaction in urban Zambia. In: P. H. Leiderman, S.K. Tulkin, and A. Rosenfeld (Eds). *Culture and Infancy.* New York: Academic Press.
39. GRAHAM, P., RUTTER, M. AND GEORGE, S. 1973. Temperamental characteristics as predictors of behaviour disorders in children. *Am. J. Orthopsychiat.*, 43:328.
40. GREENFIELD, P. 1972. Cross-cultural studies of mother-infant interaction: Towards a structural-functional approach. *Human Develop.*, 15:131.

41. GREGORY, I. 1965. Anterospective data following childhood loss of a parent. *Arch. Gen. Psychiat.*, 13:110.
42. HERTZIG, M.E., BIRCH, H.G., THOMAS, A., AND MENDES, O.A. 1968. Class and ethnic differences in the responsiveness of preschool children to cognitive demands. *Monogr. Soc. Res. Child Develop.*, 33:1.
43. HOLT, L.E. 1894. *The Care and Feeding of Children.* New York: D. Appleton.
44. HULL, C.L. 1943. *Principles of Behavior.* New York: Appleton-Century-Crofts.
45. KAGAN, J., AND KLEIN, R.E. 1973. Cross-cultural perspectives on early development. *Amer. Psychol.*, 28:947.
46. KARDINER, A., AND LINTON, R. 1939. *The Individual and His Society.* New York: Columbia University Press.
47. KIEV, A. 1972. *Transcultural Psychiatry.* New York: Macmillan.
48. KILBRIDE, J.E. AND KILBRIDE, P.L. 1975. Sitting and smiling behavior of Baganda infants: The influence of culturally constituted experience. *J. Cross-Cult. Psychol.*, 6:88.
49. KLEIN, R.E., LASKY, R.E., YARBROUGH, C., HABICHT, J., AND SELLERS, M.J. 1977. Relationships of infant/caretaker interaction, social class, and nutritional stature to developmental test performance among Guatemalan infants. In: P.H. Leiderman, S. Tulkin, and A. Rosenfeld (Eds). *Culture and Infancy.* New York: Academic Press.
50. KLEINMAN, A. 1978. A clinical relevance of anthropological and cross-cultural research. *Amer. J. Psychiat.*, 135:427.
51. KLUCKHOHN, C., AND MURRAY, H. (Eds). 1948. *Personality in Nature, Society and Culture.* New York: Alfred A. Knopf.
52. KONNER, M. 1977. Infancy among the Kalahari Desert San. In: P. Leiderman, S. R. Tulkin, A. Rosenfeld (Eds). *Culture and Infancy,* New York: Academic Press.
53. KONNER, M. 1978. Social and personality development: An anthropological perspective. In: M. E. Lamb (Ed.). *Social and Personality Development.* New York: Holt, Rinehart and Winston.
54. LAMBO, T.A. 1956. Neuropsychiatric observations in the western region of Nigeria. *Brit. Med. J.*, 2:1388.
55. LAMBO, T.A. 1960. Concept and practice of mental health in African cultures. *East Afric. Med. J.*, 37:464.
56. LECHTIG, A., DELGADO, H., LASKY, R.E., KLEIN, R.E., ENGLE, P.L. YARBROUGH, C. AND HABICHT, J. 1975. Maternal nutrition and fetal growth in developing societies: Socioeconomic factors. *Am. J. Dis. Childn.*, 129:434.
57. LEIDERMAN, P.H., AND LEIDERMAN, G.F. 1977. Economic change and infant care in an East African agricultural community. In: P. H. Leiderman, S.R. Tulkin and A. Rosenfeld (Eds). *Culture and Infancy.* New York: Academic Press.
58. LEIDERMAN, P.H., TULKIN, S., AND ROSENFELD, A. (Eds). 1977. *Culture and Infancy.* New York: Academic Press.
59. LEIGHTON, S., AND KLUCKHOHN, C. 1947. *Children of the People. The Navaho Individual and His Development.* Cambridge: Harvard University Press.
60. LESTER, B.M., KOTELCHUK, M., SPELKE, E., SELLERS, M.J. AND KLEIN, R.E. 1974. Separation protest in Guatemalan infants: Cross-cultural and cognitive findings. *Develop. Psychol.*, 10:79.
61. LEVINE, R. 1970. Cross-cultural study in child psychology. In: P. Mussen (Ed.). *Carmichael's Manual of Child Psychology.* New York: Wiley.
62. LEVINE, R. 1977. Child rearing as cultural adaptation. In: P.H. Leiderman, S.R. Tulkin, and A. Rosenfeld (Eds.). *Culture and Infancy.* New York: Academic Press.
63. LEWIS, M. AND FREEDLE, R. 1973. Mother-infant dyad: The cradle of meaning. In: P. Pliner, L. Krames, T. Alloway (Eds.). *Communication and Affect.* New York: Academic Press.
64. LEWIS, M. AND ROSENBLUM, L.A. (Eds.). 1974. *The Effect of the Infant on its Caregiver.* New York: Wiley.
65. LEWIS, M. AND WILSON, C.D. 1971. Infant development in lower-class American families.

Paper presented at the Meeting of the Society for Research in Child Development, Minneapolis, April.

66. MALINOWSKI, B. 1972. *Sex and Repression in Savage Society.* New York: Harcourt, Brace.

67. MASLOW, A.H. 1937. Personality and patterns of culture, In: R. Stragner (Ed.). *Psychology of Personality.* New York: McGraw-Hill.

68. McCANDLESS, B.R. AND TROTTER, R.J. 1977. *Children: Behavior and Development.* New York: Holt, Rinehart.

69. MEAD, M. 1928. *Coming of Age in Samoa.* New York: Morrow.

70. MEAD, M. 1930. *Growing up in New Guinea.* New York: Morrow.

71. MEAD, M. 1931. Primitive children: Cross cultural studies. In: C. Murchison (Ed.). *A Handbook of Child Psychology.*, Worcester, Mass.: Clark University Press.

72. MEAD, M. 1936. The use of primitive material in the study of personality. *Character and Personality*, 3:1.

73. MEAD, M. 1952. Some relationships between social anthropology and psychiatry. In: F. Alexander and H. Ross (Eds.). *Dynamic Psychiatry.* Chicago: University of Chicago Press.

74. MEAD, M. AND BATESON, J. 1942. *Balinese Character.* New York Academy of Science, Special Publications 2.

75. MILLER, N.E. AND DOLLARD, J. 1949. *Social Learning and Imitation.* New Haven: Yale University Press.

76. MINDE, K. 1974. The first 100 cases of a child psychiatric clinic in Uganda: A follow-up investigation. *East Afric. J. Med. Res.*, 1:95.

77. MINDE, K. 1975. Psychological problems in Ugandan school children: A controlled evaluation. *J. Child Psychol. Psychiat.*, 16:49.

78. MINDE, K. 1976a. Child psychiatry in developing countries: Some lessons learned. *East Afric. J. Med. Res.*, 3:149.

79. MINDE, K. 1976b. Child psychiatry in developing countries. *J. Child Psychol. Psychiat.*, 17:79.

80. MINDE, K. 1977. Children in Uganda: Rates of behavioural deviations and psychiatric disorders in various school and clinic populations. *J. Child Psychol. Psychiat.*, 18:23.

81. MINDE, K. 1978. The impact of social, psychological and physical illness on the child and his family II: Some clinical research considerations. *Canada's Ment. Hlth.* 26:17. Suppl No. 1.

82. MUGYENYI, P., FARRANT, W., AND MINDE, K.K. 1973. The effects of institutionalization upon the development of Ugandan infants: A controlled evaluation. *Ugandan Med. J.*, 2:104.

83. MUNROE, R.H., AND MUNROE, R.L. 1972. Obedience among children in an East African society. *J. Cross-Cult. Psychol.*, 3:395.

84. MUNROE, R.L., AND MUNROE, R.H. 1975. *Cross-cultural Human Development.* Belmont, Ca.: Wadsworth Publishing Co.

85. OKEAHIALAM, T.C. 1975. The handicapped child in the African environment. In: R. Owor, V.L. Ongom and B. G. Kirya (Eds). *The Child in the African Environment: Growth, Development and Survival.* Proceedings of the 1974 Annual Scientific Conference of the East African Medical Research Council, Nairobi. East African Literature Bureau.

86. PIAGET, J. 1936. *The Origins of Intelligence in Children.* New York: International Unversities Press.

87. PLESS, I.B., AND ROGHMANN, K.K. 1971. Chronic illness and its consequences: Observations based on three epidemiological surveys. *J. Pediat.*, 79:351.

88. RUTTER, M. 1971. Parent-child separation: Psychological effects on the children. *J. Child Psychol. Psychiat.*, 12:233.

89. RUTTER, M. 1974. Functional disorders and educational underachievement. *Arch. Dis. Child.*, 49:249.

90. RUTTER, M. 1975. *Helping Troubled Children.* Hammondsworth: Penguin.
91. RUTTER, M., COX, A., TUPLING, C., BERGER, M., AND YULE, W. 1975. Attainment and adjustment in two geographic areas: I. The prevelance of psychiatric disorder. *Brit. J. Psychiat.*, 125:493.
92. RUTTER, M. 1977. Brain damage syndromes in children: Concepts and findings. *J. Child Psychol. Psychiat.*, 18:1.
93. SCHAFFER, H.R., AND EMERSON, P.S. 1964. The development of social attachments in infancy. *Monogr. Soc. Res. Child Develop.*, 29, Ser. No. 94, 5.
94. SEARS, R.R. 1948. Personality development in contemporary culture. *Proceedings of the American Philosophical Society.* 92:363.
95. SEARS, R.R., MACCOBY, E.E., AND LEVIN, H. 1957. *Patterns of Child Rearing*, Evanston, Ill.: Row, Peterson.
96. SEIDEL, U.P., CHADWICK, D., AND RUTTER, M. 1975. Psychological disorders in crippled children: A comparative study of children with and without brain damage. *Dev. Med. Child Neurol.*, 17:563.
97. SIGAL, J.J., CHAGOYA, L., VILLENEUVE, C., AND MAYEROVITCH, J. 1973. Later psychosocial sequelae of early childhood illness (severe group). *Amer. J. Psychiat.*, 130:786.
98. STEINHAUER, P., MUSHIN, D.N., AND RAE-GRANT, Q. 1974. Psychological aspects of chronic illness. *Pediat. Clinics of N. Amer.*, 21:825.
99. SUPER, C.M. 1976. Environmental effects on under development: The case of African infant precocity. *Develop. Med. Child Neurol.*, 18:561.
100. TERMAN, L.M. 1916. *The Measurement of Intelligence.* Boston: Houghton, Mifflin.
101. THOMAS, A., BIRCH, H., CHESS, S., HERTZIG, M.E., AND KORN, S. 1963. *Behavioral Individuality in Early Childhood.* New York: New York University Press.
102. THOMAS, A. AND CHESS, S. 1977. *Temperament and Development* New York: Brunner/Mazel.
103. Thomas, A., Chess, S. and Birch, H.G. 1968. *Temperament and Behavior Disorders in Children.* New York: New York University Press.
104. THOMAS, A., CHESS., S., SILLEN, J. AND MENDES, O. 1974. Cross-cultural study of behavior in children with special vulnerabilities to stress. In: D.F. Ricks, A. Thomas, M. Roff (Eds.). *Life History Research in Psychopathology Vol. III.* Minneapolis: University of Minnesota Press.
105. TIZARD, B. AND REES, J. 1975. The effect of early institutionalization on the behaviour problems and affectional relationships of family reared children. *J. Child Psychol. Psychiat.*, 16:61.
106. TULKIN, S.R. 1977. Social class differences in attachment of ten month-old infants. *Child Develop.*, 44:171.
107. TULIN, S.R. 1977. Social class differences in maternal and infant behavior. In: P.H. Leiderman, S.R. Tulkin and A. Rosenfeld (Eds.). *Culture and Infancy.* New York: Academic Press.
108. WATSON, J.B. 1918. *Psychology from the Standpoint of the Behaviorist.* Philadelphia: Lippincott.
109. WATSON, J.B. 1928. *Psychological Care of Infant and Child.* New York: W.W. Norton.
110. WERNER, E. 1972. Infants around the world: Cross-cultural studies of psychomotor development from birth to two years. *J. Cross-Cult. Psychol.*, 3:111.
111. WHITING, B.B. (Ed) 1963. *Six Cultures: Studies in Child Rearing.* New York: Wiley.
112. WHITING, B.B. 1973. Rapid social change: threat or promise? *The Neglected Years: Early Childhood.* United Nations Children's Fund.
113. WHITING, J.W.M. 1977. A model for psychocultural research. In: P. H. Leiderman, S. R. Tulkin and H. Rosenfeld (Eds). *Culture and Infancy.* New York: Academic Press.
114. WHITING, J.W.M., AND CHILD, L.L. 1953. *Child Training and Personality. A Cross-cultural Study.* New Haven: Yale University Press.
115. WITTKOWER, E.D., AND PRINCE, R. 1974. A review of transcultural psychiatry. In: S. Arieti (Ed.). *American Handbook of Psychiatry.* New York: Basic Books.

116. WOLKIND, S., AND RUTTER, M. 1973. Children who have been "in care"—an epidemiological study. *J. Child Psychol. Psychiat.*, 14:97.
117. YARROW, L. 1961. Maternal deprivation: Toward an empirical and conceptual re-evaluation. *Psychol. Bull.*, 58:459.
118. YATKIN, U.S., AND MCLAREN, D.S. 1970. The behavioural development of infants recovering from severe malnutrition. *J. Ment. Def. Res.*, 14:25.

15

UPBRINGING IN THE SUPER-RICH

MICHAEL H. STONE, M.D.

Associate Clinical Professor of Psychiatry,
Cornell University Medical College, New York

INTRODUCTION

One would suppose that persons whose wealth was at the multimillionaire level would be so content and so few in number as to be of no interest to psychiatry. Despite the old adage, "Money does not bring happiness," many imagine that it does. Although people seeking consultation with a psychiatrist do not constitute a random sample of the population, clinical experience with the "super-rich" would lead one to suspect that the adage is correct as stated.

In this chapter we will examine some of the patterns of child-rearing peculiar to this small but influential group. Emotional and social disturbances common among those of its members who become ill will then be discussed, along with the special techniques of psychotherapy that are often necessary in dealing with the super-rich and their children. Persons of considerable wealth are, as mentioned by Aronson and Weintraub (1), over-represented among the caseload of psychiatrists in private practice; further, their life-style sets the tone for a large segment of the population. For these reasons, it behooves the clinician to be familiar with the social patterns—both the healthy and the maladaptive—among the very wealthy.

In certain respects, emotional problems occurring in children of the wealthy are similar to those noted in children of the famous and the politically influential—as described by Main (10) and by Weintraub (15). Here we will concentrate upon problems related more directly to wealth.

325

Among the more prominent features distinguishing child-rearing patterns in the wealthy from those encountered in other classes are 1) preoccupation with form and 2) reliance on a large household staff. Another potential source of difficulty lies in the often faulty preparation the child receives for dealing with the large amounts of money at his disposal.

Matters of Form

Concern about manners, rules of etiquette and the formation of a pleasing social façade, while hardly restricted to upper-class parents, is at times carried to extremes in families of the very wealthy. This is true whether the wealth has been inherited through many generations or has been acquired more recently. Bion (2) has commented upon the role of the aristocracy in any culture; namely, the aristocracy serves as a repository of the rules about good breeding and good form, as well as of the history of the culture itself. Aristocracy sees itself as the guardian of tradition.

In 20th century Western society, with its high literacy rate and easy access to books and the media, there is a less pressing need for members of the highest social class to fulfill such roles: The means of disseminating cultural values and norms of behavior are now multiple and widespread. In some families of the super-rich, parents emphasize matters of form and discourage the expression of negative feelings in a way that eventually strikes their children as curiously out of synchrony with the times and certainly discrepant with the values taught to the vast majority of their less-well-off schoolmates. In families that happen to enjoy both wealth and emotional health, parental emphasis on form need not be pathogenic from a psychiatric point of view. The child who has almost nothing to complain about, even if criticism of family members has been forcefully bred out of him, will not grow up feeling stifled. The psychiatric community has little experience with such fortunate children; we can only guess at their number, but I suspect it would be quite small.

In the wealthy families whose children become our patients, the appearance of the "happy family" is not backed up by substance. Communication is often sparse and superficial. Repression of hostile feelings (viz., of being unloved, neglected, unwanted) may be so strong, and loyalty to the image of the "good" family so intense, as to constitute serious impediments to resolution by psychotherapy. Certain young patients from these families will tend, once the repression has been lifted, to withhold expression of the negative sentiments for months, out of fear either of "retribution" from the parents or of loss of face for "tattling" on some member of the family circle.

The Household Staff

Families of great wealth regularly have a large household staff, whose availability and presence intensify the prevailing family atmosphere. Life in the harmonious household will be all the more pleasurable because the tasks that ordinarily interfere with the parents' ability to spend time with their children are performed by others. But a bleak house may become even bleaker: Almost all of the mother's usual functions may become delegated to a nanny, with mother-child interaction reduced to the minimum.

Father-child interaction may be reduced to the vanishing point. In some homes of the super-rich the only older males available to the children are hired male attendants and companions. The impact of parental deprivation will depend to some extent on the degree such behavior departs from the norms of other wealthy families to which the child is exposed. In many upper-class English homes of the 19th and early 20th centuries, children had only a few minutes contact each day with their mothers (6). There may have been little outward resentment of this, however, because the pattern represented a time-honored tradition. Now, especially in America, where a true aristocratic tradition is lacking, it is no longer possible for wealthy parents to rely so heavily upon the services of others without heaping up tremendous resentment.

In many families of the very wealthy, especially where the parents themselves had little emotional rapport with their own parents, the mothers parentify their husbands, devoting inordinate time and attention to them, and correspondingly little to their children. The husbands, in these instances, are being utilized as mother-surrogates, making up for the deprivation experienced years before by their wives (14).

Parental deprivation in certain families of the super-rich may be carried to an extreme seldom encountered, paradoxically, except among the very poor. This is discernible not only in our ongoing work with patients from wealthy backgrounds, but also from case descriptions in the psychoanalytic literature. For example, the first clinical vignette in Helene Deutsch's paper on the As-If Personality (4) concerns a young woman from an aristocratic European family raised chiefly by a group of three or four nannies working in shifts around the clock. In the hyper-conventional atmosphere of this household, the patient had been carefully instructed as a child to "love, honor and obey" the parents, even though the latter were actually seen only on rare occasions. Comparable to the situation of Deutsch's patient is that of a patient whom I reported on earlier (13): As a child this patient had been cared for by a large number of nurses and other household personnel on an immense estate bordered only by a still larger estate belonging to a cousin. She never saw the "townspeople" until she was 12. Her own parents went away to Europe for about half the year every year; one year it happened that the mother was away for six months, not abroad, but in a sanatorium for treatment of a nervous breakdown. The patient grew up assuming that her mother had been away on "vacation," as usual, learning 20 years later and quite by chance about the mother's illness. Since her father was often away on business and completely preoccupied with it when he was home, she experienced just as serious a deprivation of father as of mother. The strong depressive cast to the personality noted in a number of patients reared in similar circumstances is reminiscent of the anaclitic depression in the institutionalized children observed by Spitz (11). These syndromes may be engendered in large part by the serious parental, particularly maternal, deprivation in early life.

In those families of the super-rich where it is meaningful to speak of maternal deprivation, narcissistic character disorders are usually noted in the mothers. Great wealth may attract great beauty, and some women who enjoy the latter are vain, self-centered and more accustomed to receiving adulation than to bestowing tender concern toward others, including their own children. As mothers, these women tend to be aloof, particularly toward their daughters, in relation to whom intense competitive feelings may emerge as the daughters reach adolescence.

Case example

A girl of 17 sought psychiatric consultation because of depression and difficulty concentrating on her studies. She was the only child of a wealthy industrialist, who had died two years earlier. Her mother, a former model, was a frivolous woman who still spent much of her waking day fussing over her appearance. She had rarely spent much time with the patient at any point in the latter's development. Almost all child-rearing and household tasks had been delegated to servants.

The patient had enjoyed a warm relationship with her father. His death was doubly devastating since the loss was compounded by her having been left with a mother whom she scarcely knew. A year after the death of the father, the mother remarried and moved to a different city with her new husband, leaving the patient behind to be cared for by the old household staff in the home where she grew up. The mother rapidly became immersed in "society" and professed not to have time to visit or be visited by her daughter.

Management of money

Certain problems that arise in children of the very wealthy appear to be expressions of an archaic mode of role-differentiation between the sexes. The boys, for example, ordinarily receive ample instruction in business matters as they grow up; some are carefully trained to manage large sums of money early on, with the expectation of one day occupying positions of financial power in the community. Daughters from the same families, however, often receive no instructions at all in handling the large estates they come to control with their brothers.

The impact of such neglect on later development depends, of course, on the prevailing atmosphere within the family and on the overall emotional health of the child.

Case examples

A divorced woman in her late twenties sought psychoanalytic treatment after a series of ungratifying relationships with men. She was the only child of a wealthy Southern banking family. Her parents' marriage had been stable though unsatisfactory, especially for her mother, who felt "widowed" because of her husband's long working hours. Each parent, nevertheless, had always maintained a cordial and affectionate relationship with the daughter. The father kept tight reins over the family's finances, partly out of a conscious effort not to spoil their child. The family lived well but not lavishly, and the patient had no idea until she was nearly 20 that her parents were rich. The father assumed that, because she was a girl, his child would never have any "head" for money, and as a result never acquainted her with the sums she actually had at her disposal. She lived modestly on her own earnings as a dance-instructress, becoming aware only in the middle of her analysis that she could have spent ten times what she earned, merely by availing herself of a large trust fund of whose existence and size her father had never told her. Suspecting there might be such a trust, she finally questioned him very timorously on the subject. However, by the time she learned of her own not inconsiderable wealth, she had already become so frugal in her habits that she made no changes in her style of life. The patient, who functioned fairly effectively in both social and occupational spheres, felt only minimal resentment at having been kept in the dark so long about sums already in her name. She identified with her father's viewpoint, stating that she never was any good at mathematics and that it was probably all for the best that her father exerted this degree of control over her money.

Whereas the preceding example concerned a psychoneurotic patient growing up in a mildly schismatic family, the following example concerns a "borderline" patient from a severely schismatic family.

The patient entered psychotherapy at 18 because of difficulty concentrating on her studies during her first year at college. She had also been depressed over a romantic disappointment. Aggravating these problems was her abuse, over several years, of marijuana and various psychotomimetic drugs.

Her family was one of the wealthiest in the United States. Her father, an industrialist, was away from the home much of the time during her childhood, and during her adolescence suffered a protracted illness, of which he died when the patient was 15. Almost until his death, he shut himself up in his own quarters, conducting business from his sickbed and allowing almost no visits from the patient or any of her three brothers. Her mother, a well-functioning but aloof and narcissistic woman, had been estranged from the father for many years, though continuing to live under the same roof. The patient was raised by a succession of governesses, and had scarcely more contact with her mother than with her father.

Her brothers, all considerably older than herself, had received from their father, before his long illness, rather ample instructions regarding the nature and size of the family's holdings. The father saw to it they learned about investments, real-estate management, and the like, whereas all such topics were scrupulously avoided with his daughter.

The patient's attitude about money was frivolous; her management of it was chaotic. She alternated between periods of Spartan self-abnegation and wild spending. In either phase she alienated friends and acquaintances, offending some by absurd displays of thriftiness (in which she would stint on food) and others through inappropriate gifts, which aroused envy instead of gratitude. The pathetic heights reached during these outbursts of generosity included the impulsive purchase for her fiancé of a Rolls-Royce which he had been admiring in a dealer's showroom. Although he himself came from an affluent family, he was so unnerved by this act (he was unsure whether it represented crassness or craziness, but was alarmed by either possibility) that he broke off the engagement.

Inner Discipline

Closely related to the problems of managing money noted in some children of the super-rich is a problem in the area of self-discipline. In the vast majority of families, work is a necessity for one or both parents, and children must perform various chores if the household is to function smoothly. Much of what most people do all day long is quite purposeful. In this "work-ethic" environment, education of the children is also viewed as a necessity so that the children may maintain or improve their condition during adult life.

In families of great wealth, however, these norms do not always prevail. The children do not have to do chores or find employment for survival reasons; the focus in their education may be on "refinement" rather than on the acquisition of necessary skills. Here, again, less is expected of the daughters in some of these families than of the sons.

One encounters on occasion children whose parents neither worked nor pursued any social or artistic interests, while, in addition, remaining largely aloof from the role of parenthood. In some instances these parents have never attended a school function in which their children took part, have never given a compliment for any scholastic or athletic endeavor, and have seldom given a word of encouragement of any kind. What one sees in the children is an alarming lack of inner discipline for either recreational or occupational pursuits. One also notes in them, even in adolescence, a chronic sense of boredom or emptiness, along with a lowered self-esteem. The latter appears related to a style of family life in which these children were never able to secure for themselves the feeling that they mattered to anyone.

Case examples

School authorities had recommended psychotherapy for a high-school girl of 17 because of declining performance and marijuana abuse. Her multimillionaire father had never worked; both parents had substantial incomes from investments. Both led superficial lives devoted to parties, gambling, and travel. These activities kept them too "busy" to involve themselves in any significant way in the care of their four children. The two sons were sent to academic schools; the daughters to "finishing" schools that emphasized matters of grooming and etiquette. The only strong interest that ever surfaced in the patient was in horsemanship, but neither parent had ever attended the riding shows in which she participated.

By the time she entered psychotherapy she presented no more than a shell of a personality. Devoid of strong interests, hobbies (her enthusiasm about horses having already waned), religious or ethical values, or commitments of any kind, she wandered in and out of relationships, had casual sexual affairs with either sex and came only sporadically to her sessions. Because of her lack of motivation, her impenetrable politeness, and the tenuousness of all her relationships, including the one with her therapist, treatment never got beyond the starting point. Efforts to interest her in the notion of working toward some goal or persevering in some interest failed. Occasionally she would mention a dream during her sessions, the content of which invariably centered on one of two themes: loneliness, or a homosexual embrace with a friend or older woman. The implications of the latter provoked in her considerable anxiety. After a year and a half of thrice-weekly therapy (alternatingly supportive and expressive in nature), she made a hasty and inappropriate marriage and abruptly left treatment. Meeting her at a chance encounter two years later, I learned that the marriage had lasted only six months. She remembered who I was but did not recall my name.

Though outwardly sicker than the patient of the preceding example, a schizoaffective woman of 24 made a gradual recovery over a ten-year span in psychotherapy: Equally lacking in discipline at the outset, she was nonetheless highly motivated to "amount to something." She had also come from a home of extraordinary wealth and equally extraordinary parental indifference. But she identified strongly with a grandfather who had been an inventor, manufacturer, and later, the founder of the family fortune. Actively discouraged by her mother from pursuing any interests, she remained determined to achieve fame in some creative endeavor. Unfortunately, she had little talent and was very disorganized in her efforts either to manage her daily life or to master a profession. She had assumed graduate studies were out of the question for her, as though she could not "afford" tuition.

The first two years in treatment were largely spent in exhorting her to learn the details of her financial situation. After losing innumerable documents and forgetting on many occasions to contact the executors of her estate, she finally became aware that she had more than enough funds to permit a course of study. She then began to work toward a degree in the history of art, taking only a few courses at a time. To foster discipline, the focus in treatment shifted at this time to her school assignments and her schedule. The sessions took on a tutorial quality: Homework assignments were discussed and help was given in the organization of research papers. Since she originally felt that becoming an art historian was a pale second to becoming a famous artist, she was often at the point of quitting. Psychotherapeutic work now centered on her grandiosity and simultaneous self-depreciation. As these attributes became less marked and as her capacity for perseverance and self-regulation gradually increased, she managed eventually to complete her studies and to find a gratifying position.

PSYCHIATRIC DISORDERS AMONG THE SUPER-RICH

How the prevalence of serious emotional disorders among the very wealthy compares with that seen in the rest of the population is not known. Manifest schizophrenia is noted more frequently in the lower socioeconomic groups than in the upper (9). With respect to the more subtle disorders, let alone to the notion of emotional well-being, accurate measures on a sociological plane are not available, apart from such surveys as the Midtown Manhattan Study (12). These, in turn, are not informative for the class of individuals under examination here. The remarks that follow should not be construed as indicating that wealth predisposes to emotional illness, even at the characterological level. It is suggested, however, that psychiatric disorders among children of the super-rich, when detected by clinicians in various locales, fall for the most part into one of three categories. This has been so in my own series of patients, as well as in the patients described by Wixen (16) and Grinker (7).

The most frequently noted disorders are the following: 1) depression, 2) narcissistic character disorder, and 3) sociopathy.

Depression

The depressive syndromes encountered in this group are often related to the unusual degrees of parental (especially maternal) deprivation, as illustrated in some of the preceding clinical examples. Chronic feelings of emptiness, ennui, and boredom are prominent features, seen more often than other types of dysphoric feeling-states, such as sadness or suicidal preoccupation.

Some patients present with severe eating disturbances that appear to be "depressive equivalents" (3), not necessarily accompanied by the affect of sadness. These disturbances include anorexia nervosa, anorexia alternating with bulimia or bulimia with bouts of forced vomiting (but without antecedent food-avoidance). I am excluding from the discussion instances of such eating disorders where there is a positive family history of serious affective illness (viz., unipolar depression), since in these cases the eating disturbances might have occurred even in the absence of early deprivation. It is precisely the existence of these severe depressive syndromes without the positive family history that is so interesting, since it speaks to the profundity of early deprivation that one sometimes finds in children who, superficially, seem blessed with every advantage.

Narcissistic Character Disorders

Under ideal conditions a child will mature in relation both to the outside world and to his inner concept of himself. In the first instance we are speaking of the object-relational path of development; in the latter, of the "narcissistic" path of development. Normal narcissism, if we may use the term in this abstract and non-pejorative sense, will be expressed as a mixture of appropriate self-regard, realistic self-appraisal and enlightened self-interest. There will be a balance between the capacity for intimacy, a concern for others—and the normal-narcissistic attributes.

Under adverse circumstances one may see, instead, the emergence of what Kernberg (8) has defined as pathological narcissism. In the presence of hereditary predisposition to the classical psychoses, the tendency toward extreme forms of narcissism would appear to be augmented still further.

Pathological narcissism includes the following features: (a) grandiose fantasies that are particularly unrealistic (in contrast to the more realistic fantasies of the normal child, who longs for attention and control over the figures of his adult world); (b) an inability to depend on others, particularly, to preserve genuine love and gratitude in the face of criticism from someone close; (c) an excessive and wholly unrealistic demandingness; (d) coldness and aloofness (when not actively engaged in "charming" others) and a tendency to disregard others except as possible suppliers of emotional needs; and (e) an insatiable desire for admiration and for the exclusive possession of all that is valuable in the world (8, p. 272).

If one adds to this catalog of abnormal narcissistic manifestations the qualities of vanity, superficiality and the coexistence of low self-esteem along with grandiosity, one captures the personality profile seen again and again among the young members of the super-rich households who seek psychiatric treatment.

Lacking in many of the homes of the super-rich child—and adolescent patients—was the parental interest ordinarily demonstrated, as Freudenberger and Overby have mentioned (5), " . . . by telling children stories, by listening to their conversation with others, or by listening *to* them."

Case example

The 17-year-old depressed girl from one of the earlier vignettes had been, like her mother, a high-school beauty-queen. Many features of pathologic narcissism were present in her personality. She was preoccupied with her appearance to the extent of spending three to four hours every morning before the mirror, making herself up. Her acquaintances experienced her as flighty, supercilious and self-centered. Although she often fancied herself a "queen," intense feelings of inferiority were evoked in the course of a romantic relationship with an intellectual young man, in comparison to whom she felt self-conscious and stupid. Efforts to treat her depression and narcissistic character disorder were hampered by her impatience with the slow and uncomfortable process of self-revelation in analytic psychotherapy.

Sociopathy

The inclusion of sociopathy in this section is not meant to imply that the very wealthy are more prone to antisocial behavior than persons of other socioeconomic levels; however, when sociopathic personality features are encountered in the children of the super-rich, they may prove uncommonly refractory to treatment. Wealthy parents, if they themselves are disdainful of social norms, may go to extraordinary lengths to nullify the usual corrective processes mobilized by society to contain or counteract antisocial behavior.

In an earlier paper, I mentioned the example of a young man who passed bad checks amounting to tens of thousands of dollars, all ultimately taken care of by his wealthy father to circumvent an arrest—and the supposed stain on the family's honor (13). In a more recent example, an adolescent boy with a long record of breaking into houses, theft, drug abuse and sale of narcotics was, upon being apprehended, just at the point of going to jail, when his father, a man of enormous wealth and influence in the community, persuaded the judge to have his son sent instead to a psychiatric facility (where he continued to conduct his drug business unhampered). Less flagrant examples are legion; the phenomenon partakes of the "V.I.P." syndrome described so well in the articles of Main and Weintraub. Some practical measures for dealing with sociopathy in this context are offered in the following section.

SPECIAL PROBLEMS IN TREATMENT

Children of the very wealthy constitute one of several specially privileged groups in our culture; when they have emotional disorders of any kind, they often become "V.I.P." patients, particularly if the illness requires placement in a hospital setting. The families of such children may attempt to control—and at times undermine—the treatment regime. The parents may wish for consultation with a "top" person or may insist, in the case of a hospitalized child, on conferring with the director about routine matters ordinarily handled by the therapist or the staff. Main and Weintraub both emphasize the need to put the patient's best interests ahead of one's own feelings. One must develop a sense of proportion about when to give in and when to stand firm. If a family threatens to interrupt treatment unless permitted to meet with the "top person," at a time that might be most disadvantageous to the patient, it is much better to swallow a bit of pride and make the arrangement. If the family urges the use of vitamin "X" in the treatment of their schizophrenic child, that is the time to be firm about what is and is not known to be effective in such conditions. The therapist needs to be in touch with the feelings this class of patients will often stir up in him, especially, envy and contempt, lest they interfere with the establishment of a proper treatment relationship (13).

When parental deprivation appears to have been the chief factor contributing to a depressive disorder in a young patient, the therapist will often have to rely on more active techniques than mere interpretation. It may be necessary to actualize in various ways the need for a concerned and empathic parent. The patient described earlier, who never moved off her family's estate till she was 12, also never took a meal with her parents nor had either of them inspect her schoolwork. Her feelings of abandonment about all these years of indifference could not be resolved by verbal methods alone; when this became clear, we took to scheduling her sessions at 4 o'clock and sharing tea and biscuits. Written assignments and term papers were now gone over quite methodically during her hours, special strategies were suggested for getting through difficult courses, and so forth. It was only after many months of altering the therapeutic work so as to provide this nurturing experience, that she began to improve in her scholastic performance and to develop some enthusiasm for a particular line of study.

The last example also illustrates the kind of modifications in therapy that may be required in order to deal with the problem so common to this group of patients: lack of inner discipline and goals. As therapists our lives are ordinarily characterized by discipline and a high sense of purpose. We must be willing to let these qualities show a bit more than usual, so that the patient who is deficient in these qualities may more readily identify with them and incorporate them into his own life. This element in the therapy is often so important with such patients that the verbal and interpretive work done in the sessions becomes, instead of the primary force in the process of recovery, a kind of tender trap—by which we make the patient into a captive audience of our more disciplined character structure. We force the patient, as it were, to imbibe, gradually, our sense of enjoyment and pride in our work. This is no easy task with children of the very wealthy. However desperately they may need to find gratifying work in order to feel useful or good about themselves, they seldom need to work for the money and may therefore be poorly motivated to work. Besides enhancing this identificatory process, of course, we must often give concrete help and encouragement with the scholastic or occupational problems our patients are experiencing.

Serious narcissistic character deformations among children of the super-rich pose even more challenging problems in therapy than do similar traits in people of average means. Once a highly narcissistic patient learns that he cannot count on his therapist automatically to supply his inordinate needs for praise and attention, he will tend to become discouraged about treatment and contemptuous if the therapist. But if other problems compel his remaining in treatment, and if there are no resources available for gratifying these wishes in other ways, the patient may continue, reluctantly at first, meantime permitting the pathologically narcissistic traits to be explored and eventually modified. The very wealthy, on the other hand, find it all too easy to escape the unpleasant aspects of exploratory psychotherapy. My efforts to treat one highly narcissistic adolescent failed, for example, partly because of his capacity to dodge unpleasant topics in our sessions by "taking off'' at a moment's notice to play tennis in Monaco, ski in Switzerland or go yachting off the Bahamas. His parents maintained six homes and it was not always easy to trace his whereabouts in order to arrange our schedule. The family's wealth seemed to convert a merely difficult psychiatric problem into an unmanageable one.

Sociopathic character disorders, notoriously resistive to our efforts even under the best of circumstances, may also become harder to treat in the presence of great wealth. The young man who passed bad checks, for example, made no improvement until his father was finally persuaded to stop making the checks good and to allow his son to spend time in jail, if that is what the authorities decreed. The one day he actually spent in jail had a more salutary effect upon his sociopathic tendencies than had the many months spent, unwillingly at that, in therapy. Afterwards, he began to take his characterological defects seriously and made significant progress in his treatment. Because the wealthy are so accustomed to having their own way, it often requires an unusual degree of firmness and incorruptibility on the part of the therapist if any headway is to be made with sociopathic traits in children of the super-rich.

In treating children of the super-rich, it will usually be important for the therapist to form a strong alliance with the most reasonable close relative, once it becomes clear who that person is. Whereas the therapist by himself may be powerless to prevent inappropriate spending, frivolous canceling of sessions, abuse of drugs, or repetitive antisocial acts, a parent or, at times, an older sibling may be able to assist greatly in curbing such behavior. This kind of family work, ordinarily avoided in classical psychoanalysis, may be necessary not only with latency-age children or early adolescents, but with those in their late teens and early twenties as well. The intervention by the father in the example just above accomplished what was not being accomplished in the traditional two-person therapeutic relationship.

CONCLUDING REMARKS

There is a tendency in psychiatry to assign prognostic value to the nosologic categories in common use. Many mistakes will arise if one does so across the board for each category: Not all cases of "schizophrenia" have a poor prognosis; "character disorder" is not always a better thing to have than a schizophrenic or manic "psychosis." Other variables that influence outcome, such as motivation, social and occupational assets, psychological-mindedness, self-discipline and even one's long-range goals (or lack of them) can so modify the clinical picture that a schizophrenic patient in whom these other variables are largely favorable will often outperform a patient with a severe character disorder, whose reality-testing has always been intact, but whose motivation, discipline etc. have been poor. These points are driven home dramatically in psychotherapeutic work with children of the very wealthy: Here, these characterologic and other nonspecific features seem to dominate the picture from the standpoint of prognosis. As an example, two young women with depressive episodes have been discussed above. The one kept on the family estate until she was 12 had a schizoaffective illness, punctuated by many brief psychotic episodes. According to traditional diagnostic norms she was much sicker than the anorectic girl who bought her boyfriend the expensive car and whose condition was "borderline." But the first girl was highly motivated for psychotherapy, followed any advice (including advice about medications) carefully, and although deficient in inner discipline at the outset, was able to build upon what she had, and eventually became much more autonomous. Her "less sick" counterpart was less motivated, more narcissistic, tended to sabotage efforts to help her, and continued, despite her millions, to lead an empty and ungratifying existence.

REFERENCES

1. ARONSON, H. AND WEINTRAUB, W. 1968. Social background of the patient in classical psychoanalysis. J. Nerv. and Ment. Dis., 146:91-98.
2. BION, W. 1959. Experiences in Groups. New York: Basic Books.
3. DA FONSECA, A. F. 1963. Affective equivalents. Brit. J. Psychiat., 109:464-469.
4. DEUTSCH, H. 1942. Some forms of emotional disturbance and their relationships to schizophrenia. Psychoan. Q., 11:301-321.
5. FREUDENBERGER, H. AND OVERBY, A. 1969. Patients from an emotionally deprived environment. Psychoan. Review, 56:299-312.
6. GATHORNE-HARDY, J. 1973. The Unnatural History of the Nanny. New York: The Dial Press.
7. GRINKER, R. R., JR. 1977. The poor rich: the children of the super-rich. Presented at the 113th Annual Meeting of the American Psychiatric Association, Toronto, May 3rd.
8. KERNBERG, O. F. 1975. Borderline Conditions and Pathological Narcissism. New York: Jason Aronson.
9. KOHN, M. 1973. Social class and schizophrenia. Schizophr. Bull., 7:60-79.
10. MAIN, T. F. 1957. The ailment. Brit. J. Med. Psychol., 30:129-145.
11. SPITZ, R. 1946. Anaclitic depression. Psychoan. Study of the Child, 2:313-342.
12. SROLE, L., LANGER, T. S., MICHAEL, S. T., OPLER, M. K. AND RENNIE, T. A. C. 1962. Mental Health in the Metropolis: The Midtown Manhattan Study. New York: McGraw-Hill.
13. STONE, M. H. 1972. Treating the wealthy and their children. Internat. J. Child Psychother., 1:15-46.
14. STONE, M. H. AND KESTENBAUM, C. J. 1975. Maternal deprivation in the children of the wealthy. Hist. of Childhood Q., 2:79-106.
15. WEINTRAUB, W. 1964. The V.I.P. syndrome: A clinical study in hospital psychiatry. J. Nerv. and Ment. Dis., 138:182-193.
16. WIXEN, B. 1973. Children of the Rich. New York: Crown Publishers.

16

INTERGENERATIONAL EXCHANGE: TRANSFERENCE OF ATTITUDES DOWN THE GENERATIONS

Rita R. Rogers M.D.

Clinical Professor of Psychiatry, University of California, Los Angeles;
Chief, Division of Child Psychiatry, Harbor General Hospital,
Torrance, California

INTRODUCTION

It is a truism that the personalities of our parents and grandparents are inextricably entwined with our own: The subject constitutes one of the central themes—perhaps *the* central theme—of Western myth and literature. The clinician dealing with pathology finds himself repeatedly exploring the subtle processes of imitation, identification, and incorporation called intergenerational transmission. How is it that the ethos of our fathers becomes part of us? How is it that we acquire their attitudes toward pleasure and pain, work and leisure, life and death? How do their experiences determine ours?

Some answers are obvious, of course, and observation gives us others. We can roughly divide the parent-child intercourse into direct communications—the words and deeds through which the parent tells the child about himself, his forefathers, and his attitudes—and indirect communications. Indirect communications often are those the clinician must explore; they are the means through which the parent seeks to define himself and his offspring.

The intimate conversation is never unaffected by the impact of external events: Anything that seriously alters one's external circumstance effects profound shifts in one's internal realities. The parent must make constant adjustments to maintain his balance in a world of flux; the intimacy of their lives means that his offspring must change too. The psychiatrist naturally wishes to explore these fluctuations.

The external change we must examine most carefully is the tremendous contemporary shift in family structure and modes of communication. Today's children grow up constantly assaulted by the alien. Their world is much larger than that of their parents. Television and other forms of mass communication alter the traditional modes of experience and perception, and we are only beginning to discern how this has altered the modes of transmitting information between the generations.

BETWEEN PARENT AND CHILD

It is perhaps best to begin by describing as clearly as possible the traditional relationship—the balance of power—between parent and child. Human children, comparatively helpless as they are, are profoundly dependent. Their parents are their world—their models, their protectors, their teachers, their sources of nurture and stability. Most children desire strength in their parents. They seek models to imitate. Most desire a parental framework to grow within and rebel against.

A parent conveys to his offspring not only his way of perceiving the world but also his own spectrum of emotions—his anticipations and frustrations, hopes and guilts. Perhaps the most poignant and universal adult experience is sadness at promise unfulfilled—the years, as Wordsworth has it, bring "the inevitable yoke"—and this sadness, in varying disguises, is the most common element in parent-child relationships. The parent sees his early self in the child; he remembers his youthful zest and power. The child's expectations rekindle his own, and the adult's sense of loss can be painful enough to provoke a turning away and renunciation. He assigns the blame—or the uncompleted task—to his offspring.

This is perhaps the most obvious way our parents live on in us. Its variations produce some of the most painful conflicts between the generations. The child expects mastery from the parent; the parent must cope every day with his lack of it.

The parent may convey unrealistic expectations to his child; sometimes an entire generation—this is a common element in a way—is put in the position of avenging parental injuries or completing parental tasks. Adults, after all, conceive of themselves as part of a group. Their personal vulnerabilities are enmeshed with those of the group; they identify themselves with the group's triumphs. Particular events are internalized as powerful con-figurations that give the group structure and unity; when the events are those that make the group feel powerless, the individual members' sense of strength and mastery is dealt a serious blow, and the hurt, distorted by time and passion, may be transmitted over several generations, until finally a new generation is compelled to the action that will heal it.

The responses of the younger group will be conflicted. Their elders must cope with situations they cannot master; the children bitterly resent the weakness of their ancestors. In this century we have seen a nation's youth become ferocious warriors, embracing the cause of their ancestral hurt with exaggerated passion. The young resent the burden placed upon them but they are unable to reject it. They shoulder the burden partly because of direct communications from their parents, but the stronger message is in-direct, and in political situations often unaccompanied by any kind of reality testing. Israel and Palestine are cases in point (1).

A group situation is, of course, an extension of individual ones. On an individual level, clinicians frequently see yet another response to a parent's feelings of failure. The parent attempts to regain his youth by merging with the strong new generation; he seeks, in effect, to make the child the father of the man. The child usually finds this intolerable. For example, a patient, the eldest and most cherished daughter of a physician, rejected her father when she was 15; at that time he divorced her mother, leaving her and his four children, moving to a singles' apartment building, and plunging into a pseudo-youthful bachelor's life. He attempted to use his daughter as a model, listening to the rock music she enjoyed, dressing modishly by her standards, dating young women only slightly older than she, and in general trying to be her contemporary. This was, in part, an effort to maintain his relationship with her, but it was also his way of dealing with his new freedom and his regrets for the youth he had left behind. She was bitterly angry: She felt too young to be a model for him; more importantly, the parent-child balance had been seriously disturbed. The impression of strength that parents give and their role as models are important factors in the parent-child alliance: They gratify the child's always reemerging and never fully satisfied need for nurture. The child cannot nurture the parent: The child is too young for the role and he cannot cope with signs of parental weakness.

Even in this most basic parent-child relationship, there are aspects left unexamined. Clinicians have many examples of the ways a parent's dreams affect his dependent child; we know less about how the child's behavior affects the parent. In the case just described, most of us, like the daughter, would see her behavior as a response to his; we are not equally ready to

explain how his change from father and provider into that of a young bachelor might have been affected by the behavior of the girl and her siblings.
We know even less about how external events affected the behavior of both
parent and child and how the milieu that surrounded them was integrated
into their personalities. It is particularly important in examining parent-
child relationships to remember that they do not exist in a void; their lives,
now more than ever, are partly shaped by the world around them, a point
I will discuss more fully below.

PARENT AND CHILD AS PATIENTS

All parents and children are both allies and enemies. The generations
constantly affect one another and their relationship always is in a state of
change, always subject to external events and to the inner representations
of those events. The child's experiences from infancy through adulthood
determine how he integrates himself into his immediate milieu and into the
larger world. This is true for everyone; it is especially noticeable in families
where serious emotional problems injure the adults. Children's reactions to
these problems may reverberate through several generations. The adult not
nurtured in infancy—the adult who as a small child was neglected, deprived
of affection, or treated distantly—might not remember the experiences, but
will be formed by them nevertheless. The most common product of this kind
of infancy is an adult with a severe, unrecognized craving for nurturing that
inhibits his own ability to nurture. Children who suffer from damaging
situations often are doomed to repeat them. Indirect communications—the
behavior of an alcoholic parent, for example, or the rage of a frustrated
one—often are accompanied by contradictory direct communications. The
child continues the conflict into his adulthood and may pass it to his own
children. This kind of inheritance is particularly obvious among the children
of mentally disturbed parents.

A child of a parent who requires psychiatric hospitalization usually blames
himself—a child, after all, sees himself as the center of the universe—and
searches within himself for the causes of the parental turmoil. Unfortunately, his attitude often is reinforced by the adults around him: He is
encouraged not to let his behavior aggravate the parent's condition. The
child's response is to assume that minor transgressions are the cause of the
parent's illness. As an illustration: A patient, the father of four children by
three different marriages, was certain that he would eventually be hospitalized in a mental institution and that none of his children would care. He
was careful not to give his children material possessions, acting on the theory

that if he did, they would maintain contact with him after his hospitalization only for mercenary reasons. This patient's mother, after years of severe mental illness, had finally been hospitalized in a state institution. The patient, then a child, had been relieved. The only son, he was repeatedly asked by his mother to kiss her—something he was reluctant to do. She had told him this would cure her. His conflict and distress shaped his adult life.

THE LESSONS TAUGHT

I have discussed thus far the situations that revolve specifically about the roles parent and child play for one another. But as every child and parent knows, the great parental role is that of teacher. The parent educates the child in a number of areas, both directly and indirectly, and the lessons he teaches form the child's personality. This is true in the most basic sense: The parent teaches the child about gender identity and sexual roles, about his relationship to his body in sickness and in health, and many other things. Parental teaching affects every aspect of the growing child's life. The formation of character is the parent's primary role in his relationship with his child. The therapist often must deal with the lessons taught by parents.

Learning the Male Sexual Role

A 50-year-old patient suffered severely from his ambiguity concerning his masculine role, his relationship to authority, and his position as a father. His mother was a woman of superior intellect and accomplishments; she had looked down upon his less-educated father as a product of a class lower than hers. The patient, her only son, admired her but felt overpowered, not only by her but by his three elder sisters. As a child he craved leadership from his father and even tried to find strengths in the older man to admire, but the father always was overshadowed by the powerful mother. This was particularly emphasized when the son contracted a severe illness and became helplessly dependent on his mother. She tended him efficiently; the father became even more shadowy and ineffectual.

As an adult, the patient craved powerful, leaderlike men; he also wanted tenderness from them, which created severe disappointments in his professional life. He attempted to endear himself to his supervisors in childish, subservient ways that served only to undermine his position. His relationships with women were different but even more disappointing. He wanted strong, determined, leading women—and felt they despised him. As a father, he was tender and caring, but he could not accept any real dependency from his son: His uncertainty about his father made him ambiguous about his own role as father. He was, for example, financially secure, but he made sure that the money for his son's education came from sources other than himself; he simply could not see himself as giving and strong.

At the time this man was a patient, his son was a college student who already showed marked traces of his father's ambiguity. An extremely intelligent boy, he abandoned his college career, seeking situations and relationships where he could lean on other people emotionally. He tried to advance himself by appeals to emotion rather than by his not inconsiderable ability. The problems had been transmitted to a third generation.

Learning to Be a Mother

The way a woman mothers is exquisitely influenced by the behavior of her own mother. Women who become mothers have no choice but to model themselves on the mother they remember, and in the process, good and bad qualities are magnified. The situation becomes particularly intense when women are determined not to repeat the sins of their own mothers. The more they try to avoid the mothering style they know, the more they see themselves as replicas of their own mothers. They fear their children will hate them as they hated their mothers, and their anguish and resentment against themselves are very great.

A bright, attractive, and very efficient woman patient is a case in point. As a child she had been ashamed of her mother's inability to speak English and her "backward ways." She modeled herself on a neighbor she admired. The mother, resenting her own feelings of being neglected, frequently threatened her daughter with the words, "Wait until you have a child; then you will know what it feels like."

The woman was married late in life to a man she did not love. She bore only one child, a daughter, of whom she was extremely overprotective. She smothered the child with attentions to her physical security. At the same time, she was completely unable to show tenderness to the girl or to nurture her emotionally. The young daughter quickly perceived her mother's vulnerability about her role. She accused the mother of wanting to get rid of her. Although this was a form of emotional reaching out, the statement was, unfortunately for the daughter, true. In psychotherapy, the woman admitted that she actually did want to get rid of her daughter; guilt prevented her from doing so. She acknowledged that she could not send the girl to boarding school—she would fear the child's return too much.

As one watched the little girl play, one saw her identification with her mother, and one also saw the remnants of the mother's negative identification with the girl's grandmother. The little girl sent her dolls to live with relatives; assuming the role of mother, she pointed out to the dolls that she was much better at other things, such as running an office, than at mothering.

Choosing a Vocation

Parents influence their children's vocational choices in both positive and negative ways. A patient I saw provides a good illustration. She was a 50-year-old school teacher who had been reared by a non-professional but very successful mother. The mother had not thought much of her daughter in general, and she had thought even less of the child's intellectual abilities. She had been cold with the patient, limiting contact with her mostly to sermons. The daughter's response was an attempt to prove her mother wrong. She became a school teacher, but since she had incorporated her mother's low esteem for herself, she was a poor one.

She extended the emotional complex to her own daughter, rearing her in the anticipation of intellectual failure. Her daughter attended college but did poorly there. When she finished her undergraduate work, she refused to go to graduate school; instead, she returned to an undergraduate program. Her anger against her mother prevented her from obtaining a professional qualification. She made herself as different from her mother as possible, assuming different clothes, weight, hairstyle, and life-style. But she was tied to her mother as her mother had been to her grandmother: She needed to prove the older woman wrong and she was suffocated by her guilt about that need.

In a somewhat similar case, a lawyer conveyed to her daughter that the daughter was not clever and would never be a success. The daughter was overweight, a condition related to her mother's treatment of her—the mother had emphasized slenderness and weighed the girl daily—but early in her teens she sought and found sexual encounters that served as a substitute for the emotional closeness she lacked. She finally married, anticipating and receiving rejection from her husband matching that she had received from her mother.

This young woman had a daughter and she was preoccupied with the girl's weight. She succeeded in getting the child involved in an athletic activity that involved constant weighing, since acceptance in the activity depended on maintaining a certain weight. The child eventually was rejected, having exceeded the weight limitation, and the mother's own turmoils were acutely reactivated. In therapy she acknowledged that the child's life did not depend on an activity that required a particular weight. She recognized that she had involved her daughter in the activity mostly because of her own unresolved frustrations at her mother's treatment of her. She had wanted to be different from her mother but she was trapped by her old wounds and succeeded in recreating in the new generation the situation that had caused them.

Sickness and Health

Attitudes toward the body are transmitted from parent to child in a complex conglomeration of biology and feeling. The genetic link between generations is accompanied by intense feelings about the physical aspects of life. Communications about and attitude toward the body are styled and patterned early in childhood, and the style is transferred from generation to generation. It is natural that this be so. Parents are, of course, concerned with their children's physical welfare; children who crave attention soon learn that their bodies are the most useful sources of attention-getting devices. At the same time, children learn styles and attitudes—somatic expressions of emotion—that are peculiar to their parents. Obvious examples of indirect communication are the angry mother who claims she has a headache or the parent who doesn't want to do something and claims he is "under the weather." Any example of a person's saying not, "I am sad, I crave affection," but, "I am ill" falls in this category.

Further, proclivities, not to mention actual dysfunctions, are genetically transmitted. Disease becomes a fine vehicle for the expression of strong interpersonal feelings.

One of the more obvious examples of this is the case of a 36-year-old woman treated by a gastroenterologist for colitis. She revealed to her psychiatrist that she was preoccupied with her fear of dying of cancer of the colon. She confided that the fear caused her to awake trembling in the night. Her mother had died of the disease, and the patient had witnessed the older woman's suffering with horror.

This patient had had a difficult relationship with her mother; she disliked the older woman and felt disliked in return. The expression of the conflict was chiefly somatic. Since her early childhood, the patient, who suffered from psychogenic megacolon, had withheld bowel movements, to the mother's dismay. The parental treatment for this was enemas and laxatives. Both parents, whenever they considered the child fussy or ill-tempered, administered the medicines. The household apparently fused all the members' moods, feelings, and problem-solving attempts around the evacuation of the bowels, and the girl's dysfunction augmented the preoccupation. It is understandable that the patient became obsessed with—and feared inheriting—her mother's cancer.

On the other hand, misinformation about genetic transmission of disease—and common misinformation about "psychosomatic illness"—lead to a different problem not infrequently encountered. The patient in this case was an obese but attractive young woman who came for consultation because of her frequent aches and pains. Her emotional conflict between cravings for dependency and a need for independence offered fertile ground indeed for the explanation of her pains as psychosomatic. But during psychotherapy it was discovered that her mother had suffered from rheumatoid arthritis and that she herself had been diagnosed as having the disease, information she had withheld from the psychiatrist, as she had dismissed it herself. In dealing with the communications between the generations, attention to physical details and expressions about them is crucially important.

THE MODERN AGE

Until relatively recently the formation of a child's character went on within the confines of a fairly small group—the family and the immediate community. The communication among individuals was more intense than it now is, the impact of alien groups less severe. Generations communicated with words and deeds: The words were stories, the deeds were the actions children performed as they were introduced to the activities of their parents and grandparents. The contemporary world and especially contemporary mass communications have vastly altered this state of things. Family patterns have changed. Psychiatry has not yet come to grips with these changing patterns, nor has it defined the new family structures.

Certain effects are obvious. Children's communications with their parents have been drastically limited; the impact of a heterogenous, alien world has drastically increased. A large portion of the young middle class passively absorbs information about the lives of imaginary characters presented to them every day by the television. Children frequently know more about the details of television characters' lives than they do about those of their parents; they absorb and remember complex interactions—all imaginary—that have nothing to do with their actual lives. The more people watch television, the less they talk. The children's fantasies derive not from tales of their parents and grandparents, but from stories presented to them daily. What are we to make of this? What is the effect of the children's receiving stimuli that have no relation to them or to their families? To what extent are expectations for life, freedom, pleasure, and all the rest, influenced by the television?

Indications thus far are that viewing is extremely selective. A study of patients and non-patients who watched the tremendously popular series "Roots" on television in 1977 showed that what people absorb is based largely on their own internal realities(2). The series, based on a book by Alex Haley, depicted the struggles of generations of a black family in America, from early days in slavery through the Civil War and freedom. Some reactions among the study group: A woman who had given up her illegitimate son for adoption 17 years previously was most moved by the hero's mother's realization that she would never see her son again. Although the scene was far eclipsed by other parts of the drama, the patient, tortured by remorse, found it the most meaningful part of all. The fictional mother was a shadowy, glamorized figure; the patient's inner reality nevertheless related most closely to her plight. Another patient, whose fantasy was that she had impregnated herself and that her only child was therefore wholly hers, was fascinated by a birth scene. An obese, unhappy 14-year-old, whose slender mother considered her a "foreign body," saw the most important part of the movie to be the tender kindship exhibited by black children in their nursery; her longing for acceptance and membership in a family group dictated what she saw in the drama.

So a high selectivity prevails in the responses to the ubiquitous stimulus of television. These dramatic exposures serve to stimulate unresolved dilemmas and concerns in individual members of the audience. Communications with parents and grandparents stimulate similar concerns, but usually those communications are geared to the needs of the child; they serve not as action performed upon him but as interaction between people. Television interrupts that interaction in ways still not fully understood. Surely television distances a child from his ancestors; it may distort his relationship to them. The models presented to most middle-class children are those of a nuclear family; since television is, like every other popular medium, a profitable concern, its emphases and ideals are overwhelmingly materialistic. A society in which elders are imitated and their ideals incorporated by the rising generation must be profoundly influenced by a pervasive value system of this kind; we do not yet know how much. Clearly the modes of intergenerational communication are in a state of flux; we now are attempting to define or at least observe new modes.

At present, new structures and modes of communication cannot be defined as good or bad. Children now are being introduced early to a world full of information; in many cases, children understand a world their parents cannot comprehend, and this must influence the parent-child alliance. Contemporary children might be compared to the children of migrants, who, understanding the new world and its ways, served as models for and leaders of their parents.

CONCLUSION

Intergenerational exchange is an integral part of the patterns of human existence; it affects all aspects of life. We know some of the traditional communication modes; we now are faced with defining the new modes created by the industrial world. There are shifts occurring in intergenerational roles as there are shifts in the traditional hierarchical structures. Easily followed rules and mores are disappearing, but humans still crave direction and leadership. The rituals that served as organizers of human existence and cushions for its difficulties seem to be disappearing. Expressions of hunger for a new order are everywhere. The task now is to define the new structures and combine them with the best of the old so that we can then define and assist the ever-continuing work that goes on between the generations.

REFERENCES

1. ROGERS, R.R. 1976. The emotional contamination between parents and children, *Am. J. Psychoanalysis*, 36:3, 267.
2. ROGERS, R.R. 1977. Selective interpretation of mass media communications. (unpublished paper).

CLINICAL ISSUES

17

A REVIEW OF THE PREVALENCE OF PSYCHIATRIC DISORDER IN CHILDREN UNDER FIVE

Marianne Kastrup, M.D.

Research Associate, Institute of Psychiatric Demography, Aarhus Psychiatric Hospital, Risskov, Denmark

and

Johannes Nielsen, M.D.

Chief of Service, Cytogenetic Laboratory and Consultant of the Samsø Project, Institute of Psychiatric Demography, Aarhus Psychiatric Hospital, Risskov, Denmark.

INTRODUCTION

In the last couple of generations the psychiatric concept of childhood has undergone a succession of changes (83). Initially, the focus was on the past and efforts were made to trace adult disorder to childhood. Later, the focus was on the future with the main interest in prevention of problems by treating them at their incipiency. In recent years, the focus has mainly been on the present, with increasing concern in discovering and treating mental problems in children, not only because of what they might lead to but also because of the suffering and the distress they might cause at present.

The interest in studying the size of the problem of mentally disturbed children is a relatively recent development (72). Presently, the planner of mental health services may pose such questions as: "What is the demand for child psychiatric services? How does it differ from the need? What types of services are necessary to provide sufficient treatment facilities for child psychiatric patients?"

353

The child psychiatrist may ask, "How many children suffer from psychotic or less severe disorders to a degree that it causes distress to the child or its family? Are the nature and the severity of these disorders related to the child's sex, social background, family conditions, place of residence, etc.? In what way are the problems a function of the child's age?"

The general practitioner may ask, "What is the probability that I will see a disturbed child in my consultation? How frequently may I encounter a specific mental symptom among normal children and what is the significance of its presence? What kind of psychiatric disorders are preferably treated by professionals other than child psychiatrists?"

Prevalence studies have addressed themselves to such problems by analyzing the frequency of psychopathological behaviour in unselected populations of children, the variation in frequency depending upon the social and family background, the change in manifestations according to age group, the need for child psychiatric services estimated in the light of findings from such studies, the utilization of available services, and elucidation of factors determining referral to psychiatric treatment.

PROBLEMS IN STUDYING PREVALENCE

The term "prevalence" is used in different ways—alone, as "point prevalence," or as "period prevalence." These terms all aim to estimate the number of persons with a defined disorder at a given time in a given population (75, 111, 117, 141). When "prevalence" is used alone it should indicate "point prevalence," which refers to the number of persons with the disorder at a given point in time in a given population. The concept "period prevalence" should preferably not be used, since it is the sum of point prevalence and incidence.

In prevalence studies, the cross-sectional method is the method of choice. The advantages, as well as disadvantages, of the method and the problems encountered when studying prevalence have been thoroughly described by others (44, 50, 88, 105, 106, 153, 158). Even though different prevalence studies of mental disorders in childhood may have employed the same methodology, it is difficult to compare the findings due to the absence of a satisfactory standardized and widely recognized classification and categorization of child psychiatric disorders. Theoretical knowledge will inevitably lag behind unless clear categorization exists on the basis of which observation may be assembled. The urgent need for an agreed upon frame of reference in evaluating and differentiating between the various mental disorders in children has previously been emphasized (20, 28, 108, 155, 169, 171, 172).

The diagnostic problems are more pronounced in younger children. The categorization of the non-psychotic disorders is particularly difficult, since a sufficient body of knowledge is lacking (99, 208), but several attempts have been made to cluster symptoms (51, 180, 206). In children younger than five it is possible to distinguish certain broad categories. Childhood psychoses, primarily consisting of infantile autism, hyperkinetic syndrome, and certain specific delays of development are fairly well described, but comprise only a limited proportion of the total number of disorders. The greatest proportion comprises children with emotional disorders, conduct disorders, combinations of these disorders, transitory reactions, and various non-classifiable syndromes.

CHILDHOOD PSYCHOSES

In the W.H.O. proposal for a classification of childhood disorders (169, 171, 172) psychoses are divided into infantile, disintegrative, and schizophrenic. Many other approaches have been made and many other terms have been used with reference to childhood psychoses, indicating the diagnostic confusion in the field (10, 15, 38, 40, 123, 135, 150, 159, 162, 196, 200).

Whether infantile autism actually is a precursor of childhood schizophrenia is a subject of considerable debate. Kanner (85), who originally described the hitherto unrecognized syndrome (80), has stressed that infantile autism has passed from non-recognition to overrecognition. Rutter et al. (173) and Kolvin et al. (98) employed diagnostic criteria similar to, but somewhat broader than, those of Kanner and agreed that psychotic symptoms appearing at a very early age represent a clinical entity different from schizophrenia of later childhood. They found that psychoses in children show two peaks, one before the age of three and one around age 11. Onset between those age periods is quite rare.

Psychotic disorders in children are serious but infrequent (34, 82). Thus, four cases of "infantile psychosis" were found among 8,300 admissions by Fontes (46), while Bender (7) reported that 12 percent of children admitted over a 20-year period suffered from schizophrenia. Most epidemiological field surveys of childhood autism deal with prevalence over the entire range of childhood (8, 64, 90, 140).

One of the best known surveys (113, 114) was carried out in Middlesex, England. A screening of all children between the ages of eight and ten residing in the area at a given day was carried out in order to identify those with autism. It was found that 2.1 per 10,000 had a nuclear autism syndrome and another 2.4 per 10,000 showed several features of autism, increasing the prevalence to a total of 4.5 per 10,000.

An almost similar finding was reported in the Camberwell, England, survey, estimating age-specific prevalence rate for childhood autism at 4.8 per 10,000 (202), although children below age five were not included.

In a survey in the Aarhus county, Denmark, Brask (17) studied case histories of children between the age of two and 14 on a given day in all psychiatric hospitals, pediatric or neurological wards, mental retardation services or any of the 20 treatment centers accepting psychotic children. On the basis of this, a clinical judgment was made whether or not the child was psychotic. The main finding was that the age-specific prevalence of the autistic syndrome was 4.3 per 10,000. In all autistic children, abnormal behaviour had appeared before the age of six and in 75 percent before the age of three; however, only 15 percent belonged to the group of early infantile autism described by Kanner.

In Wisconsin, Treffert (191) obtained information on all children aged three to 12 seen for treatment or evaluation during a five-year period with a diagnosis of childhood schizophrenia. The sample was divided into: group A, comprising classic infantile autism excluding organicity; group B, comprising serious psychotic disorder with a later onset; and group C, comprising probable psychoses complicated with demonstrable organicity, deafness, aphasia or other evidence of brain damage. Group A is of particular interest as this group had an average age of 5.1 years. The total age-specific prevalence was estimated at 3.1 cases per 10,000, of which group A only accounted for 0.7 per 10,000.

A high male:female ratio of 3.4:1 in infantile autism was observed by Treffert and others (1, 35, 81, 114). Treffert (191) discussed certain characteristics of children with infantile autism. These children differed significantly from the other two groups in terms of educational level of parents, a finding that has been supported by a number of authors (35, 81, 96, 114, 149, 170). Eisenberg and Kanner (41) and Rimland (149) found that families not only tended to be on a high educational level but also seemed to be obsessive, cold and intellectual. Other studies have not supported this hypothesis (35, 136).

In the development of autism some kind of cognitive defect probably plays an important role, but little is known concerning the biological defects. Kolvin (96) found a significantly greater occurrence of cerebral dysfunction among children with infantile psychoses than among children with psychoses of later onset. Perinatal complications also seem to be a risk-factor (113, 186), even though the findings are far from conclusive (81). A differentiation between early and late onset also shows that mothers of early onset psychotic children show low neuroticism and extraversion (96) whereas a low frequency of schizophrenia or other mental disorders was apparent in that group.

In summary, we find that different epidemiological studies have shown very similar prevalence rates with four to five children per 10,000 suffering from childhood autism. Some studies have found that almost half of the children manifest a typical autistic syndrome and the rest have many different features without exhibiting the classic symptoms of autism. Further studies are, however, needed regarding the prevalence of the syndrome in very young children.

HYPERKINETIC SYNDROME

The term "hyperkinetic syndrome" has often been used synonomously with such terms as "minimal brain damage," "minimal dysfunction," "choreiform syndrome," and "brain damage syndrome." Different investigators have, however, used the terms differently, employing varying inclusion criteria. A comparison of research findings is consequently difficult. This is further complicated by the fact that many authors consider brain damage to be included in the hyperkinetic syndrome. Most hyperkinetic children do, however, not suffer from any structural brain abnormality (197) and many of them do not present any neurological symptoms.

Rutter (165) has recently reviewed the current status in the field of brain damage, concluding that, despite the fact that biological factors frequently play a part in the aetiology, the syndrome is not a brain damage syndrome. The evidence that genetic factors play a role is tentative (22), and one of the main problems at present is to analyse what way the hyperkinetic syndrome differs from the wide range of conduct disorders. Hyperkinetic children are characterized by never being still, being easily distracted and spending only few moments on any activity. This implies that they are generally unable to manage in school and are therefore brought to professional attention. Consequently, prevalence surveys of this disorder have primarily concentrated on school age populations (137, 173, 184), even though the disorder has usually been manifest since the age of three or four.

Analyses on hyperactivity in the early years of childhood are sparse (21), primarily concentrating on clinical samples (189). Schleifer et al. (179) studied the nursery behaviour and tested the cognitive style and motor impulsivity in hyperactive preschoolers of normal intelligence and matched controls. Only one-third of the hyperactive sample was assessed as more than moderately active by "blind" raters and only the very active children seemed to be truly hyperactive, resembling school-age children referred to treatment.

Due to the variations in the diagnostic criteria and methods of case findings, the observed prevalence rates have varied from 1 to 200 per 1,000 but in all studies boys outnumber girls by a factor of 4-6 to 1. The prognosis of the young hyperactive children is relatively poor (21, 63, 73) and the findings of Campbell et al. (21) indicate that children hyperactive in preschool years continue to have difficulties in elementary school.

LANGUAGE AND SPEECH DISORDERS

Studies of speech disorders have frequently been based upon children referred to treatment (76). It is, thus, the most severe cases which have been studied. Until recently, delay in speech or language was not considered a real problem until the child reached school age. The prevalence of a marked language delay when starting school among physically healthy children of normal intelligence has been reported to be around 1 per 1,000 (77, 173). Many more children have articulation defects but without serious impairment of their use of language; this condition is probably as prevailing as one in every 20 children (163). The prevalence of delayed language development is substantially higher among mentally retarded children and children with cerebral palsy and developmental disorders. A higher prevalence is also found among socially and culturally deprived children due to lack of stimulation.

Because of the wide range of normal development and speech and language, many clinicians tend to postpone any treatment of a delay. The confusion concerning the definition of the disorder among preschool children has also contributed to the lack of prevalence surveys in this age group (164). This is unfortunate, since preschool years are agreed to be the optimal period for acquiring language (175).

One of the few attempts to assess the frequency of deficient language development was carried out by Stevenson and Richman (185). They delineated abnormality arbitrarily, using two criteria in evaluating 36-month-old children: Abnormality was defined as expressive language age less than or equal to 30 months, i.e., six months behind chronological age, and expressive language less than or equal to two-thirds of chronological age. Based on these criteria they reported that the prevalence of the conditions among three-year-old children amounted to 31.2 and 22.2, respectively, per 1,000. The rate of language delay not associated with any general retardation was found to be 5.7 per 1,000. Boys outnumbered girls, though not significantly, which is in accordance with most other studies. The observed prevalence may partly be explained by the fact that a certain number of the normally intelligent children may initially show a delay, with rapid change before the age of five.

From a sample of normal children of similar age, Randall et al. (139) estimated the prevalence to be 6.2 per 1,000 for those deviating more than two standard deviations in both comprehensive and expressive language and a prevalence of 12.5 per 1,000 deviating more than two standard deviations in expressive language. In Germany, Hellbrügge et al. (67) studied four-to-six-year-olds, observing that 27 percent stammered or lisped, 20 percent spoke unclearly and 11 percent were unable to make whole phrases. Based on three-to-five-year-old children referred to treatment, Ingram (77) found a prevalence of 0.7 per 1,000 and the National Institute of Neurological Diseases and Strokes estimated that one in every 170 children suffered from a developmental disability affecting the development of language (175).

ENURESIS AND ENCOPRESIS

Whether enuresis should be classified as a psychiatric disorder is questionable, but referral to psychiatric service of a group of children suffering from the disorder is indicated (57). Many (177) favour the view that the rate of psychiatric disorders is higher in children with enuresis than in other children. Rutter et al. (174) demonstrated an association between the presence of enuresis and psychosocial disorders and in the Newcastle survey a relatively higher frequency of behaviour disorders was also reported (122). Some claim that children with secondary enuresis are more likely to be mentally disturbed than children with primary enuresis (62, 174) and both found psychiatric problems were closely associated with children suffering from enuresis diurna as well as nocturna. The associations are not reverse, however, and enuresis must not be considered a sign of mental disorder.

Lack of bladder control is a physiological phenomenon in infancy. The age from which to name the condition enuresis is not agreed upon; Macfarlane et al. (115) mention an age of 21 months, whereas others (86) do not talk about enuresis nocturna till the age of three. The prevalence of enuresis has frequently been estimated in school children. Oppel et al. (132, 133) observed enuresis every night in 21 percent of three-to-five-year-olds and at least once a week in further 43 percent, with a significant preponderance of boys. Blomfield and Douglas (11) found, among 5,386 children at age four, a prevalence of bedwetting amounting to 13.6 percent of boys and 10.6

percent of girls of which 3.7 percent and 3.2 percent, respectively, were regular bedwetters. Rutter et al. (174) estimated the prevalence of enuresis at age five as 13.4 percent in boys and 13.9 percent in girls, whereas Hellbrügge et al. (67) found that 20.4 percent of boys and 26.0 percent of girls aged four to five were enuretic. Forrester et al. (47) reported of enuresis nocturna in 20.7 percent of four-to-five-year-old boys and 17.3 percent of girls.

Generally, girls acquire bladder control earlier than boys, but studies have shown that the boy: girl ratio lies around 1 between the age of four and six, increasing again after school age. Enuresis diurna is much less frequent; Oppel et al. (133) found that 12 percent still had enuresis diurna at the age of four. At age five, 2 percent had enuresis diurna once a week and 8 percent once a month (37).

Encopresis may also be considered a developmental problem and here, too, the age at which lack of control is considered abnormal varies (69). Some authors claim the age limit lies around two years (3), whereas others (138) find it unrealistic to talk about faecal incontinence as an abnormal phenomenon before the age of four. The time of acquiring control is socially and culturally determined (2) and only limited information is available concerning the prevalence of this disorder during early years of childhood.

BEHAVIOUR PROBLEMS

The vast majority of mental disorders in children younger than five are constituted by the vaguely defined group of behaviour problems (163). These disorders have two important characteristics: They represent quantitative deviations from normal development and many of their manifestations may be seen as a response to specific situations (210).

Analysis of the prevalence and the nature of mental disorders has frequently been based upon selected groups of children, such as hospital populations, children referred to treatment, or children belonging to a specific social group or community (4, 12, 53, 68, 74, 78, 102, 103, 128, 152, 183, 201, 203). Based on case register information, Wing et al. (201) found that, in a two-year period, 39.5 boys and 21.1 girls per 10,000 younger than four were referred to psychiatric services in Aberdeen. In Baltimore, the corresponding figures were 24.8 and 15.0 per 10,000 and in Camberwell, 76.5 and 24.5 per 10,000.

In prevalence studies of the rural population on the Danish island of Samsø Nielsen and Nielsen (128a) found a prevalence of past and present mental illness of 0.3 percent for children under four, 4 percent for children aged five to nine, and 14 percent for children aged nine to 14. The average annual referral rate of children to the community psychiatric service on Samsø during a 20-year-period 1957-76 was 0.2 percent for children under four, 1.8 percent for children aged five to nine and 1.1 percent for the age group 10-14 (128b).

A number of factors, including the attitude of the parents, the availability of services, the symptomatology, and the socio-cultural norms, determine who is referred to treatment (43, 45, 49, 52, 54, 173, 178, 201, 203, 205). Still, children brought to professional attention are found to represent the most severe cases (112, 173).

Surveys of children referred to treatment may also explain the tendency to pay attention to the presence of individual psychopathological items without duly recognizing that similar symptoms may occur quite extensively in the general population. The presence of isolated items seems, however, to have limited psychopathological significance (84, 104, 178). Most symptoms deviate only quantitatively from normality. Thus, most disorders are not diagnosed on the basis of the occurrence of single items but on the basis of a multiple symptomatology of a handicapping or persisting nature (173). In other words, we have many symptoms but few disease entities.

Numerous studies have reported a high frequency of isolated psychological symptoms in young children (56, 66, 67, 115, 118, 127). During early years of childhood, worries and fears are predominant. They may be associated with dangers of the dark leading to sleeping difficulties or nightmares (66), or they may be associated with food, resulting in poor appetite and food fads (67). Difficulties in controlling anger and frustration are also common (56), as well as temper tantrums as a way of expressing anger.

Epidemiological Field Surveys

We know that to a considerable degree individual symptoms are part and parcel of growing up; consequently, in order to get a more comprehensive picture of the frequency of behaviour disorders, epidemiological field surveys are needed. Several large-scale surveys have been undertaken (e.g., 173, 178). Investigations have primarily concentrated on children of school age, partly due to the interest in an early detection of maladjusted children. A classical survey of a random sample of school children was undertaken in the U.S.A. by Lapouse et al. (107). Their considerations concerning problems of definition, case finding procedure and delineation of disorders have had much impact on the field. Lapouse et al. (107) and Lapouse (105) observed a remarkably high prevalence of behaviour problems. Their conclusions that behaviour disorders are best defined as disorders deviating from prevailing norms and associated with functional impairment are also valid in children under five. They doubted whether the presence of individual deviations is truly indicative of psychiatric disorders or whether these deviations may be considered as transient phenomena in normal development.

The question arises: How does one identify the behaviourally disturbed preschool child in an epidemiological field survey? In recent years, increasing interest has developed in screening large groups of children, using a multitude of different rating scales or checklists. Unfortunately, most screening devices have originally been chosen for older children (32, 33, 55, 134, 173, 178, 181, 182, 199). Another drawback with reference to very young children is that most screening devices use teachers as suppliers of information either alone or in combination with parents.

Comparatively few rating scales for preschool children have emerged (5, 30, 59, 94, 95, 147, 194). In this age group parental reports are the main source of information. The shortcomings of these in terms of fallible memory, distortion of answers, and interpretations of the significance of certain symptoms represent another difficulty (27, 61, 151). These shortcomings are particularly important in surveys of very young children, due to their great variation in behaviour and the lack of opportunity to cross-validate the parental reports with others.

Bearing these difficulties in mind, it is understandable that a limited number of researchers have concentrated on this particular age group. Richman and Graham (147) developed a valid and most useful instrument aimed at detection of preschool children at risk. It comprises 12 questions on behaviour items (BSQ) known to give rise to difficulties. Based upon parental reports, each item is rated 0, 1 or 2, corresponding to no, little or marked difficulty. The sum of the scores produces a total score and cut-off points of 10 or more suggests a risk of showing a behaviour problem. A behaviour checklist (BCL) using the same 12 items but filled in directly by the parents was developed. BCL was found to be less discriminative than BSQ, i.e., producing more false positives and false negatives; BSQ identified 100 percent of moderately to severely disturbed, BCL 82 percent.

This device has been employed in several important surveys. In Richman et al.'s study (148), a random sample of 705 families in a London borough with three-year-old children was contacted. Among this group, 111 children showed a score of 10 or more; of those 111, 10 children had, furthermore, a language delay. The problem group and a control group of similar size were clinically assessed, showing 10 percent false negatives, i.e., not selected by BSQ, but assessed to have clinical symptoms. Adding these, the overall prevalence of behaviour problems was estimated at 7 percent having moderate to severe disturbances and an additional 15 percent having mild problems. Overall, boys had higher rates than girls of moderate to severe problems; the difference, however, was not significant. Further, the difference in rate according to social class was not significant.

A breakdown in individual items revealed that the most frequent problem was night wetting seen in 36.8 percent of the total population, poor appetite (17.2 percent), day wetting (16.9 percent), waking at night (14.3 percent), overactivity (13.7 percent), fears (12.8 percent), difficulty in settling at night (12.5 percent), faddy eater (11.7 percent). Boys were significantly more likely to be overactive, wetting at night and day and soiling. Girls, on the other hand, were more likely to show fears.

The results suggest that the frequency of preschool children with behaviour and emotional disorders is comparable to that seen in later childhood (173).

Minde and Minde (124) used the same scale in a survey of 240 children registered for junior kindergarten in Toronto and representing a good cross-section of the area's population. The parents filled in the behaviour checklist describing the behaviour over the previous three or four weeks. The cut-off point was set at 10 points. A structured interview was also given to 125 randomly selected children from the total sample. Both screening devices found eight out of 125 (6.4 percent) as deviant, but in only five cases were the same children selected. As regards the individual items, 64 percent were reported as having difficulties in settling down at night, 52 percent were reported as having eating problems, 38 percent had temper tantrums, 33 percent had problems in relationship with others, 29 percent were difficult to manage, 28 percent showed fears, 19 percent showed worries and 16 percent had difficulties in concentration. A roughly equal number of boys and girls exhibited symptoms.

Coleman et al. (29) used the same questionnaire in a survey of 100 three-year-old children attending nursery schools in a London borough. They found that 65 percent showed fears, 53 percent had difficulties in relationship with others, 41 percent had worries, 41 percent were management problems, 36 percent were unwilling to go to bed and 29 percent had temper tantrums.

In all three surveys, the authors investigated the stability of symptoms. Richman (146) screened the problem group and the control group after one year. She found that individual symptoms at three did not predict outcome at four, but that the problem group was more likely to have behaviour problems after one year than the control group. A similar method was used by Minde and Minde (124). The high score children were found to have lost more symptoms than they had gained, whereas the reverse was true for the other groups. A strong consistency in parental ratings was present, suggesting that very young children may have more in common with older children than one has previously assumed and that certain abnormal behaviours are relatively stable already among children of kindergarten age. Also, Coleman et al. (29) reported that a significant change with age in symptoms was concentrated in those symptoms that may be seen as developmental phenomena.

The consistency of the behavioural symptoms was also the topic of one of the surveys which has had the greatest impact (115). A representative sample of every third child born in Berkeley, California during the period from January 1, 1928 to June 30, 1929 was followed. The 252 children were divided into two matched groups. Intensive intervention took place in one group, whereas no intervention took place in the other group; the reported findings refer to the latter. Data were collected through a simple open questioning technique in which non-structured maternal reports were classified according to empirically designed scales. These were divided according to descriptive criteria, making it possible to compare intensity, frequency and age distribution of the individual symptoms.

Although the occurrence of symptoms was reported as problem incidence rather than prevalence, the study deserves mentioning in this review. As regards the occurrence of symptoms, five tendencies were observed: 1) Problems whose frequency fell with increasing age, e.g. speech disorders and problems in toilet training. 2) Problems might increase in frequency with increasing age, a trend observed consistently only in nail-biting. 3) A third pattern was that symptoms increase gradually to an optimum and thereafter fall, as was seen in lying and lack of appetite. 4) The fourth pattern, which was the most common, showed two peaks, one around six and a second around the start of puberty. 5) Finally, certain problems, such as extreme sensitivity, seemed to have little relation with age.

An analysis of the age of the highest incidence revealed that important factors are the developmental aspect of problems, periods of tension, sex differences in the age in which problems emerge, and the emergence of coping devices.

At each age level the authors listed behaviour problems shown by more than one-third of the children. At 21 months, the problems in boys were enuresis, restlessness and temper tantrums, in girls enuresis, food finickiness, thumb-sucking, specific fears and temper tantrums; at three years of age, the problems were food finickiness, overactivity, specific fears and temper tantrums in boys, and the same symptoms, together with somberness, in girls. At three and a half, boys showed overactivity, specific fears, temper tantrums, lying, oversensitivity and negativism, and girls showed food finickiness, overactivity, specific fears, temper tantrums, oversensitivity, physical timidity, and jealousy. At four there was only one change in the behaviour pattern of boys—negativism was no longer prevailing; girls at this age no longer showed food finickiness and physical timidity.

Many problems differed significantly in boys and girls. At age 21 months, boys showed a greater frequency of enuresis diurna, irritability and excessive emotional dependence; at age five, boys showed a higher frequency of temper tantrums. Girls showed a higher frequency of excessive modesty and specific fears at age three, of somberness at age four, and of physical timidity at age five. Analysis of the correlation between certain behaviours at different ages showed that, although problems tended to be present for varying periods of time, change rather than persistence was of the greater significance.

GENERAL HEALTH CONTROLS

Another approach to the question of detecting children with behavioural and developmental problems is through studies associated with the prophylactic health controls.

In Sweden, general health examinations of four-year-old children have been made since 1960, and among four-year-olds in Lund (91, 92, 93), 22 percent were well adjusted, 25 percent exhibited slight behavioral symptoms and 38 percent had symptoms motivating parental advice. In 10 percent referral to child guidance clinics seemed indicated and 4 percent were in need of immediate expert help. Twenty-three percent of children from Dalby, Sweden, needed no help, 63 percent needed advice or treatment within the frames of the child guidance clinic and 14 percent were referred to psychiatric/psychological treatment (70). In Gothenburg (60), 13 percent of four-year-old children were estimated to have a behaviour differing from what was expected; 6 percent had a minor behaviour deviation, 4 percent needed advice from psychologists/psychiatrists and 3 percent needed long-term psychiatric care. Vuille (192, 193) estimated that 23 percent of four-year-olds in Uppsala had behaviour disorders and 14 percent needed treatment, and of suburban Stockholm children aged four (101, 187) about one-third exhibited mental problems of a severity needing referral to a psychologist/psychiatrist.

An improvement of the effectiveness of the psychological screening programs was found necessary (129, 130). The authors stressed that field investigations frequently show considerably higher prevalence figures than those reported in the Swedish health controls, partly due to the fact that the latter not only aim at establishing prevalence figures of disturbed mental health, but also concern themselves with active management of the problems.

Another important experiment was started in Enebakk, Norway (13, 14), aiming at early intervention and change of deviance. Of the four-year-old children, 41 percent showed some kind of psychological problems requiring more help than what was routinely given. One-fifth of the children came from families with nervous disorders, about one-tenth from families with social problems and, finally, one-tenth of the children also had a developmental delay.

FACTORS DETERMINING PREVALENCE

To generalise, most surveys estimate the prevalence of significant mental disorders in children to be between 5 and 15 percent. These crude figures are by themselves not so important; they must be considered in relation to the children's total functioning. The degree of impairment is particularly important (163), since the presence of any abnormality is not necessarily associated with impairment in terms of suffering, social restriction, interference with development, or effects on others.

The significance of disorder is a function of a number of variables. We know that the appropriateness of most behaviour patterns is related to the age of the child and that abnormality has meaning only when age is taken into consideration. We also know that the frequency and the nature of psychic problems differ in boys and girls (9, 87, 115, 145, 173, 178). This difference is observed in children brought to professional attention, but a preponderance of boys exhibiting behavioural problems is also reported in field surveys. Many hypotheses have been proposed in order to explain this difference, but it is generally agreed that it is a combination of biological differences and social stereotypes we observe to an exaggerated degree in disturbed children (42, 119).

Family conditions and life circumstances are also factors of great importance. The association between psychiatric illness in parents and in children has been thoroughly investigated (e.g. 48, 58, 144, 157, 203, 207). This relationship is also observed in field surveys (79). Marital discord and divorce are associated with an increase in psychological problems in children (145, 157, 195), as are very young mothers, single-parent families, and very large families. Children who have been in care also have a higher occurrence of behaviour problems (209); further, multiproblem families seem to produce a higher risk of behavioural deviations (190). Ordinal position has been investigated and is still a matter of much debate, and that only children have a particularly high prevalence has not yet been confirmed. Some (115, 178) report that a preponderance of behavioural problems are observed in elder children.

Socio-cultural and environmental factors are important. Much research has been carried out to analyse the influence of social class (65, 120, 203), but no clear-cut results have yet been reported. An understanding of the many cultural variations in assessment of normality is essential when estimating the prevalence of mental disorder, but low social class per se is not found to be associated with a special high prevalence. On the other hand, some studies have shown that children from deprived areas have more psychiatric problems (25, 26) than children from rural areas, but no difference has been shown between children from deprived areas and from settled working-class areas.

The urban-rural difference has traditionally been studied in terms of delinquency rates. Recently, there has been an increasing interest in analysing child psychiatric symptoms as a function of area differences (87, 109, 167). The most comprehensive and well-known studies have been carried out in U.K. (161, 167), concluding that the higher prevalence of deviances in urban as opposed to rural children aged 10 might possibly be explained by a higher proportion of family discord, broken homes, high turn-over rate of staff and pupils in schools, and larger families in overcrowded houses. The question of housing, particularly the relation between mobility, health and economy in modern suburban communities, is important (71, 143, 187). It has been suggested that living in high rise buildings is particularly damaging to the young child.

EARLY DETECTION AND PROGNOSIS

Two further questions need to be considered: Is it possible to identify mental disorders or children at high risk at a very early age and treat them before the problems turn into severe disorders? May we use the early behaviour of children as a predictor of later problems?

The assumption that it is possible to predict later problems from early behaviour is primarily based on retrospective studies of persons with apparent mental problems and significant preponderance of mental disorders in childhood compared with those of a control group (24, 121, 160). Prospective studies are necessary to solve the question, but a few investigations have related early behaviour to the development of problems. Chamberlin (24) concluded that early behaviour in the home does not per se predict later behaviour to a degree that it is feasible to identify children at risk. Early symptoms are thus not good prognosticators. From observations of infant behaviour it is not possible to distinguish troubled from less troubled children (166, 189). Korsch (100) commented that no behaviour at very early years may characterize children at risk for later maladaptation and stressed that until now the epidemiological approach for identifying children at risk has generally lead to disappointment. Prevention of mental problems through an early identification is tentative.

Consistency of behaviour over time is greater within the same setting than across settings (23, 29, 124, 173, 178). Even though most symptoms seem to change from one age to another, children who exhibit many symptoms at one age also tend to do so at a later age (29, 88, 89, 115, 146, 148, 198). Some authors, including Richman (146) and Westman et al. (198), indicate that behaviour at age three or four may have predictive value. Other authors favour the view that emotional dysfunction at school start is a very good prognosticator of later maladjustment (16, 32, 39, 110, 115, 126, 131, 154).

With regard to the general outcome of mental disorders of early child-hood, it seems quite favourable—perhaps more so for girls than for boys (36, 204). Well-defined syndromes, such as autistic syndrome or hyperki-netic syndrome, have a fairly poor prognosis, irrespective of the kind of treatment given (18, 73, 116). Emotional disorders tend to have the best outcome (210), whereas the conduct disorders may turn chronic and develop into more serious personality disorders (152, 160). Some authors have found a reduction in observed problem behaviour among treated children com-pared with those not treated (125), whereas others claim that improvement is hardly influenced by treatment, the improvement rate being around two-thirds in both groups (178).

PROVISION OF SERVICES

The above-mentioned findings and the fact that most children at some time during their development show signs of disturbed behaviour have given rise to doubt as to the need and desirability of treatment. Rutter and Gra-ham (168) and Scott et al. (176) stressed that prevalence does not equate demand and reported that, even among children with a psychiatric disorder sufficiently marked or prolonged to cause handicap to the child itself or distress to the family or community, only about one-third required treat-ment. One-third might possibly require treatment, and one-third need only advice or diagnosis.

A common view expressed by Buckle and Lebovici (19) is that professional intervention is justified only if the disorder persists long enough to authorize a prognosis of lifelong disorder. Others favour the view that all children with psychological problems merit help and that the aim—no matter what the condition—is to reduce suffering (142).

With the inadequate provision of services prevailing in most countries (97, 176, 210), referral to treatment of all children with psychological problems is beyond available means. Consequently, it is of utmost importance to work towards a balance between need and demand. Here, prevalence surveys may provide the necessary relevant information for actions to ensure the identification and treatment of mental health problems in very early childhood.

REFERENCES

1. ANNELL, A. 1963. The prognosis of psychotic syndromes in children. *Acta psychiat. Scand., 39*, 235.
2. ANTHONY, E.J. 1957. An experimental approach to the psychopathology of childhood: Encopresis. *Brit. J. med. Psychol., 30*, 146.
3. BAKWIN, H. AND BAKWIN, R. 1953. *Clinical Management of Behaviour Disorders in Children*. Philadelphia: W.B. Saunders.
4. BALDWIN, J. 1968. Psychiatric illness from birth to maturity: An epidemiological study. *Acta psychiat. Scand., 44*, 3.
5. BEHAR, L. AND STRINGFIELD, S. 1974. A behaviour rating scale for the preschool child. *Develop. Psychol., 10*, 601.
6. BELL, R.Q., WALDROP, M.F. AND WELLER, G.M. 1972. A rating system for the assessment of hyperactive and withdrawn children in preschool samples. *Amer. J. Orthopsychiat., 42*, 23.
7. BENDER, L. 1958. Genesis in schizophrenia during childhood. *Acta paedopsychiat., 1/2*, 101.
8. BENDER, L. 1974. The family patterns of 100 schizophrenic children observed at Bellevue, 1935-1952. *J. Autism & Child. Schizop., 4*, 279.
9. BENTZEN, F. 1963. Sex ratios in learning and behaviour disorders. *Amer. J. Orthopsychiat., 33*, 92.
10. BERES, D. 1956. Ego deviation and the concept of schizophrenia. *Psychoanal. Stud. Child., 11*, 164.
11. BLOMFIELD, J.M. AND DOUGLAS, J.W.B. 1956. Bedwetting prevalence among children aged 4-7 years. *Lancet, 1*, 850.
12. BOESEN, V. AND BREMS, O. 1969. Det. børnepsykiatriske klientel i et praksis forskningsprojekt. The child psychiatric patients in a research project in general practice. *Ugeskr. Laeg., 135*, 2405.
13. BOGEN, B., SOLUM, L., STORVIK, O. AND SOMMERSCHILD-SUNDBY, H. 1972. *Helsestasjonen i Støpeskjeen*. Oslo: Universitetsforlaget.
14. BOGEN, B. AND SUNDBY, H.S. 1976. *Helsestasjonen alltid i Støpeskjeen*. Oslo: Universitetsforlaget.
15. BOMBERG, D., SZUREK, S. AND ETEMAD, J. 1973. A statistical study of a group of psychotic children. In: S. Szurek and I. Berlin (Eds.), *Clinical Studies in Childhood Psychoses*. New York: Brunner/Mazel.
16. BOWER, E. 1960. *Early Identification of Emotionally Handicapped Children in School*. Springfield, Ill.: Charles C Thomas.

17. BRASK, B.H. 1967. Om behovet for hospitalspladser til psykotiske bᶠrn. The need for hospital beds for psychotic children: An analysis based on a prevalence investigation in the county of Århus. *Ugeskr. Laeg.*, *129*, 1559.

18. BRASK, B.H. AND DAHL, V. 1959. The prognosis of mental disorders in children. *Acta psychiat. Scand.*, *34*, suppl. 136, 266.

19. BUCKLE, D. AND LEBOVICI, S. 1960. *Child Guidance Centres.* Geneva: W.H.O.

20. CAMERON, K. 1955. Diagnostic categories in child psychiatry. *Brit. J. med. Psychol.*, *28*, 67.

21. CAMPBELL, S.B., ENDMAN, M.W. AND BERNFELD, G. 1977. A three-year follow-up of hyperactive preschoolers into elementary school. *J. Child. Psychol. Psychiat.*, *18*, 239.

22. CANTWELL, D.P. 1975. Genetics of hyperactivity. *J. Child Psychol. Psychiat.*, *16*, 261.

23. CHAMBERLIN, R.W. 1976. The use of teacher checklists to identify children at risk for later behavioural and emotional problems. *Amer. J. Dis. Child.*, *130*, 141.

24. CHAMBERLIN, R.W. 1977. Can we identify a group of children at age 2 who are at high risk for the development of behaviour or emotional problems in kindergarten and first grade? *Pediatrics*, Suppl. *59*, 971.

25. CHAZAN, M. AND JACKSON, S. 1971. Behaviour problems in the infant school. *J. Child Psychol. Psychiat.*, *12*, 191.

26. CHAZAN, M. AND JACKSON, S. 1974. Behaviour problems in the infant school: changes over two years. *J. Child. Psychol. Psychiat.*, *15*, 33.

27. CHESS, S., THOMAS, A. AND BIRCH, H.G. 1966. Distortions in developmental reporting made by parents of behaviourally disturbed children. *J. Amer. Acad. Child. Psychiat.*, *5*, 226.

28. CHILAND, C. 1977. Problems in child psychiatric epidemiology contributions from a longitudinal study. In: P.J. Graham (Ed.). *Epidemiological Approaches in Child Psychiatry.* London: Academic Press.

29. COLEMAN, J., WOLKIND, S. AND ASHLEY, L. 1977. Symptoms of behaviour disturbance and adjustment to school. *J. Child Psychol. Psychiat.*, *18*, 201.

30. COLLIGAN, R.C. AND O'CONNELL, E.J. 1974. Should psychometric screening be made an adjunct to the pediatric preschool examination? *Clin. Pediat.*, *13*, 29.

31. COWEN, E.L., DORR, D., CLARFIELD, S., KRELING, B., McWILLIAMS, S.A., POKRACKI, F., PRATT, M.D., TERRELL, D. AND WILSON, A. 1973. The AML: a quick-screening device for early identification of school maladaptation. *Amer. J. Comm. Psychol.*, *1*, 12.

32. COWEN, E.L., PEDERSON, A., BABIGIAN, H.M., Izzo, L.D. AND TROST, M.A. 1973. Long-term follow-up of early detected vulnerable children. *J. Cons. Clin. Psychol.*, *41*, 438.

33. COWEN, E.L., TROST, M.A., IZZO, L.D., LORION, R.P., DORR, D. AND ISAACSON, R.V. 1975. *New ways in School Mental Health.* New York: Human Sciences Press.

34. CREAK, M. 1963. Childhood psychosis: A review of 100 cases. *Brit. J. Psychiat.*, *109*, 84.

35. CREAK, M. AND INI, S. 1960. Families of psychotic children. *J. Child. Psychol. Psychiat.*, *1*, 156.

36. CUNNINGHAM, J.M., WESTERMAN, H.H. AND FISCHHOFF, J. 1956. A follow-up study of patients seen in a psychiatric clinic for children. *Amer. J. Orthopsychiat.*, *26*, 602.

37. DEJONGE, G.A. 1973. Epidemiology of enuresis: A survey of the literature. In: I. Kolvin, R. Mackeith, and S.R. Meadow (Eds.). *Bladder Control and Enuresis.* London: SIMP, Heinemann.

38. DEMYER, M., CHURCHILL, D., PONTIUS, W. AND GILKEY, K. 1971. A comparison of five diagnostic systems for childhood schizophrenia and infantile autism. *J. Autism & Child.Schizop.*, *1*, 175.

39. DOUGLAS, J.W.B. AND MULLIGAN, D.G. 1961. Emotional adjustment and educational achievement—the preliminary results of a longitudinal study of a national sample of children. *Proc. roy. Soc. Med.*, *54*, 885.

40. EISENBERG, L. 1972. The classification of childhood psychosis reconsidered. *J. Autism Child. Schizop.*, *2*, 338.

41. EISENBERG, L. AND KANNER, L. 1956. Early infantile autism. *Amer. J. Orthopsychiat.*, 26, 556.
42. EVANS, E.G.S. 1976. Behaviour problems in children. *Child: Care, Health and Development*, 2, 35.
43. EWALT, P.L., COHEN, M. AND HARWATZ, J.S. 1972. Prediction of treatment acceptance by child guidance clinic applicants. *Amer. J. Orthopsychiat.*, 42, 857.
44. FALKNER, F. 1973. Long term developmental studies: A critique. *Res. Publ. Ass. nerv. ment. Dis.*, 51, 412.
45. FAVEZ, F. AND BETTSHART, W. 1976. Comparison statistique entre des cas de rupture et des cas de traitement dans un service de psychiatrie d'enfants—A statistical comparison between disrupted cases and treated cases in a psychiatric service. *Soc. Psychiat.*, 11, 171.
46. FONTES, V. 1958. Schizophrenia infantile. *Acta Paedopsychiat.*, 25, 183.
47. FORRESTER, R.M., STEIN, Z. AND SUSSER, M.W. 1964. A trial of conditioning therapy in noctural enuresis. *Develop. Med. Child. Neurol.*, 6, 158.
48. FRIEDMAN, R.J. 1974. MMPI characteristics of mothers of preschool children who are emotionally disturbed or have behaviour problems. *Psychol. Rep.*, 34, 1159.
49. FURMAN, S.S., SWEAT, L.G. AND CROCETTI, G.M. 1965. Social class factors in the flow of children to out-patient psychiatric facilities. *Amer. J. publ. Hlth.*, 55, 385.
50. GARMEZY, N. AND DEVINE, V.T. 1977. Longitudinal vs. cross-sectional research in the study of children at risk for psychopathology. In: J.S. Strauss, H.M. Babigian, and M. Roff (Eds.). *The Origins and Course of Psychopathology*. New York: Plenum Press.
51. GARSIDE, R.F., BIRCH, H., SCOTT, D. McI., CHAMBERS, S., KOLVIN, I., TWEDDLE, E.G. AND BARBER, L.M. 1975. Dimensions of temperament in infant school children. *J. Child Psychol. Psychiat.*, 16, 219.
52. GATH, D. 1968. Child guidance and the general practitioner. *J. Child Psychol. Psychiat.*, 9, 213.
53. GATH, D., COOPER, B., GATTONI, F. AND ROCKETT, D. 1977. *Child Guidance and Delinquency in a London Borough*. London: Oxford University Press.
54. GILBERT, G.M. 1957. A survey of "referral problems" in metropolitan child guidance centers. *J. Clin. Psychol.*, 13, 37.
55. GLIDEWELL, J.C., DOMKE, H.R. AND KANTOR, M.B. 1963. Screening in schools for behaviour disorders: Use of mothers' reports of symptoms. *J. Educ. Res.*, 56, 508.
56. GOODENOUGH, F.L. 1931. *Anger in Young Children*. Minneapolis: University of Minnesota Press.
57. GRAHAM, P. 1973. Enuresis: A child psychiatrist's approach. In: I. Kolvin, R.C. MacKeith, and S.R. Meadow (Eds.). *Bladder Control and Enuresis*. London: SIMP, Heinemann.
58. GRAHAM, P. AND GEORGE, S. 1972. Children's response to parental illness: Individual differences. *J. psychosom. Res.*, 16, 251.
59. GRAHAM, P., RUTTER, M. AND GEORGE, S. 1977. Appendix C. Temperamental characteristics schedule. In: A. Thomas, and S. Chess, *Temperament and Development*. New York: Brunner/Mazel.
60. GÖTEBORGSFÖRSÖKET 1972. Hälsekontroll av 4-åringar—Health controls of 4-year olds. *Läkartidningen*, 69, 1893.
61. HAGGARD, E.A., BREKSTAD, A. AND SKARD, Å.G. 1960. On the reliability of the anamnestic interview. *J. abnorm. soc. Psychol.*, 61, 311.
62. HALLGREN, B. 1956. Enuresis. *Acta psychiat. Scand.*, 31, 379.
63. HALVERSON, C.F. JR. AND WALDROP, M.F. 1976. Relations between preschool activity and aspects of intellectual and social behaviour at age 7½. *Develop. Psychol.*, 12, 107.
64. HARPER, J. AND WILLIAMS, S. 1975. Age and type of onset as critical variables in early infantile autism. *J. Autism Child Schizo.*, 5, 25.
65. HARRISON, S.I., McDERMOTT, J.F., WILSON, P.T. AND SCHRAGER, J. 1965. Social class and mental illness in children. *Arch. Gen. Psychiat.*, 13, 411.

66. HEALY, A. 1972. The sleep patterns of preschool children. *Child Behaviour*, *11*, 174.
67. HELLBRÜGGE, T., BARTL, G., BRACK, U., WITTROCK, J. AND SCHUK, H. 1974. Häufigkeit, Art und soziale Bedingleit von Verhaltensstörungen im Vorshulalter. *Mschr. Kinderheil. 122.* 532.
68. HENNINGSEN, B.J. 1974. Ambulant børnepsykiatri Childpsychiatric out-patients. *Ugeskr. Laeg.*, *136*, 1519.
69. HERSOV, L. 1976. Fecal soiling. In: M. Rutter and L. Hersov (Eds.). *Child Psychiatry*. London: Blackwell.
70. HOLST, K., KÖHLER, L. AND KÖHLER, E.-M. 1970. Undersökninger av 4-åringar—Investigations of 4-year olds. *Läkartidningen*, *67*, 3673.
71. HOOPER, D., GILL, R., POWESLAND, P. AND INEICHEN, B. 1972. The health of young families in new housing. *J. psychosom. Res.*, *16*, 367.
72. HOWELLS, J.G. (Ed.) 1965. *Modern Perspectives in Child Psychiatry*. London: Oliver & Boyd.
73. HUESSY, H.R., METOYER, M. AND TOWNSEND, M. 1973. 8-10 year follow-up of 84 children treated for behavioural disorder in rural Vermont. *Acta Paedopsychiat.*, *40*, 230.
74. INDENRIGSMINISTERIET 1954. Ministry of Internal Affairs: De profylaktiske børneundersøgelser—The prophylactic health controls. *Ugeskr. Laeg.*, *116*, 740.
75. INGHAM, J.G. AND MILLER, P. McC. 1976. The concept of prevalence applied to psychiatric disorders and symptoms. *Psychol. Med.*, *6*, 217.
76. INGRAM, T.T.S. 1959. Specific developmental disorders of speech in childhood. *Brain*, *82*, 450.
77. INGRAM, T.T.S. 1963. Delayed development of speech with special reference to dyslexia. *Proc. roy. Soc. Med.*, *56*, 199.
78. ISAGER, T. 1976. Distrikts børnepsykiatri-District child psychiatry. *Ugeskr. Laeg.*, *138*, 2396.
79. JONSSON, G. AND KÄLVESTEN, A.-L. 1964. *222 Stockholmpojkar*. Stockholm: Almquist & Wiksell.
80. KANNER, L. 1943. Autistic disturbances of affective contact. *Nerv. Child.*, 2, 217.
81. KANNER, L. 1954. To what extent is early infantile autism determined by constitutional inadequacies? *Proc. Ass. Res. Nerv. & Ment. Dis.*, *33*, 378.
82. KANNER, L. 1958. History and present status of childhood schizophrenia in the U.S.A. *Acta Paedopsychiat.*, *25*, 138.
83. KANNER, L. 1960. Child Psychiatry: retrospect prospect. *Amer. J. Psychiat.*, *117*, 15.
84. KANNER, L. 1960. Do behavioural symptoms always indicate psychopathology? *J. Child. Psychol. Psychiat.*, *1*, 17.
85. KANNER, L. 1965. Infantile autism and the schizophrenias. *Behav. Sci.*, *10*, 412.
86. KANNER, L. 1972. *Child Psychiatry*. 4. ed. Springfield, Ill: Charles C. Thomas.
87. KASTRUP, M. 1977. Urban-rural differences in 6 year olds. In: P.J. Graham (Ed.). *Epidemiological Approaches in Child Psychiatry*. London: Academic Press.
88. KLACKENBERG, G. 1971. A prospective study of children. *Acta Paediat. Scand.*, Suppl., *224*, 1.
89. KLACKENBERG, G. 1974. Förskoleålderens föränderlige symptom bild—The change in symptom pattern of preschool age. *Soc. Med. Tidsskr.*, *51*, 88.
90. KNOBLOCH, H. AND PASAMANICK, B. 1975. Some etiologic and prognostic factors in early infantile autism and psychosis. *Pediatrics*, *55*, 182.
91. KÖHLER, L. 1973. Physical examination of four-year-old children. *Acta paediat. Scand.*, *62*, 181.
92. KÖHLER, L. 1973. Health control of four-year-old children. An epidemiological study of child health. *Acta paediat. Scand.*, suppl. *235*.
93. KÖHLER, L. AND LINDQUIST, B. 1972. Barnhälsovården—före och efter skolans början Child health care before and after the school start. *Läkartidningen*, *69*, 6049.
94. KOHN, M. AND ROSMAN, B.L. 1972. A social competence scale and symptom checklist for the preschool child. *Develop. Psychol.*, *6*, 430.

95. KOHN, M. AND ROSMAN, B.L. 1973. A two factor model of emotional disturbance in the young child: Validity and screening efficiency. *J. Child. Psychol. Psychiat.*, *14*, 31.
96. KOLVIN, I. 1971. Psychoses in childhood. In: M. Rutter (Ed.). *Infantile Autism: Concepts, Characteristics and Treatment*. Edinburgh and London: Churchill Livingstone.
97. KOLVIN, I. 1973. Evaluation of psychiatric services for children in England and Wales. In: J.K. Wing and H. Häfner (Eds.), *Roots of Evaluation. The Epidemiological Basis for Planning Psychiatric Services*. Oxford: Oxford University Press.
98. KOLVIN, I., OUNSTED, C., HUMPHREY, M., McNAY, A., RICHARDSON, L., GARSIDE, R., KIDD, J. AND ROTH, M. 1971. Studies in the childhood psychoses. I-VI. *Brit. J. Psychiat.*, *118*, 381, 385, 396, 403, 407, 415.
99. KOLVIN, I., WOLFF, S., BARBER, L.M., TWEDDLE, E.G., GARSIDE, R., SCOTT, D. McI. AND CHAMBERS, S. 1975. Dimensions of behaviour in infant school children. *Brit. J. Psychiat.*, *126*, 114.
100. KORSCH, B.M. 1977. The answer is no. *Pediatrics*, suppl. *59*, 1063.
101. LAGERKVIST, B., LAURITZEN, S., OLIN, P. AND TENGVALD, K. 1975. Four-year-olds in a new suburb: The need for medical and social care. *Acta paediat. Scand.*, *64*, 413.
102. LAMBERT L., ESSEN, J. AND HEAD, J. 1977. Variations in behaviour ratings of children who have been in care. *J. Child Psychol. Psychiat.*, *18*, 335.
103. LANDONI, G., PENNING, R., MERINS, G. AND BETTSCHART, W. 1973. Étude de la clientèle d'un service de guidance infantile—A study of the patients in a child guidance clinic. *Soc. Psychiat.*, *8*, 1.
104. LAPOUSE, R. 1965. The relationship of behaviour to adjustment in a representative sample of children. *Amer. J. Publ. Hlth.*, *55*, 1130.
105. LAPOUSE, R. 1966. The epidemiology of behaviour disorders in children. *Amer. J. Dis. Child.*, *111*, 594.
106. LAPOUSE, R. 1967. Problems in studying the prevalence of psychiatric disorder. *Amer. J. Publ. Hlth.*, *57*, 947.
107. LAPOUSE, R., MONK, M.A. AND STREET, E. 1964. A method for use in epidemiologic studies of behaviour disorders in children. *Amer. J. Publ. Hlth.*, *54*, 207.
108. LAVIK, N.J. 1973. The classification problem in child and adolescent psychiatry. *Acta psychiat. Scand.*, *49*, 131.
109. LAVIK, N.J. 1977. Urban-rural differences in rates of disorder. In: P.J. Graham (Ed.), *Epidemiological Approaches in Child Psychiatry*. London: Academic Press.
110. LIEM, G.R., YELLOTT, A.W., COWEN, E.L., TROST, M.A. AND IZZO, L.D. 1969. Some correlates of early-detected emotional dysfunction in the schools. *Amer. J. Orthopsychiat.*, *39*, 619.
111. LIN, T.-Y. AND STANDLEY, C.C. 1962. *The Scope of Epidemiology in Psychiatry*. Geneva: W.H.O.
112. LOBITZ, G.K. AND JOHNSON, S.M. 1975. Normal versus deviant children. A multimethod comparison. *J. Abnorm. Child. Psychol.*, *3*, 353.
113. LOTTER, V. 1966. Epidemiology of autistic conditions in young children. I. prevalence. *Soc. Psychiat.*, *1*, 124.
114. LOTTER, V. 1967. Epidemiology of autistic conditions in young children. II. Some characteristics of the parents and children. *Soc. Psychiat.*, *1*, 163.
115. MACFARLANE, J.W., ALLEN, L., AND HONZIK, M.P. 1962. *A developmental Study of the Behaviour Problems of Normal Children between 21 months and 14 Years*. 2.ed. Berkeley and Los Angeles: University of California Press.
116. MACLAY, I. 1967. Prognostic factors in child guidance practice. *J. Child Psychol. Psychiat.*, *8*, 207.
117. MacMAHON, B. AND PUGH, T.E. 1970. *Epidemiology*. Boston: Little, Brown.
118. MASSLER, M. AND MALONE, A.J. 1950. Nailbiting: A review. *J. Pediat.*, *36*, 523.
119. McCONVILLE, B.J. 1975. The future for child psychiatry. Mandate for change. *Canad. psychiat. Ass. J.*, *20*, 209.
120. McDERMOTT, J.F., HARRISON, S.I., SCHRAGER, J., WILSON, P., KILLINS, E., LINDY, J.,

AND WAGGONER, R.W. 1967. Social class and mental illness in children. *J. Amer. Acad. Child. Psychiat.*, *6*, 309.

121. MELLSOP, G.W. 1972. Psychiatric patients seen as children and adults: Childhood predictors of adult illness. *J. Child Psychol. Psychiat.*, *13*, 91.

122. MILLER, F.J.W., COURT, S.D.M., WALTON, W.S. AND KNOX, E.G. 1960. *Growing up in Newcastle-upon-Tyne*. Oxford: Oxford University Press.

123. MILLER, R.T. 1975. Childhood schizophrenia: a review of selected literature. In: S. Chess and A. Thomas (Eds.), *Annual Progress in Child Psychiatry and Child Development*. New York: Brunner/Mazel.

124. MINDE, R. AND MINDE, K. 1977. Behavioural screening of preschool children: A new approach to mental health. In: P.J. Graham (Ed.), *Epidemiological Approaches in Child Psychiatry*. London: Academic Press.

125. MITCHELL, W.S., ROTHWELL, B. AND BURTENSHAW, W. 1975. Mothers and their disturbed preschool children: an intervention study. *Child: Care, Health and Development*, *1*, 389.

126. MULLIGAN, G., DOUGLAS, J.W.B., HAMMOND, W.A. AND TIZARD, J. 1963. Delinquency and symptoms of maladjustment: the findings of a longitudinal study. *Proc. roy. Soc. Med.*, *56*, 1083.

127. NEWSON, J. AND NEWSON, E. 1968. *Four-Years-Old in an Urban Community*. Middlesex: Penguin Books.

128a NIELSEN, J. AND NIELSEN, J.A. 1977. Eighteen years of community psychiatric service in the island of Samsφ. *Brit. J. Psychiat.*, *131*, 41.

128b NIELSEN, J. AND NIELSEN, J.A. 1978. Personal communication.

129. NILSSON, C., SUNDELIN, C. AND VUILLE, J.-C. 1976. General health screening of four-year-olds in a Swedish county. *Acta Paediat. Scand.*, *65*, 663.

130. NILSSON, C., SUNDELIN, C. AND VUILLE, J.-C. 1977. General health screening of four-year-olds in a Swedish county. *Acta Paediat., Scand.*, *66*, 289.

131. O'NEAL, P., AND ROBINS, L.N. 1958. The relation of childhood behaviour problems to adult psychiatric status: a 30-year follow-up study of 150 subjects. *Amer. J. Psychiat.*, *114*, 961.

132. OPPEL, W.C., HARPER, P.A. AND RIDER, R.V. 1968. Social psychological and neurological factors associated with nocturnal enuresis. *Pediatrics*, *42*, 627.

133. OPPEL, W.C., HARPER, P.A., AND RIDER, R.V. 1968. The age of attaining bladder control. *Pediatrics*, *42*, 614.

134. PETERSON, D.R. 1961. Behaviour problems of middle childhood. *J. Cons. Psychol.*, *25*, 209.

135. PIGGOT, L.R. AND SIMSON, C.R. 1975. Changing diagnosis of childhood psychosis. *J. Autism Child. Schizo.*, *5*, 239.

136. PITFIELD, M. AND OPPENHEIM, A.M. 1964. Childrearing attitudes of mothers of psychotic children. *J. Child Psychol. Psychiat.*, *5*, 51.

137. PRECHTL, H. AND STEMMER, C. 1962. The choreiform syndrome in children. *Develop. Med. Child. Neurol*, *4*, 119.

138. QUAY, H.C. AND WERRY, J.S. (Eds.) 1972. *Psychopathological Disorders in Childhood*. New York: Wiley.

139. RANDALL, D., REYNELL, J. AND CURWEN, M. 1974. A study of language development in a sample of 3-year-old children. *Brit. J. Dis. Communication*, *9*, 3.

140. REES, S.C. AND TAYLOR, A. 1975. Prognostic antecedents and outcome in a follow-up study of children with a diagnosis of childhood psychosis. *J. Autism Child Schizo.*, *5*, 309.

141. REID, D.D. 1960. *Epidemiological Methods in the Study of Mental Disorders*. Geneva: W.H.O.

142. Report of the Joint Commission on Mental Health of Children 1973. *The Mental Health of Children: Services, Research and Manpower*. New York: Harper & Row.

143. RICHMAN, N. 1974. The effects of housing on preschool children and their mothers. *Dev. Med. Child. Neurol., 16*, 53.
144. RICHMAN, N. 1976. Depression in mothers of preschool children. *J. Child Psychol. Psychiat., 17*, 75.
145. RICHMAN, N. 1976. Disorders in preschool children. In: M. Rutter and L. Hersov (Eds.), *Child Psychiatry.* Oxford: Blackwell.
146. RICHMAN, N. 1977. Short term outcome of behaviour problems in 3-year-old children. In: P.J. Graham (Ed.), *Epidemiological Approaches to Child Psychiatry.* London: Academic Press.
147. RICHMAN, N. AND GRAHAM, P.J. 1971. A behavioural screening questionnaire for use with 3-year-old children. *J. Child Psychol. Psychiat., 12*, 5.
148. RICHMAN, N., STEVENSON, J.E. AND GRAHAM, P.J. 1975. Prevalence of behaviour problems in 3-year-old children. *J. Child Psychol. Psychiat., 16*, 277.
149. RIMLAND, B. 1965. *Infantile Autism.* London: Methuen.
150. RIMLAND, B. 1971. The differentiation of childhood psychoses. *J. Autism. Child. Schizo., 1*, 161.
151. ROBBINS, L. 1963. The accuracy of parental recall of aspects of child development and of child-rearing practices. *J. Abn. Soc. Psychol., 66*, 261.
152. ROBINS, L.N. 1966. *Deviant Children Grown Up.* Baltimore: Williams & Wilkins.
153. ROBINS, L.N. 1970. Follow-up studies investigating childhood disorders. In: E. Hare and J.K. Wing (Eds.), *Psychiatric Epidemiology.* Oxford: Oxford University Press for the Nuffield Provincial Hospitals Trust.
154. ROBINS, L.N. 1972. Follow-up studies of behaviour disorders in children. In: H.C. Quay and J.S. Werry (Eds.) *Psychopathological Disorders of Childhood.* New York: Wiley.
155. RUTTER, M. 1965. Classification and categorization in child psychiatry. *J. Child Psychol. Psychiat., 6*, 71.
156. RUTTER, M. 1966. Behavioural and cognitive characteristics of a series of psychotic children. In: J.K. Wing (Ed.), *Early Childhood Autism.* Oxford: Pergamon.
157. RUTTER, M. 1966. *Children of Sick Parents: An environmental and Psychiatric Study.* Maudsley Monograph No. 16, Oxford: Oxford University Press.
158. RUTTER, M. 1970. Discussion of follow-up studies investigating childhood disorders. In: E. Hare and J.K. Wing (Eds.), *Psychiatric Epidemiology.* Oxford: Oxford University Press for the Nuffield Provincial Hospitals Trust.
159. RUTTER, M. 1972. Childhood schizophrenia reconsidered. *J. Autism. & Child. Schizop., 2*, 315.
160. RUTTER, M. 1972. Relationships between child and adult psychiatric disorders. *Acta psychiat. Scand., 48*, 3.
161. RUTTER, M. 1973. Why are London children so disturbed? *Proc. roy. Soc. Med., 66*, 1221.
162. RUTTER, M. 1974. The development of infantile autism. *Psychol. Med., 4*, 147.
163. RUTTER, M. 1975. *Helping Troubled Children.* Middlesex: Penguin Books.
164. RUTTER, M. 1976. Speech delay. In: M. Rutter and L. Hersov (Eds.), *Child Psychiatry.* London: Blackwell.
165. RUTTER, M. 1977. Brain damage syndromes in childhood. Concepts and findings. *J. Child Psychol. Psychiat., 18*, 1.
166. RUTTER, M., BIRCH, H.G., THOMAS, A. AND CHESS, S. 1964. Temperamental characteristics in infancy and the later development of behavioural disorders. *Brit. J. Psychiat., 110*, 651.
167. RUTTER, M., COX, A., TUPLING, C., BERGER, M. AND YULE, W. 1975. Attainment and adjustment in two geographical areas: I. The prevalence of psychiatric disorders. *Brit. J. Psychiat., 126*, 493.
168. RUTTER, M. AND GRAHAM, P. 1966. Psychiatric disorder in 10- and 11-year old children. *Proc. Roy Soc. Med., 59*, 382.

169. RUTTER, M., LEBOVICI, S., EISENBERG, L., SNEZNEVSKIJ, A.V., SADOUN, R., BROOKE, E. AND LIN, T.-Y. 1969. A triaxial classification of mental disorders in childhood. *J. Child Psychol. Psychiat.*, *10*, 41.
170. RUTTER, M. AND LOCKYER, L. 1967. A five to fifteen-year follow-up study of infantile psychosis. *Brit. J. Psychiat.*, *113*, 1169.
171. RUTTER, M., SHAFFER, D. AND SHEPHERD, M. 1973. Preliminary communication. An evaluation of the proposal for a multiaxial classification of child psychiatric disorders. *Psychol. Med.*, *3*, 244.
172. RUTTER, M., SHAFFER, D. AND SHEPHERD, M. 1975. *A multiaxial classification of child psychiatric disorders.* Geneva: W.H.O.
173. RUTTER, M., TIZARD, J. AND WHITMORE, K. 1970. *Education, Health and Behaviour.* London: Longman.
174. RUTTER, M., YULE, W. AND GRAHAM, P. 1973. Enuresis and behavioural deviance: Some epidemiological considerations. In: I. Kolvin, R. MacKeith and S.R. Meadow (Eds.) *Bladder Control and Enuresis.* London: SIMP, Heinemann.
175. SCHWARTZ, A.H. AND MURPHY, M.W. 1975. Cues for screening language disorders in preschool children. *Pediatrics*, *55*, 717.
176. SCOTT, D.McK., KOLVIN, I., TWEDDLE, E.G. AND McLAREN, M. 1976. Psychiatric care of children and adolescents. In: A.A. Baker (Ed.), *Comprehensive Psychiatric Care.* London: Blackwell
177. SHAFFER, D. 1976. Enuresis. In: M. Rutter and L. Hersov (Eds.) *Child Psychiatry.* London: Blackwell.
178. SHEPHERD, M., OPPENHEIM, B. AND MITCHELL, S. 1971. *Childhood Behaviour and Mental Health.* London: University of London Press.
179. SCHLEIFER, M., WEISS, G., COHEN, N., ELMAN, M., CVEJIC, H. AND KRUGER, E. 1975. Hyperactivity in preschoolers and effect of methylphenidate. *Amer. J. Orthopsychiat.*, *45*, 38.
180. SCHMIDTCHEN, S., ONDARZA, G.V. AND DAHME, B. 1974. Faktorenanalytische Untersuchung von Verhaltensstörungen bei Kinder. *Praxis der Kinderpsychologie und Kinderpsychiatrie*, *23*, 270.
181. SINES, J.O., PANKER, J.D., SINES, L.K. AND OWEN, D.R. 1969. Identification of clinically relevant dimensions of children's behaviour. *J. Cons. Clin. Psychol.*, *33*, 728.
182. SPIVACK, G. AND SPOTTS, J. 1965. The Devereux child behaviour scale: Symptom behaviours in latency age children. *Amer. J. Ment. Defic.*, *69*, 839.
183. STAHL, B. 1968. Projects for research in general practice in greater Copenhagen and the county of Ringkøbing. *Acta psychiat. Scand.*, suppl. *203*, 69.
184. STEWART, M., PITTS, F., CRAIG, A. AND DIERNF, W. 1966. The hyperactive child syndrome. *Amer. J. Orthopsychiat.*, *36*, 861.
185. STEVENSON, J. AND RICHMAN, N. 1976. The prevalence of language delay in a population of three-year-old children and its association with general retardation. *Develop. Med. Child. Neurol.*, *18*, 431.
186. TAFT, L.T. AND GOLDFARB, W. 1964. Prenatal and perinatal factors in childhood schizophrenia. *Develop. Med. Child. Neurol.*, *6*, 32.
187. TENGVALD, K., LAGERKVIST, B., LAURITZEN, S. AND OLIN, P. 1974. Fyraåringan i en ny förort. Four-years-old in a new suburb. *Soc. Med. Tidsskr.*, *51*, 99.
188. THOMAS, A. AND CHESS, S. 1977. *Temperament and Development.* New York: Brunner/Mazel.
189. THOMAS, A., CHESS, S. AND BIRCH, H.G. 1968. *Temperament and Behaviour Disorders in Children.* New York: New York University Press.
190. TONGE, W.L., JAMES, D.S., AND HILLAM, S.M. 1975. *Families without Hope.* Kent: Headley Brothers Ltd.
191. TREFFERT, D.A. 1970. Epidemiology of infantile autism. *Arch. Gen. Psychiat.*, *22*, 431.
192. VUILLE, J.-C. 1971. Uppspårande av somatiske avvikelser ock psykologiska

problem.—Detection of somatic deviations and psychological problems. *Läkartidningen, 68,* 456.
193. VUILLE, J.-C. 1971. Den almänna hälsokontrollen av fyraåringar—The general health control of 4-year-olds. *Läkartidningen, 68,* 449.
194. WALKER, D.K. 1973. *Socioemotional Measures for Preschool and Kindergarten Children. A Handbook.* San Francisco: Jossey-Bass.
195. WARDLE, C.J. 1961. Two generations of broken homes in the genesis of conduct and behaviour disorders in childhood. *Brit. Med. J., 2,* 349.
196. WENAR, C., RUTTENBERG, B., DRATMAN, M. AND WOLF, E. 1967. Changing autistic behaviour. *Arch. Gen. Psychiat., 17,* 26.
197. WERRY, J.S. 1972. Organic factors in childhood psychopathology. In: H.C. Quay and J.S. Werry (Eds.), *Psychopathological Disorders of Childhood.* New York: Wiley.
198. WESTMAN, J.C., RICE, D.L. AND BERMANN, E. 1967. Nursery school behavior and later school adjustment. *Amer. J. Orthopsychiat., 37,* 725.
199. WIMBERGER, H.C. AND GREGORY, R.J. 1968. A behavior checklist for use in child psychiatry clinics. *J. Amer. Acad. Child. Psychiat., 7,* 677.
200. WING, J.K. (Ed.) 1966. *Early Childhood Autism. Clinical Educational, and Social Aspects.* Oxford: Pergamon.
201. WING, L., BALDWIN, J.A. AND ROSEN, B.M. 1972. The use of child psychiatric services in three urban areas: An international case-register study. In: J.K. Wing and A.M. Hailey (Eds.), *Evaluating a Community Psychiatric Service.* London: Nuffield Provincial Hospitals Trust, Oxford University Press.
202. WING, L., YEATES, S.R., BRIERLEY, L.M. AND GOULD, J. 1976. The prevalence of early childhood autism: comparison of administrative and epidemiological studies. *Psychol. Med. 6,* 89.
203. WOLFF, S. 1961. Social and family background of preschool children with behaviour disorders attending a child guidance clinic. *J. Child Psychol. Psychiat., 2,* 260.
204. WOLFF, S. 1961. Symptomatology and outcome of preschool children with behaviour disorders attending a child guidance clinic. *J. Child Psychol. Psychiat., 2,* 269.
205. WOLFF, S. 1967. Behavioural characteristics of primary school children referred to a psychiatric department. *Brit. J. Psychiat., 113,* 885.
206. WOLFF, S. 1971. Dimensions and clusters of symptoms in disturbed children. *Brit. J. Psychiat., 118,* 421.
207. WOLFF, S. AND ACTON, W.P. 1968. Characteristics of parents of disturbed children. *Brit. J. Psychiat., 114,* 593.
208. WOLKIND, S. AND EVERITT, B. 1974. A cluster analysis of the behavioural items in the preschool child. *Psychol. Med., 4,* 422.
209. WOLKIND, S. AND RUTTER, M. 1973. Children who have been in care—an epidemiological study. *J. Child Psychol. Psychiat., 14,* 97.
210. W.H.O. 1977. Child mental health and psycho-social development. *Technical report series 613,* Geneva:W.H.O.

18

UNEXPECTED DEATH IN INFANCY

H. HARTMANN, M.D.

Professor of Forensic Medicine

and

G. Molz, M.D.

Professor of Perinatal Morphology,
Gerichtlich-Medizinisches Institut der Universität, Zürich

INTRODUCTION

The mortality rate varies during different stages of human life (Figure 1). The first mortality peak is during the first months. In this period, the proportion of unexpected deaths is high (Figure 2), with most deaths resulting from natural causes. Accidental and homicidal deaths occur during the whole of childhood, while suicide is extremely rare in the young child (15). Unexpected infant death has to be reported to the coroner; an autopsy should always be performed, because it is impossible to elucidate the cause through postmortem external examination only.

DEATHS FROM NATURAL CAUSES—SUDDEN INFANT DEATH SYNDROME

Between the ages of two weeks and one year almost half of the children who die at home are found dead unexpectedly (7). The Sudden Infant Death Syndrome (SIDS), also called "crib death" or "cot death," has been recognized as a specific clinicopathological entity and the major cause of death after the neonatal period (2). A satisfactory *definition* for the syndrome is difficult in view of the unknown etiology and the inadequate knowledge about the pathogenic mechanism. The current working definition is that derived from the 1969 conference on this syndrome:

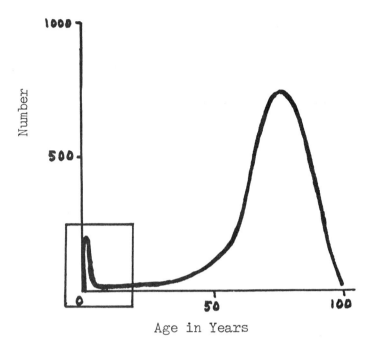

FIGURE 1. Mortality Rate (City of Zurich, 1971-75)

The sudden death of any infant or young child which is unexpected by history, and in which a thorough postmortem examination fails to demonstrate an adequate cause of death (27).

Epidemiology

The *incidence* of SIDS is two to three deaths per 1000 live-births (16). This rate has been found to be identical for regions with Western civilization standards, including the United States and Canada as well as Great Britain and Western Europe. The annual death rate from SIDS has been estimated to lie between 8,000-10,000 SIDS in the United States (3), about 2,000-3,000 in Great Britain (29) and 2,000-4,000 in Western Germany (22). In the city of Zurich, Switzerland (population 385,000), the incidence is 1.1 per 1,000 live-births. During the period from 1964 to 1977, of the 57,864 live-births (29,631 males and 28,233 females), 67 infants (41 males and 26 females) died unexpectedly between one week and one year of age (13). Although the

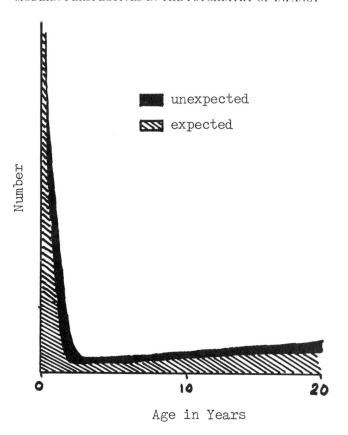

FIGURE 2. Mortality Rate of Children (City of Zurich, 1971-75)

rate is low, SIDS was a leading cause of death after the neonatal period in the last three years.

Sex, Age and Multiple Birth

Most of the studies have indicated a higher frequency of SIDS in males than in females. This possibly reflects only the general male preponderance in mortality and infectious disease morbidity in infants (2). In our own series we see a similar predominance. Out of the 141 cases of SIDS, 89 (61 percent) were male infants. In the control group, out of the 752 clinically ill infants dying at a comparable age and during the same period, 437 (58 percent) were male infants (13).

The highest death rate occurs in infants less than six months of age (11). The peak incidence is between two and four months. Rarely, cases have been reported in infants younger than one week. Beckwith (2) noted the youngest case at the age of four days. A significant relationship was found with twin delivery (8); the risk of SIDS in a twin appears to be over twice as high as that in a singleton.

Relationship to Sleep

One of the striking features of SIDS is that it attacks without warning. In the typical case an apparently healthy infant is put to bed. Some time later the baby is found dead. There is almost no evidence that a struggle has taken place. The infant is still in the same position as when last seen alive. SIDS probably occurs during normal sleeping periods and is not associated with an audible cry. Bergman (3) reported that in over one-third of his cases adults were sleeping in the same room as the infant but heard no noises from him.

Beckwith (2) also stated that several dozen times a vigilant adult was in an immediately adjacent area. Although sleep is an almost universal part of the story of SIDS, some of the victims die during feeding or in a stroller. These infants are observed to become stiff, stop breathing and become cyanotic (12).

Findings at Autopsy

Careful necropsy and intensive histological examination, as well as investigations in virology, bacteriology, immunology and vitreous humour chemistry, reveal many abnormalities.

Forrest Hay and Emery (9) pointed out the important role of microscopy in their experience with over a thousand SIDS deaths. Most reports indicate that a cause of death can be demonstrated at autopsy in one- to two-thirds of the cases (33). Fatal infectious diseases such as myocarditis or meningitis are reported. The major lesions are found in the respiratory tract in form of tracheobronchitis and bronchiolitis. These findings indicate that the infants were not completely healthy before death but had minimal defects which contributed to their deaths.

One-third to half of the infants have only minor changes. Outstanding among these findings are intrathoracic petechiae in the visceral serosal surfaces of the lungs, pericardium and thymus. Petechiae also may be found on the parietal surfaces of the chest. Blood does not clot in the heart and vessels. Pulmonary congestion and edema, along with minor microscopic inflammatory inflitrates, may be present in the lung. The thymus is usually large in size and shows minimal stress effects.

Recently, Naeye (17, 18) demonstrated as *new findings* hypertrophy and hyperplasia of smooth muscle fibers in the media of small pulmonary arteries, increased weight of the right cardiac ventricle and abnormal retention of brown fat in the vicinity of the adrenals. In addition, 63 percent of the victims had a reduced and 23 percent an enlarged volume of glomic cells in their carotid bodies. Naeye also reported abnormal hepatic hematopoesis. These findings are still under discussion (19).

The concept of *"near miss for SIDS"* is based on observations of infants found to be limp, apneic, cyanotic and with marked bradycardia. Most of the infants recovered after resuscitation, but some of the babies subsequently died suddenly. Based on the reversible "near miss," cyanotic-apneic spells have become an important focus of current research (12). In addition, attempts are underway to discover infants at risk.

High-risk Infants

Much work has been done by Carpenter and Emery (4, 5, 6) creating a multistage scoring system for identifying infants at risk of SIDS. The scoring at birth considered mother's age and blood group, urinary infection or polyhydramnion during pregnancy, duration of labour, prematurity, birth order, breastfeeding. Increasing age of the mother, blood group A, and breastfeeding were associated with *low* risk. The post-neonatal score collected data about the first month of life in the babies who died during this period. An important variable was a history of cyanotic attacks and feeding difficulties.

In 1973, Steinschneider (26), monitoring five infants who were referred because of cyanotic episodes, discovered protracted apnea during sleep. Two of the five, siblings, died suddenly afterwards and their autopsies revealed findings typical of SIDS. In his subsequent findings, Steinschneider found that prolonged apneic spells occurred more frequently when respiratory-tract infections were present. In recent studies (26A), it has become evident that infants at risk for prolonged sleep apnea were born of mothers whose urinary estrogens at 40 weeks gestation were significantly lower than in controls.

Shannon et al. (24) observed abnormal regulation of sleeping ventilation on examining the response to carbon-dioxide breathing in infants with prolonged sleep apnea who had needed resuscitation. These infants failed to change tidal volume adequately during carbon-dioxide breathing. They postulated a defect in the regulation of alveolar ventilation.

Reaction of Parents to SIDS

The sudden and unexpected loss of an apparently healthy infant produces a tremendous shock. Parents feel responsible for the sudden death. The emotional trauma can be very great. First of all, parents must be convinced that the death was not their fault and was not caused by suffocation. Valdés-Dapena (31) and Beckwith (2) have made a habit of giving an explanation to the parents immediately upon completion of the autopsy, informing them of the diagnosis and telling them some of the facts about SIDS. Most parents want to know why their baby died. We discuss our findings as soon as the autopsy and laboratory analyses are completed, trying to answer their questions about SIDS and about the prognosis for a subsequent child. In our personal experience, follow-up contact is very helpful. Among 141 families in which a case of SIDS occurred, 41 subsequent infants were born. Except for one, all are alive and healthy.

Treatment

Treatment of the apneic, cyanotic infant is obviously ventilation. Gunteroth (12) reported his experience with a home monitor in a half-dozen "near misses" and recommended monitoring equipment until six months of age.

ACCIDENTAL DEATHS

Road Traffic Accidents (20, 21)

Road accidents account for two-thirds of all accidental childhood deaths. Children are most likely to be killed as pedestrians between the ages of three and 10 years (80 percent trying to cross the road; one-half during unexpected maneuvers). In the age group seven to 15, bicycle riders have the highest risk of fatal accidents (50 percent wheel off in a side road; 20 percent hits on straight road; 15 percent intersection collisions). The number of children killed as passengers is five times smaller than the number of pedestrian fatalities. Small children under the age of six years are significantly safer in rear seats, especially in a restraint system which is designed to suit their size (25). School children are well protected on rear or front seat by belt wearing.

The injuries sustained by road traffic accidents are heavier in children than in adults because a larger proportion of the body of a child pedestrian is hit at the first impact. Most critical are head injuries, which are frequently observed in children. The main recommendations to prevent children from road traffic deaths are the following:

> Small children without adult attendance must be kept away from roads. As car passengers they should not be allowed to sit in front.

> School children have to receive practical and individual road safety education. The effect of theoretical and general safety education is small. Before the age of 14 no child should be allowed to ride a bicycle on a public road.

> Car passengers have to use restricting systems designed for children.

> Roads frequently used by children must have safe crossing facilities and low speed limits. Safe playgrounds separated from traffic should be available.

Home Accidents

Up to the age of five years children are more likely to be killed by home accidents than by traffic accidents.

Suffocation is said to be the most common cause of accidental death in babies or small children. Unfortunately, this diagnosis is frequently ruled by the coroner without autopsy. The omission brings grief and self-accusation to the parents, who are already psychologically traumatized by the sudden loss of the child. Since their guilt feelings are aggravated by such a verdict, no "asphyxia by suffocation" verdict should be accepted without careful analyses (past history, scene investigation, autopsy, special examinations). A great number of the cases prove to belong to the unexpected baby death. Nevertheless, some suffocations are not disputable. They occur by aspiration of food or foreign bodies, by plastic bags or sheets covering mouth and nose, by burying the face in a smooth and moist pillow etc.

Fatal *burns and scalds* occur mostly in the age group under two and are observed in connection with fire, hot water or oil from different origins. Medical examination has to carefully differentiate the real accident from child abuse. The same caution has to be taken in case of alleged fatal *fall* from bed, cot, high chair, swaddling table or stairway. Detailed description of the fall with reconstruction of its biomechanics is required, taking into consideration height, nature of the floor, weight and injuries of the child.

Intoxication occurs in all stages of infant life, but the number of children affected declines with increasing age. Fortunately, the outcome in a great many cases is much better than estimated by anxious parents. Therefore, clinical examination in suspected poisoning should exclude such harmless cases before initiating intensive treatment and/or expensive chemical analyses. As a precaution, the doctor should immediately take a sample of blood and urine in a glass cylinder and store it in the refrigerator. In Switzerland, the following toxic agents are most frequently implicated in fatal intoxications of children: carbon monoxide (open fire, incomplete combustion of gas or fuel in closed rooms); drugs (narcotics, antidepressants, other psychoactives); sewer gas in rural toilets; mushrooms (amanita phalloides). In the U.S., aspirin and lead ingestion (old, deteriorated housing) play an important role.

Drowning occurs in babies (bath tub) or in children who do not know how to swim (private swimming pool). After such an event, responsible people risk being charged for negligence and being sued. No baby should be left alone in a bath tub! Pools have to be protected with a fence to prevent unauthorized entrance.

HOMICIDAL DEATHS

The most frequent situations of homicidal death in children are ill-treatment (cruelty and neglect-battered child syndrome), infanticide, sexual offence, kidnapping, and killing with parental suicide. During such a crime the child may be killed intentionally or accidentally. While the medical expert has to assess the injuries as to their origin (how? by what means?) and their consequences, the judge has to decide whether the death is accidental, manslaughter, or murder.

The Battered Child Syndrome

This syndrome (1, 10, 14, 23, 28, 30, 32) occurs at all levels of the social scale but more frequently in the lower income group. It is estimated that 3 in every thousand children suffer from serious injury by abuse. (See chapter 20 for a detailed account of this syndrome).

Infanticide

Although the literal meaning of *infanticide* comprises a deliberate killing of a child of any age and by anybody, the term is mostly used only for the *killing of a newborn by the mother*. A charge before a jury or a court needs clearest evidence of the felony; stillbirth, inviability (prematurity, diseases or malformation), or accidental death have to be definitely excluded. Live birth is demonstrated by fully expanded lungs and by the presence of air in the bowels. The pathologist has then to search for injuries suggestive of infanticide. This felony is practicable without leaving external traces, for instance by smothering with a plastic bag or drowning. But in most cases sufficient signs of mechanical violence will be evident (nail marks, scratches, bruises, signs of asphyxiation). They have to be carefully estimated and distinguished from inadvertent injuries during labour. The conclusion of the medical expert is based finally on the correlation of his findings with the description of the circumstances of the birth given by the mother. Temporary insanity of the mother during labour or childbirth must be taken into consideration by an experienced forensic psychiatrist, especially if the question of neglecting the newborn arises as a cause of death.

Sexual Assault

During a *sexual assault*, death may be accidental or homicidal. Different causes are possible (strangulation, stab, cut, etc.), but frequently the situation clearly indicates progress of the felony. Sometimes unique and bizarre findings may mislead the doctor, especially if he lacks experience. He has to be careful in the interpretation of local injuries: Children suffering from pin worms may have scratches on the external genitalia and the anus unrelated to a sexual crime. The mucosa of the vestibule also may be injected and swollen from simple rubbing by the child.

Examining a little child after a sexual assault requires much patience and tact from the practitioner. The real history is difficult to obtain. Feelings of fear, shame, defence tend to push it away. Fantasy may play a tricky role. The doctor must learn the terms the child understands for things like penis, vagina, sperm. Swabs should be dried quickly on a slide (gauze-swabs are worse than those taken with a platinum loop). Testing for sperm and prostatic fluid including blood typing, as well as search for venereal diseases, requires a specialized laboratory.

SUICIDAL DEATHS

Under the age of 10 years suicide is extremely rare. In Switzerland only one case has been observed in the last decade. Up to the age of 14 years, the number is still small. Boys predominate in a ratio of approximately 5 to 1 over girls. Hanging is well to the fore. Some situations are complex and point to an accident, e.g. during a tying game or sexual play. In those cases the manner of death can only be determined by psychological autopsy. The real boom of suicide occurs in puberty. Frequent motives are lover's grief, school or home problems, early mental disease. The decision to commit suicide and the performance are frequently abrupt and transitory in juveniles. Therefore, the chance of prevention is high, if somebody realizes the danger in time.

REFERENCES

1. ANDERSON, W.R. AND HUDSON, R.P. 1976. Self-inflicted bite marks in battered child syndrome. *Forens. Sci.*, 7, 71.
2. BECKWITH, J.B. 1977. *The Sudden Infant Death Syndrome.* U.S. DHEW Publ. No. (HSA) 77-5251.
3. BERGMAN, A.B. 1973. Sudden infant death syndrome. *Am. fam. physician*, 8, 95.
4. CARPENTER, R.G. AND EMERY, J.L. 1974. Identification and follow up of infants at risk of sudden death in infancy. *Nature, 250,* 729.
5. CARPENTER, R.G. AND EMERY, J.L. 1977. Final results of study of infants at risk of sudden death. *Nature, 286,* 724.
6. CARPENTER, R.G., GARDNER, A., McWEENY, P.M. AND EMERY, J.L. 1977. Multistage scoring system for identifying infants at risk of unexpected death. *Arch. dis. childh.*, 52, 606.
7. EMERY, J.L. 1973. Classifying and recording unexpected deaths in infants. *J. clin. Path.*, 26, 386.
8. FEDRICK, J. 1974. Sudden unexpected death in infants in the Oxford record linkage area. *Brit. J. prev. soc. Med.*, 28, 164.
9. FORREST HAY, I. AND EMERY, J.L. 1976. Cot death. *Lancet*, I, 146.
10. GEORGE, J.E. 1973. Spare the rod: A survey of the battered-child syndrome. *Forens. Sci.*, 2, 129.
11. GUILLEMINAULT, C. AND ARIAGNO, R. 1977. Sudden infant death syndrome. *Bull. europ. Physiopath. resp., 13,* 591.
12. GUNTEROTH, W.R. 1977. Sudden infant death syndrome (crib death). *Am. Heart J., 93,* 784.
13. HARTMANN, H. AND MOLZ, G. 1977. Unexpected death in infancy. *Hexagon Roche, 5,* (2) 1.
14. KEMPE, C.H. 1971. Paediatric implications of the battered baby syndrome. *Arch. dis. childh., 46,* 28.
15. LYONS, M.M. 1972. Pediatric forensic pathology. *J. Med.* (New York), 72, 816.
16. MANDELL, F. AND BELK, B. 1977. Sudden infant death syndrome. The disease and its survivors. *Postgrad. Med. 62,* 193.
17. NAEYE, R.L. 1974. Hypoxemia and the sudden infant death syndrome. *Science, 186,* 837.
18. NAEYE, R.L. 1974. Pulmonary-arterial abnormalities in the sudden-infant-death syndrome. *New Engl. J. Med.*, 289, 1167.
19. NAEYE, R.L. AND FISHER, R. 1976. Cardiac and other abnormalities in the sudden infant death syndrome. *Scientific Proc. Ped. Path. Conf.*, Boston.
20. *Proceedings of the International Meeting on Biomechanics of Trauma in Children* 1974. Lyon.
21. *Proceedings of the 6th Conference of the International Association of Accident and Traffic Medicine* 1977. Melbourne.
22. SCHMIDT, G. 1971. Der plötzliche Kindestod in Westdeutschland. *Stud. Generale, 24,* 1144.
23. SCHMITT, B.D. AND KEMPE, C.H. 1975. *Child Abuse. Management and Prevention of Battered Child Syndrome.* Basle: Ciba-Geigy Ltd.

24. SHANNON, D.C., KELLY, D.H. AND O'CONNELL, K. 1977. Abnormal regulation of ventilation in infants at risk for sudden-infant-death syndrome. *New Engl. J. Med. 297*, 747.
25. SPRENGER, H. AND WALZ, F. 1977. Unfalluntersuchung: Rücksitzpassagiere und Kinder. *Eidgenössische Polizeiabtlg, Bern.*
26. STEINSCHNEIDER, A. 1972. Prolonged apnea and the sudden infant death syndrome: Clinical and laboratory observations. *Pediatrics 50*, 646.
26a STEINSCHNEIDER, A. 1977. Sleep apnea and the sudden infant death syndrome. U.S. DHEW Publ. No. (NJH) 77-1436.
27. BERGMAN, A.B., BECKWITH, J.B. AND RAY, C.G. 1969. *Sudden Infant Death Syndrome.* Proceedings of the Second International Conference on Causes of Sudden Death in Infants. Seattle: University Washington Press.
28. *Symposium of Battered Child Syndrome* 1973. *Beitr. gerichtl. Med., 31*, 92.
29. TEARE, D. AND KNIGHT, B. 1971. Der Tod in der Wiege. *Stud. Generale, 24*, 1131.
30. TRUBE-BECKER, E. 1973. Die Kindesmisshandlung und ihre Folgen. *Pädiat. Praxis, 12*, 389.
31. VALDÉS-DAPENA, M. 1975. The sudden infant death syndrome—1975; and up-date for pathologists. *Bull. Int. Acad. Path., 16*, 15.
32. WILCOX, D.P. 1976. Child abuse laws: Past, present and future. *J. Forens. Sci., 1*, 71.
33. WORKING PARTY FOR EARLY CHILDHOOD DEATHS IN NEWCASTLE 1977. Newcastle survey of deaths in early childhood 1974/76, with special reference to sudden unexpected deaths. *Arch. dis. Childh., 52*, 828.

19

MOURNING FOR YOUNG CHILDREN

Hugh Jolly, M.D., F.R.C.P.

Physician-in-Charge,
Department of Paediatrics,
Charing Cross Hospital, London

INTRODUCTION

I first became concerned with the needs of bereaved parents and the lack of help they had received when, in the course of my ordinary work as a paediatrician, I found myself constantly coming in contact with parents who, having lost a child, had received so little help that mourning was incomplete and the family was suffering from a preventable load of stress. The majority of these parents had lost their child as a stillbirth.

STILLBIRTH

In Great Britain there are at present about 7000 stillbirths each year. However, the subject has received scant attention in research literature. For example, a major text in the field published in 1972 (3) contains no reference to stillbirth. When I have questioned obstetricians, paediatricians and midwives about the procedural policy in their hospital for dealing with the dead baby and helping the parents, I am usually met by an embarrassed answer, indicating a total lack of knowledge as to what happens; it is only rarely that I learn of a policy of active help for the parents.

Death has replaced sex as the taboo subject and until recently doctors and nurses received no training in the handling of death. In many respects, the doctor's medical training has decreased his natural ability to help at this time, because it is aimed at curing. Consequently, the death of his patient is felt as personal failure for which he feels guilty, while the needs of relatives are, to a considerable extent, swamped by personal feelings. Bourne (2) has evidence showing the reluctance of family doctors to remember the patients who have had a stillbirth. On the other hand, nurses are better equipped to help because their training has emphasized caring rather than curing, so that their feelings of guilt are lessened.

Mourning takes weeks or months to complete, but completion is difficult to reach if, in the first place, the person being mourned has not been seen after death. In the case of stillborn babies, mourning is yet more difficult if the baby has never been seen at all. But in many hospitals the baby is removed at once before the mother has any opportunity to see, let alone hold, her baby.

Countless mothers have described to me what it is like to go through pregnancy and end with nothing to show for it—a non-event. The feeling of loss is all the greater if you end with a vacuum, having earlier felt your baby living and moving inside you. One mother described how she tried to sit up to see her dead baby but was pushed back by the nurse, who not only would not allow her to see her baby but refused to tell her the sex. To this day she does not know whether she had a son or a daughter.

One mother was told, "What you haven't seen you don't miss." I was frequently told what it felt like not to have a grave to visit. Some went to the cemetery looking for a grave, only to find a barren strip of land instead of the headstone they had hoped for. "*The baby was buried in a communal grave before we realized. We were informed of the position of the grave, but on visiting it with flowers were made more desolate because there was only a flat stretch of ground there, with no feeling of visiting our son. We felt he had been buried like so much rubbish, in fact with no acknowledgement of his much wanted brief existence.*"

One mother of a newborn baby was unusually anxious. It was only discovered after this baby's birth that her previous baby had been stillborn. I remember talking to her and learning how her husband, in order (as he believed) to spare her feelings, had never told her where the baby was buried. The next day I was able to talk to him and his wife. He could understand his wife's needs and told her the name of the cemetery which they then planned to visit as soon as she left the hospital. Her anxiety over the new baby largely vanished.

A devout Catholic mother, having recovered her feelings sufficiently to wish to plan the funeral arrangements for her stillborn baby, found that she was too late—the hospital authorities had already burnt her baby. In the light of this experience, it is hardly surprising that one mother told me of the fear, shared by her husband and herself, that their dead baby would be used by the hospital for experimentation.

In 1975 I wrote about stillborn babies in two of my regular articles in *The Times* (5, 6). These produced a flood of letters. Many of the writers described how this was the first time they had ever been able to express their feelings. One mother wrote, "Your article made me feel for the first time since it happened that my feelings are not so unnatural as I had feared." Another wrote, "My husband and I never speak of it as it is too painful and even our children do not know of it." Another letter read, "Eventually my first husband and I were divorced; we both agree that the break up originated from the inability to cope adequately with the loss of our child."

One father was kept out of the labour ward while his wife was delivering their stillborn baby and described himself as being "locked" in another room. After the delivery he was allowed to go to the labour ward and, on the way there, he passed the open door to the wash-up room. There lying on the draining board among some dirty tea cups was his baby.

One mother wanted to steal babies from prams; another described how the baby's brother thought that she had gotten rid of the baby. The vast majority of those who wrote emphasized their wish to have seen their dead baby even if the baby was malformed. Those who had not seen their baby were particularly bitter.

This apparent callousness and lack of understanding for the feelings of the bereaved parents extends beyond the hospital. In England, when registering the baby's death, the father has, until recently, received a document for the undertaker headed in bold type "Certificate for Disposal (Stillbirth)." Many parents have described to me their distress on receiving a document permitting them to "dispose" of their much loved and wanted baby. It is traumatic enough to have the anachronism of registering the baby's birth and death at the same moment. Three years of pressure on the Registrar-General have now resulted in a more humane certificate in which the word "disposal" has been omitted.

All mothers feel a sense of failure when they have been delivered of a dead baby. The poignancy of their feelings was summed up for me by one mother when she told me she felt she had created death. Another said she had not given birth, but death.

One mother, whose baby was known by the medical staff to be dead, told me of a charade acted by the staff whereby they listened to the baby's heart during labour and said everything was going on fine. When, without warning, the baby was born dead, she screamed, and was immediately given an injection to knock her out. When she came round from this, she went into hysteria.

Management of Stillbirths

What can be done to ease this load of sorrow and help parents to be able to mourn their stillborn babies so that they can recover from their emotional distress? In the first place, parents must be told if the baby is known to have died *in utero*. In fact, most mothers will be aware of this already from cessation of movements. Mothers have also described to me how a dead baby feels stiff during the process of birth. The atmosphere among the labour ward staff is bound to be different when the baby is known to be dead before delivery; the staff should be able to share their sorrow with the parents. I emphasize parents because it is essential for the father also to be present in order to support his wife in their mutual grief.

Once the baby has been delivered, the parents should be helped (not forced) to see and to hold their dead baby (10). Since this requires previous discussion and training of staff, I make a point of talking about it with all new staff in order that they can be prepared for a stillbirth, which they may first encounter with little time to work out what to do. I am constantly amazed by the sensitive manner in which young, inexperienced doctors can handle the situation if prepared beforehand. The baby should be brought to the parents wrapped in a comforting blanket rather than in the clinical green cloths normally used for receiving newborn babies.

In one instance, a young house officer was able to sit on a mother's bed holding the dead newborn baby wrapped in a blanket. Gradually, he was able to encourage the mother to feel the baby's foot through the blanket and eventually to feel the whole baby. Finally, she was able to look at her baby without the surrounding blanket and to handle him.

On another occasion, a young woman obstetric house surgeon delivered a single girl of a stillborn baby without any relative present. The mother didn't want to see her baby so the doctor removed him from the ward. Ten minutes later the mother asked for her baby and the doctor brought him back. She sat on the mother's bed, placing the baby beside her. Slowly she was able to get the mother to feel the baby's hands and feet and then to touch him all over. At this point the doctor left the room because, as she later told me, she felt superfluous. She returned ten minutes later to find the mother holding her baby in her arms. This she did for one hour, during which time she was joined by the baby's father and her sister. Together they were all able to mourn the dead baby.

Even if a baby is deformed, he should be seen by the parents. If they are not allowed to do so they will be haunted by imagining the monster they have created, which is always worse than the real thing. Even the most severely deformed baby can be sensitively shown to parents so that their feelings of horror are reduced by the skillful use of drapes to cover the deformed parts for a time.

Parents should be helped to plan the funeral so that it takes place when the mother is well enough to attend. The other children in the family, whatever their ages, should also take part. This funeral should not be confined to those legally termed stillborns—28 weeks gestation or more—but should take place for younger babies if this is the wish of the parents. In such cases, a certificate from the hospital doctor for the undertaker is all that is required.

Some parents prefer a funeral service in the hospital chapel, leaving the hospital authorities to arrange the burial or cremation afterwards.

How to help the mother while she remains in the hospital is another important question. There is a tendency to arrange for her to be discharged from hospital with great rapidity, but this is not necessarily the best arrangement. Discharge should be worked out on an individual basis. Rapid discharge is sometimes motivated by the staff's discomfort, but there is much they can do to help if the mother stays in the hospital during this stage, especially if early discharge means leaving a mother to brood on her own at home.

It is not a good idea for the mother to spend all day alone in a single room in hospital. Permission should be obtained from her so that the other mothers in the ward can be told of her loss and can talk appropriately to her. This is usually preferable to sending her off to a gynaecological ward to prevent her from meeting mothers of healthy newborn babies.

We make a point of offering the father a portable bed in his wife's room so that even if he is away at work during the day he can always be with her during the otherwise lonely hours of the night.

Every member of staff must be trained to understand the feelings of the parents and their need for time to mourn. They must know that the most hurtful suggestion possible is to recommend having another baby quickly in order to "replace" the dead one. No baby can replace a dead one, who will remain a permanent member of the family even though no longer living. It is rare to find later that the stillborn baby has not been named by the parents.

Ongoing help must be provided by someone trained—a doctor, nurse, social worker, health visitor, minister or priest. Such help will enable parents to work through their grief, thereby reducing the length of the period of depression and guilt which is an inevitable accompaniment of bereavement. It helps if parents have agreed to an autopsy so that they can be told whether their baby was normal and, if not, of possible future genetic risks.

A child quoted in Nanette Newman's *Lots of Love* helps all this to make sense: *"When my daddy was driving, we saw a fox lying on the road and nobody stopped. You should always stop and say goodbye to dead things."*

The feelings of loss described with a stillborn baby also take place when a mother has a miscarriage or termination of pregnancy or when she gives up her baby for adoption. For this reason these losses are discussed in the next section. When taking the medical history from a pregnant woman, it is essential to learn if any such losses have occurred, since feelings of bereavement will be enhanced during pregnancy and especially when the new baby is born. If the mother is warned of this natural experience, her distress will be lessened. Failure to help leads to needless maternal anxiety and guilt with the newborn baby.

What I have so far described pertains to most Westernized nations; more "primitive" societies are likely to have traditional ceremonies in which the mutual grief of the tribe sustains the parents in their loss. Nevertheless, the more I talk to mothers, the more I become aware of the similarity of their feelings. Recently, a Muslim Yoruba woman from Nigeria was delivered in our hospital of a stillborn baby. I talked out her grief with her and found her feelings of loss to be identical with those of English women. I saw her later the same morning with her Muslim husband and she was a changed woman. He told me (and his wife) that she would forget; I was quite incapable of conveying to him the feelings of loss which she had described to me a few hours earlier. Had I only met the parents together, I would never have learned the wife's real feelings and might have been convinced by her forceful husband's statement that women from Nigeria didn't feel the same and that she would soon forget.

However, a Jewish woman delivered of a stillborn baby was the one mother who told me how her religion had removed all her problems regarding the funeral and burial. She believed that a stillborn baby had to be buried in the coffin of another woman, although, in fact, this is not a Jewish rite. She also knew that, being a woman herself, she would not be permitted to attend the funeral.

In an attempt to provide further help on a wider scale a group of interested workers have produced the draft of a leaflet which it is suggested could be given to parents who have suffered the loss of a stillborn infant (1, see Appendix).

Miscarriage

For some years, when taking a medical history on any child referred to me, I have asked the parents whether they have lost a child or sustained a miscarriage. On learning of a miscarriage I always put the same question to them: "I get the feeling that we doctors do not know what it is like for a mother to experience a miscarriage—do you mind if I ask you about it?" Parents have often expressed grief at being asked but never resentment. The answer is almost always the same. First, they speak of the physical pain, which is often described as the same as or even worse than the pain of full-term labour; secondly, they speak of the feeling of loss and subsequent emptiness for which help has seldom been offered. I imagine that the severity of the labour pains results, in part, from the fact that the cervix is unripe and therefore less easily dilated and partly from the grief which accompanies the realization of the impending loss of a much wanted baby.

These feelings of loss are accentuated during subsequent pregnancies and immediately after delivery. It is, therefore, essential that the history taken in the antenatal clinic covers miscarriage so that mothers can be helped to be aware that it is natural for feelings of grief for the lost baby to be accentuated at this time.

Termination of Pregnancy

It is possibly even more essential to learn of a previous termination when taking a pregnant woman's history in the antenatal clinic. When a previous pregnancy was aborted, the woman may feel a sense of guilt, as well as enhanced feelings of grief and loss, during this pregnancy. It is also important to enquire if the father of the terminated pregnancy is the same as the father of the present baby and to establish whether the present father knows of the previous termination. These issues can easily be raised on the first antenatal visit when the subject is first mentioned, but it is extremely difficult to bring them up on subsequent visits. As a paediatrician, I have often found myself in a helpless situation with a couple showing anxiety about their new baby. The antenatal notes record a previous termination but give no indication whether that baby's father was the same as the present and whether he, in fact, knows of the termination. I am, therefore, like someone gagged because I can make no reference to the termination, although it may well be the cause of the anxiety over the new baby.

Termination of pregnancy can create guilt feelings even if it is only contemplated but not carried out. In these days, when consideration of termination is not uncommon, later guilt feelings are felt by the mother when she looks at the baby she might have destroyed, even if the possibility of termination was considered only momentarily. Awareness of this possibility and an appropriate discussion will go far to set a mother's mind at rest.

Neonatal Death

The loss of a baby in the neonatal period is likely to cause greater grief than a stillborn baby because the child has been known as a person. On the other hand, the period of grief with a stillborn baby may be longer and less complete if the baby has not been seen or handled.

Particular attention must be paid to the needs of parents whose babies require intensive care in a special unit where they are nursed in incubators and ventilators, surrounded by intensive monitoring equipment so that they are hardly visible. Parents must be encouraged to touch the baby in the incubator, since if the baby dies without the parents' making contact, they will feel like the parents of a stillborn who do not see the baby. We have found that mothers of babies nursed naked in intensive care are helped by being offered the opportunity to dress their dead baby. In a sense, this may be the most normal activity they have been able to preform for their baby. Many are intensely grateful for a photograph of their dead baby—their one tangible memory.

Crib Deaths

There can be few greater shocks than putting a normal baby to sleep in his crib only to find him dead a few hours later. Most parents will attempt to resuscitate the baby and rush him to hospital. The casualty doctor should undertake emergency resuscitation procedures, unless it is so obvious that the child is dead and that the parents accept this fact that such procedures would be inappropriate.

After this procedure it is important to sit down with the parents and record a full medical history. Nothing is more distressing for parents than to be questioned only by the coroner's officer. After taking the history, the doctor should examine the dead baby in another room, unless it is clear that the parents would prefer to be present. Bacterial swabs, a blood culture and a lumbar puncture should be performed in an attempt to identify the cause of death.

Most of this work will be undertaken by the paediatric house physician who is called to casualty. It is our policy for him to arrange to see the parents again the next day in order to tell them the autopsy results. He does this with a senior social worker who is especially experienced in the problem and arranges ongoing help for the parents.

In relation to the care of future children born to parents who have sustained a crib death, it is interesting that they prefer that they should sleep in the parental bed rather than in a crib. If there were any truth in the smothering theory, it would seem that such parents might be more frightened by having their babies in bed with them.

Death of an Older Child

To understand the needs of parents in this situation, it is necessary to discuss first the care of the dying child. This requires an understanding of a child's views on death.

Every child thinks about death. He learns of relatives who have died and meets it in animals, especially if he has pets. But even earlier, as soon as he is old enough to feel attached to another person, he becomes aware of the possibility of losing that person. Fear of death, originating in the fear of losing something loved, is a basic human emotion which arises spontaneously in a child without being instilled from outside. Children, therefore, cannot be shielded from the idea of death, as some parents might wish; they can only be helped to accept it as part of the cycle of life. In fact, being more matter-of-fact than their parents, children are realistic enough to know that if everyone went on living there would soon be no room left on the earth for new babies.

Once a child can talk he will ask about death, just as he will ask about sex, though it will be some time before he appreciates that death is irreversible. Consequently, some of his words and reactions may seem callous by adult standards. It is essential to be aware of the stage of understanding reached by the child. The mother of a toddler might be unnecessarily hurt by his common remark to her when cross:: "I wish you were dead." This means, of course, that he wishes his mother to go away temporarily but to be available to return as soon as the child gives instructions.

It takes the child many conversations before he understands about death. It is essential to be accurate and honest, never using stupid phrases like "lost" instead of dead. Obviously, if grandpa is "lost," you should get moving at once and find him! Similarly, to refer to someone who has died as having gone to sleep is bewildering for a child, who may fear he will be taken away in his sleep. He may also be distressed if he didn't say goodnight to grandpa before he went to "sleep." To refer to death as being taken by God to live with him will also frighten a child that he too may be "taken."

Adult emotions, when talking about death, are coloured by fear of the unknown. This complicates matters for the young child still at the stage when he believes that adults know everything. Even the most religious parent is ignorant about death and a possible afterlife.

Fortunately, the child does not need exact answers. He wants assurance that his parents are neither worried nor preoccupied by fear of death. A child can understand that death causes disintegration of the body, especially if he keeps pets. How many children have wanted to dig up the pet they buried to see how much he has disintegrated? How parents react will depend on their own beliefs, but they should convey that the memory and the influence of a person live on after death, so death is not the end of that individual.

Reactions of Children to Bereavement

A small child may regard death as a kind of magical punishment, especially if it involves a brother or sister, towards whom he is bound to have had feelings of anger and jealousy. At times he may consider that the death is caused by his own destructive thoughts. In order to compensate, he may behave extra well, as if attempting to reverse the situation and bring the dead person back to life. Alternatively, he may behave badly in order to draw punishment on to himself, thereby lightening his load of guilt.

Parents of such children may feel angry that their child is not grieving appropriately, whereas he is grieving in a manner which fits his concept of death. The greatest disaster may occur when parents, lost in their own grief, fail to understand and share the grief felt by their children when bereaved. On one occasion, a surviving brother whose feelings of grief were ignored by his parents committed suicide. Children must be given the time and the opportunity to talk about their loss. They are very likely to feel they are being compared unfavourably with their lost sibling who may become immortalized—to their detriment. The surviving children should be reminded of the good things they did for the one who has died. They should also be told that, of course, it is normal for children to quarrel and this had nothing to do with the sibling's death.

Adult fears of death are bound up with the fear of no longer existing. Children are frightened of pain at the moment of death. This is evident from their questions and their drawings. If asked to draw death they are likely to create scenes of fighting with bombs, guns and bows and arrows. Red is the predominant colour. It is clear that their ideas have been influenced by television.

A child who loses a pet needs time for mourning in order to recover from the distress of bereavement. Rushing out to the pet shop for a replacement is totally unsuitable. Moreover, immediate replacement might make the child believe that the loss of any loved one could be neutralized in this way.

Talking to the Child with a Potentially Fatal Illness

When taking with a fatally ill child, it is essential to listen carefully to the child in order not to miss any of his questions. If, in effect, he is asking, "Am I going to die?" the first reply should be "What made you ask?" This should be explained to all student nurses during their first day on a children's ward so that they do not gloss over the vital question if it comes their way. After giving the child the opportunity to answer, the nurse is usually best advised to tell the child that he is asking such important questions that she is going to call the head nurse or the doctor to answer them.

When a child with leukaemia or cancer asks if he is going to die, I explain that the illness is trying to kill him. Consequently, I am having to give him powerful drugs to kill the illness. In this way I can lead on to the side effects of cytotoxic drugs, especially loss of hair.

Parents are sometimes reluctant to tell a dying child the truth, but a child is helped by knowing the facts. He can soon tell if his parents are lying and will want to know why, in relation to the most important question he has ever asked, he is not told the truth.

One of a child's reactions, if not told the truth by parents or staff, is likely to be that death must be even worse and more painful than he had imagined; therefore, he is right to be frightened.

Upon learning the truth, children can be seen to relax. Parents and child can begin to talk again to each other and to share feelings which previously they were all experiencing alone. To an extent they may begin the process of mutual mourning. A teenage girl with inoperable sarcoma was able to help her parents accept her impending death with peace and dignity.

In peacetime there are few opportunities for heroism. Dying is an opportunity for heroic behaviour to which a child is likely to respond if helped.

ADOPTION

The mother who gives up her baby for adoption needs the opportunity and understanding to allow her to mourn the loss of her baby. It helps if she has handled her baby before he goes away to be adopted, but on no account must she be forced to care for her child or to breastfeed the infant, as happens in some hospitals. We find that if a mother asks not to see her child, she often, eventually, makes her way to the nursery when no one is looking.

Following adoption, the bereaved mother needs sensitive and expert on-going help. If this is not provided, she is likely to become pregnant again quickly, without ever coming to understand her own needs and how they arose.

HANDICAPPED CHILD

Telling the parents the facts relating to a child, such as a Down's syndrome baby, whose handicap is recognized at birth requires an understanding of their needs. These parents have to be helped to mourn the loss of the perfect child they expected before they can come to terms with the handicapped child they have.

The news should be given early—not later than the second day—to both parents at the same time by the consultant in charge. They should be given the facts sympathetically but without excessive emotion. The one request I have heard repeatedly from parents of handicapped infants is, "Please teach your medical students not to preface their remarks by saying they have bad news to tell or referring to a tragedy—this is for us to decide."

SUMMARY

Mourning for young children differs according to the age of the child when death occurs. Seeing and handling the dead child are as vital with stillborn babies as in any other bereavement. Mourning is also necessary for the baby given away for adoption and for the perfect baby expected when a handicapped child is born instead.

Mourning takes time; otherwise it becomes compounded so that everything else around the bereaved person also seems dead. Guilt is part of the process of mourning. At first this is directed towards working out what could have been done to prevent the death. Later, guilt is felt when the bereaved individual begins to experience enjoyment again, and then feels that this is disrespectful to the dead person.

Subsequent children can never replace the lost infant, since the lost child remains a permanent member of the family who is talked about and remembered. This is essential for the safety of the marriage. Parents should also be aware that the feeling that it is unnatural to outlive one's own child is almost universal among bereaved parents.

REFERENCES

1. BEARD R. W., BECKLEY J., BLACK D., BREWER C., CRAIG Y., HILL A.M., JOLLY H., LEWIS E., LEWIS H., LIMERICK S., LISTON J., MORRIS D., SCRIVEN D., AND WILSON R. 1978. Help for parents after stillbirth. *British Medical Journal, 1*, 172.
2. BOURNE, S. 1968. Psychological effects of stillbirths on women and the doctors. *J. roy. Coll. gen. Pract., 16*, 103.
3. HOWELLS, J.G. 1972. *Modern Perspectives in Psycho-Obstetrics*. Edinburgh: Oliver & Boyd.
4. JOLLY, H. 1975. Telling a child about death. *The London Times*, August 13.
5. JOLLY, H. 1975. How hospitals can help parents to bear the loss of a baby. *The London Times*, November 5.
6. JOLLY, H. 1975. The heartache in facing the facts of a stillborn baby. *The London Times*, December 3.

   The above three articles are reproduced in *More Commonsense About Babies and Children* Jolly, H. 1978 Pelham Books (hardback) and Sphere Books (paperback).

7. JOLLY, H. 1976. Stillbirth—A new approach. *Nursing Mirror, 143*, 40.
8. JOLLY, H. 1977. Loss of a baby. *Aust. Nursing J., 7*, 40.
9. JOLLY, H. 1976. Family reactions to stillbirth. *Proc. Roy. Soc. Med., 69*, 835.
10. JOLLY, H. 1978. Loss of a baby. *Australian Paed. J., 14*, 3.
11. LEWIS, E. 1976. The management of stillbirth. Coping with an unreality. *Lancet, 2*, 619.
12. NEWMAN, N. 1974. *Lots of Love*. London: Collins.
13. SCHIFF, H. S. 1977. *The Bereaved Parent*. New York: Crown.

APPENDIX:
HELP FOR PARENTS AFTER STILLBIRTH

LEAFLET FOR PARENTS WHOSE CHILD WAS STILLBORN

These notes have been prepared to help you following your baby's death.

Information for Parents Who Have Had a Stillborn Child

The death of a baby before or during birth is an overwhelming disappointment, bringing grief and distress to the parents, doctors, and nurses. In spite of recent advances in medicine and obstetrics which have reduced the number of newborn babies that die, about 1 in 100 babies born in England and Wales is stillborn.

What is Stillbirth?

Stillbirth is the death of a baby in the last three months of pregnancy or during labour.

Why Did Your Baby Die?

Sometimes a reason for the baby's death is found at post-mortem examination, but very often no cause is found. Post-mortems are not done routinely on stillborn babies but should be done to try to find out why your baby died. This may be important to help your doctor to advise you about your next pregnancy.

Was Your Baby's Death Anybody's Fault?

Everybody is upset when a stillbirth occurs. Parents, doctors, and nurses experience a sense of failure, loss, and grief, and wonder if the tragedy could have been avoided. Parents, especially mothers, are likely to blame themselves; there is also a strong tendency for parents to blame the doctors and nurses. This is part of the grief and depression many people feel after suffering such a personal loss. It may help to talk to a doctor, a midwife, or a health visitor about your thoughts and feelings. Talking with other mothers often helps.

Is It More Difficult to Give Birth to a Stillborn Baby?

It is very distressing to carry a dead baby inside you. Although labour and delivery are the same for live and stillbirths, they may feel different because of the sense of waste in giving birth to a dead baby.

Should You See and Hold Your Baby?

This is never an easy decision and even though it is painful it is worth thinking about. You and your husband have every right to see and hold your baby if you so wish. This may seem strange to some parents, although it is an obvious desire for others. The experience of holding your baby even though he is dead may make him a more real person to remember and in this way may help you and your husband.

What Will Happen to My Milk?

Mothers are often surprised and distressed to find that they produce milk even though their baby has died. You may find that for medical reasons you will not be given drugs to dry up your milk. You will stop producing milk quite quickly, but do not express the milk even if you feel uncomfortable, as expressing will stop the milk drying up. Your midwife or health visitor will be able to advise you how to relieve discomfort at this time.

Registering the Baby's Death

A stillbirth has to be registered with the registrar of births and deaths and the hospital will tell you what you have to do. It will help you to talk about your baby if you give him or her a name.

Funeral and Burial Arrangements

If you so wish, the hospital can arrange for your baby's burial without charge. Parents often find a funeral service and marking the grave or the place of cremation helpful to them in their loss.

Parents' Grief

Whenever someone we love dies, we go through a period of grief and mourning. This also happens after a stillbirth, although parents may feel they are grieving for a child they have never known, especially if they have never seen the baby, because a stillbirth leaves the parents with an emptiness and a bewildering sense of a non-event. People grieve in different ways. After the first shock some people want to talk about the tragedy repeatedly while others want to withdraw into themselves. Some feel angry; others reproach themselves, and many women after a stillbirth feel inadequate and a failure as a woman. Many are excessively concerned over their other children, while some find themselves unable to cope with them. These are normal reactions which generally lessen in time. Most important is to recognise that it is better to let yourself grieve and express your sorrow. When parents feel depressed, talking to another parent who has suffered a stillbirth can help and so can talking to others whom they feel are understanding, such as a doctor, chaplain, social worker, or health visitor. It can help to make a marriage deeper and stronger if parents share their grief.

Children's Reactions to Stillbirth

Children are sensitive and share the family's loss. They may not understand or talk about death in the same way as an adult. Stillbirths are especially difficult for them because the baby they expected has disappeared. They may not be able to talk about their fears and the younger ones cannot understand explanations. They need to be reassured of their parents' love and affection, however difficult it may be for parents at the time. It helps to explain the facts to them and allow them to express their feelings of sadness, anger, or bewilderment. Children are often less afraid of death than adults and are more upset by disappearance. It is less frightening for children to be told the truth than to leave them in ignorance at the mercy of their imagination. Children in the family are sometimes bewildered that the brother or sister they were expecting is not coming after all and they may need to be reassured they were not the cause of the baby's death. Some children become difficult instead of showing their grief, while others may only allow their distress to come out later. Help is available from your family doctor, who may refer you to a paediatrician, a medical social worker at the hospital, or to a child guidance clinic.

What about Another Pregnancy?

Your obstetrician or family doctor will advise you about this, but it is advisable to wait a few weeks or even longer before starting another baby. Don't let yourself be pushed into having another baby but wait until you are ready. People are often unaware of how deeply and for how long some parents can mourn a stillborn child. Neighbours, friends, and relatives may not understand your grief and are often embarrassed to talk to you about the baby. The deep feelings that are brought to the surface by a stillbirth often lead to family disagreements that you should not take too seriously. You should discuss with your family doctor where to have your next baby. You may be happier to return to the obstetrician you already know, but do not feel guilty if you find you prefer to go elsewhere if you have unpleasant memories of the events surrounding your loss.

Anxieties during Your Next Pregnancy

You are bound to be anxious about your next baby. Make sure that your family doctor knows what has happened and see him as frequently as you need to. Explain to friends and relatives that you may need them any time you feel worried. The right company or even a chat on the telephone can calm fears. If you have other children they may become anxious during your next pregnancy, and, although they may not show it, they may need the opportunity to talk about it. There is a great sense of joy and relief when the next baby is born safely, alive, and well, but there can be unexpected and bewildering reactions. Some react either by being totally absorbed in the baby or by feeling unreal and unable to care for him. Some parents overprotect the new baby. It is not uncommon and quite normal for parents to find themselves crying for the baby that died and grieving anew while loving and cuddling their newborn baby.

Reactions of Others to the Next Baby's Birth

Most people are delighted when you have your next baby and often assume that you will then forget that you ever had a stillbirth. Don't let these reactions interfere with your enjoying your new baby.

R.W. BEARD	AVRIL M. HILL	JUDY LISTON
JANET BECKLEY	HUGH JOLLY	DAVID MORRIS
DORA BLACK	EMMANUEL LEWIS	DAN SCRIVEN
COLIN BREWER	HAZLANNE LEWIS	RICHARD WILSON
YVONNE CRAIG	SYLVIA LIMERICK	

20

THE BATTERED YOUNG CHILD

Selwyn M. Smith, M.B., B.S., M.D., F.R.C.P. (C), D.A.B.P.N., M.R.C. Psych., D.P.M.

Associate Professor of Psychiatry,
Faculty of Health Sciences, School of Medicine
University of Ottawa;
Psychiatrist in Chief, Royal Ottawa Hospital

and

Domingo Pagan, B.S., M.D., D.A.B.P.N. (Child Psychiatry)

Clinical Instructor,
Faculty of Health Sciences, School of Medicine
University of Ottawa;
Staff Psychiatrist, Family Court Clinic,
Departments of Forensic and Child Psychiatry;
Staff Psychiatrist, Department of Child Psychiatry
Royal Ottawa Hospital, Ottawa, Ontario, Canada

HISTORICAL BACKGROUND

Literature and art are replete with varied and sundry accounts of the historical maltreatment and battering of children. William Blake touchingly intimates the terror of abandonment in childhood (3), but the dread terror of abandonment pales before the actual horror of battering.

Significantly, the battering of children has aroused public concern and action only in recent times (see Table 1).

TABLE 1
Historical Survey of Child Abuse (52)

1860	Ambrose Tardieu	Described the medico-social phenomenon of maltreated children.
1888	Samuel West	Described familial periosteal swellings (atypical rickets)
1899	National Society for the Prevention of Cruelty to Children	Founded in New York State
1946	John Caffey	Described a "new syndrome" of recurrent subdural haematomas in association with fractured long bones.
1953	F. Silverman	First to suggest that trauma was responsible for Caffey's Syndrome.
1955	Woolley and Evans	First to suggest the parents were responsible for child abuse.
1962	Kempe and Colleagues	Coined the emotive term Battered Child Syndrome.
1963	Index Medicus	The subject heading, Child Abuse, first appears as an official listing in the source book of medical literature.
1966	British Paediatric Association	Issues Warning Memorandum and offers definition and guidelines for treatment.
1968	Reporting laws	U.S.A. and other countries (United Kingdom excepted) pass mandatory reporting legislation.

1972	Selwyn Smith and colleagues	Describe psychiatric, psychological and social characteristics of baby batterers.
1973	Tunbridge Wells Study Group	Publishes recommendations for improving management of the problem.
1975	Children's Act	New legislation passed in United Kingdom making further provisions for children. Breaks with the concept of "parenthood means ownership" of the child.
1977	J. Densen-Gerber and colleagues	Bring to the American public's attention the widespread practice of sexual exploitation of children. Responsible for legislation prohibiting pornography involving children.

In the last two decades, child abuse has received increasing attention from professional and public agencies. Throughout the ages, literature is fraught with numerous examples of the oppression and barbarous maltreatment of children. Such maltreatment, dressed in the clothing of ignorance and superstition, of social and political invalidation, of economic exploitation, of discipline, of pedagogy, and of religious fervour, was manifested in psychological and physical degradation, mutilation, infanticide, murder and abandonment.

In 1860, Ambroise Tardieu, a French specialist in forensic medicine, published a medico-legal study of abuse and maltreatment of children. In 1888, Samuel West read a paper titled, "Acute Periosteal Swellings in Several Young Infants of the Same Family Probably Rickety in Nature," before the Medical Society of London (58). This was clearly a case description of a battered child that had been misdiagnosed. In 1946, American radiologist John Caffey published several articles dealing with a puzzling new syndrome characterized by "the roentgen disclosures of fresh, healing and healed multiple fractures in the long bones of infants whose principle disease was chronic subdural hematoma." Later Caffey suggested parental violence as the etiological factor, a suggestion offered by several other investigators (6, 7, 8, 9).

DEFINITION

In 1962, Kempe et al. (24) reported the results of a nationwide survey in the United States of non-accidental injury to children in a one-year period; they found 302 cases of abuse from 71 hospitals and 447 cases from 77 district attorneys and proposed the term "battered child syndrome" to characterize "a clinical condition in young children who have received serious physical abuse, generally from a parent or foster parent." They suggest that this syndrome "should be considered in any child exhibiting evidence of fracture of any bone, subdural hematoma, failure to thrive, soft tissue swelling or skin bruising, in any child who dies suddenly, or where the degree and type of injury are at variance with the history given regarding the occurrence of trauma" (p. 17).

Subsequently, the literature has become replete with synonyms for the "battered child syndrome." Some of these terms have addressed themselves to underlining issues of etiology, medical intervention and management, treatability, public complacency and legal definition. Suffice it to say that child abuse, if broadly defined, encompasses the battered, the neglected and the persecuted child; Fontana et al. (15) have proposed the term, "maltreatment syndrome in children," suggesting that "a maltreated child often presents itself without obvious degree of being battered but with the multiple minor physical evidences of emotional and, at times, nutritional deprivation, neglect and abuse," and adding that "a battered child is only the last phase of the spectrum of the maltreatment syndrome" (p. 1389). The United States Child Abuse Prevention and Treatment Act, passed in April, 1975, defines child abuse as "the physical or mental injury, sexual abuse, negligent treatment or maltreatment of a child under the age of 18, by a person who is responsible for the child's health or welfare, under circumstances which indicate that the child's health or welfare is harmed or threatened thereby."

It is difficult to arrive at a consensus of opinion concerning definition. Child neglect, in the legal sense, constitutes all those conditions listed in law under which a court may find a child neglected or in need of protection. The term child neglect covers the abused and battered child, as well as the child whose parents are unable or unwilling to adequately care for them.

Child abuse and battering are at the end of a neglect continuum, which ranges from neglect due to ignorance on the part of the parents to deliberate maltreatment. It is not always possible to distinguish the point at which neglect becomes abuse. Abuse can take the form of a direct physical attack, severe or unusual discipline, the deprivation of basic needs such as food, or any other action that could cause immediate physical or mental damage to a child. The term child battering is usually confined to one type of abuse, namely, direct physical injury to the child, resulting from intentional use of excessive force by an adult.

Unfortunately, confusion and lack of definition have limited communication among those working in the field and fostered misunderstanding among those who wish to define the problem more clearly. Many of the terms applied to describe the phenomenon of child abuse are euphemistic expressions that maintain public complacency. In contrast to medical and social definitions, non-accidental injuries are classified by police under such headings as murder, attempted murder, manslaughter, infanticide, wounding, assault and cruelty. Clarity of definition is further hampered by the fact that courts determine the definition. Since courts of law are influenced by the public, the definition will change from time to time and be dependent on the emotional climate in a particular area.

The publicity and attendant legislation associated with child abuse have not diminished the gravity of the problem. For example, in the United States, attention given to child abuse in the medical literature was followed by the rapid institution of laws which required the reporting of child abuse and which protected the reporting agent against legal risk. This resulted in a rash of reporting of child abuse cases which was not paralleled by orderly, well financed and efficient treatment programs and which, unfortunately, has been associated with instances of abuse of family privacy and of danger to the particular child. The ambiguous concept of emotional neglect, as well as the failure to deliver promised intervention and effective treatment, underlies the ineffectiveness of the child abuse laws. There is increasing concern that professional scrutiny has led to increased sensitivity coupled with inappropriate responses (treatment measures).

CLINICAL MANIFESTATIONS

It is obvious that early diagnosis and treatment are essential. Despite the subtle and broad definitions of child abuse, child abuse or battering does not present great diagnostic difficulty. "It is not often appreciated that many individuals responsible for the care of infants and children . . . may permit trauma and be unaware of it, may recognize trauma but forget or be reluctant to admit it, or may deliberately injure the child and deny it" (48, p. 413). Certainly, this statement implicates parental stonewalling and denial as a factor confronted in the diagnostic consideration of child abuse, but professional inertia may collude with the former factor to circumvent early diagnosis and treatment. A firm, frank and compassionate confrontation will often facilitate communication about abusive child-rearing, in general, and child abuse (battering), in particular.

The classic picture consists of a multiplicity of lesions in varying stages of healing. However, the diagnosis of child abuse should be considered in any child presenting with soft tissue injury, skeletal fracture, subdural hematoma, failure to thrive, sudden death, etc., especially when there is a delay in seeking medical advice on the part of the parents and a dissonance between the history and the clinical findings.

The overwhelming majority of battered children are below the age of three years. In the National Society for the Prevention of Cruelty to Children Study, approximately 90 percent of the battered children were three years or younger. Furthermore, this study suggested a statistically significant tendency for younger children to be at greater risk of severe injury (37). Other studies (35, 46, 50) support these observations, and suggest that any injury in a young child should prompt consideration of child abuse in the diagnostic assessment (see Figure 1).

Soft Tissue Injury

Bruises, abrasions and lacerations are practically ubiquitous in the battered child. Although bruises are common in young children, the distribution, as well as the presence of lesions in varying stages of healing, is the significant factor in determining child abuse. Often the lesion is suggestive of the method or implement used. For example, examination of the chest may reveal fingertip bruise marks as a result of forcefully gripping and shaking the child, which may be associated with fractures of the underlying ribs; punctate burns are secondary to burning with cigarettes; the "fluid level" sign is associated with dipping in hot fluids; burns of the buttocks and perineum are associated with being seated on hot stoves or radiators, or being dipped into hot fluids; there may be impressions of an electric cord, lash or belt buckle, or impressions of a bite (29, 51).

Bruising of the abdomen is common, but may often be minimal. It is associated with severe intra-abdominal injury and should prompt further examination, since rupture of abdominal organs is the second most common fatal injury, after head injury (11).

Cameron, Johnson and Camps (10) consider that laceration of the mucosa of the lip from the alveolar margin of the gum is pathognomonic. This injury, which was present in 50 percent of their cases, resulted from a blow on the mouth or other efforts to silence a screaming or crying child.

Bruising of the scalp and forehead is associated with underlying injury

HEAD INJURY:
Skull fracture; subdural hematoma; subarachnoid hemorrhage; intracranial hemorrhage; rarely, severe intracerebral injury may be associated with an absence of external signs.

OPHTHALMIC INJURY:
Injuries to the eyelid; posterior subcapsular cataracts; retinal separation; lens displacement; retinal hemorrhage; sub-conjunctival hemorrhage.

VISCERAL INJURY:
Gastric or intestinal per-forations; liver, spleen or kidney lacerations; rupture of abdominal viscera; intestinal obstruction; severe intestinal injury may be associated with a paucity of external signs.

BONE INJURY:
Radiologic appear-ance of lesions in vary-ing stages of healing; shearing and elevation of the periosteum with subperiosteal calcification in subperiostal hemorrhages; fracture of the clavicle; multiple rib fractures; fracture of the long bones; fractures of spine and pelvis are uncommon; metaphyseal defects.

SOFT TISSUE INJURY:
Bruises, abrasions and lacerations are ubiquitous and may consist of lesions in varying stages of healing or may assume the form of highly suspicious lacerations of the mucosa of the lip from the alveolar margin of the gum or subgaleal hematoma.

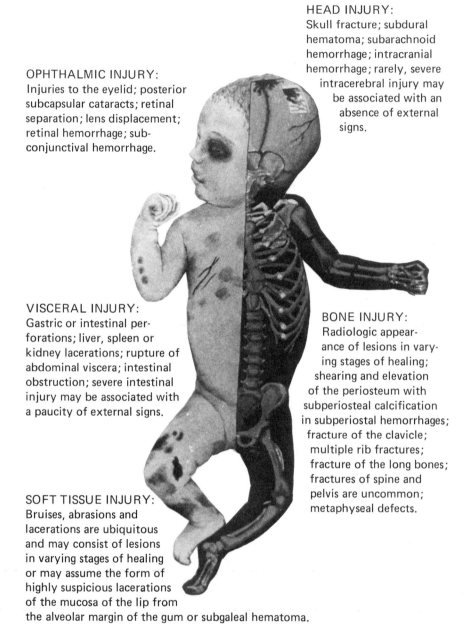

FIGURE 1. Physical Manifestations of Child Battering

of the skull and brain, but this injury may not be overtly apparent. A clue to diagnosis is provided by the presence of a subgaleal hematoma. "The most likely cause of childhood subgaleal hematoma is a vigorous hair pull by the grip of an enraged adult" (19).

Sussman (56) has described four characteristics which distinguish skin lesions in the battered child syndrome from other skin lesions: 1) The lesions are often concentrated in clusters on the trunk and buttocks and, to a lesser extent, on the head and proximal segments of extremities. 2) The lesions are morphologically similar to the implements used to inflict trauma. Hands, belt buckles, straps, ropes, burning cigarettes or matches, or other instruments, which have been identified as weapons used to traumatize a child, produce bleeding and characteristic straight, curvilinear, circular or jagged lesions. 3) Bleeding into the skin is purpuric—and almost never petechial—and it is distributed among the abrasions and scratches. 4) The skin lesions are of different ages and, in this respect, bear some similarity to the bony pathology.

Ophthalmic Injury

Injuries to the eyelid, posterior subcapsular cataracts, peripheral choroido-retinal atrophy, retinal separation, lens displacement, preretinal and retinal hemorrhages, sub-conjunctival hemorrhages, sub-hyaloid hemorrhages, etc. have been reported as manifestations (29).

Mushin (36) and Harcourt and Hopkins (20), in describing a series of battered baby cases with ocular damage, stress the frequency of permanent visual impairment in this condition, and underline the necessity for a complete ophthalmic examination in all such cases.

Visceral Injury

Gastric or intestinal perforations with intestinal obstruction, liver, spleen or kidney lacerations, pseudo cyst of the pancreas, rupture of the liver, and abdominal viscera with tearing of the mesentery have also been described. As mentioned above, severe intestinal injury may be associated with a paucity of external signs, and the subsequent delay in diagnosis may contribute to morbidity and mortality.

Head Injury

Head injury is very common. Fracture of the skull and associated brain damage are the commonest cause of death in child abuse cases. The child may be struck directly in the head, may be swung through the air against a hard surface or may be violently swung and/or shaken and develop a subdural hematoma. It is important to note that the last method, probably the least common, may not be associated with external signs of injury to the head.

Bone Injury

Radiographic examination is mandatory in the battered child syndrome. The danger of missing the diagnosis of the battered child is far greater than the risk of x-ray exposure and a skeletal survey is warranted in a child where battering is suspected. Needless to say, in fatal cases a skeletal survey is a prelude to formal autopsy.

The important diagnostic point consists of the radiologic appearance of lesions in varying stages of healing. Silverman (49) has reviewed the radiological aspects at length and shown that films taken too early after the initial trauma may fail to detect changes in the long bones. Since it is the healing process that is seen in many cases, rather than the acute trauma of fracture, he has suggested that x-rays should be repeated in two-three weeks if the original films are negative. "To the informed clinician the bones tell a story the child is too young or too frightened to tell" (11).

Radiographic lesions consist of: epiphyseal separation; shearing and elevation of the periosteum with subperiosteal calcification in subperiosteal hemorrhages; rib fractures (commonly multiple and seen as a line running down near the psterior angles of the ribs and revealing themselves radiographically as a "beading effect" when callus formation has had time to occur); fractures of the clavicle; chipping of the corners of the epiphyses of large joints; metaphyseal fracture-like defects (translucent zones on radiography); metaphyseal fragmentation.

Although radiological changes are rarely confused with many other conditions, Silverman (49) has listed several entities that should be considered in the differential diagnosis. These include: epiphyseal separation from known trauma, scurvy, syphilis, osteogenisis imperfecta, infantile cortical hyperostosis, osteoid osteoma, fatigue fractures, "Little League elbow," neurogenic sensory deficit, and congenital indifference to pain.

Other Clinical Manifestations

Manson (33) was the first to describe the association of celiac syndrome (malabsorption) and parental abuse. Koel (30) has suggested that failure to thrive and baby battering are on a continuim, and Bullard et al. (5) in their study of 13 infants with failure to thrive syndrome, unexplained by organic disease, found the mothers to be lacking in self-esteem and unable to assess their babies' needs and their own work realistically. Dine (13) has reported an unusual variant of child abuse, by describing a child who presented with bizarre neurological signs; the mother had given this child her own tranquilizer (perphenazine). Joos (22) has mentioned that child abuse in a very subtle form is encountered almost daily by the pediatric allergist when he sees children suffering from severe allergic rhinitis or asthma, in which environmental allergens, such as household pets, play a prominent role. Fiser, Kaplan and Holder (14) have detailed how a battered child can mimic the pseudo paralysis of congenital syphilis.

Although there have been no long-term prospective studies on the consequences and sequelae of child abuse, Martin (34) studied 42 abused children during a three-year period. Even though all of the children have not been followed the full three years, the study reveals significant findings about the abused children and their development. Martin's study has shown that permanent damage to the brain is a frequent sequela of physical abuse. Forty-three percent of his series showed neurological abnormalities at follow-up examination. Sixty-six percent of these children had obvious neurological impairment—hemiparesis, focal signs, optic atrophy and pathological primitive reflexes. The remaining one-third had more subtle signs, which included various "soft" neurological findings with minimal brain dysfunction. Of these 18 children with neurological dysfunction, only 50 percent had a history of skull fracture or subdural hematoma, demonstrating that brain damage may be related to less dramatic trauma. Although nearly 50 percent of the brain-damaged children had normal intelligence, Martin suggested that their handicaps might preclude success at school.

EPIDEMIOLOGY

Prevalence

The true extent of child abuse is not known, since many cases are not reported or go unrecognized. In the United States, it has been predicted that between 1973 and 1982 there will be one and a half million reports of child abuse, 50,000 deaths, 300,000 permanent injuries, and 1,000,000 potential abusers. Rosenfeld and Newburger (45) state that in 1967 fewer than 7,000 cases of child abuse came to the attention of the authorities, but in 1974 there were more than 200,000 cases reported. In Canada, the rate is estimated to be 250 cases per million population (1). In England, Oliver et al. (39), in a careful study, have estimated that the likely rate of severe attacks on children under five years of age is 10 per 100,000 population, or 2,450 severely battered children per annum (see Table 2).

The major problem in trying to determine the extent of child abuse has been establishing the ratio between the number of actual cases and the number of reported cases. The actual number of cases depends on the effectiveness of the reporting system in any given area. The report of the New York State Assembly Select Committee on Child Abuse of April, 1972, for example, noted that, in 1966, there were some 400 reported cases of suspected child abuse in that state alone. By 1971, when New York's reporting system had become more effective, the annual total had climbed to 3,200 cases.

Difficulties in obtaining accurate statistics include the following: *incomplete and misinterpreted facts* due to ignorance of what to look for and what to ask, shortage of time, fear of arousing anger, litigation or alienation in a client or patient, a wish to maintain confidentiality, incapacity to face the concept of open aggression by parents, and deception by parents; *available but uncollected information* due to the mobility of the families involved, deliberate changes of doctor or hospital to cover successive assaults, inaccurate identification of the child concerned, lack of standardization of records, and failure to make one person responsible for collection; and *unavailable information* due to the privacy of homes and to the tradition of helping and protecting the parent, which may obscure the needs of the child (47).

It is our view that current statistics underestimate the problem. Improvement could readily be made if child welfare organizations referred a suspected case to experienced medical personnel for confirmation and computer recording of the diagnosis. It is also of interest that, in the United States, where mandatory reporting of child abuse cases has been in existence for a number of years, conflicting estimates still occur. Unfortunately, even if reliable statistics were available, efficient management of the problem would not necessarily occur. In terms of morbidity and mortality, conservative estimates strongly suggest that child abuse is a problem of major concern to society.

Causative Factors

The dynamics of violence in society, and particularly within the family, are complex and multifaceted. The analysis of family violence requires analysis of attributes and attitude of the parents, of characteristics of the child,

TABLE 2

Proportions of children seen in routine medical practice who are the victims of violence or ill-usage at the hands of their parents or guardians (47)

Study	Country	Setting	Results
Laucer et al. (1974)	U.S.	Admissions to San Francisco General Hospital	3 percent of total admissions are due to child abuse
Kempe (1969)	U.S.	Children under 5 seen in Emergency Room	15 percent of the children seen are the victims of child abuse
Kempe (1971)	U.S.	Children under 2 seen with fractures	25 percent of the children seen are the victims of child abuse
Fried (1973)	Canada	Young children and babies with fractures	15 percent of the children seen are the victims of child abuse
Fried (1973)	Canada	Young children and babies seen with trauma in the Hospital Emergency Room	25 percent of the children seen are the victims of child abuse
Okell (1971)	U.K.	Children under 3 attending the Casualty Department	6.7 percent of total children are victims of physical abuse; 8.9 percent are victims of obvious neglect
British Medical Journal (1973)	U.K.	Casualties in children under 2 years	10 percent of total children are victims of physical abuse
British Medical Journal (1973)	U.K.	Fractures in children under 2 years	25 percent of total children are victims of physical abuse
Jackson (1972)	U.K.	London children seen with physical Injury at King's College Hospital, London	18 percent of total children are victims of physical abuse
Ounsted et al. (1974)	U.K.	Paediatric referrals to Park Hospital, Oxford	11 percent of total children are victims of physical abuse

and of environmental factors. Typically, the parents are seen as the vectors of transmission of violent behaviour, although more recently the role of the mass media, notably television, is being investigated as an instigator of violent behaviour (57). The parents are often portrayed as the victims of environmental factors associated with parental stress and frustration, which lead them to perpetuate their roles as vectors of violence. Furthermore, both parents and children are viewed as stressed and unsupported by changing family structures (for example, the breakdown of the extended family, the single-parent family, the working mother, etc.), by the general deterioration of social responsibility, and by the institutionalization of care. In the latter regard, the institutionalization of health care demands a humane and open relationship between caring agencies. Particularly in child abuse cases, the legislative impact of the reporting statutes must be coupled with competent and cooperative interrelationships among the courts, the mental health agencies and the social agencies.

Another cultural determinant impinging on the issue of family violence is the issue of corporal punishment. Historically, corporal punishment has been used as a means of managing the behaviour of children by parents, schools and police authorities. The advent of child protection and advocacy attitudes has called much attention to this issue. In terms of biological and psychological perspectives, Prescott (42) has suggested that crimes of violence and child abuse are associated with deprivation of physical affection and repression of developing sexual behaviour, stating "I am now convinced that the deprivation of physical sensory pleasure is the principal root cause of violence . . . pleasure and violence have a reciprocal relationship." This is a noteworthy observation in the light of other hypotheses relating violent behaviour to disturbed parent-child perception and interaction. In addition, various biological determinants, such as constitutional or inheritable defects, congenital and acquired brain damage, and drug-induced behavioural alteration, come into play; one can well imagine the potential dire consequences of interaction between a brain-damaged child and his parent or a brain-damaged parent and his child.

The literature does not support the view that a particular personality profile exists for the abusive parent. Yet, despite the frustrations of parenting, the majority of parents do not commit violence on their children. The psychology of violence and of abusing parents suggests that multiple factors are involved in the causation of violence on children. The literature is replete with particular models of causation of child abuse.

Violence towards children represents a social derivative of biological, psychological, and cultural interaction; theories as to causation must, therefore, be framed in terms of these factors. A variety of models have been established to assest in the understanding of child abuse—a psychodynamic model, a personality or character trait model, a social learning model, a family structure model, an environmental stress model, a social-psychological model, and a mental illness model (21). While none of these models is complete in itself, each contains a central core of determinants that have been considered as basic to causation.

Smith and his colleagues (50, 51) have described in detail the psychosocial characteristics of parents who battered 134 children. In this study it was found that abuse was associated with youthful parenthood. The parents were also poorly prepared for taking on the responsibility of rearing a dependent child. There was an infrequent occurrence of battering by older parents with large families, suggesting that child abuse diminished with parental age. Battering parents were also predominantly from the lower social classes.

An important factor was a lack of family cohesiveness. In more than one-third of these cases, the mother was living with some other man. Half the mothers had married before the age of 20 and three-quarters had conceived premaritally—a combination particularly likely to lead to marital breakdown. Other predictors of divorce included short aquaintance before marriage, disagreement in child-rearing, dissatisfaction with the partner's handling of the child, and neurotic and personality dissorders. The evidence strongly suggested that battered children would eventually grow up in broken homes and be at risk of social and educational maldevelopment.

Smith's disturbing findings that the rates of occurrence of premarital conception and illegitimacy were two and three times, respectively, higher than the general population rates and appeared to be important precursors of child abuse accorded with Resnick's (44) data showing that the inconvenience of an unwanted and illegitimate child is the most common motive responsible for child murder.

Three-quarters of the mothers and two-thirds of the fathers in Smith's study had abnormal personalities. The less severe types of personality disturbance were more commonly found among the mothers who, in general, had features of emotional immaturity and dependence. Nearly half were of subnormal intelligence. In many cases, child abuse occurred as an ineffectual method of controlling a child's behaviour. Techniques of teaching appropriate child-rearing skills, based realistically on the mothers' low intelligence, need to be applied as a method of correcting such ineffectual parental care.

In contrast to the mothers, the fathers were of normal intelligence. One-third of them were labeled psychopaths, a finding that contrasted strikingly with Kempe's (26) generalization that psychopathy is a feature in only two percent of battering parents. Nearly one-third of the fathers (and a significant proportion of mothers) had criminal records, usually for larceny. Nine percent of the fathers had committed crimes of violence and five percent had been convicted for serious sexual offences. Recidivism was also a striking feature of child abusers. The capriciousness of the legal system towards parents who battered babies was highlighted by the finding that, although one-fifth of the battered children's siblings had also previously been abused, only one parent had been charged with cruelty or neglect. It appears clear, therefore, that criminality and recidivism, particularly if associated with a psychopathic personality disorder, should caution against an optimistic outcome. When these factors are present, invoking a care order is essential if further battering incidents are to be prevented.

Another subgroup among the parents were those with neurotic illness, nearly half the mothers being in this group. The usual symptomatology present was an admixture of depression and anxiety. One-third reported having an unhappy childhood. Such neurotic mothers (in contrast to psychopathic fathers) confessed to harming their children and expressed a willingness to discuss their difficulties further. From a treatment point of view, such mothers will respond to symptomatic relief combined with a program of social learning.

A separate and fortunately small group of parents were those with psychotic illness. These parents tend to inflict bizarre injuries, in keeping with their delusional and hallucinatory experiences. Their management must deal primarily with the underlying mental illness.

Henry (21) has reviewed the literature dealing with the psychological aspects of child abuse. Varied methodologies and models—utilization of the case history, the listing of descriptive characteristics and typologies of child abusers, the use of predictive scales, and infrequent utilization of controls in the study of psychosocial characteristics of abusing (battering) parents—characterize most previous studies. Criticisms of the varied methodologies relate to the retrospective nature of the studies, the resulting lack of testable hypotheses emanating from the studies, and the absence of control groups.

Henry cautiously presents the following conclusions regarding the psychological aspects of child abuse:

> 1) Socioeconomic status may contribute to psychological characteristics.

2) Role reversal may be occurring in an abuse situation, with the result that the perpetrator may appear relatively lacking in remorse and may even appear somewhat righteous.
3) Parents who abuse their children are often relatively young, namely, under 25.
4) Recidivism is common.
5) The intellectual functioning of the parents is usually in the normal range.
6) Abusive parents often were themselves victims of abuse in their childhood.
7) Mental illness may be a contributing factor, but rarely is psychotic illness a precipitating factor.
8) Characteristics of the child, such as mental defectiveness, medical illness, or being the product of an unwanted pregnancy, may correlate with abuse but are neither necessary nor sufficient causes for abuse.
9) No consistent and homogeneous personality profile of an abusive parent has been identified.
10) The conceptualization of typologies acknowledges the lack of an identifiable personality profile of an abusive adult, but allows for categorization of abusers and for a potentially more fruitful method of studying their psychological characteristics.
11) The emergence of scales within existing psychometric tests promises some hope for a more efficient detection of potential abusers and for early treatment (40).

LEGAL ASPECTS

In the United States, during the last decade, all of the states enacted child abuse reporting statutes; interestingly, all of the states had prior child abuse and neglect statutes providing for criminal sanctions for the battering and neglect of children and for the termination of parental rights. The reporting statutes have resulted in a dramatic increase in child abuse reporting, but such statutes have not been accompanied by a corresponding and effective increase in programs designed to deal with the problems or by effective organization and coordination of the varied agencies which deal with the problem. In the United States, the National Center for Prevention and Treatment of Child Abuse and Neglect (31) reports that, in 49 out of 50 states, reporting of suspected abuse is mandatory; the one exception (New Mexico) simply has a child abuse reporting statute. The upper limit on age of children covered by these statutes ranges from 12 (Georgia) to 18 in most states. Some statutes cover any person who is mentally retarded regardless of age (Washington). Every state in the Union grants immunity to persons required to report; 39 states have removed the evidentiary problem of privileged communications in cases of child abuse, and the great majority have removed the privileged status of communications between husband and wife and doctor and patient; 28 states have established some form of central registry for keeping track of suspected cases of child abuse; 29 states provide criminal sanctions for failure to report (31).

Historically, the child has been the property of the parents, especially of the father; Roman law (*Patria Potestas*) gave the father absolute control over his children. Subsequently, in English law, the concept of the parent's (father's) absolute right to the children prevailed, but over several centuries the concept evolved that custody involved not only rights to the child, but responsibility for the care of the child. In 18th century England, the doctrine of *parens patriae* emphasized that the crown should protect all those who had no other protector and allowed the court to assume jurisdiction over the welfare of children.

In England, the Guardianship of Infants Act (1925) proclaimed the equality of the mother and father with respect to custody. In the United States, parallel developments occurred which caused a gradual erosion of the father's rights, but sentimentalism and the mystique of motherhood accompanied a developing cultural assumption that the woman was better suited to caring for children. In the United States, *Finlay* v. *Finlay* (13a), in 1925, affirmed the court's duty to proceed and act as *parens patriae* in order to do what is in the best interest of the child. The concept of the *best interest of the child* appeared in the statutes of almost all the states, subsumed a process of elimination of a particular parent in a custody dispute, and reflected an accompanying emphasis on the mother's right to custody rather than an emphasis on consideration of the child's needs.

Numerous investigators have stressed the primary importance of evaluating the child's emotional and developmental needs in custody disputes. Anna Freud, whose concepts of developmental lines, sequences of development, and characteristics of the child's mind are amplified in *Beyond The Best Interests of The Child (18)*, has attempted to shape legal decision-making along lines which will enhance and nourish the internal environment of the child. This work defines "the least detrimental alternative" as "that specific placement and procedure for placement which maximizes, in accord with the child's sense of time and on the basis of short-term predictions given the limitations of knowledge, his or her opportunity for being wanted and for maintaining on a continuous basis a relationship with at least one adult who is or will become his psychological parent" (18, p. 53).

Custody disputes promote the psychological abuse of children, highlight

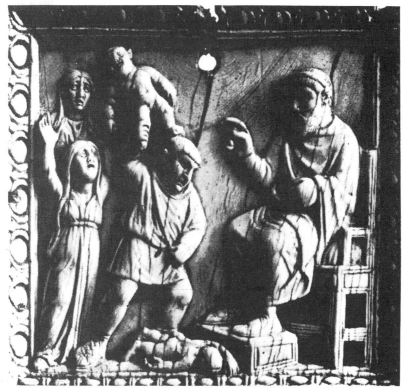

FIGURE 2. "Massacre of the Innocents," Ivory Relief. (From Schiller, G. *Iconography of Christian Art.* Vol. 1, 1971. London: Lund Humphries Publishers, Ltd.)

the legal impotency of the child, and emphasize the child's disadvantage in interactions with adults. The interaction between the abusive parent and the battered child is notably different from the custody dispute, but perhaps there are common cultural attitudes toward children that shape the etiology and course of these seemingly dissimilar situations.

Another peripheral issue impinging on the issue of child abuse is the issue of corporal punishment. In this regard, every society has normative values regarding violence and children have historically been victims of violence in the guise of discipline, education, and treatment. The past whipping of children on Innocents Day in Christian countries (Figure 2), as part of religious education and observance and the thrashing of epileptic children to drive out the devil (43) are prominent examples.

Today, parents are given license to beat their children in the pursuit of discipline, namely, corporal punishment. Furthermore, there has been much debate regarding the suitability and value of corporal punishment for children in the educational system; the legal doctrine *in loco parentis* has been cited as a doctrine which permits the teacher to stand in place of the parent and use corporal punishment to secure appropriate behaviour. In the United States, the Supreme Court ruled that the imposition of corporal punishment can never violate the eighth amendment prohibition against cruel and unusual punishment, and essentially distanced the federal courts from corporal punishment issues, leaving the further resolution of the issue at the local level (21a).

If one believes that abusing parents are "quick to apply the rod," then one must be prepared to view their behaviour in the light of broader cultural sanctions regarding the corporal punishment of children. Consider the abusing parent in the light of the biblical injunction, "spare the rod and spoil the child," in the light of the widespread use of corporal punishment, in the light of conflicting expert opinion on the utility of corporal punishment, and in the light of legal sanctions of corporal punishment. The majority of the states in the United States allow corporal punishment by statute or by case law, while federal legislation defining or regulating corporal punishment within the states does not exist.

Despite the view that a child belongs to himself in the care of his parents, the social recognition and enforcement of his rights have lagged. Law reform may address itself to this lag by extending more adult rights to children and/or by recognizing particular developmental needs for children. The former is characterized by the codification of due process for minors or by guaranteeing children the right to request medical care without parental request. A noteworthy example of the latter is Foster's (17) legal prescription for a *bill of rights* for children.

> A child has a moral right and should have a legal right:
> 1) To be regarded as a person within the family, at school and before law.
> 2) To receive parental love and affection, discipline and guidance, and to grow to maturity in a home environment which enables him to develop into a mature and responsible adult.
> 3) To be supported, maintained, and educated to the best of parental ability, in return for which he has a moral duty to honor his father and mother.
> 4) To receive fair treatment from all in authority and to be heard and listened to.
> 5) To earn and keep his own earnings and to be emancipated from the parent-child relationship when that relationship is broken down

and he has left home due to abuse, neglect, serious family conflict or other sufficient cause, and when his best interest would be served by the termination of parental authority.

6) To be free of legal disabilities or incapacity save where such are convincingly shown to be necessary and protective of his actual best interest.

7) To seek and obtain medical care and treatment and counselling.

8) To receive special care, consideration and protection in the administration of law and justice so that his best interests are always a paramount factor (p. xiii).

The recognition and codification of children's rights might notably address itself to a prevailing ambivalence regarding the nature and value of children, and might serve as a prescription against normative and permissive cultural attitudes of violence against children.

Criminal proceedings are designed to punish an offender, and conviction may offer little by way of prevention or treatment of child abuse, except that a conviction may effect removal of the abusive parent. Furthermore, in the area of child battering, criminal proceedings may be fraught with evidentiary problems; namely, battering occurs in the privacy of the home and often a defendant and/or spouse is not a competent and compellable witness in cases of violence against children in such situation. In addition, guilt must be established beyond a reasonable doubt; the demonstration of the battering or the death of the child does not answer the question of who committed the offense. Addressing this problem, as well as affording an example of the general ambivalence toward children, the Canadian Criminal Code statutes regarding cruelty to animals offer a dramatic comment, namely, the defendants under such statutes are obliged to demonstrate that they did not commit the offense: "Evidence that a person failed to exercise reasonable care . . . of an animal . . . thereby causing it injury . . . is in the absence of any evidence to the contrary, proof that such injury was caused or was permitted to be caused wilfully or was caused by wilful neglect" (11a). This is a reversal of onus to that seen in child-battering prosecution. Interestingly, the Society for the Prevention of Cruelty to Children, founded in New York City in 1871, traces its origin to the case of Mary Ellen, a girl who was maltreated by her adoptive parents and who was removed from her adoptive parents via the aid of the Society for the Prevention of Cruelty to Animals on the grounds that as a member of the animal kingdom her case could be adjudicated via cruelty to animal law (16).

Finally, the protection of the child from abuse requires clarification and refinement of existing statute and of legal process. The problems posed by

an adversary system in the management of the abused child are characterized by needs for: refinement of the definition of "children requiring intervention"; clarity of focus in terms of the child's needs versus parental
supervision; protection of the family from overzealous and insensitive reporting; the confidentiality, accessibility, and effective utilization of medical
records, especially psychiatric reports; clear lines of communication between the family court and criminal court in overlapping jurisdiction; and
the utilization and function of advocacy representation for the child.

TREATMENT

The initial thrust of treatment consists of a rapid definition of the problem, the identification of family dynamics and stressors, and the protection
of the child. The multiplicity of lesions lend themselves to a multidisciplinary
team approach utilizing a varied and wide array of medical specialities in
the endeavour of diagnoses; for example, the services of a radiologist, dentist, ophthalmologist, neurologist, etc. are useful and often necessary for
the correct identification of child abuse. One must then be prepared to make
a rapid and complete assessment of the individual family dynamics and
stressors,—to evaluate the occurrence of abusive experience within the family; to evaluate the parental family history and make note of particular and
present life stressors within the family; evaluate the psychological state of
mind of the parents and especially note the presence or absence of psychiatric illness; evaluate the parental attitudes toward the child; determine the
child-rearing practices within the family; evaluate the parental response to
the abuse; evaluate the ego strengths of the family members; and evaluate
the support system within and without the family. Finally, one must be
prepared to protect and shelter the particular child. Ideally, such evaluation
and management occur with a balance of firmness and compassion; the
machinery of evaluation and management should not punish or alienate an
already burdened family situation.

Psychotherapeutic Considerations

The sight of a battered child elicits varied and intense feelings of anger,
fear, sadness, etc. which bear on the clinical situation at hand. Effective
management and treatment may be unduly and unfavorably influenced by
the associated countertransference reactions. Various investigators have explored and reviewed the negative countertransference reactions elicited in
work with violent patients and the resultant disruption of an empathic ther-

apeutic relationship. The translation of feelings of anger, fear, sadness, revulsion, etc. into varied reactions—outward rejection of the patient, fantasies of destructive behavior directed against the therapist, denial with resultant breakdown in the history-taking process, a facilitation of the patient's potential for violence, an identification with the patient accompanied by a lack of confrontation of the actual and potential violence in the patient, a presumed revivification of the therapist's own conflicts about aggression—have all been discussed in the literature (32). In addition, a common fantasy in working with battering parents or parents who have killed a child is the "ogre fantasy," namely, that the parents are a different species or kind of person; this fantasy is easily dispelled by confrontation with the parents.

The initial evaluation should concern itself with an evaluation of parental pathology. Despite the fact that the majority of battering parents do not exhibit a psychiatric illness in the standard sense, a small percentage of parents appear to suffer from severe psychiatric disorders, e.g. schizophrenia, postpartum disorders, depressive illness, alcohol and drug abuse, which require more intensive and prolonged psychiatric care. Such care may require a vigorous and protective attitude toward the child, a realistic deferral of assignment of the family treatment by the usual child protective agencies, and a postponement of a more leisurely, prolonged process of relearning and altering patterns of maladaptive child rearing. Yet, if we view parenting as a process of growth and development, then we might view treatment of the abusive parent as a process of exploring and reorganizing child-rearing attitudes and techniques along more rewarding lines for both the parent and the child. We must be prepared to confront, explore, and abandon stereotypes of the battering parent in order to maximize the therapeutic relationship in a context of relearning when such a process of relearning is indicated.

A significant area of intervention that appears to receive little attention is the psychotherapeutic treatment of the child. Typically, the emphasis of treatment is placed on protection from further physical assault for the child or on psychotherapeutic treatment of the parent. However, battering usually occurs during critical periods of psychosexual, separation-individuation, motor, language and cognitive development. Battering represents, at the very least, a developmental interference and, at most, a vector for brain damage. Furthermore, battering usually occurs in an ambience of emotional and physical deprivation, so that long-term effects must be considered. There is evidence to link battering, as well as deprivation, to the perpetuation of violence in subsequent generations, to the later appearance of antisocial behavior, and to the later picture of mental handicap, brain damage or mental retardation. Furthermore, what are the more subtle effects of battering on personality structure when gross pathology is not subsequently observed? The internalization of the battering experience and the transgenerational transmission of such experience require further exploration. Indeed, the developmental and/or personality defects associated with the battering experience require further clarification.

A total psychotherapeutic approach for battered children might include: early identification of high risk infants and families with associated supportive therapeutic programs; the establishment of therapeutic day care settings and day nurseries; conjoint play therapy for the parent and child; individual psychotherapy for children with histories of battering at latency age via a therapeutic school setting, etc. In short, a comprehensive therapeutic effort is needed, affording a diagnostic and potentially corrective experience, associated with more appropriate educational planning in the face of neurotic conflict, personality disorder, borderline or psychotic disturbance, brain injury with specific learning disabilities, mental retardation, etc., which often occur in the battered child.

Treatment Modalities

The long-term management of treatment is obviously directed by the manner and nature of the initial intervention. Two modes of intervention have been portrayed in the literature—one can be characterized as an authoritarian approach and the other as a supportive approach.

The authoritarian approach can be characterized by the following viewpoint. Polansky and Polansky (41), in reporting to the Joint Commission on Mental Health for Children, questioned the ability of therapists to achieve personality change in battering parents which would assure the welfare of the children. Their skepticism led them to view physical abuse of children as "an area in which social, medical and legal action must be authoritative, intrusive and insistent" (p. 76). In this report they are also highly critical of the efficacy of casework.

Because of these conclusions, Polansky and Polansky (41) suggested the following seven (abridged) recommendations, "some of which may seem rather shocking to people unaccustomed to viewing with general detachment the sufferings of children outside their own families."

1) In the presence of clear evidence of child abuse a child should be removed from the parental home.
2) Following removal of the injured child the nonguilty parent should be forbidden to remove any other children they have from intensive court surveillance.

3) Parents found responsible for child battering should be punished by a lengthy prison term rather than probation.

4) Children neglected or abandoned by their parents should be promptly removed from the home with the expectation that they will not be returned for a considerable period of time.

5) In the presence of failure to thrive, the child must be returned to a suitable clinic for regular medical checkup. Failure by the parent or social agency to carry this out should result in legal actions.

6) Sterilization should be made available to any married person who wants it and should be made available free for those unable to pay.

7) It should become a general legal principle that no woman should have to bear a child whom she really does not want.

By way of contrast, the therapeutic approach of Kempe (25) and his colleagues (55) illustrates the supportive approach. Over the last few years, Kempe et al. have attempted to treat the deprived parent by "mothering," so that emotional dependency on the child and isolation are lessened and feelings of trust are developed. In order to achieve this goal, Kempe and Helfer (27) have experimented with the use of innovative therapeutic techniques. These include the following:

1) Parent-aids—these are foster grandparents whose job it is to simply cuddle hospitalized children.

2) Twenty-four-hour lifeline services—these operate on the lines of the samaritans. Telephone contact with the parents is available seven days a week.

3) Homemaker services—these provide support and treatment for battering mothers who are unable to cope with the demands of their small children.

4) Crisis nurseries—these provide "a place where a child can be safely placed for no other reason than the mother's relief."

5) Mothers Anonymous—this is a self-help group modeled along the lines of Alcoholics Anonymous and founded in 1970 by a 29-year-old mother known as Jolly Kay who had almost strangled one of her two children.

Other treatment approaches emphasize a reliance on social agency management versus psychiatric management; individual psychotherapy for abusive parents versus group psychotherapy; psychotherapy settings; separation of the child from the family via hospitalization, child care center placement or foster placement; hospitalization and treatment of the entire family; interpretive versus supportive psychotherapy, etc. (51).

Interestingly, Kempe (28) has drawn an interesting parallel between inadequate parenting and marital breakdown. "Society has worked out a way to manage failure in marriage; it is called divorce. We should be prepared to accept failures in totally unregulated, random parenthood by permitting, without social stigma, either voluntary or involuntary termination of parental rights for children from those parents who cannot, for one reason or another, give them the minimal physical and emotional support they deserve.''

Practical Management

Essentially, the aim of management is to ascertain the causes of family malfunction and overcome them. The dual aim underlying treatment is to protect the child and hopefully rehabilitate the parents. The emphasis on management must be to protect the child and accept that these two aims cannot always be reconciled.

Following an abuse incident, the child should be admitted to the hospital. Hospitalization takes the steam out of the situation and provides a safe place for the child. The family and siblings should be encouraged to visit the hospital as this will afford an opportunity to gather important information. Medical, nursing and social work staff involved in the assessment of a child abuse situation must show special understanding, tact, and skills in conducting interviews with the parents. Because of this, we recommend a specialized hospital-based team, comprised of a pediatrician, a psychiatrist, a nurse, a social worker and a psychologist, to achieve these aims. An initial confrontation with the parents often results in antagonism and removal of the child from hospital, with a failure to achieve crucial information that will assist in decision-making.

The physician's task is to obtain a detailed history from the parents, focusing on the child's developmental milestones and problem areas in parent-child interaction. The parents' method of child-rearing should be discussed. Injuries should be clearly described and recorded by photographs. It is important to exclude those rare conditions that may occasionally mimic child abuse by requesting hematological and biochemical investigations as well as skeletal surveys and other relevant tests. Information should also be sought from the family practitioner, other hospitals, and police. Enquiries should be made from social agencies as to the child's possible previous involvement and whether there have been previous causes for concern. Child abuse registers, if available, should be searched for evidence of previous abuse. Serial electroencephalograms are helpful in monitoring the effects of head injury. Psychological testing will not only provide a baseline of a child's behaviour and intelligence level, but will assist in exploring parental claims that their child is "difficult to handle." The child's height and weight, accurately measured under standardized conditions, should be plotted on percentile charts.

Most parents, if skillfully handled, gain confidence in the specialized medical team's approach. When this stage is reached, the parents relax sufficiently to give a detailed description of their family, marital and other problems. A psychiatrist, assisted by an experienced social worker, should arrive at a diagnosis, with an understanding of the family dynamics, in a space of two or three weeks. Coupled with background information obtained from a variety of sources, immediate long-term management of the child and his family can then be planned. In the majority of cases, child abusers can be managed by identifying and modifying those factors that cause and release their anger. However, in a minority of cases, a detailed psychodiagnostic evaluation establishes that the likelihood of the parents' responding to treatment is remote. In such cases, strong consideration must be given to permanent removal of the child from his parent's care. The pediatrician or the psychiatrist, as the leader of the medical team, should notify the statutory agency of his opinion and be prepared to provide written or oral evidence to substantiate it. He should not shirk this important duty. Separating an abused child from his family is usually considered a last resort that is harmful to the "therapeutic situation." The converse is, however, often the case. Removal from a battering situation is usually beneficial, provided substitute foster care that provides adequately for the child's needs can be obtained. Attempts should not be made to rehabilitate the parents at the expense of the safety of the child. This, unfortunately, frequently occurs. Family supervision by social workers, whether it is voluntary or imposed by a court order, does not overcome the inherent difficulty in managing this hard core group of cases, namely, that no supervisor can be with a child or his family for more than a fraction of the time.

CONCLUSION

If one accepts the premise that child abuse is behaviour having biological, psychological, cultural and social determinants, then one can attempt to design and implement preventive approaches to this problem. However, despite the fact that much is voiced about the welfare and rights of children, the truth is that child welfare and children's rights are low priority items in terms of sensitive legislative reform and adequate health planning.

If one also accepts the premise that parenting is a developmental stage, then it is not hard to envision comprehensive education programs which will engage the parent-to-be and deal with the child prior to conception. In this regard, a psychological assessment could be part of the prenatal program, and birth could represent an important arena for educative and preventive programs.

Finally, if one accepts the complexity of dealing with child abuse after the fact, then one will not easily subscribe to any one particular approach, but will attempt to individualize each family, and attempt to achieve balance between an authoritarian and supportive approach.

REFERENCES

1. ANDERSON, J. 1976. Extent of the problem. In: *Child Abuse and Neglect. A Report to the Canadian House of Commons.* Ottawa: Printing and Publishing Supply and Services, Canada.
2. ARIES, P. 1962. *Centuries of Childhood.* New York: Vintage Books.
3. BLAKE, WILLIAM. "Songs of Innocence and of Experience" and "Verses and Fragments From the Rosetti and Pickering Manuscripts." In: *The Portable Blake,* Penguin Books.
4. BOWLBY, J. (Ed.) 1952. *Deprivation of Maternal Care.* New York: Schocken Books.
5. BULLARD, D.M., GLASER, H.F., HEAGARTY, M.C., AND PIVCHIK, E.C. 1967. Failure to thrive in the "neglected child." *Amer. J. Orthopsych.,* 37.
6. CAFFEY, J. 1946. Multiple fractures in the long bones of infants suffering from chronic subdual hematoma. *Am. J. Roentgen. Rad. Ther.,* 56, 163-173.
7. CAFFEY, J. 1946. Infantile cortical hyperostoses. *J. Pediat.,* 29, 541-549.
8. CAFFEY, J. 1957. Some traumatic lesions in growing bones other than fractures and dislocations: clinical and radiological features. *Br. J. Radiol.,* 30, 225-238.
9. CAFFEY, J. 1972. The parent-infant stress syndrome. (Caffey-Kempe Syndrome. The battered baby syndrome.) *Amer. J. Roentgen Rad. Ther. Nucl. Med.,* 114, 218-229.
10. CAMERON, J.M., JOHNSON, A.R.M. AND CAMPS, F.R. 1966. The battered child syndrome. *Medicine, Science and Law,* 6, 2.
11. CAMERON, J.M. 1970. The battered baby. *Brit. J. Hosp. Med.,* 4, 769.
11a Canadian Criminal Code. 1973. Section 402. Ottawa: Information Canada.
12. DERDEYN, A.P. 1976. Child Custody Contests in historical perspective. *Amer. J. Psych.,* 133, 1369.
13. DINE, M.S. 1965. Tranquilizer poisoning: an example of child abuse. *Pediatrics,* 36, 782.
13. FINLAY V. FINLAY 1925. 148 NE 624.
14. FISER, R.H., KAPLAN, J. AND HOLDER, J.C. 1972. Congenital syphilis mimicking the battered child syndrome. *Clip. Ped.,* 11, 3o5.
15. FONTANA, V.J., DONOVAN, D. AND WONG, R.J. 1963. The maltreatment syndrome in children. *N.E.J. Med.,* 269, 1389.
16. FONTANA, V.J. 1971. *The Maltreated Child. The Maltreatment Syndrome in Children.* Springfield, Ill.: Charles C Thomas.
17. FOSTER, H.H. 1974. *"Bill of Rights" for Children.* Springfield, Ill.: Charles C Thomas.
18. GOLDSTEIN, J., FREUD, A. AND SOLNIT, A.J. 1973. *Beyond the Best Interests of the Child.* New York: Free Press.
19. HAMLIN, H. 1968. Subgaleal hematoma caused by hair pull. *J.A.M.A.,* 204, 339.
20. HARCOURT, B. AND HOPKINS, D. 1971. Ophthalmic manifestations of the battered baby syndrome. *Br. Med. J.,* III, 398.
21. HENRY, D.R. 1978. The psychological aspects of child abuse. In: S.M. Smith (Ed.), *The Maltreatment of Children.* Lancaster, England: Medical and Technical Publishing Co.
21a INGRAHAM V. WRIGHT, 45 U.S.L.W. 4364 (April 19, 1977).
22. JOOS, T.H. 1969. Child abuse: A different point of view. *Pediatrics,* 45, 511.

23. JUSTICE, B. AND JUSTICE, R. 1976. *The Abusing Family.* New York: Human Sciences Press.
24. KEMPE, C.H., SILVERMAN, F.N., STEELE, B.F., DROEGENMUELLER, W., AND SILVER, H.K. 1962. The battered child syndrome. *J.A.M.A.*, 181, 17.
25. KEMPE, C.G. 1968. Some problems encountered by welfare departments in the management of the battered child syndrome. In: R.E. Helfer and C.H. Kempe (Eds.), *The Battered Child.* Chicago: University of Chicago Press.
26. KEMPE, C.H. 1969. The battered child and the hospital. *Hosp. Prac.*, 4, 44.
27. KEMPE, C.H. AND HELFER, R.E. 1972. *Helping the Battered Child and His Family.* Philadelphia and Toronto: J.B. Lippincott.
28. KEMPE, C.H. 1973. Position paper for hearings of the subcommittee on children and youth of the committee on labor and public welfare. U.S. Senate, March 31. Unpublished.
29. KNIGHT, B. 1977. The battered child. In: C.G. Tedeschi, W.G. Eckert and L.G. Tedeschi (Eds.), *Forensic Medicine. Toronto: W.B. Saunders Co.*
30. KOEL, B.S. 1969. Failure to thrive and fatal injury as a continuum. *Amer. J. Dis. Child.*, 118, 565.
31. LIGHT, R.J. 1973. Abused and neglected children in America: A study of alternative policies. *Harvard Educ. Rev.*, 43, 556.
32. LION, J.R. AND PASTERNAK, S.A. 1973. Countertransference reactions to violent patients. *Amer. J. Psych.*, 130, 207.
33. MANSON, G. 1964. Neglected children and the celiac syndrome. *J. Iowa Med. Soc.*, 54, 228.
34. MARTIN, H. 1972. The child and his development. In: C.H. Kempe and R.E. Helfer (Eds.), *Helping the Battered Child and His Family.* Oxford: J.B. Lippincott Co.
35. McHENRY, T., GIRDANY, B.R., AND ELMER, E. 1963. Unsuspected trauma with multiple skeletal injuries during infancy and childhood. *Pediatrics*, 31, 903-908.
36. MUSHIN, A.S. 1971. Ocular damage in the battered baby syndrome. *Br. Med. J.*, III, 402.
37. National Society for the Prevention of Cruelty to Children. 1976. *At Risk: An Account of the Work of the Battered Child Research Department, NSPCC.* London: Routledge and Kegan Paul.
38. OLIVER, J.E. AND TAYLOR, A. 1971. Five generations of illtreated children in one family pedigree. *Brit. J. Psych.*, 123, 81.
39. OLIVER, J.E., COX, J., TAYLOR, A. AND BALDWIN, J.A. 1974. *Severely Ill-Treated Young Children in North-east Wiltshire.* Research Report No. 4. Oxford Record Linkage Study. Oxford Regional Health Authority.
40. PAULSON, M.J., AFIFI, A.A., THOMASON, M.L., AND CHALEFF, A. 1974. The MMPI: A descriptive measure of psychopathology in abusive parents. *J. Clin. Psychology*, 30, 387.
41. POLANSKY, N.A. AND POLANSKY, N.F. 1968. The current status of child neglect in this country. In: *Report at Task Force 1. Joint Commission on the Mental Health of Children.* Washington, D.C.
42. PRESCOTT, J.W. 1975. Body pleasure and the origins of violence. *Bulletin of the Atomic Scientists*, November, 1975, pp. 10-20.
43. RADBILL, S.X. 1968. A history of child abuse and infanticide. In: R.E. Helfer and C.H. Kempe (Eds.), *The Battered Child.* Chicago: University of Chicago Press.
44. RESNICK, P.J. 1969. Murder of the newborn: A psychiatric review of neonaticide. *Amer. J. Psychiat.*, 126, 1414.
45. ROSENFELD, A.A. AND NEWBURGER, E.H. 1977. Compassion vs. control. Conceptual and practical pitfalls in the broadened difinition of child abuse. *J.A.M.A.*, 237, 2086.
46. SCHLOESSER, P.T. 1969. The abused child. *Bull. Menninger Clin.*, 28, 260-268.
47. SCOTT, P.D. 1977. Non-accidental injury in children. *Brit. J. Psych.*, 131, 366.
48. SILVERMAN, F.N. 1953. The roentgen manifestations of unrecognized skeletal trauma in infants. *Amer. J. Roent., Rad. Ther. and Nuc. Med.*, 69, 413.
49. SILVERMAN, F.N. 1968. Radiologic aspects of the battered child syndrome. In: R.E. Helfer and C.H. Kempe (Ed.), *The Battered Child.* Chicago: University of Chicago Press.

50. SMITH, S.M. AND HANSON, R. 1974. One hundred and thirty four battered children: A medical and psychological study. *Br. Med. J.*, III, 666-670.
51. SMITH, S.M. 1975. *The Battered Child Syndrome.* London and Boston: Butterworths.
52. SMITH, S.M. 1978. Child abuse. In: R. Gaind and B. Hudson (Eds.), *Current Themes in Psychiatry.* London: MacMillan.
53. SMITH, S.M. (Ed.). 1978. *The Maltreatment of Children.* Lancaster, England: MTP Press Limited.
54. SPITZ, R. 1965. *The First Year of Life.* New York: International Universities Press.
55. STEELE, B.F. AND POLLOCK, C.P. 1968. A psychiatric study of parents who abuse infants and small children. In: R.F. Helfer and C.H. Kempe (Ed.), *The Battered Child.* Chicago: University of Chicago Press.
56. SUSSMAN, S.J. 1968. Skin manifestations of the battered child syndrome. *J. Red.*, 72, 99.
57. U.S. Department of Health, Education and Welfare. 1972. *Television and Social Behavior. A Technical Report to the Surgeon General's Scientific Advisory Committee on Television and Social Behavior.*
58. WEST, S. 1888. Acute periosteal swellings in several young infants of the same family, probably rickety in nature. *Br. Med. J.*, I, 856-857.

21

DEPRESSION IN THE YOUNG CHILD

Julian Katz,
F.R.C. Psych., F.R.A.N.Z.C.P.,D.P.M.

Associate Professor of Child Psychiatry,
University of Sydney, Australia

INTRODUCTION

The recognition of mental or emotional disturbance in childhood is a relatively new dimension in psychiatry, but the presence of such disturbance is now a well-accepted fact. The recognition of the presence of mood disorder in children has come about more slowly, and the diagnosis of depression in childhood is still regarded by some as controversial. Bowlby (4), noting the frequency with which the reality and pathogenic implications of grief in early childhood have been overlooked, says there seems to be a widespread need by adults to deny any state in a child smacking of depression and to take steps, often with some success, to persuade the child that he is not unhappy. Furman (10), discussing a related topic, namely the age at which children develop an ability to mourn, comments on the pain evoked in adults when exposed to the poignancy of a child's mourning for a parent. The adult frequently wishes the child should not be faced with the pain of mourning and then has difficulty in acknowledging the evidence of this pain. The need on the part of parents to deny depression feelings in children is shown in the following incident.

Case History

Chris, a bright, active encopretic five-year-old, usually very playful but obstinate, came into the consulting room after hearing his mother

435

whisper "He's doing it at school now," dropped into a chair, and, quite unlike his usual self, was apathetic and sad. He denied anything was wrong, but became tearful when his mother's remark was mentioned. Throughout the session he was sad and withdrawn, wanly smiling with a shrug of the shoulders at any suggestions. When his mother came to collect him, she reacted to the remark that he seemed depressed today with an emphatic "Nonsense, he will do anything for attention. He is probably tired, that's all," at which Chris jumped off his chair, yelling he was going to the canteen, and rushed out of the room, managing in the process to sweep the toys off the table and to scatter papers in the waiting room. "That's my boy," said mother, "never depressed. I sometimes wish he were."

This almost universal denial is shown also by the fact that children are seldom brought for consultation for symptoms that distress them, though they are frequently brought because of symptoms that distress others. Parents who would not hesitate to get help for a phobic or obsessional disturbance, a learning problem or behaviour difficulty do not think of requesting help for a persistently unhappy child. It is only in recent years that depression in children has been given a professional respectability by its inclusion in the classification proposed by the Group for the Advancement of Psychiatry in its reports on *Psychopathological Disorders in Childhood* (11).

DEFINITION

Although depression in children is being recognised with greater frequency, efforts to define and elucidate the condition have proved to be difficult and have given rise to a good deal of controversy. The various usages of the word depression have added to the difficulties of definition and classification. The word conveys many states of mind, from a common emotional experience resulting from a lowering of spirits or unhappiness to a severe and debilitating illness. Describing an illness by a commonly used word for a common emotion has given rise to the risk of regarding all depression as a disease requiring medical treatment.

Although depression in adults is a common psychiatric problem, and the signs and symptoms have long been known, there is still a substantial lack of agreement on the essential differences between the various forms of depressive illness met with in clinical practice. The differentiation of endogenous and reactive, bipolar and monopolar, neurotic and psychotic depression is far from satisfactory and presently the basis of much discussion.

During childhood, where maturational change and developmental factors greatly influence the picture, it is not surprising that the clinical manifestations seen in adults may not be found. This is particularly so in regard to manic-depressive psychosis or psychotic depression. Anthony and Scott (2) claim that manic-depressive psychosis, as a *clinical* entity, has yet to be demonstrated in early childhood. But there is good reason to believe in its existence as a *psychodynamic* entity. Other authors(1,9), however, have suggested that the possibility of manic-depressive psychosis in children may still have to be considered.

Hill (12) points out that depression can be regarded as a disease, a reaction, or a posture—or it can be all three. Depression is a *disease* in the sense that its manifestations are deviations from normal behavioural and biological functions. It is a *reaction* in the sense that it is a response to a crisis situation, usually involving a loss and resulting in a decline of self-esteem. But, as Hill points out, the clinician's skill is best shown when he understands the patient's depression as a *posture*, the symptoms of which are a form of communication. The patient's posture conveys the sum total of his feelings, fears and needs. The total posture pattern is a complex form of communication conveying emotional meaning and may evoke in the practitioner, as a participant-observer, protective responses of sympathy and solicitude, provided his emotional sensitivity is sufficiently attuned to the message. It is such empathic responses on the part of the observer that account for the diagnosis of depression in young infants. In young children it is more profitable to regard the condition as an affective reaction rather than a disease, and to view it in terms of the child's developmental status.

THE CONCEPT OF DEPRESSION

In order to cut through the tangled skein of psychodynamic theories and the various genetic, neurophysiological investigations put forward to elucidate the origins, status and clinical manifestations of depression, Anthony and Benedek (3) have come to regard the concept of depression as a phenomenon of human life and an integral part of human existence. This is essentially a psychobiological view and regards the depressive affect at all stages of development in the human life cycle as normal, ubiquitous and inevitable. There is a constant interplay between the various overlapping components which together make up the total individual. These include the genetic and biological aspects of the individual, which have neurophysiological and endocrinological ramifications in the body, as well as the basic psychological (personality) makeup of the individual and his reactive responses to the prevailing conditions in which he finds himself.

Anxiety and Depression

As far as clinical manifestations go, depression and anxiety have much in common. If we view depression as an affect with the same conceptual status as the affect of anxiety, much of the literature on depression in children can be integrated in a meaningful way. Both are basically unpleasant subjective feelings, very much integral parts of normal human development. Both, furthermore, have survival value. Whereas anxiety represents a basic reaction to danger, depression is a basic reaction to loss of supply and sustenance. Anxiety tends to activate the organism; in moderation it may facilitate perception, speech and fantasy. This brings about a fight-flight response to deal with the threat.

In young infants and children anxiety produces behaviour calculated to call out protective responses on the part of caretakers. During infancy it is usually the negative affect—an unpleasurable state produced by hunger, pain or other discomfort—that activates behaviour calling for attention and care on the part of the mother or other caretaker. If there were no such response to the infant's unhappy state, he could not survive. Although this interaction plays a part in mother-infant bonding, positive or pleasurable affects are also necessary for satisfactory bonding and for ensuring maternal care. These are evoked by the baby's eye contact with the mother, vocalisations and gurglings and smiles.

Engel (8) has shown the psychobiological basis of both these primary affects of unpleasure in infancy—anxiety and, as he terms it, conservation-withdrawal. He has described in some detail the psychic, behavioural and physiological accompaniments of these affects. The loss of support and comfort of the nurturing person or "love object" brings about the conservation-withdrawal response. This occurs regularly in the course of growing up. He regards the conservation-withdrawal mechanism as the counterpart of the biological arousal process, which in its more intense form gives rise to anxiety. In its intense form the conservation-withdrawal mechanism gives rise to depression. Response of either type may be enhanced and facilitated in some individuals by virtue of some genetic and biochemical factors. As a result, such individuals may be predisposed to the later development of depressive reactions. The conservation-withdrawal mechanism is a universal experience in the face of loss and drives the individual to immobility and unresponsiveness; the person experiences lassitude, fatigue, loss of energy, and a feeling of helplessness and hopelessness. There is a reduction of physiological and metabolic activities and a loss of muscle tone. Like anxiety, the depressive reaction is, in certain circumstances, a normal and appropriate affective response. It may be considered abnormal when it occurs in inappropriate circumstances or persists for an undue length of time, or when a child (or the caretaker) is unable to make the necessary and appropriate adaptation to it. The individual's capacity to tolerate depression plays a part in determining the extent to which it can be endured before there is a breakdown in adaptation.

THE PSYCHOPATHOLOGY OF CHILDHOOD DEPRESSION

The origins and development of depression are complex, with roots in genetics, biological maturation, and environmental experience. The study of the psychodynamics of childhood depression is intimately related to theories of early ego (personality) development and the growth of object relations—that is, the development and maintenance of interpersonal relations. These theories have been reviewed in their historical context by Malmquist (14) and Anthony (3). Earlier psychodynamic formulations were reconstructions from analytic treatment of depressed adults and were seen in terms of psychoanalytic theory of instincts. Such concepts as introjection, turning against the self, narcissistic injury, loss of object, and ambivalence were used in the development of theories of object relations.

The relationship of early childhood experiences to adult psychopathology is crucial to the understanding of mental illness generally. There is a considerable consensus of opinion as to the relevance of early infantile experience to the predisposition of later depression. A crucial question is the degree to which the symptomatology in the adult represents a direct repetition of the original developmental process. Many otherwise very different constructions see similarities between adult depressive illness and the infantile responses to actual or threatened object loss. It is hypothesized that disturbances in the development of satisfactory object relations predispose the individual to adult illness.

The Depressive Position

Melanie Klein (21) has made the postulate of the "depressive position" basic to her theory of depression. This is regarded as a normal phase of development occurring during the middle of the first year. Before this, the infant is subject to many primordial anxieties from instinctual conflicts—conflicts arising out of the growing awareness of the difference between self and not-self, between feelings of satisfaction and of frustration in experiences related to the feeding situation, nursing care, etc. The infant's anxiety is handled by mechanisms of splitting into good and bad parts or "part-objects," which are then dealt with by the processes of projection and introjection. The "depressive position" comes about as a result of the infant's awareness that the satisfying part-object and frustrating part-object are one and the same and that the object of its love and the object of its hatred are the same object. With this goes the development of ambivalence and guilt feelings.

Klein saw the depressive position as being crucial to the child's future emotional development. Much of the psychopathology of later life was seen as a result of failure to work through this position. Klein implies that there is a "pining" for the loved good object and postulates that a common ego defense mechanism is the "manic" defense, which is specifically directed against the feeling of pining for the lost object and the pain that feeling causes.

Segal (21) points out that the depressive position is never fully worked through and that the anxieties pertaining to ambivalence and guilt, as well as situations of loss which reawaken depressive experiences, are always with us. Good satisfying experiences help establish good internal objects in the infant which later safeguard against the development of depressive illness. Although the infant is not regarded as "suffering" from depression during this period, this theory implies that the unconscious content of adult depression revealed in dreams and fantasies is similar to the infant's experience. It also implies that inadequate working through of the depressive position results in predisposition to later depression.

Winnicott (22) presents views which are similar but not identical to those of Klein. He sees the depressive position as the attainment of a state in early development in which the infant relates to the whole mother in an ambivalent way. The state can best be described as one in which "concern for the object" develops. Winnicott regards the depressive position not as a phase but as an achievement. If all goes well in mother-infant relations during the "holding phase" and weaning, this phase should take place during the second half of the first year, but it may take longer to be established. Some people never attain it.

The attainment of the depressive position signifies a development from the state of ruthless demandingness to a state of concern for the "caretaker object"—the mother—and, in particular, concern about the effects of the infant's instinctual demands on the mother. There is, in fact, now a capacity to feel guilt and a desire to make restitution. Winnicott suggests that if the individual has attained this state, his reaction to loss is one of grief or sadness. If he fails to do so, the child "wet blankets" his whole inner world and functions at a low level of vitality. The child's mood will be one of depression.

Both Winnicott and Klein assume that the depressive reaction can only occur when a certain stage of development is reached, characterised mainly by a capacity for "whole object relationships" and associated with ambivalent feelings towards the object.

Central to the theory of the depressive position is the role of aggression and ambivalence. Sandler and Joffe (20) point out that while conflict over ambivalence is an important source of mental pain and, therefore, a possible source of the depressive response, it is only one of a number of possible sources of pain, and that the depressive response is by no means specifically and uniquely related to it.

The Depressive Constellation

Benedek (3) presents a theoretical reconstruction of infantile depression relating to subsequent depressive experience which has some resemblance to Klein's depressive position, but is based on the psychobiological transaction in the mother-infant unity. Psychic representation in the infant evolves under the influence of periodic events, starting with need and ending with satiation or satisfaction: for example, hunger-feeding-satiation; bowel tension-evacuation-relief. The depressive constellation is a construct representing the negative pole of the mother-infant interaction, basically in connection with experiences in alimentation. The negative affect which Benedek calls depressive constellation starts when the sensation of hunger activates crying and continues until the baby feels close to the breast. The positive pole of the affective experience develops with satiation of hunger. With the hunger cry begins the process by which the infant introjects the memory traces of frustrated feelings of hunger associated with the frustrating mother. The negative traces lead to the structuring of feelings of badness: bad self = bad mother. When the infant is satiated and soothed, the image becomes one of feeding: soothing good mother = satiated good self. With competent and adequate mothering there is a positive outcome to the mother-infant interaction which leads to the development of confidence. This functions like an emotional shelter, thus becoming a factor in the infant's ability to learn to wait.

The polarity of the confidence-depressive constellation in infant's experience is reminiscent of Erikson's (8a) trust versus mistrust phase in the oral stage of development. The depressive constellation is associated with ambivalence and feelings of anger, which, when excessive, affect the infant's "self" as well as its relation with mother.

Depressive Reaction

In their consideration of the depressive reaction in young children, Sandler and Joffe (19,20) found that it occurred in circumstances in which the child was faced with threats to its well-being. An essential aspect of this is a feeling of having lost, or being unable to attain, something essential to its integrity and well-being. This was combined with a feeling of being helpless and hopeless—a virtual "giving up"—reminiscent of Engel's conservation-withdrawal mechanism.(8).

Generally it has been assumed that the loss experienced by the depressed child or adult is the loss in reality or in fantasy of an important love object, but it may equally be a loss of a previous state of self. With respect to the loss, Sandler and Joffe put more emphasis on the loss of a previous state of self than on the fact of a lost object per se. When a love object is lost, what is really lost is the state of well-being implicit, psychologically and biologically, in the relationship with the object. The young child who suffers physical or psychological deprivation before object representation has been adequately structured may show a depressive response to the loss of psychophysical well-being. Even the older child who has learned to distinguish between self- and object-representations may react with depression to a developmental crisis such as the birth of a sibling, which is not so much primarily object loss as a feeling of having been deprived of an ideal state of having sole possession of mother. Not all varieties of unhappiness can be equated with a depressive reaction. If, however, the response is characterised by feelings of helplessness and passive resignation, the child may be considered to be depressed.

Basic Depressive Reactions

Mahler (13) considers that systematised affective disorders do not occur in childhood, because the immature personality structure of the infant and child is not capable of producing a state of depression, such as seen in the adult. Nevertheless, she maintains that grief, as a basic ego reaction, does prevail in childhood. In considering the dynamic interrelationship of object-loss, separation, anxiety and depression, she states that more often than not what is referred to as object loss is not real object loss but fantasy loss—"intrapsychic" loss of an object. She claims that real object loss does not occur frequently enough to account for the widespread proclivity towards depressive moods or depressive illness. It must be loss in fantasy—that is to say, intrapsychic conflict of a particular type—which brings about the occurrence of depression as an affect and results in a proclivity towards a basic depressive mood.

Mahler envisages this intrapsychic conflict as arising during an inadequate working through of the separation-individuation phase of development, because of some difficulty in the mother-child interaction. The child reacts with a depressive response, seen as "a basic affective reaction, very much as anxiety is." As a result, the child's "confident expectation" of need satisfaction is undermined, as is its self-esteem and basic trust, with a resulting sense of helplessness. On the basis of identification with the "aggressor" (i.e. mother), there is a turning of the aggression against the self.

Attachment and Loss

Bowlby's (5,6) well-known contributions to the theory of separation, loss and mourning in infancy and childhood have relevance for the psychopathology of depression. He regards the infant's tie to his mother or mother substitute as not being primarily the result of his dependence on the mother for need gratification. He points out that the survival of the infant is assured by the formation of emotional bonding between the mother and infant. The process of attachment starts at birth, the infant having several behavioural systems such as sucking, clinging, crying and smiling calculated to bring about the attention of the mother or other caretaking adult. This attachment behaviour is seen as a class of behaviour distinct from feeding or sexual behaviour and of equal significance in human existence.

Bowlby and others have described a sequence of events occurring when a child is separated from mother under the headings of protest, despair and detachment. Protest is seen as being related to separation anxiety, despair to grief and mourning and detachment to defence. These are best seen as phases of a single process. Grief is an amalgam of anxiety, anger and despair, when the love object is feared irrevocably lost. Violent and angry feelings frequently erupt against the departed. Grief differs from separation anxiety in that, with the latter, hope persists that the loss is retrievable. Mourning is a complex psychological process which sees the individual through the disturbed and disorganised reaction to form an adjustment. If not adequately worked through, it may lead to pathological behaviours. The reaction to loss of an object in childhood not only is seen as analogous to grief and mourning in adulthood, but can also predispose the individual to later psychopathology with depression as an important outcome.

The response of children to the mental pain of separation or frustration varies from angry protest to passive resignation. Normally, aggression is mobilised and directed against the source of pain. This is well shown by the observations of Bowlby on the separation of young children from their mothers. The aggression may then be used to alter the circumstances or relieve suffering to some degree and so lead to progressive adaptation. Or it may be directed against the self and so lead to disturbances in development. The depressive response appears to be associated with underlying aggression. Analysis of depressive reactions in children frequently uncovers feelings of impotent and ineffectual rage. But the outward manifestation is a state of helpless resignation and inhibition. In children who do not act out the aggression, it becomes inhibited or directed against the self; the child feels himself to be disliked or hated, denigrated and generally bad and unsatisfactory. There is often a constant vacillation between hatred of self and hatred of object.

The role of the superego in producing depressive reactions plays an important part in many theoretical approaches. On the one hand, feelings of guilt arising in the superego may result in the oppression; on the other hand, this affective state may arise through repressed aggression. But the role of the superego in depression in children has been a source of controversy, with little consensus as to when superego functions commence or attain maturity.

MANIFESTATIONS OF DEPRESSION IN YOUNG CHILDREN

The multifarious clinical manifestations of depressive response in young children have defied classification. Not all children react similarly to external and intrapsychic events; there are many factors which determine why some children react to frustration and loss, or any other form of mental pain, with depressive reaction, while others remain angry or unresigned. Constitutional predisposition must be one of these factors.

There are many defensive manoeuvres a child may carry out to deal with primary affects of unhappiness to prevent their emergence in consciousness. The most common are denial and reversal of affect. The depressive feelings are reversed and obscured by excitement, clowning, and overactivity. In unguarded moments the child's facial expression may give away the underlying depressive affect.

Individuals develop various mechanisms for dealing with depressive affect. The method of choice will depend upon the individual's genetic-constitutional makeup, maturation, and development. The variety of mechanisms has given rise to the concept of depressive equivalents or disguised forms of depression. Before adequate therapeutic measures can be instituted, these methods of presentation must be recognised. Without this realisation much of the patient's communications may be missed.

Depression During Infancy

In infants, "ego" is "body ego" and affects are expressed in bodily terms. Spitz (17) has described two sorts of "emotional deficiency disease" in infants: partial affective deprivation or anaclitic depression, and complete emotional deprivation or hospitalism (marasmus). The picture is of a sad, weepy infant with lack of contact with the environment. Motor retardation, poor responses to stimuli, loss of appetite, loss of weight, and generally retarded development are seen in these infants. Spitz named the condition depression because the symptomatology and facial expression of these children were similar to that found in depressive adults. A condition for the development of anaclitic depression is that the infant should have had a good relationship with its mother prior to separation. If the process has not gone too far, recovery may be stimulated by "tender loving care."

Although anaclitic depression had been described as a syndrome in its own right, related to object loss, it can be regarded as a basic psychophysiological reaction to deprivation. We might remember in this context Margaret Ribble's (15) observations on the lack of adequate mothering in infancy as a cause of withdrawal and stupor in infants. Children suffering from organic deficiency diseases like infantile pellagra, kwashiorkor malabsorption, and "failure to thrive" syndromes show, in addition to the specific symptoms of the illness, the same general withdrawal and appearance presenting a clinical picture of a depressive reaction. Generally, in chronic childhood illnesses, management of a depressive reaction may have to be considered in the treatment of the whole child. In infancy the depressive reaction is often shown by eating and sleeping disturbances, colic, crying and head banging. It is frequently found that mothers of such infants are depressed and/or anxious.

Depression in the Preschool Child

Preschool children present a more variable clinical picture, The overall mood is one of sadness and unhappiness or irritability. The child shows a degree of withdrawal and either constant or intermittent lack of interest in his surroundings. He may appear bored, discontented, and not easily satisfied, with little capacity for enjoyment. In general, he communicates a sense of rejection and of feeling unloved. Sleep disturbances and upset in appetite are common, as are rocking and other repetitive activities. There may be bursts of overactivity or the child may be constantly on the go. Contact with the child is difficult. Habit disorders like enuresis, encopresis and nail biting are common.

Depression in the School-aged Child

In older children the picture can be even more varaiable and depressive equivalents more frequent. The underlying depressed mood may only show from time to time to the acute observer. Behavioural problems replace depressive feelings. There is a persistence of infantile temper tantrums; disobedience and provocative behaviour may frequent result in physical punishment, for which the child seems sometimes to be begging. School performance falls off; in fact, there may be loss of interest in learning, truancy and running away from home; accident-proneness and other self destructive behaviours may be evident.

The child himself has feelings of inferiority and is convinced that he is in some way bad and therefore unacceptable. These feelings frequently lead him into antisocial and aggressive acting-out behaviour which results in vicious cycles of rejection and more violence, reinforcing his belief in his own badness. Some children will express their feelings of inferiority by drawing attention to their ugliness or stupidity. Failure in school is often put down to increasing laziness and, indeed, the child shows less and less desire for any constructive activity. Generally he appears bored, although in some instances he will reveal to the observer the underlying mood of sadness and hopelessness which, however, he may still deny. It is only when there is some evidence of the underlying depressive reaction that the behavioural or psychosomatic symptoms can be regarded as being associated with the depressive affect (7,18).

SUICIDE DURING CHILDHOOD

The suicide rate among preadolescent children remains fairly low which may, in part, be the result of the child's inability to carry out his own self-destruction. However, suicidal threats occur not infrequently and should be regarded as a plea for help by a child struggling with an unbearable burden. Some cases of accidents or accidental poisoning may similarly reflect a call for help by a child trying to cope with his underlying depressive feelings.

FAMILY BACKGROUND

In the majority of instances, the family's reaction is an important factor in the child's behaviour. Depression in one or both parents is a frequent finding in the family history. Apart from a genetic factor which may be involved, depression in a parent may markedly affect the emotional atmosphere of the family. Infants and young children, particularly, may be as emotionally deprived by a depressed parent as by an absent one. We now realize that, in the case of an otherwise healthy but persistently vomiting and whining infant, one must look for depression in the mother.

TREATMENT

Whatever the age of the child, the proper management of his depression requires an adequate understanding of his development and the environmental situation in which he is placed. In general, treatment must be family oriented to encourage the development of a sustained, supportive, emotional environment. Older children may require individual psychotherapy. Stimulant drugs should be avoided. Tricyclic antidepressants, although not always effective, may be useful in the control of symptoms such as sleep disturbances, especially in older children. However, they should be used in combination with some form of psychotherapy for the child and the family.

CONCLUSION

There is general agreement that depression as a clinical entity, as seen in the adult, has not been demonstrated during childhood. On the other hand, depression as a basic affect or mood is a universal and ubiquitous experience throughout the life cycle and may be seen at any age. Anxiety and depression are basic affects which in a certain range of expression may be regarded as normal. But they can become manifest as a clinical entity when some predisposing factors or environmental circumstances promote them.

Depression as an existential fact cannot be eliminated, but certain experiences are known to enhance the frequency and depth of later depressions and, indeed, other mental difficulties. We need to look into the possibility, therefore, of protecting young children from these experiences. These include a large range of experiences that, one way or another, threaten the well-being and integrity of the child by undermining and disrupting harmonious parent-child interaction. These can be environmental privations, deprivations of emotional support and of psychological stimulation. The list of causes of family disruption is long, but generally includes parental loss from death, separation or desertion; parental depression and parental rejection; and chronic illness in the child or either parent.

When, as is often the case, it is not possible to protect the child from certain happenings, the child and the family must be helped to cope with their feelings and their problems with a minimum of emotional crippling. This requires adequate psychiatric or other counselling care through periods of stress. More needs to be done to ensure adequate preparation of individuals and families to anticipate and cope with the variety of developmental and accidental crises they may be subjected to.

REFERENCES

1. ANNELL, ANNA-LISA 1967. Manic depressive illness in children and effect of treatment. *Acta Paedopsychiat.*, 36, 292-301.
2. ANTHONY, E.J. and SCOTT, P. 1960. Manic-depressive psychosis in childhood. *J. Child. Psychol. Psychiat.*, 1, 53-72.
3. ANTHONY, E.J. and BENEDEK, T. 1975. *Depression and Human Existence*, Boston: Little Brown.
4. BOWLBY, J. 1960. Grief and mourning in infancy and early childhood. *The Psychoanalytic Study of the Child*, 15, 9-52.
5. BOWLBY, J. 1969. *Attachment and Loss. Vol. 1. Attachment.* London: Hogarth.
6. BOWLBY, J. 1973. *Attachment and Loss, Vol. 2. Separation: Anxiety and Anger.* London: Hogarth.
7. BURKE, H.C. and HARRISON, S.I. 1962. Aggressive behaviour as a means of avoiding depression. *Amer.J.Orthopsychiatry.*, 32. 416-422.
8. ENGEL, G.L. 1962. Anxiety and depressive withdrawal: the primary affects of unpleasure. *Int. J. Psychoanal.*, 43. 89-97.
8a. ERIKSON, E. H. 1950. *Childhood and Society.* New York: W. W. Norton.
9. FROMER, E.A. 1968. Depressive illness in childhood. In: A. Coppen and A. Walker (Eds.) *Symposium: Recent Developments in Affective Disorders.*
10. FURMAN, R.A. 1964. Death and the young child. *Psychoanalytic Study of the Child*, 19, 321-333.
11. GROUP FOR THE ADVANCEMENT OF PSYCHIATRY. 1966. *Psychopathological Disorders in Childhood.* Report No. 62.
12. HILL, D. 1968. Depression: disease, reaction, or posture? *Amer. J. Psychiat.*, 125, 4, 445-457.
13. MAHLER, M.S. 1961. Sadness and grief in infancy and childhood. *The Psychoanalytic Study of the Child*, 16, 332-351.
14. MALMQUIST, C.P. Childhood depression: A clinical and behavioural perspective in depression in childhood. In: J. Schulterbrandt and A. Ruskin (Eds.) New York: Raven.
15. RIBBLE, M.A. 1943. *The Rights of Infants.* New York: I. U. P.
16. ROCHLIN, G. 1965. *Grief and Discontent.* London: J. & A. Churchill.
17. SPITZ, RENE A. 1965. *The First Year of Life.* New York: International Universities Press.
18. TOOLAN, J.M. 1962. Depression in children and adolescents. *Amer. J. Orthopsychiat.*, 32, 404-415.
19. SANDLER, J. and JOFFE, W.G. 1965. Notes on childhood depression. *Int. J. Psa.*, 41, 352-351.

20. SANDLER, J. and JOFFE, W.G. 1965. Notes on pain, depression and individuation. *The Psychoanalytic Study of the Child*, 20, 394-424.
21. SEGAL, H. 1964. *Introduction to the Work of Melanie Klein*. London: Heinemann.
22. WINNICOTT, D. W. 1965. *Collected Papers*. London: Tavistock Press.
23. WINNICOTT, D. W. 1965. *The Maturational Process of the Facilitating Environment*. London: Hogarth.
24. ZETEL, E.R. 1960. Symposium on Depressive Illness. *Int. J. Psa.*, 41. 476-480.

22

THE RECOGNITION OF
INFANTILE PSYCHOSIS

Barbara Fish, M.D.

Professor of Psychiatry,
Division of Child Psychiatry and Mental Retardation;
Associate Member, Mental Retardation Research Center,
University of California, Los Angeles

INTRODUCTION

General Definition

The term infantile psychosis encompasses a range of severe, pervasive disorders of development and total personality functioning, which involve characteristic distortions of the timing, rate, and sequences of many aspects of development, resulting in poorly integrated motor and visual-motor skills, and peculiar and erratic patterns of cognitive and social-affective functioning.

Infantile psychosis is a generic term which refers to psychoses occurring before three and a half to five years of age. It includes psychoses associated with known organic brain syndromes (OBS) and a group without localizing signs of brain pathology. In the latter, symptoms suggestive of central nervous system (CNS) dysfunction are often present to a varying degree, but the nature of any underlying brain disorder has not yet been identified.

This work was supported in part by Public Health Service grant MH-30897 from the National Institute of Mental Health, and by a grant from the Harriett Ames Charitable Trust, New York.

Brief History of Changing Concepts and Terminology

Until the 1930s, dementia praecox or schizophrenia was diagnosed in children under 16, using much the same standards as were being applied to adult patients. This literature has been reviewed elsewhere (13,19,22,65,73,88).

Authors, beginning with Potter(65), emphasized that prepuberty schizophrenia was not so rare, although hallucinations only occurred after six years, and delusions after nine years; further, they began to identify patients under four years of age. Despert (19,20) noted that symptoms in children were less differentiated and more variable than in adult schizophrenics, and that speech was frequently psychotic and non-communicative, despite a normal rote vocabulary.

Bender (4,5) pointed to the erratic and variable disorganization of all patterned behavior in childhood schizophrenia. This included immature muscle tone and motility, poor integration of visual-motor and proprioceptive perceptual patterning, in addition to defects in language, the sense of personal identity, and relatedness to others. Her "pseudodefective" subgroup had onsets before two years, and included some children who had no recognizable words(6).

Kanner initially considered infantile autism to be "the earliest possible manifestation of childhood schizophrenia"(41, 42). He considered the "aloneness" and "obsessive insistence on sameness" as the two pathognomonic symptoms(39), substituting the term "aloneness" for the autistic withdrawal in schizophrenia to emphasize that this could occur without any prior history of social relatedness.

Benda(3) and Bender(7) stated that Kanner's key symptoms of withdrawal, stereotyped behavior, and severely retarded speech would encompass many severely retarded children with organic brain disorders, as well as the most retarded schizophrenic children with onsets under two years. Much later, Kanner himself expressed dismay that the term autism was being applied too loosely to a vast and heterogeneous group of severely impaired children.

Since then, there have been two major schools of thought concerning infantile psychosis. One set of investigators has observed a continuity between a subgroup of infantile autistics and later schizophrenia. This group (e.g., Bender (5,8,9,11), Campbel(14), Fish(23,25,28,30,32,33), Goldfarb (34,35,57), Ornitz (59,60,62,63), Ritvo (70,71), and Shapiro (81,82,83,84), attempts to exclude, or to study separately, those autistics who have diagnosable OBS. Others (e.g., Kolvin (48,49), Knobloch (46), Rutter (50,51,

74,75,76,78,79), and Schain (80), have considered infantile autism simply as a behavioral syndrome, and have included varying numbers of profoundly retarded and grossly brain-damaged children in their samples. Many of the seeming contradictions between the different studies of infantile psychosis stem from these different points of view and the resulting differences in selection criteria.

Until sufficient data are available to delineate etiological subdivisions of infantile psychosis, some conventions must be adopted in order to compare studies of different populations. The categories and criteria outlined below are those in the current version of the American Psychiatric Association's Committee on the Diagnostic and Statistical Manual, Third Edition (DSM-III, December, 1977) (1). These criteria approach those in the current ninth revision of the International Classification of Disease (ICD-9). The final published versions of both may differ somewhat from the following.

DSM-III CRITERIA FOR PSYCHOSES IN CHILDHOOD (I.E., "PERVASIVE DEVELOPMENTAL DISORDERS")

General Discussion of the Classifications

Using the multiaxial system of the DSM-III, the behavioral syndromes of infantile psychosis and mental retardation are noted on Axis I, under Mental Disorders. Any associated organic brain disorder is noted on Axis III, using the ICD-9-CM codes.

The diagnostic criteria for infantile autism in the DSM-III have been drawn largely from Rutter's work (77,78,79). DSM-III has also adopted the convention that schizophrenia in childhood must meet the criteria for schizophrenia in adults, although these criteria are as ill-adapted to the facts of development in childhood in 1979 as they were during the decades prior to Potter's 1933 discussion. The strict criteria for both of these disorders should make for greater reliability in diagnosis. However, this system will also result in the necessity for diagnosing a much larger number of very young psychotic children as "Atypical childhood psychosis," and creates other problems discussed below (under A DIVISION OF INFANTILE PSYCHOSES INTO "SCHIZOTYPAL" AND NEUROLOGICAL SUBGROUPS).

The operational definitions for the critical symptoms are based on earlier work by the author (27,31,32), and recently have been modified for use in the U.C.L.A. Clinical Research Center for the Study of Childhood Psychosis, in collaboration with Ornitz, Ritvo, and Tanguay.

Infantile Autism (DSM-III: 299.0x)

Necessary and sufficient symptoms.

(a) through (d) are required for the diagnosis.

(a) *Autistic withdrawal*: The child is aloof, distant, showing only mechanical responsiveness and no sustained emotional relatedness to the examiner or others. Appears preoccupied; facial, behavioral, and attentional responses to the examiner or others are oblique and delayed, and frequently require forceful stimuli. The most severely withdrawn may appear oblivious of others and avoid eye contact.

(b) There is a *severe impairment in verbal and nonverbal communication*. Speech is significantly retarded; the child may be mute or only use jargon. If words are used, speech is predominantly non-communicative, consisting of distorted syntax, immediate and delayed echolalia. It often has little apparent connection with the current context of play or conversation.

Communication by gesture, appropriate facial expression, and the non-verbal aspects of speech (intonation, stress, phrasing, and rhythm) also are severely impaired.

(c) There are bizarre responses to the environment, which include either:

1) *Abnormal, stereotyped preoccupations* with odd objects or minor details of the environment, which significantly preclude more age-appropriate organized goal-directed activity. The child rigidly repeats a limited repertoire of behaviors, manipulates objects without regard for their physical properties or usual functions, and does not combine and exploit objects in age-appropriate patterned play. There may be preoccupation with tactile or visual details, repetitive spinning or flicking at objects, or perseverative stacking or lining up of objects in stereotyped ways.

2) *Complex ritualistic behaviors*. Simple everyday routines, or an apparently haphazard arrangement of toys or other objects, or idiosyncratic ritualistic movements and behavior patterns are reproduced in precisely the same manner, over and over, down to the most minute, irrelevant detail.

(d) Symptons (a) through (c) have developed prior to 30 months of age.

Schizophrenia (DSM-III: 295.xxx)

Necessary and sufficient symptoms.

This diagnosis requires the presence of a *formal thought disorder* typical of schizophrenia, which should be documented by a verbatim example. Speech is incoherent to a significant degree, with confused sentences, distorted syntax, and illogical and idiosyncratic associations and reasoning. In a few psychotic children, language is sufficiently complex to be able to diagnose schizophrenia before the age of five, even according to this criterion.

The characteristic hallucinations and delusions listed in the DSM-III as alternative criteria for diagnosing schizophrenia in adults have not been reported in children under nine years.

Atypical Childhood Psychosis (DSM-III: 299.8x)

Necessary and sufficient symptoms.

(a) through (c) must be present:

(a) A gross and sustained disturbance in emotional relationships, manifested by such symptoms as the lack of an appropriate affective interaction, asociality, lack of empathy, and inappropriate, impersonal clinging.

(b) Three of the following should be present:

1) Acute, excessive and seemingly illogical anxiety; catastrophic reactions to everyday occurrences; unexplained panics.

2) Diminution, rigidity, distortion, and peculiarity of affect, including lack of appropriate fear reactions, unexplained rages, and extreme mood lability.

3) Sustained resistance to change in the environment, including ritualistic and repetitive behavior.

4) Peculiar motility disturbances, including hyper- or hypoactivity, peculiar posturing, peculiar hand or finger movements.

5) Abnormalities of speech, such as question-like melody, monotonous voice.

6) Abnormal sensory and perceptual experiences seen in over- or undersensitivity to sensory stimuli, e.g., hyperacusis.

7) Self-mutilation: Biting, hitting, severe head banging.

(c) Onset of the full syndrome during childhood and after 30 months of age.

A DIVISION OF INFANTILE PSYCHOSES INTO "SCHIZOTYPAL" AND NEUROLOGICAL SUBGROUPS

Essential Features of a Clinical Diagnostic Entity: Limitations of the DSM-III Criteria for Psychotic Disorders in Children

Diagnoses in psychiatry, as in the rest of medicine, should be based on categories which, first of all, are defined by explicit criteria, and, secondly, have been shown to have a more or less predictable course(90). The DSM-III definitions are based on explicit criteria, and, in this respect, they represent some improvement over the DSM-II definition for childhood schizophrenia. However, the criteria for *infantile autism* will select a heterogeneous group of children. Many will be profoundly retarded children whose organic brain disorders may be diagnosable in infancy. In others, the OBS may only become apparent later.

Features Which Differentiate "Schizotypal" and Neurological Subgroups Within the DSM-III Categories of Infantile Psychosis

Follow-up studies have demonstrated that some psychotic children under five years, who would be diagnosed autistic or atypical childhood psychosis in the DSM-III, later develop a clinical picture which meets all the current criteria for schizophrenia. Explicit criteria, with tested reliability and predictive validity, are needed to identify this subgroup of infantile psychosis. However, the clinician must use currently available data in order to guide parents and educators of young psychotic children today; one cannot wait another 10 or 20 years before formulating tentative predictions of outcome for concerned parents.

The following guidelines are drawn largely from published studies which were recently reviewed (30), including a longitudinal prospective study of preschizophrenic infants who are now 18 to 25 years of age. More recent follow-up data by Campbell et al. (14) and Shapiro and Huebner (84), of the infantile psychotics studied by Fish et al. (33), have confirmed the usefulness of these subgroups.

"Schizotypal" features

These characteristics identify those infantile psychotics who show an increased incidence of schizophrenia, borderline schizophrenia, or disabling schizoid or paranoid personality disorders in later life. Before five years, they may show infantile autism *or* atypical childhood psychosis. At a mean age of three and a half, half of those studied by Fish et al. (33) had typically psychotic speech; 80 percent of the remainder developed such speech within the next five years. All would have fit the DSM-III criteria for infantile autism when they were first seen. The "schizotypal" features consist of atypically irregular patterns of neurological and psychological functioning which apparently reflect an early dysregulation of many aspects of development (30).

(a) *An intra-test profile of functioning which is unlike the usual patterns in chronic organic brain disorders.*

1) *On developmental testing, the infant passes more advanced tasks,*

which represent higher cognitive functions, at near-normal levels, while failing simpler or more primitive tasks—e.g., a four-month-old infant rolled over and pivoted at an eight-month-level, but could not sit as well as a four-month-old by the time he was six months ("Charles") (26); a ten-month-old manipulated and combined objects almost at age level, but was unable to sit as well as a four-month-old ("Peter") (23); a 16-month-old swiftly copied a two-block tower, approximately at age level, but could not transfer objects from one hand to the other, like a six-month-old; a three-year-old responded adeptly to the formboard and adapted quickly at age level when the board was rotated, but was unable to build a four-block tower as well as an 18-month-old.

The "peaks of performance" included in the classic British "nine points"(15) referred to comparable phenomena. Such patterns of nonverbal functioning are analogous to the disturbance of older schizophrenic patients, who fail easy items on an intelligence test and then succeed on more advanced items during the same session.

In contrast to these schizotypal or preschizophrenic infants, *higher* cognitive functions are usually depressed *first* in infants with brain damage, whereas postural development or simple combinatory skills become retarded only when the damage is more severe. Therefore, if the "peaks" were success with the formboard and blocks in a child with retarded speech, this disparity alone would *not* differentiate a schizotypal from a brain-damaged infantile autistic.

2) *Abilities which are clearly demonstrated at one moment are not exploited or used adaptively.* A 16-month-old, who quickly built a two-block tower, returned to aimless wandering and dangled a string for the rest of the examination. A three-year-old said, "Man arm torn," and then lapsed back into his usual incoherent and incomprehensible speech. A four-year-old read unfamiliar words in a professional journal, accurately sounding them out phonetically, but did not utilize the simplest of familiar words to express what were apparently urgent desires. Similar examples abound in the earliest descriptions of childhood schizophrenics (5,19,20,40).

(b) *A fluctuation of development over time, unlike the course of ordinary retardation, precocity, or degenerative disorders.* There are transient retardations of development, sometimes with the temporary loss of a previous ability, followed by transient acceleration. For example, the infant may raise his head very early but not sit for months; or he stands as soon as he sits but seems fearful, unstable, and won't walk for months; or head control may be lost (10,23,55). Such fluctuations in gross-motor and visual-motor skills may be so mild that they are missed, unless they are recorded accurately at the time(30). Early speech is lost in about half of schizotypal infantile psychotics, without a return to previous levels (28).

In a prospective study of infants born to schizophrenic mothers, disorganized development, in which physical growth paralleled the changing rate on Gesell testing, was significantly related to the severity of psychiatric disorder at 10 years(30). This included those children independently diagnosed as schizophrenic at 10 years, and those who became psychotic in adolescence (Fish, unpublished data, 1978). In studies by others, a subgroup of psychotic children without OBS shows definite growth failure, with bone age or height falling below the tenth percentile (21,85).

Profiles typical of organic brain disorder: No unusual high points or fluctuations in development

Other autistic infants are profoundly retarded from birth, without unusual high points or acceleration. They usually do not acquire any words by three or four years, and gain, at most, a 30-40 developmental quotient on some performance tasks (33/"Group A," 61). Gross motor development may not be retarded.

Infantile autistics of this type usually show increasing retardation as they mature. Although some simple skills may be acquired, many never acquire speech, or reach only the most rudimentary levels (14,33).

Characteristics of Infantile Psychosis Related to the Incidence of Organic Brain Disorders

In the classification by Fish et al. (33) of infantile psychotics seen at two to five years of age, all would have fit the DSM-III criteria for autism. At that time, only the higher functioning children were diagnosed as DSM-II childhood schizophrenics. Those with no high performance skills were diagnosed psychosis with mental retardation.

The importance of differentiating infantile psychotics with schizotypal features from those with presumptive organic brain disorders is demonstrated on Table 1. These 10 major studies of infantile psychosis reported enough data to analyze the incidence of OBS in their samples. Two studies of childhood schizophrenia with onsets after two to five years, which provided similar data, are listed for comparison.

It is clear from Table 1 that, once Bender and Kanner presented criteria for diagnosing infantile psychosis, populations were identified which differed from later onset childhood schizophrenia. The groups with infantile psychosis have four to 10 times as many with performance IQs under 50 as the

TABLE 1

Organic Brain Disorders in Infantile Psychotics Compared to Later Onset Childhood Schizophrenics

Source	Publication Year	Age At Onset (Year)	N	% With Organic Brain Syndrome		% With Epilepsy		% With Severe Obstetric Complications	% With Full Scale or Performance IQ's <50	
				Definite	Total Possible	When First Seen	Of Later Onset			
Schizophrenia										
Kolvin	1971	5-15	33	27	31	12(-16?)	—	12	3	Full
Bender	1972	2-10	50	2	12	8	4	8	10	Full
Infantile Psychosis										
Bender	1972	<2	50	8	16	10	6	28	36[a]	Full
Fish	1968,1976[b]	<2	38	3	3	3	0	18	37[c]	Performance
Goldfarb	1961	<5	26	4	15	4	—	23	—[d]	
Kanner	1953	≤2	100	1	1	0	1	0	—	
Creak	1963	—	100	14	14	5	7	—	—	
Lotter	1967	≤4.5	32	19	31	12	—	22	59	Performance
Kolvin	1971	<3	46	39	54	19(-22?)	—	35	51	Performance
Rutter	1967, 1970	≤5	63	35	63	3	28	—	46	Performance
Schain	1960	—	50	54	—	42	—	6	—(100?)	Performance
Knobloch	1975	<2	50	100	100	74	—	56	60(<35)	Performance

[a]16% with Full Scale IQ on the WISC ≤90.
[b]All children examined between 2 and 5 years of age. Includes additional unpublished (1976) data.
[c]66% With Verbal IQ's <50.
[d]54% with a Full Scale IQ on the WISC <75; 35% with a Full Scale IQ ≤90.

childhood schizophrenics, two to four times as many with severe obstetrical complications. The verbal impairment in most samples of infantile psychosis is even greater. In seven studies, most children were untestable on verbal measures; in Fish's two- to five-year-olds, 66 percent had verbal IQs under 50 prior to treatment. Only Bender's and Goldfarb's groups have children with average verbal IQs.

Infantile psychosis with and without OBS

Table 1 also demonstrates that there are two major subgroups of infantile psychosis which differ in their degree of cognitive impairment and the incidence of organic brain disorders. Bender (4,5,9), Kanner (39,40,42), Goldfarb (34), and Fish (33, and 1976 unpublished data) (in the United States), and Creak (15,16,17) (in the United Kingdom) began with the concept of childhood schizophrenia as a disease entity analogous to adult schizophrenia, or even continuous with it (9,30). Therefore, these five authors attempted to diagnose infantile psychosis which resembled schizophrenia, and excluded children with known neurological disorders. As a result, the incidence of organic brain disease in these studies (with the partial exception of Creak's group) is not much higher than the incidence of OBS in later onset childhood schizophrenics. Relatively few developed convulsions by adolescence (or adulthood, in Creak's and Bender's series). Two of Creak's (16) patients had neurolipoidosis at autopsy. None of Bender's (8) four patients, who had died by 40, had brain disease at autopsy.

The second group of investigators, Lotter (52,53), Kolvin (48,49), and Rutter (74,75,78,79) (in the United Kingdom), and Schain(80) and Knobloch and Pasamanick (46) (in the United States), considered autism to be a syndrome defined only by behavioral criteria. Therefore, they disregarded possible etiologic factors and included children whether or not they had organic brain disorders. The "definite" and "possible" OBS included epilepsy, meningitis, toxoplasmosis, neurolues, lead encephalopathy, spastic dyplegia, etc. Their rates of OBS are two to 100 times higher than those in the first group. The incidence of later epilepsy in Rutter's group is four to five times higher than in Creak's or Bender's groups.

Different rates of familial schizophrenia

Since these groups have such different rates of OBS, one would not expect them to have similar genetic histories for schizophrenia. This is borne out by the data in Table 2. In Bender's and Fish's groups, the rates of parents hospitalized for schizophrenia are lower than for schizophrenic children

TABLE 2

Schizophrenic Relatives of Infantile Psychotics Compared to Later Onset Childhood Schizophrenics

Source	Publication Year	Probands		Parents Hospitalized for Schizophrenia		Siblings With Autism (A) or Schizophrenia (S)	
		Age at Onset (Year)	% In SES Class V	N	% Schizophrenia	N	% Affected
Schizophrenia							
Kolvin	1971	5-15	19	64	9.4	56	1.8 (S)
Bender	1972, 1976$_a$	2-10	52	100	12.0	87	13.8 (S)
Infantile Psychosis							
Bender	1972, 1976$_a$	<2	38	100	7.0	44	4.5 (A,S)
Fish	1968, 1976$_b$	<2	24	70	5.7	48	8.3 (S)
Meyers & Goldfarb;	1962;	<5	18	84	2.4 (-21?)$_c$		
Goldfarb	1968						
Kanner	1953	≤2	10 (IV&V)	200	0	131	2.3 (A)
Creak & Ini	1960	—	2	120	1.7 (-2.5?)	135	0 (2.2?)$_c$
Lotter	1967	≤4.5	13 (IV&V)	60	0 (1.7-8.3?)$_c$	62	0 (4.8?)$_c$
Kolvin	1971	<3	2	92	1.1	68	0
Rutter & Lockyer	1967	<5	3	126	0	85	0 (2.4?) (A)

a Parents with nonschizophrenic psychoses in earlier report (1972) eliminated (Bender, oral communication, 1976).
b Includes additional unpublished (1976) data on the next 20 psychotic children admitted to the nursery.
c See text for details.

with later onsets, but they are significantly higher than the prevalence in the general population.

Meyers and Goldfarb (57) reported that 21 percent of parents were schizophrenic, but only 2.4 percent were hospitalized. The remainder included "borderline, pseudoneurotic, and compensated schizophrenics" whom others might consider "schizoid personalities." In Lotter's (53) group, no parent "was known to be schizophrenic," but hospital notes were available on only four of six who were hospitalized, and Lotter warns of "the difficulty of obtaining reliable information" on disorders not requiring hospitalization. A careful reading of their vignettes suggests that one to five (e.g., 1.7 percent to 8.3 percent) of these parents might be suspected of having acute psychotic or chronic borderline disorders in the "schizophrenia spectrum" (45). Given the small sample size and the dilution by an indeterminate number with neurologic disorder, Lotter's data are insufficient to make a strong case either for *or* against an increased risk for schizophrenia in these relatives.

The rates of OBS are lower in Lotter's and Creak's groups than in Kolvin's and Rutter's, but they are still two to six times higher than the incidence of OBS in the children studied by Bender and Faretra, and by Fish. One would not expect children with OBS to have families with increased rates of schizophrenia. Hence, it is misleading to calculate familial rates of schizophrenia in populations diluted by a large but indeterminate number of children with OBS. One should not be surprised to find more familial schizophrenia in populations in which organic brain disorders have been excluded more successfully.

Although the studies by Kanner, Creak and Ini, Lotter, and Rutter and Lockyer report no increase in parents hospitalized for schizophrenia, the rates for definite or possible autism in the siblings of the probands is 50 times higher than the incidence in the general population. The disparity between the increased sibling rates for autism and the normal rates for schizophrenia in the parents has yet to be explained.

Different socioeconomic distributions

These populations also differ with regard to their socioeconomic class composition. The families of the infantile psychotics described by Bender and Faretra (9) and Fish (1976, unpublished data) have two to three times more class V families than the general population, and more than Goldfarb's (35) and Lotter's (53) groups. Ritvo et al. (70), similarly, found as many class IV and V families among their psychotic sample as in their non-psychotic controls. The groups studied by Kanner (42), Creak and Ini (17), Rutter and Lockyer (79), and Kolvin et al. (48) have almost no families in class V. It has been well established (47) that there is an increased prevalence of schizophrenia in this lowest socioeconomic group. The large number of such families in the series of Bender and Faretra and of Fish is consistent with their increased familial rates of schizophrenia. The exclusion of class V families from the other studies, whatever the reasons, has apparently eliminated one source of families with high rates of schizophrenia that was available to the Bellevue studies of Bender and Faretra, and Fish.

Different outcomes: Later schizophrenia or simple cognitive and neurological defect

It is not surprising that these different subgroups of infantile psychosis also have different outcomes. In Kanner's group (44), 44 percent of the "speaking" group were psychotic at follow-up in adolescence. Unfortunately, few authors have followed up psychotic children into adulthood. Kanner (43) followed up only the first 11 cases but gave no diagnoses. Rutter's (75) report of a mail follow-up, at a mean age of 21.7 years, provided information on social adjustment and the additional cases of epilepsy, but no other neurologic data and no psychiatric diagnoses.

The few groups followed into adulthood are listed in Table 3. Annell (2) and Bennett and Klein (12) included schizophrenics with onsets under five years, but their follow-up diagnoses are not reported separately for the early-onset cases.

In Bender and Faretra's (9) and Dahl's (18) series, the incidence of schiz-

TABLE 3
Childhood Schizophrenics Independently Diagnosed Schizophrenic as Adults

Source	Publication Year	Age at Onset (Year)	N	% Schizophrenic As Adults (Age Range, Year)
Annell	1963	<2-9	19	85 (15-23)
Bennett and Klein	1966	3.5-10	12	100 (40-45)
Bender and Faretra	1972	<2-10	100	94 (22-45)
		<2	50	90 (22-45)
Dahl	1976	<2- <14	17	53[1] (20-40)
		<2	10	50 (-90?)[2] (20-40)

[1] One-third of these diagnosed as having chronic "atypical psychosis". "Same characteristics as the schizophrenics," including hallucinations, but less florid symptoms and lower intellectual function.
[2] See text for details

ophrenia in adulthood was almost as high for the children with onsets of psychosis before two years of age as it was for those with later onsets. Other psychiatrists had diagnosed 90 percent of Bender's early-onset cases as adult schizophrenics. Ten percent were considered to be organically defective. Bender's detailed report indicates that twice as many childhood schizophrenics (63 percent) remained chronically disabled and institutionalized, compared to schizophrenics first admitted as adolescents or adults (33 percent). Children with an onset of psychosis before two years had the highest rate (72 percent) of chronic hospitalization, compared to 54 percent for the childhood schizophrenics with onsets between two and 11 years.

While only 50 percent of the infantile psychotics in Dahl's (18) series were diagnosed as unquestionably schizophrenic in hospitals when adults, four additional patients (40 percent, for a possible total of 90 percent) appear to be in the "schizophrenia spectrum." Their independent hospital diagnoses were as follows: one with "schizophreniform psychosis" (at age 15) and "schizophrenia (pseudoneurosis)" (at 18); one with psychosis secondary to oligophrenia (at 15 to 22) and schizophrenia (at 28); one with schizoid character disorder; and one with "psychosis infantilis antea" (whom Dahl personally diagnosed as having borderline schizophrenia [written communication, December, 1976].

It is obvious that the limited criteria for infantile autism in the DSM-III will select heterogeneous groups of infantile psychotics composed of varying admixtures of children with major neurological impairment, as well as other children whose course and genetic background are more closely related to adult schizophrenia. The author considers the latter group to be at the most severe extreme of chronic, "process" adult schizophrenia (30). Since they have a lower rate of parental schizophrenia and a higher rate of obstetrical complications than later-onset childhood schizophrenics (Tables 1 and 2) (9), one can speculate that brain damage adds to their cognitive deficits (69), and may even precipitate their earlier onset of symptoms (86).

CHARACTERISTIC FEATURES AND COURSE OF INFANTILE PSYCHOSES

A Spectrum of Early Developmental Deviations

Deviant development, often from birth, and a variety of disturbed behaviors occur before the onset of psychosis in the vast majority of infantile psychotics. The characteristic features at each level of development in the life of a psychotic child depend on the child's maturing abilities and the nature and severity of the disease. There is a spectrum of deviations in development, with gradations in severity (25,28,30,32,33). This ranges from the most retarded infantile autistics at the extreme of severity to preschizophrenics who only have schizoid or paranoid personality disorders during childhood. These latter have the least early developmental and cognitive impairment and are at the mildest extreme of this developmental spectrum. This spectrum of developmental disorders and personality deviations is summarized on Table 4.

The most severe infantile autistics, who later have the most severe cognitive impairment, most frequently have severe retardation of gross-motor skills, as well as of early visual-motor skills (25,33,52,61). Infantile autistics, on the other hand, who have schizotypal features, are more likely to show spurts in early development and milder retardation. They are more likely to develop speech which is complex enough to reflect psychotic disorganization later on. "Atypical childhood psychotics" show less early retardation than do autistics, and therefore show more complex ritualistic behaviors and more complex fantasies and preoccupations. The DSM-III criteria for schizophrenia in childhood require even higher cognitive functioning. Speech complex enough to reflect a formal thought disorder with incoherence or "derailment" may sometimes occur before five years. It is more likely to become evident in the later course of children with infantile autism or atypical childhood psychosis, if they have milder cognitive impairment. Some preschizophrenics, who have personality disorders in childhood, show irregular patterns of early development, which are similar to those in atypical childhood psychosis and schizophrenia in childhood, but milder in degree (30).

Infantile Autism

The very young autistic infant frequently is overly quiet and apathetic. Muscle tone, crying, and activity are decreased, and there is no postural accommodation to being picked up. Others are excessively irritable, rigid, and tense, with irregular patterns of sleeping, feeding, and elimination. Vasovegetative control may be excessively labile or underresponsive (5,11). Children were flushed and perspiring, or had blue, cold extremities. There might be excessive fever with minor infections or none with severe illness. Gross-motor development often is retarded, but may be irregular or precocious (10,33).

There often is an inattentiveness to the human face and voice, a lack of response to other visual stimuli and even to pain, but an oversensitivity to other sounds (e.g., music, television commercials, vacuum clearners). In-

attention to toys is succeeded by absent or deviant reaching for and manipulation of objects. They may only be cast or flicked away, or dropped from
a limp hand. The infant usually does not develop the differentiated social
responses of the second six months; he does not comprehend or imitate
gestures, play "peek-a-boo" or "pat-a-cake," or wave bye-bye. Babbling
and the first words may develop with minimal delay in the second six months
and then be dropped, or speech may be retarded from the beginning.

These deviations appear more bizarre in the second year. The child remains mute and unresponsive, or speaks, only rarely, in echolalic fashion.
As visual-motor and perceptual development do not progress normally, the
child's strange, restricted, and stereotyped manipulation of objects and his
ritualistic behaviors become more obvious (63). These bizarre responses to
the environment represent deviations from the usual organization of attention and the ordinary responses to patterned stimulation in the environment.
The experiments of Hermelin and O'Connor (37) have elucidated the nature
of certain deficits which underlie these behaviors and which differ from the
deficits in subnormals. In severely retarded autistic children, there may be
very little change once behavior has reached this level. Others may progress in a variety of ways, including an evolution into an "atypical" psychosis or a clearly schizophrenic picture.

Atypical Psychosis and Schizophrenia in Early Childhood

Preschizophrenic infants and those who develop atypical psychoses may
show the same early deviations as the young autistic infant. However, development is more likely to be punctuated by erratic accelerations with more
evidence of precocity. These infants also may be overly responsive and very
demanding of attention; they may seem to be alert and sociable, although
usually with increased sensitivity and difficulty in imitative and gestural
play.

Disturbed behavior usually becomes prominent in the second year. The
child may show an increased withdrawal; he may show an increased panic
and desperate clinging to the mother; or there may be abrupt, unmodulated
shifts between extremes of affective expression; flat, underresponsive affect,
with little variation in facial or vocal expression, alternates with silly gig-
gling, explosive crying, or undifferentiated states of irritability, excitement,
panic or rage. These acute shifts in affect are precipitated by minimal,
ordinarily irrelevant changes in the environment or arise inexplicably, without any external stimulus discernible to the examiner (32). The severity of
these behaviors results in chaotic, frantic behavior, which usually baffles

TABLE 4

Developmental Symptoms at Various Ages in Infantile Psychoses and Other Severe Childhood Disorders

Symptoms (Sx)	Age in Years[1]	Infantile Autism		Atypical Childhood Psychosis	Childhood Schizophrenia	Severe Schizoid Personality Disorders With Schizotypal Sx in Childhood
		With OBS	Schizotypal			
A. *Physiological Instability*	0—	0/+	0/+	+	+	+
Fluctuating skeletal growth	0—	0	0/+	+	+	+
B. *State Behavior*						
1. Unusually irritable	0—	0/+	0/+	0/+	0/+	+
2. "Abnormally quiet"[2]	0—	0	+	+	+	+/0
C. *Affect*						
1. Irritable, labile	0—	0	0	+	+	+
2. Blunted to flat	1 mo.—	*+	*+	+	+	+/0
3. Incongruous	6 mos.—	0	0/+	+	+	0
4. Severe panic/rage reactions	2—	0	0	+	+	+/0
D. *Motor Development (Gross & Fine)*						
1. Retarded development	0—	+	+	+/0	+/0	+/0
2. Stereotypic movements	1—	+	+	+/0	+/0	0
3. "Soft" neurologic signs	1—	+	+	+	+	+
4. Fluctuating development; peculiar intratest profile	0-2	0	0/+	+	+	+
E. *Perceptual Development*						
1. Retarded development	0—	+	+	+	+	+
2. Bizarre, stereotypic preoccupation with objects	6 mos.—	*+	*+	+/0	+/0	0
3. Fluctuating development	0—	0	0/+	+	+	+
4. Peculiar intratest profile	6 mos.—	0	0/+	+	+	+
5. Distorted percepts[3]	4—	0	0/+	+	+	+/0
6. Hallucinations	6—	0	0	0/+	+	0
7. Hallucinations specific to schizophrenia	9—	0	0	0/+	*+	0
F. *Language Development*						
1. Retarded development (speech and comprehension)	8 mos.—	*+	*+	+	+/0	+/0
2. Poor nonverbal communication	10 mos.—	*+	*+	+	+	0
3. Noncommunicative speech	1—	*+	*+	+	+	0
4. Fluctuating development	1—	0	+	+	+	+/0
5. Peculiar intratest profile (jargon and sentences)	2—	0	0/+	+	+	+/0

TABLE 4 (continued)

Symptoms (Sx)	Age in Years[1]	Infantile Autism		Atypical Childhood Psychosis	Childhood Schizophrenia	Severe Schizoid Personality Disorders With Schizotypal Sx in Childhood
		With OBS	Schizotypal			
6. Incoherent speech	3—	0	0/+	0/+	*+	0
7. Derailed/irrelevant associations	3—	0	0/+	0/+	*+	0
8. Bizarre beliefs/fantasies; morbid preoccupations	6—	0	0	0/+	*+	+/0
9. Paranoid/Sc hneiderian delusions	9—	0	0		*+	0
G. *Social Development*						
1. Autistic withdrawal	2 mos.—	*+	*+	+	+	0
2. Ritualistic behaviors	1—	*+	*+	+	+	0
3. Abnormal, impersonal clinging	2—	0	0	+	+	+/0

[1]0— = From Birth on.
[2]Fish, B. (1977). Neurobiologic antecedents of schizophrenia in children: Evidence for an inherited, congenital neurointegrative defect. *Arch. Gen. Psychiat. 34*, 1297. (Alert, but apathetic, limp; rarely cry or move).
[3]Distorted percepts = Draw-A-Person, Bender-Gestalt, TAT, Rorschach.
*+ = presence required for diagnosis; + = frequently present; +/0 = may/not be present; 0 = usually absent

the parents. Only when emerging speech becomes clearly non-communicative and idiosyncratic is the child's psychosis clearly recognizable.

If language is less fragmented, the child may enter school, but his disturbed behavior makes normal peer interaction impossible. Academic performance is impaired or reflects his obsessive preoccupation with certain topics or fantasies. Fantasies generally involve morbid preoccupations with the body's functioning or with introjected persons or objects; they may involve exaggerated preoccupations with oral aggression, with the child's own identity, and his orientation in time and space (5).

From about five to six on, schizophrenic children may develop severe anxiety states with obsessive and compulsive phenomena, or exhibit all manner of persecutory and paranoid symptomatology, becoming withdrawn or violently aggressive and destructive. All combinations of these manifestations may occur.

Many of these children show poorly integrated patterns of motility. Awkward, "dyskinetic" motility, with a heavy-footed, wide-based gait and poorly coordinated associated movements, may remain as residues of early gross-motor retardation. They are significantly poorer than controls on finger-to-finger and finger-to-nose coordination, tests of rail-walking, and on the Lincoln-Oseretsky Battery (34). These "soft" (i.e., nonfocal) neurologic signs generally represent delayed development or poor integration of CNS functioning and do not constitute a syndrome which points to any specific localization in the CNS. Similar neurologic disorders have been found in large controlled studies of infants (56) and children (54) who were genetically at risk for schizophrenia, and in the controlled studies of children who subsequently developed schizophrenia, especially the more chronic forms (58,67,68,72,89). These soft neurologic signs persist in many adolescent (38) and adult (66,87) schizophrenics. Other deviant motor patterns include stereotyped "hand-flapping" and oscillating, whirling on the longitudinal axis, walking on tiptoe, excessive "motor compliance" (5,11,31,63,64), and catatonic posturing.

The perceptual and thought disorders, which appear later and are seen in the clinical symptoms and the psychological test responses of higher functioning psychotic children, resemble the disturbances of adolescent and adult schizophrenics. These findings have been reviewed elsewhere (31) and are familiar to most psychiatrists. Goldfarb et al. (36) found that the IQs of children who initially scored below 45 remained low, but the functioning of children who scored higher than that tended to improve with treatment. Bender (8) reported serial verbal IQs obtained over much longer spans of 20 to 35 years. While many with infantile psychosis showed deterioration, especially during chronic institutionalization, some schizophrenic children rose from verbal IQs below 80 to average or superior levels; a few rose from untestable levels before five years to scores above 70. One or more IQ tests above 70, prior to 11 years, was associated with a better outcome.

DIFFERENTIAL DIGNOSIS

Infantile Autism

In infantile autism, autistic withdrawal which begins at birth must be differentiated from a sensory deficit and from profound retardation without psychosis, which could also result in absence of responses to the environment. It may be difficult to distinguish these disorders before six months. To meet all the DSM-III criteria for autism, a child must engage in bizarre stereotypic behaviors. Complex rituals are more clearly recognized after independent locomotion and exploratory behaviors occur.

Decreased babbling in the second six months and a selective inattention to the human voice should arouse suspicion, but it is difficult to establish that *language* is significantly *retarded* before 18 months. Therefore, although many symptoms may be present earlier and one could suspect the diagnosis by six months, a child usually could not meet all the necessary criteria for infantile autism until after 18 months.

In other autistic children, the onset may be less insidious, or else mild early disturbances are overlooked. The "onset" may then be signaled by a relatively acute regression in social, vocal, and affective responses, and often in gross-motor and visual-motor development. Children who have appeared to be alert, responsive, and even precocious earlier suddenly change. Their expression becomes dull; the focus of their attention becomes oblique, vague, and non-responsive. They may suddenly go limp and become unable to chew or swallow textured food. These changes may be sufficiently marked so as to be obvious in a succession of baby pictures. This frequently occurs between eight to 10 months of age, but it may occur at any time before 30 months (24,25). Onset of psychosis after 30 months is classified arbitrarily as "Atypical childhood psychosis" in the DSM-III.

Childhood Schizophrenia

A similarly arbitrary "onset" is established by the DSM-III criteria for schizophrenia. The preschizophrenic infant may show the same disturbances from birth as the autistic infant and may have disturbed behavior continuously thereafter. However, using the DSM-III, a diagnosis of schizophrenia could not be made until speech was sufficiently complex to document a formal thought disorder. Some schizophrenic children have typical disturbances of syntax and meaning, with clearly psychotic speech, as soon as they speak in three- to four-word sentences. This is rare before two years.

Children who lapse into psychotic speech after a period of relatively normal communication usually have had early developmental symptoms. In the largest series (9), onsets of schizophrenia after two years clustered between three and a half to four years, and five to six years, with another peak at nine to 10 years. A minority (30 percent) of the late onset children previously had appeared to be relatively normal, although "overly quiet, model children." Almost all of those with onsets up to seven years had been obviously disturbed before. About 40 percent were withdrawn and autistic; 45 percent had other forms of disturbed behavior.

Most children have an insidious onset. Concerned parents may seek an early evaluation, or progressively more deviant behavior may not be recognized until the child attends school. "Onset" becomes an artifact of when psychotic material finally was elicited.

Some children have a more acute onset. They may abruptly regress in speech and behavior between three and five years of age. Even their motility may become clumsy, requiring differentiation from the organic dementias. Acute onsets in latency often appear to follow illness, injury, or a severe psychological trauma, such as loss of a parent or disruption of the home.

Bender and Faretra (9) found the most dramatic onsets in girls between four and seven years. Psychotic children with severe anxiety states, obsessive-compulsive, or paranoid symptoms must be differentiated from children with neuroses and from those with antisocial, aggressive behavior disorders.

Depending on the threshold of parental concern and the sophistication of the attending physician, infantile autism, atypical psychosis, or schizophrenia may be suspected well before three years of age. If there is little early precocity or agitation, the retardation and unresponsiveness may not be investigated until special schooling is required. Unfortunately, the irregular development in the preschizophrenic infants usually goes undocumented, and the schizophrenic child frequently is not seen professionally until grossly psychotic behavior becomes unmanageable at home, nursery, or grade school. Panic, excitement, or aggression is noticed before aloof, self-isolating behavior and a quiet preoccupation with bizarre delusions.

Early diagnosis of atypical childhood psychosis and schizophrenia in childhood would be possible if more attention were paid to the schizotypal features discussed above. The parents of the child with irregular development are usually baffled by the child's strange combination of abilities and inadequacies. However, they are usually told that the child will outgrow whatever transient lags in development are currently troubling them. This prediction proves to be true, of course, but that defect is then succeeded by other problems. The child who "outgrows" one problem only to develop symptoms in another area needs as much attention as the child with persistent retardation and severe withdrawal. The sensitive clinician can develop a lower threshold of suspicion for these subtle prepsychotic disorders. Early intervention can be instituted, based on an understanding of that particular child's developmental profile. This can interrupt destructive interactions between parent and child, and may mitigate the psychological sequelae of developmental disorganization in infants who are vulnerable to early psychosis (29).

REFERENCES

1. AMERICAN PSYCHIATRIC ASSOCIATION 1977. *Diagnostic and Statistical Manual of Mental Disorders, Third Edition.* Washington, D.C.
2. ANNELL, A. L. 1963. The prognosis of psychotic syndromes in children. A follow-up of 115 cases. *Acta. Psychiatr. Scand.*, 39, 235.
3. BENDA, C. E. 1952. *Developmental Disorders of Mentation and Cerebral Palsies.* New York: Grune and Stratton.
4. BENDER, L. 1942. Childhood schizophrenia. *Nerv. Child*, 1, 138.
5. BENDER, L. 1947. Childhood schizophrenia. *Am. J. Orthopsychiatry*, 17, 40.

6. BENDER, L. 1956. Schizophrenia in childhood—Its recognition, description and treatment. *Am. J. Orthopsychiatry, 26,* 499.
7. BENDER, L. 1959. Autism in Children with mental deficiency. *A.m J. Ment. Defic., 64,* 81.
8. BENDER, L. 1970. The life course of schizophrenic children. *Biol. Psychiatry, 2,* 165.
9. BENDER, L. and FARETRA, G. 1972. The relationship between childhood schizophrenia and adult schizophrenia. In: A. R. Kaplan (Ed.), *Genetic Factors in Schizophrenia.* Springfield, Illinois: Charles C Thomas.
10. BENDER, L. and FREEDMAN, A. M. 1952. A study of the first three years in the maturation of schizophrenic children. *Q. J. Child Behav., 4,* 245.
11. BENDER, L. and HELME, W. H. 1953. A quantitative test of theory and diagnostic indicators of childhood schizophrenia. *AMA Arch. Neurol. and Psyciatry, 70,* 413.
12. BENNETT, S. and KLEIN, H. R. 1966. Childhood schizophrenia: 30 years later. *Am. J. Psychiatry, 122,* 1121.
13. BRADLEY, C. 1941. *Schizophrenia in Childhood.* New York: MacMillan Company.
14. CAMPBELL, M., HARDESTY, A. S., BREUER, H. and POLEVOY, N. 1978. Childhood psychosis in perspective: A follow-up of 10 children. *J. Am. Acad. Child Psychiatry, 17,* 14.
15. CREAK, M. 1961. Schizophrenic syndrome in childhood: Report of a working party. *Br. Med. J., 2,* 889.
16. CREAK, M. 1963. Childhood psychosis: A review of 100 cases. *Br. J. Psychiatry, 109,* 84.
17. CREAK, M. and INI, S. 1960. Families of psychotic children. *J. Child Psychol. Psychiatry, 1,* 156.
18. DAHL, V. 1976. A follow-up study of a child psychiatric clientele with special regard to the diagnosis of psychosis. *Acta. Psychiatr. Scand., 54,* 106.
19. DESPERT, J. L. 1938. Schizophrenia in children. *Psychiatr. Q., 12,* 366.
20. DESPERT, J. L. 1941. Thinking and motility disorder in schizophrenic child., *Psychiatr. Q., 15,* 522.
21. DUTTON, G. 1964. The growth pattern of psychotic boys. *Br. J. Psychiatry, 110,* 101.
22. EISENBERG, L. 1957. The course of childhood schizophrenia. *AMA Arch. Neurol. and Psychiatry, 78,* 69.
23. FISH, B. 1957. The detection of schizophrenia in infancy. *J. Nerv. Ment. Dis., 125,* 1.
24. FISH, B. 1960. Involvement of the central nervous system in infants with schizophrenia. *Arch. Neurol., 2,* 115.
25. FISH, B. 1961. The study of motor development in infancy and its relationship to psychological functioning. *Am. J. Psychiatry, 117,* 1113.
26. FISH, B. 1963. The maturation of arousal and attention in the first months of life: A study of variations in ego development. *J. Am. Acad. Child Psychiatry, 2,* 253.
27. FISH, B. 1968. Methodology in child psychopharmacology. In: D. H. Efron, et al. (Eds.), *Psychopharmacology, Review of Progress, 1957—1967.* Washington, D.C.: Public Health Publication.
28. FISH, B. 1971. Contributions of developmental research to a theory of schizophrenia. In: J. Hellmuth (Ed.), *Exceptional Infant, Volume 2, Studies in Abnormalities.* New York: Brunner/Mazel.
29. FISH, B. 1976. An approach to prevention in infants at risk for schizophrenia: Developmental deviations from birth to 10 years. *J. Am. Acad. Child Psychiatry, 15,* 62.
30. FISH, B. 1977. Neurobiologic antecedents of schizophrenia in children: Evidence for an inherited, congenital neurointegrative defect. *Arch. Gen. Psychiatry, 34,* 1297.
31. FISH, B. and E. R. RITVO E. R. In press. Psychoses in childhood. In: J. D. Noshpitz and I. Berlin (Eds.), *Basic Handbook of Child Psychiatry.* New York: Basic Books.
32. FISH, B. and SHAPIRO, T. 1965. A typology of children's psychiatric disorders: I. Its application to a controlled evaluation of treatment. *J. Am. Acad. Child Psychiatry., 4,* 32.
33. FISH, B., SHAPIRO, T., CAMPBELL, M. and WILE, R. 1968. A classification of schizophrenic children under five years. *Am. J. Psychiatry, 124,* 1415.

472   MODERN PERSPECTIVES IN THE PSYCHIATRY OF INFANCY

34. GOLDFARB, W. 1961. *Childhood Schizophrenia.* Cambridge, Massachusetts: Harvard University Pres.
35. GOLDFARB, W. 1968. The subclassification of psychotic children: Application to a study of longitudinal change. In: D. Rosenthal, and S. S. Kety, (Eds.), *The Transmission of Schizophrenia.* London, Pergamon Press.
36. GOLDFARB, W., GOLDFARB, N. and POLLACK, R. C. 1969. Changes in IQ of schizophrenic children during residential treatment. *Arch. Gen. Psychiatry, 21,* 673.
37. HERMELIN, B. and O'CONNOR, N. 1970. *Psychological Experiements with Autistic Children.* Oxford, England: Pergamon Press.
38. HERTZIG, M. A. and BIRCH, M. G. 1968. Neurologic organization in psychiatrically disturbed adolescents. *Arch. Gen. Psychiatry, 19,* 528.
39. KANNER, L. 1943. Autistic disturbances of affective contact. *Nerv. Child, 2,* 217.
40. KANNER, L. 1946. Irrelevant and metaphorical language in early infantile autism. *Am. J. Psychiatry, 103,* 242.
41. KANNER, L. 1949. Problems of nosology and psychodynamics of early infantile autism. *Am. J. Orthopsychiatry, 19,* 416.
42. KANNER, L. 1953. To what extent is early infantile autism determined by constitutional inadequacies? In: *Genetics and the Inheritance of Integrated Neurological Patterns, Res. Publ. Assoc. Res. Nerv. Ment. Dis. 33,* 378.
43. KANNER, L. 1973. Follow-up study of eleven autistic children originally reported in 1943. In: L. Kanner, (Ed.), *Childhood Psychosis: Initial Studies and New Insights.* New York: Wiley.
44. KANNER, L. and EISENBERG, L. 1955. Notes on the follow-up studies of autistic children. In: P. H. Hoch, and J. Zubin, (Eds.), *Psychopathology of Childhood.* New York: Grune and Stratton.
45. KETY, S. S., ROSENTHAL, D., WENDER, P. H. and SCHULZINGER, F. 1968. The types of prevalence of mental illness in the biological and adoptive families of adopted schizophrenics. In: D. Rosenthal, and S. S. Kety, (Eds.), *The Transmission of Schizophrenia.* London: Pergamon Press.
46. KNOBLOCH, H. and PASAMANICK, B. 1975. Some etiologic and prognostic factors in early infantile autism and psychosis. *Pediatrics, 55,* 182.
47. KOHN, M. L. 1968. Social class and schizophrenia: A critical review. In: D. Rosenthal and S. S. Kety, (Eds.), *The Transmission of Schizophrenia.* London: Pergamon Press.
48. KOLVIN, I., OUNSTED, C., HUMPHREY, M. ET AL. 1971. Six studies in the childhood psychoses. *Br. J. Psychiatry, 118,* 381.
49. KOLVIN, I., OUNSTED, C. and ROTH M. 1971. Six studies in the childhood psychoses. V. Cerebral dysfunction and childhood psychoses. *Br. J. Psychiatry, 118,* 407.
50. LOCKYER, L. and RUTTER M. 1969. A five- to fifteen-year follow-up study of infantile psychosis—III. Psychological aspects. *Br. J. Psychiatry, 115,* 865.
51. LOCKYER, L. and RUTTER, M 1970. A five- to fifteen-year follow-up study of infantile psychosis: IV. Patterns of cognitive ability. *Br. J. Soc. Clin. Psychol., 9,* 152.
52. LOTTER, V. 1966. Epidemiology of autistic conditions in young children. I. Prevalence. *Soc. Psychiatry, 1,* 124.
53. LOTTER, V. 1967. Epidemiology of autistic conditions in young children. II. Some characteristics of the parents and children. *Soc. Psychiatry, 1,* 163.
54. MARCUS, J. 1974. Cerebral functioning in offspring of schizophrenics. A possible genetic factor. *Int. J. Ment. Health, 3,* 57.
55. MASSIE, H. N. 1978. The early natural history of childhood psychosis: Ten cases studied by the analysis of family home movies of the infancies of the children. *J. Am. Acad. Child Psychiatry, 17,* 29.
56. MEDNICK, S. A., MURA, M., SCHULZINGER, F. and MEDNICK, B. 1971. Perinatal conditions and infant development in children with schizophrenic parents. *Soc. Biol., 18,* S103.
57. MEYERS, D. and GOLDFARB, W. 1962. Pyschiatric appraisals of parents and siblings of schizophrenic children. *Am. J. Psychiatry, 118,* 902.

58. O'NEAL, P. and ROBINS, L. N. 1958. Childhood patterns predictive of adult schizophrenia: A 30-year follow-up study. *Am. J. Psychiatry, 115,* 385.
59. ORNITZ, E. M. 1969. Disorders of perception common to early infantile autism and schizophrenia. *Compr. Psychiatry, 10,* 259.
60. ORNITZ, E. M. 1973. Childhood autism. A review of the clinical and experimental literature (Medical progress). *Calif. Med., 118,* 21.
61. ORNITZ, E. M., GUTHRIE, D. and FARLEY, A. H. 1977. The early development of autistic children. *J. Autism Child. Schizo., 7,* 207.
62. ORNITZ, E. M. and RITVO, E. R. 1968. Perceptual inconstancy in early infantile autism. *Arch. Gen. Psychiatry, 18,* 76.
63. ORNITZ, E. M. and RITVO, E. R. 1976. The syndrome of autism: A critical review. *Am. J. Psychiatry, 133,* 609.
64. ORNITZ, E. M. and E. R. Ritvo, 1976. Medical assessment. In: E. R. Ritvo, B. J. Freeman, E. M. Ornitz, and P. Tanguay, (Eds.), *Autism: Diagnosis, Current Research and Management.* New York: Spectrum Publications.
65. POTTER, H. W. 1933. Schizophrenia in children. *Am. J. Psychiatry, 12,* 1253.
66. QUITKIN, F., RIFKIN, A. and KLEIN, D. F. 1976. Neurologic soft signs in schizophrenia and character disorders. Organicity in schizophrenia with premorbid associality and emotionally unstable character disorders. *Arch. Gen. Psychiatry, 33,* 845.
67. RICKS, D. F. and BERRY, J. C. 1970. Family and symptom patterns that precede schizophrenia. In: M. Roff, and D. F. Ricks, (Eds.), *Life History Research in Psychopathology, Volume 1.* Minneapolis: University of Minnesota Press.
68. RICKS, D. F. and NAMECHE, G. 1966. Symbiosis, sacrifice and schizophrenia. *Ment. Hyg., 50,* 541.
69. RIEDER, R. O., BROMAN, S. H. and ROSENTHAL, D. 1977. The offspring of schizophrenics II: Perinatal factors and IQ. *Arch. Gen. Psychiatry, 34,* 789.
70. RITVO, E. R., CANTWELL, D., JOHNSON, E. ET AL. 1971. Social class factors in autism. *J. Autism Child. Schizo., 1,* 297.
71. RITVO, E. R., FREEMAN, B. J., ORNITZ, E. M. and TANGUAY, P. 1976. *Autism: Diagnosis, Current Research and Management.* New York: Spectrum Publications.
72. ROBINS, L. N. 1966. *Deviant Children Grown Up.* Baltimore, Maryland: Williams and Wilkins.
73. RUBINSTEIN, E. A. 1948. Childhood mental disease in America: A review of the literature before 1900. *Am. J. Orthopsychiatry, 18,* 314.
74. RUTTER, M. 1965. The influence of organic and emotional factors on the origins, nature and outcome of childhood psychosis. *Dev. Med. Child Neurol., 7,* 518.
75. RUTTER, M. 1970. Autistic children—infancy to adulthood. *Semin. Psychiatry, 2,* 435.
76. RUTTER, M. 1972. Childhood schizophrenia reconsidered. *J. Autism Child. Schizo., 2,* 315.
77. RUTTER, M. 1974. The development of infantile autism. *Psychol. Med., 4,* 147.
78. RUTTER, M., GREENFELD, D. and LOCKYER, L. 1967. A five to fifteen year follow-up study of infantile psychosis. II. Social and behavioural outcome. *Br. J. Psychiatry, 113,* 1183.
79. RUTTER, M. and LOCKYER, L. 1967. A five to fifteen year follow-up study of infantile psychosis. I. Description of the sample. *Br. J. Psychiatry, 113,* 1169.
80. SCHAIN, R. J. and YANNET, H. 1960. Infantile Autism: An analysis of 50 cases and a consideration of certain relevant neurophysiological concepts. *J. Pediatr., 57,* 560.
81. SHAPIRO, T., CHIARANDINI, I. and FISH, B. 1974. Thirty severely disturbed children. Evaluation of their language development for classification and prognosis. *Arch. Gen. Psychiatry, 30,* 819.
82. SHAPIRO, T. and FISH, B. 1969. A method to study language deviation as an aspect of ego organization in young schizophrenic children. *J. Am. Acad. Child Psychiatry, 8,* 36.
83. SHAPIRO, T., FISH, B. and GINSBERG, G. 1972. The speech of a schizophrenic child from two to six. *Am. J. Psychiatry, 128,* 1048.
84. SHAPIRO, T. and HUEBNER, H. 1976. Speech patterns of five psychotic children now in

adolescence. *J. Am. Acad. Child Psychiatry, 15,* 278.

85. SIMON, G. B. and GILLIES, S. M. 1964. Some physical characteristics of a group of psychotic children. *Br. J. Psychiatry, 110,* 104.

86. TORREY, E. F., HERSH, S. P. and McCABE, K. D. 1975. Early childhood psychosis and bleeding during pregnancy. A prospective study of gravid women and their offspring. *J. Autism Child Schizo., 5,* 287.

87. TUCKER, G. J., CAMPION, E. W. and SILBERFARB, P. M. 1975. Sensorimotor functions and cognitive disturbance in psychiatric patients. *Am. J. Psychiatry, 132,* 17.

88. WALK, A. 1964. The pre-history of child psychiatry. *Br. J. Psychiatry, 110,* 754.

89. WATT, N. F. 1974. Childhood and adolescent routes to schizophrenia. In: D. F. Ricks, A. Thomas, and M. Roff, (Eds.), *Life History Research in Psychopathology, Volume 3.* Minneapolis: University of Minnesota Press.

90. WOODRUFF, R. A., GOODWIN, D. W. and GUZE, S. B. 1974. *Psychiatric Diagnosis.,* New York: Oxford University Press.

23

THE EARLY RECOGNITION
OF MENTAL RETARDATION

J. M. Berg, M. B., B.Ch., M.Sc., F.R.C. Psych.,
F.C.C.M.G.

*Professor of Psychiatry and Associate Professor of Medical Genetics,
University of Toronto;
Director of Genetic Services and Psychiatric Education, Surrey Place
Centre, Toronto, Canada*

INTRODUCTION

The early recognition of potential and actual disabilities, both mental and physical, has obviously beneficial implications from various standpoints. Desirable objectives, concerned with prevention, treatment and the peace of mind of affected persons and their relatives, are thus more likely to be attained. Such considerations are no less valid, and in some circumstances perhaps more so, in the sphere of mental retardation than elsewhere.

Reduction of mental ability, being a symptom and not a specific circumscribed disease, varies widely in terms of aetiology, degree and association with concomitant features. Like reduction in physical stature, it may have an essentially genetic or environmental basis; it may be anticipated before it occurs or becomes clinically apparent; it ranges from a very marked level of severity to one hardly distinguishable from the normal; and it can be the only recognizable deficiency or one manifestation in the differing patterns of anomalies which constitute distinct syndromes or disease entities.

It is the purpose of this chapter to review aspects of mental retardation related to anticipation of an increased likelihood of its occurrence prior to the event and to early recognition of individuals already affected. The major practical rationale for such prognostic and diagnostic evaluation is its significant preventive and therapeutic implications. Substantial, and even remarkable, progress has been made in these various interconnected areas in recent years and further gains are within sight.

This presentation is not intended to be exhaustive and, indeed, cannot be within the framework of a single chapter. Instead, representative issues are raised and examples are referred to in order to illustrate them. For the reader who might find it an advantage, a selected bibliography is appended suitable for further detailed reading on these, and related, issues.

RECOGNITION OF INCREASED RISKS

From time immemorial, there has been a practically universal awareness that the risk of having abnormal offspring can increase in certain circumstances. Early views often attributed these increased risks to influences of a supernatural kind, like malevolent intervention by devils or supposedly just retribution for moral transgressions imposed by wrathful gods. A wide variety of warnings also abounded over the centuries about practices to shun in order to have healthy children, such as, for example, avoidance of intercourse at or near the time of menstruation and keeping away from various unattractive sights during pregnancy. Many of these notions were based on metaphysical concepts rather than on more tenable accumulation of observed evidence in favour of the given proposition.

With the growth of scientific enquiry and advances in investigative technology, large numbers of hazards to a child not yet conceived or born have been convincingly identified. Many such hazards are connected with mental retardation and their recognition has been accompanied, to a considerable extent, by the development of suitable measures to eliminate or minimize them. These considerations apply in different situations prior to conception, prenatally, and at or after birth.

Considerations before Conception

A retarded child may be born to any couple for obscure reasons, and some indication of the likelihood of this eventuality in the general population can be derived from empirical data. Furthermore, substantial numbers of prospective parents face increased risks of having specific types of retarded offspring because of various identifiable factors directly applicable to themselves. In practice, such factors frequently are not recognized and, indeed, often cannot be in the present state of knowledge, until attention to them is drawn by the birth of an affected child. On other occasions, an increased hazard to offspring is either readily apparent or becomes so following relevant examinations, in parents who have not yet had any afflicted children. Appropriate assessment and guidance to families in each of these regards may be viewed, in a sense, as a particularly basic form of early recognition of mental retardation, because it often brings prevention within reach. These considerations are exemplified in the following discussion.

Of the various dangers of environmental origin to the developing fetus (see below), some can be counteracted suitably only before conception. For instance, protection can be achieved against the well-established deleterious consequences of maternal rubella infection early in pregnancy by determining the immune status of prospective mothers and vaccinating susceptible ones at least several months before pregnancy; vaccination during gestation is contraindicated. Less precisely clarified in humans, in terms of adverse genetic consequences including mental deficit, is parental gonadal exposure to mutagenic agents, like ionizing radiation, but precautions against avoidable exposure obviously are called for, particularly if pregnancy is a prospect.

As mentioned above, it is often not feasible to anticipate an increased risk to prospective parents of having a child with various types of mental retardation unless such a child has previously been born. The problem typically applies to many varieties of autosomal recessive, and to lesser numbers of X-linked recessive, disorders. In the former instance, each parent is a phenotypically normal heterozygous carrier of the gene concerned with a 25 percent chance in each pregnancy of having an affected offspring of either sex; in the latter case, the also phenotypically normal heterozygous maternal carrier of the relevant gene has a 50 percent chance that any son will be affected. Examples in each of these categories involving characteristic morphological cranial changes connected with mental retardation are, respectively, a form of microcephaly sometimes referred to as Seckel's bird-headed dwarfism, and a type of hydrocephaly associated with congenital stenosis of the aqueduct of Sylvius.

In other situations where potential parents are clinically healthy carriers of a gene for an autosomal, or X-linked, recessive variety of mental retardation, special tests can indicate these parental genotypes before any afflicted child is conceived. These carrier detection tests, generally biochemical in nature, can be undertaken with varying degrees of efficacy in respect, for example, to several kinds of mucopolysaccharidoses and to amino acid disorders of metabolism like phenylketonuria and argininosuccinic aciduria. A difficulty, however, with such rare disorders is the impracticability of screening potential child-bearing populations as a whole, as opposed to persons at high risk like the sibs of homozygotes or heterozygotes. If a particular section of the population can be identified as having an unduly increased frequency of heterozygous carriers for a given disorder, general screening of that group becomes more realistic. Tay-Sachs disease is a classic example of this state of affairs. Heterozygous carriers of the gene for this devastating autosomal recessive disease are about ten times more frequent among Jews of Eastern and Central European origin than among other population groups; hence "mass" screening programmes of heterozygotes appropriately can be undertaken, as indeed has happened, in the relatively readily identifiable section of the community at increased risk.

The situation with autosomal dominant varieties of mental retardation is different. Here the expectation is that the carrier of the gene for the particular condition will himself or herself be affected to a greater or lesser extent with the condition, with a 50 percent chance that any offspring also will be affected. A practical problem in these conditions is illustrated by reference to tuberous sclerosis (Bourneville's disease). Many sporadic instances are due to new gene mutation with little risk of occurrence in relatives other than children of individuals thus affected. However, because this protean autosomal dominant disease can have manifestations which range from extensive, obvious ones to slight, almost unrecognizable ones, even within the same family, special care is necessary to detect minimal features in order to predict risks of recurrence accurately.

Apart from specific gene defects of the kinds discussed above, morphologically recognizable chromosomal aberrations contribute significantly to the total number of the mentally retarded. About 0.5 percent of live births have chromosomal abnormalities, nearly all of which are connected with mental deficit. Early awareness of the raised likelihood of occurrence is invaluable, of course, both in terms of parental decisions about child-bearing and in the light of the capacity for prenatal testing of the fetus (see below). The most frequent clue providing a warning of an increased prospect of a chromosomal error, due to a non-disjunctional process, is advanced maternal age. This has a particularly striking correlation with standard (or regular) trisomy 21 resulting in the phenotype of Down's syndrome. The syndrome rises in frequency, among live births, from less than 0.1 percent below the maternal age of 30 years up to about 2.5 percent at maternal ages above 44 years, an increase of approximately 25-fold.

An important additional circumstance, independent of parental age, which markedly increases the chances of having a chromosomally, and hence mentally, abnormal child, is the presence of a balanced translocation in either parent. As such a person is clinically normal, the translocation will be detected only if a karyotype analysis is done. It is unrealistic, at present, to undertake this on all prospective parents, but a relevant family history of chromosome errors provides an indication in given instances. Particularly since cytogenetic banding techniques have been developed and applied in the 1970s, it has become increasingly apparent that many kinds of chromosomal aberrations can be transmitted by a balanced translocation carrier parent, and there has been rapidly growing documentation of these types of mental retardation. A personally investigated example concerns a phenotypically normal mother with a balanced (5p-;9p+) translocation. Two of her children had clinically different forms of severe mental retardation; the first child showed deletion of the short arm of chromosome 5(5p-, resulting in the so-called cri du chat syndrome), and the second revealed partial trisomy of the short arm of chromosome 9(9p+). If the maternal translocation state had been recognized before conception or early in pregnancy, it is almost certain that this mother would not have chromosomally abnormal, gravely impaired children.

There remains a considerable number of recognizable clinical syndromes, associated with mental retardation, which cannot be linked with confidence to a definite environmental cause, a single gene defect, or a chromosomal aberration. Examples are the eponymously designated Sturge-Weber, de Lange, Prader-Labhart-Willi and Rubinstein-Taybi syndromes, and the group of malformations known collectively as neural tube defects ranging from spina bifida and myelomeningocoele to anencephaly. If a child with any of these conditions is identified, recurrence risks can be estimated only on the basis of accumulated empirical data. For instance, if one child has been affected with de Lange syndrome or a neural tube defect, the chance of recurrence in a sib seems to be, in general, of the order of about 4 to 5 percent. The other three syndromes mentioned are nearly always sporadic, with a distinctly lower increased recurrence risk.

Many other instances of severe mental retardation also are aetiologically obscure and, unlike those referred to above, clinically undifferentiated as distinct syndromes. In these cases, too, an indication of the likelihood of repetition in families can be derived empirically; risk figures for the chance of a second child being affected similarly to an initial one usually range from about 3 to 6 percent in most studies.

Considerations during Pregnancy

Environmental perils to the fetus, particularly during the earlier stages of pregnancy, have become the subject of increasing attention and scrutiny.

A substantial number have been documented which definitely or seemingly have a distinct association with subsequent mental retardation. Some examples are shown in Table 1. The listing in the table of their nature or usual origins provides an indication of the wide ramifications of such dangers. Some of them are intimately connected with other disadvantageous circumstances, so that it can be very difficult to ascertain the precise role of each of these in producing future delay in a child's mental progress. For instance, excessive alcohol consumption may be associated with socioeconomic adversity, malnutrition and inadequate antenatal care, and the effects of thiouracil are not easily separated from those of underlying maternal thyroid disease for which the medication was used. It is noteworthy, also, as illustrated by phenylketonuria, that maternal disease of *genetic* origin can constitute an *environmental* danger to the fetus—this is just one example of the intertwined relationship between hereditary and acquired circumstances.

In terms of the theme of this chapter, the existence of any of the situations exemplified serves as a warning of the prospect of mental retardation and other disabilities in the as yet unborn child, and hence of the need to evaluate carefully that child for evidence of such consequences. More crucially important, however, is the fact that the baleful effects of the hazards referred to are eminently preventable. This can be achieved either by eliminating or avoiding the danger in the first place, or by treating the mother before fetal damage occurs.

TABLE 1

Examples of environmental hazards to the fetus connected with subsequent mental retardation

TYPE OF HAZARD	EXAMPLES	NATURE OR USUAL SOURCE
Maternal infection	Rubella Toxoplasmosis Syphilis	Viral Protozoal Spirochaetal
Maternal ingestion of chemicals	Thiouracil derivatives Mercury Chronic alcoholism	Medication Contaminated food Socio-psychiatric
Miscellaneous	Irradiation Haemolytic disease of the fetus and newborn Maternal phenylketonuria (untreated)	Medical or industrial Parental antigenic difference Maternal genetic disorder

Considerations at and after Birth

During the birth process as such, risk of damage to the central nervous system, and hence of subsequent mental retardation, essentially can be considered in two major categories. One is concerned with cerebral trauma of a direct mechanical kind and the other with cerebral anoxia or hypoxia. There is a certain degree of overlap between them and the term *birth injury* is often used in reference to both. Circumstances which are relevant in this context include: parity, multiple births, malpresentation, disproportion, too early separation of the placenta, prolapse of the umbilical cord, precipitate or prolonged labour, and premature delivery. Among important signs pointing to some of these situations are significant reduction of the fetal heart rate and meconium-staining of the amniotic fluid. The specialized knowledge of an obstetrician is, of course, frequently required to anticipate and minimize the possibilities of injury in such eventualities before and during the birth.

Once the child is born, early evidence of abnormality is often present (see section on *Postnatal Diagnosis*) as a result of preceding causal influences and events. Many new obstacles to normal mental development can arise in the months and years to come. Infections of various kinds, toxic chemical substances, head injuries and catastrophes associated with cerebral anoxia originating in the postnatal environment are among well-established causes of damage to the brain resulting in mental deficit. Like counterparts and analogous situations in prenatal life, the occurrences themselves or their deleterious consequences can be reduced significantly by judicious measures concerned with prevention and treatment. It is important to bear in mind that apparent initial recovery from such occurrences does not necessarily preclude disadvantageous long-term residual effects on mental function. These may be recognized only after continued and careful follow-up.

More subtle dangers connected with localized or generalized psychological and socioeconomic adversity have become the focus of growing attention and study. Emotional and physical deprivation due to deliberate or inadvertent neglect and abuse, for instance, can be a significant contributory factor to maladjustment and impaired mental function. Again, such situations provide both a warning of the prospects of mental damage and a summons to remedial action.

RECOGNITION OF THOSE AFFECTED

The foregoing section was concerned with the recognition of circumstances related to increased risks of mental retardation occurring before those circumstances actually produced their deleterious effects. Once the underlying causal factors, be they essentially of genetical, environmental, multifactorial or obscure origin, have come into operation, the early recognition of those affected becomes a major concern. Such diagnosis may be achieved prenatally or postnatally in different situations and is considered below in these time frames.

Prenatal Diagnosis

Current status

What may well be regarded as the most significant development of recent years, in the sphere of prevention of a growing number of types of mental retardation, has been the increasing capability of recognizing disease and malformation in the fetus sufficiently early in pregnancy to make practical intervention realistic. These endeavours are still, relatively speaking, in their infancy in that many potentially recognizable conditions cannot yet be diagnosed at all or with certainty and there remains a variable, but significant, risk component in some of the procedures. Furthermore, the practical rationale of the procedures relates to termination of pregnancies with affected fetuses rather than to the more desirable, but largely unattained, ameliorative or, better still, curative treatment. Nevertheless, despite these technical limitations and ethical concerns, there is no doubt that prenatal diagnostic measures have been a boon to many families, and facilities for undertaking them have spread rapidly in many parts of the world.

Amniocentesis

Amniocentesis via the abdominal route, usually undertaken at about 16 weeks of gestation as an outpatient procedure under local anaesthesia and in sterile conditions, is the main technique involved. Several millilitres of amniotic fluid, containing fetal cells, are thus obtained with a syringe. This provides a means for cytogenetic studies of cultured fetal cells and for biochemical as well as other investigations of the cells, both cultured and uncultured, and of the amniotic fluid as such.

The most widely used application, of much significance in regard to mental retardation, is the fetal identification of chromosomal aberrations in families at increased risk (see section on *Considerations before Conception*). Trisomy 21 (Down's syndrome) is the commonest of these aberrations, so that advancing maternal age (usually from 35 years upwards) per se is the most frequent indication for fetal karyotyping. As example of a Down's syndrome fetus identified on this basis is shown in Figure 1. Another important indication—indeed, one associated with particularly high risk—is a chromosome anomaly in either parent; this ranges from a phenotypically innocuous balanced translocation state to a sometimes clinically recognizable chromosome error compatible with fertility, such as some forms of autosomal or sex chromosomal mosaicism, and even occasionally non-mosaic chromosome excess or deletion. Other criteria for amniocentesis vary from centre to centre and include the previous birth of a chromosomally abnormal child and undue parental anxiety even in situations where the biological risk is very small. Through the use of amniocentesis, any morphologically recognizable chromosome abnormality in the fetus is detectable before the 20th week of gestation when the option of termination of the pregnancy is available to the parents in many countries.

An additional diagnostic application of fetal karyotyping should be mentioned. When a mother is known to be the carrier of the gene for a serious X-linked recessive disorder (say one connected with marked mental defect) and there is no known way of specifically detecting an afflicted fetus, a determination of fetal sex can be made. A female fetus would not have the disorder (though half of them would be expected to be carriers), whereas there is a 50 percent chance of a male being affected. Termination of a male pregnancy would remove that prospect, though at the price of an equal chance of aborting an unaffected fetus. It is a matter of debate whether or when this is justified; in the writer's view, the choice should rest squarely with the parents.

Gradually, but steadily, an increasing number of inborn errors of metabolism have become diagnosable in utero on the basis of biochemical examination of fetal cells from amniotic fluid samples obtained by amniocentesis. Many of the examinations involve enzyme assays on cultured cells and are technically subtle and complex. Thus, there may be less certainty about the accuracy of diagnosis than is generally the case with chromosome aberrations. The disorders under consideration are genetically determined (usually autosomal recessive in nature) and relatively rare. Hence, the practical rationale for testing for any of them in a given pregnancy is based on increased risks of the kinds discussed earlier, with the option of abortion if a fetus is affected. Some 30 of these disorders already have been diagnosed in utero by chemical means, with foreseeable prospects of about double that number of additional ones becoming identifiable in similar ways. Many would result in a mentally retarded child. Examples of some distinctly connected with mental deficit, in which diagnosis in the fetus has been achieved, are given in Table 2.

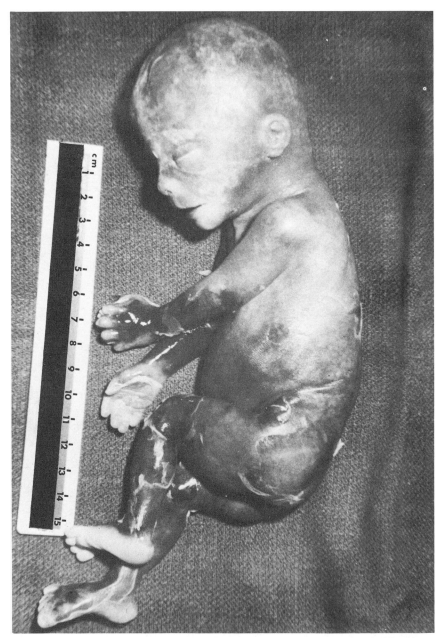

FIGURE 1. Nineteen-week Down's syndrome fetus (standard trisomy 21) identified by kary-otyping of fetal cells from an amniotic fluid sample obtained 3 weeks earlier from a 40-year-old mother (Courtesy of Dr. H. Allen Gardner, Toronto General Hospital).

TABLE 2

Examples of inborn metabolic errors connected with mental retardation which have been diagnosed in utero

TYPE OF DISORDER	EXAMPLES*
Amino acid	Argininosuccinic aciduria Maple syrup urine disease
Carbohydrate	Galactosaemia Type II glycogenosis (Pompe's disease)
Lipid	GM2 gangliosidosis (Tay-Sachs disease) Sulfatide lipidosis (infantile metachromatic leukodystrophy)
Mucopolysaccharide	Type I mucopolysaccharidosis (Hurler's syndrome) Type II mucopolysaccharidosis (Hunter's syndrome)
Miscellaneous	HGPRT deficiency (Lesch-Nyhan syndrome) Type II mucolipidosis (I-cell disease)

*Hunter and Lesch-Nyhan syndromes are transmitted in an X-linked recessive manner; the remaining 8 show autosomal recessive transmission. Because of varying terminology used in referring to these disorders, alternative designations are provided in parentheses where this seemed helpful.

A further biochemical investigation on amniotic fluid samples relevant to mental retardation is determination of the alpha-fetoprotein level in the amniotic fluid of pregnant women at increased risk of having a child with an open neural tube defect. Such mothers, up until now, have been specifically selected for testing essentially on the basis of a family history (usually a previously affected child) of neural tube defect. There are prospects that elevated maternal serum alpha-fetoprotein during pregnancy may provide a satisfactory indication for amniotic fluid testing without any relative being known to have been affected. Although a search for significantly raised alpha-fetoprotein in the amniotic fluid is a valuable diagnostic procedure, the examination is not entirely reliable because both negative and positive results can give an erroneous impression as to the fetal state in respect to a neural tube defect.

Other uses of amniocentesis related to detection and prevention or amelioration of environmentally determined disease resulting in mental retardation have been undertaken or contemplated. For example, cytomegalovirus has been recovered from amniotic fluid samples. The detection of this and other infectious agents from such samples does not seem to have, at present, a generally useful practical application.

Ultrasonography

Ultrasonography has become an important, non-invasive procedure in prenatal diagnosis. In many centres it is undertaken routinely prior to amniocentesis as a safeguard in localizing the placenta accurately. With improving equipment and expertise, ultrasound examination has substantially extended its scope as a means of recognizing abnormalities in fetal morphology. In the sphere of cerebral pathology, for instance, it is valuable in the diagnosis of anencephaly and, on the basis of biparietal measurements which can be repeated over a period of time, it may reveal significant diminution or excess of head growth. Also possibly identifiable are suspicious positions of the lateral ventricles and encephalocoele.

Fetoscopy

Direct visualization of the fetus by means of fibre optic devices, which can be accompanied by photography, raises extraordinary possibilities of recognizing external fetal malformations or anomalies indicative of particular syndromes which cannot be identified by chromosomal or biochemical examination of amniotic fluid samples. There are many such syndromes in which intellectual deficit is a feature. Three examples associated with characteristic digital abnormalities are the autosomal dominant syndrome of Apert (syndactyly) and the autosomal recessive syndromes of Laurence, Moon and Biedl (polydactyly) and of Carpenter (polysyndactyly). A photograph of fetal fingers, reproduced in Figure 2, illustrates the point.

Exposure in early pregnancy to teratogens and other environmental hazards discussed earlier also may result in external malformations as well as mental retardation. A mother thus exposed could be a suitable candidate for fetoscopy. The procedure also opens the door, as it were, to precise fetal sampling of blood, skin and other tissues, with the consequent prospect of advantageous diagnostic tests on these tissues.

Fetoscopy still has significant snags. Thus, there is the distinct danger of inducing abortion, the prospect that the relevant part of the body may not be visualized in a given instance, and the fact that absence of a particular malformation does not necessarily exclude the presence of a given syndrome. However, the procedure already has been used to good advantage and is likely to become more sophisticated and safer.

Other procedures

Other prenatal diagnostic measures of relevance to the recognition of

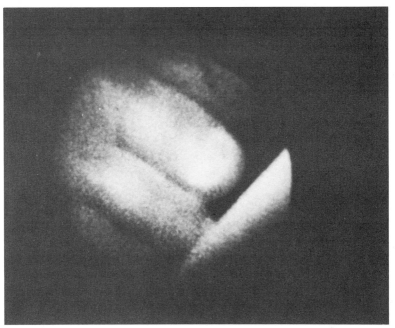

FIGURE 2. Photograph of fetal fingers visualized by fetoscopy at 17 weeks of gestation (Note: The direct *in vivo* view was clearer than in the photograph) (Courtesy of Dr. Ronald G. Benzie and *Modern Medicine of Canada*)

various forms of mental retardation have been applied, usually relatively late in pregnancy. These, including straight x-ray examination, amniography, fetography and electroencephalography, have had a distinctly circumscribed application to date because of technical limitations and/or dangers.

Postnatal Diagnosis

Once a child is born, mental retardation or the likelihood of its occurrence can be identified or anticipated on the basis of a number of considerations and observations.

Clues from history

A family, pregnancy, or personal history which raises suspicions regarding genetic and environmental hazards which have been discussed in the section of this chapter concerned with recognition of increased risks often provides the initial signal that all may not be well. Thus forewarned, the physician can undertake specific clinical, laboratory and other examinations to check whether the particular danger in a given instance produced adverse effects known to be associated with it. For example, if an infant is born to a couple who had previously had a child with one or the other enzyme defect responsible for Sanfilippo syndrome, the 25 percent recurrence risk in the new baby indicates the need for diagnostic biochemical investigation even if no clinical abnormalities are yet apparent. Similarly, known exposure to an environmental hazard, before or after birth, calls for careful diagnostic follow-up and monitoring, particularly in situations where possible developmental and related physical defects may be relatively cryptic.

Clinical findings

Though mental deficit, as such, is often difficult to pinpoint in infancy, various clinical findings at this early stage provide important evidence that the child may well be, or definitely is, affected, even though the degree is frequently not ascertainable until later. Thus, for instance, marked prematurity and substantially reduced birthweight in relation to gestational age are suspicious findings. Also, the occurrence of convulsions, of significant alterations in muscle tone, or of other signs of cerebral involvement can be distinctly helpful prognostic indicators of mental handicap. The same is true of substantial deviations from well-established norms in the size and/or shape of the head. Further, the infant who is not uncommonly described by parents as being unusually "good," in behavioural terms, may be so because his excessive sleep, rare crying, general lack of liveliness, and unresponsiveness to the environment are early manifestations of central nervous system pathology.

In addition, mental retardation is a usual, or even invariable, component of many syndromes in which a combination of morphological anomalies is sufficiently striking at the time of birth, or soon after, to enable a reasonably confident diagnosis of the given syndrome to be made promptly on clinical grounds. The syndromes of Down, of de Lange, and of Smith, Lemli and Opitz are but three of large numbers of such well-documented entities. Early recognition of these mental retardation syndromes is of great importance as a guide both to the prognosis for the affected child and to recurrence risks for relatives, even though there may be no foreseeable prospects for effective specific medical treatment.

Biochemical screening

Apart from the recognition of the probability of mental retardation in individual infants based on the considerations referred to above, special screening of newborn children in general, or of selected high-risk population groups of children, has become an increasingly applied procedure in the early detection of mental defect. Such screening largely involves the application of biochemical tests to small samples of blood and/or urine, and many jurisdictions now undertake this to a greater or lesser extent. The main focus understandably has been on disorders amenable to some degree of effective treatment.

Phenylketonuria has served as a pioneering model for these kinds of diagnostic endeavours. This inborn error of phenylalanine metabolism (now known to encompass several varieties) was discovered relatively early more than 40 years ago; it was found some 15 years later to respond favourably, in terms of prevention or diminution of deleterious mental or other consequences, to a special diet introduced in infancy. The subsequent development of the Guthrie test, a bacteriological phenylalanine assay, provided the means for centralized, mass newborn screening on a mere few drops of dried blood. Thereafter, paper chromatography and other techniques extended the scope for newborn population screening, not only for phenylketonuria and rather similar amino acid disorders, but also for a wider variety of genetically determined biochemical diseases connected with mental retardation. Among conditions, in addition to phenylketonuria, thus tested for in different countries during the first few weeks of life, on blood and/or urine samples, are: maple syrup urine disease, argininosuccinic aciduria, homocystinuria, galactosaemia and neonatal hypothyroidism. Though such diseases are uncommon, and even rare, the prospect of efficacious treatment of affected babies through early recognition by mass screening methods is a consideration entirely deserving of attention.

Other circumstances in which chemical screening of selected high-risk populations of children is indicated are connected with environmental hazards often related to adverse socioeconomic conditions. Ideally, of course, the elimination of such adversity is the solution of choice. However, that brave new world is not immediately in sight, so that other measures need to be adopted in the interim. Lead poisoning provides an important illustration. Lead has been recognized as a hazard to man for many centuries; its deleterious effects were known, for instance, to Hippocrates. In more recent years, the dangers of lead exposure for young children, not only in terms of acute encephalopathy but in terms of more insidious long-range harmful effects on mental function, have come to be appreciated. Mass screening of children living in poor environments, in which exposure often is considerable, is therefore a valuable diagnostic measure. Programmes involving blood, urinary, hair and even tooth lead screening, as well as other tests, have shown many at-risk children to be contaminated. These observations may be regarded as an early form of recognition of mental deficit amenable to treatment and, indeed, to prevention.

Developmental assessment

The discussion in this section so far has been concerned essentially with the recognition of mental retardation in infancy in the context of various telltale historical, morphological and laboratory findings. In a significant proportion of mentally retarded children such initial clues are not apparent even when a careful search is made. Early detection of mental deficit in such children is then largely dependent on a sound understanding of developmental norms and of the nature and extent of deviations from these which can be interpreted as abnormal.

These norms have been documented comprehensively and lucidly by many authorities on child development, like Gesell in the United States and Illingworth in the United Kingdom to mention but two, and need not be reviewed here. Perhaps the most important consideration to emphasize, in the light of considerable variability in individual items of developmental progress, is that early onset mental retardation is generally associated with developmental delay of differing degree in all, or nearly all, spheres, rather than in isolated ones. Related to such delay is the frequent unduly long persistence of behaviour which is typically of more limited duration in normal children. Such behaviour includes, for example, continuous indiscriminate insertion into the mouth or throwing onto the floor of anything within reach which can be handled. It seems appropriate to emphasize here also the notorious possibility of interpreting apparent developmental delay as mental retardation when the explanation for it is a specific, circumscribed abnormality like a defect in vision or hearing.

Diagnosis in older children

As the child gets older, mental retardation generally becomes more readily recognizable, particularly when it is relatively severe. Thus, certain physical manifestations of congenital mental retardation syndromes may become more obvious even if present earlier (for example, the coarse facies, stiff joints and hepatosplenomegaly in several of the mucopolysaccharidoses); or they may appear for the first time after some years (for example, the so-called adenoma sebaceum and other skin lesions in tuberous sclerosis). Also, a specific postnatal cause of mental retardation, such as cerebral infection or trauma, is usually identifiable when it occurs, and regression or lack of progress in the child's mental capacities after the event is dramatized by the contrast with previously normal function. Furthermore, even in the absence of such circumstances, mental delay becomes more evident as time goes by because of the increasing range of expected capabilities. In addition, formal psychometric testing is rather more reliable in later childhood than in infancy and, if competently undertaken with appropriate tests, advantageously supplements clinical appraisal and laboratory investigation.

During the school-age years, as earlier, care must be taken to distinguish overall mental retardation from specific disabilities, associated with impaired learning, like dyslexia or dysphasia. Further, the differentiation between behaviour disturbance of various kinds and mental deficit per se also may require special attention, a consideration which can be particularly complex because of the frequently close aetiological and clinical relationship between them. Finally, in an era often relatively enlightened and advanced in other ways, there remains a depressingly high incidence of childhood emotional deprivation, physical abuse, neglect and undernourishment. In view of that, it is perhaps fitting to end on the note that such adversity also can seriously impair mental progress and give the impression of intellectual retardation when it is not intrinsically present.

CONCLUDING COMMENTS

This chapter deliberately is focused mainly on biomedical aspects of mental retardation not generally given substantial attention in volumes appearing under a psychiatric rubric. This neglect is one reason for this focus, insufficient in itself, but there are several interlinked ones as well. Mental retardation, being a disability of the mind, is a proper professional concern *in all its aspects* for psychiatrists and individuals in related disciplines. Furthermore, those involved in work connected with early recognition of mental deficit are confronted with questions from anxious relatives not only on whether the deficit exists or not, but also why it occurs and what the likelihood of occurrence or recurrence is; well-informed answers should be available even if only to steer the enquirer towards suitable sources of further guidance. In addition, psychiatrists as such have a role in the context of serious physical, as well as mental, handicap (the conditions referred to in this chapter are very often a combination of both) because such occurrences, or fear of them, can be extremely disruptive in psychiatric terms to relatives and families.

In conclusion, it is perhaps appropriate to reemphasize the frequently crucial importance of identifying hazards to normal mental development and of early recognition of those affected, not for its own sake but because of beneficial intervention, of the kinds indicated in the text, which can then take place. Despite the many unresolved problems and uncertainties, there have been substantial advances in these various respects in recent years. More can be reasonably expected in the years immediately ahead.

BIBLIOGRAPHY

The following bibliography of recently published texts has been selected with the object of providing detailed and comprehensive coverage of topics and issues raised in this chapter. Although many other relevant and instructive works could be added, it did not seem advantageous to do so, particularly as each of the texts listed contains extensive additional references.

CLARKE, A.M. and CLARKE, A.D.B. (Eds.) 1974. *Mental Deficiency: the Changing Outlook*. 3rd edition. London: Methuen.

CROME, L. and STERN, J. 1972. *Pathology of Mental Retardation*. 2nd edition. Edinburgh: Churchill Livingstone.

ELLIS N.R. (Ed.) 1975. *Aberrant Development in Infancy*. Hillsdale, New Jersey: Lawrence Erlbaum Associates.

EMERY, A.E.H. (Ed.) 1973. *Antenatal Diagnosis of Genetic Disease*. Edinburgh: Churchill Livingstone.

FRASER, F.C. and NORA, J.J. 1975. *Genetics of Man*. Philadelphia: Lea & Febiger.

GESELL A. and AMATRUDA, C.S. 1947. *Developmental Diagnosis*. 2nd edition. New York: Harper & Row. (Note: Following the deaths of the original authors, a revised and enlarged third edition of this classic test, edited by H. Knobloch and B. Pasamanick, was produced in 1974 by the same publishers).

GRIFFITHS, M.I. (Ed.) 1973. *The Young Retarded Child*. Edinburgh: Churchill Livingstone.

HOLMES, L.B., MOSER, H.W., HALLDÓRSSON, S., MACK, C., PANT, S. S. and MATZILEVICH, B. 1972. *Mental Retardation: An Atlas of Diseases with Associated Physical Abnormalities*. New York: Macmillan.

ILLINGWORTH, R.S. 1975. *The Development of the Infant and Young Child*. 6th edition. Edinburgh: Churchill Livingstone.

JOHNSTON, R.B. and MAGRAB, P.R. (Eds.) 1976. *Developmental Disorders*. Baltimore: University Park Press.

KHANNA, J.L. (Ed.) 1973. *Brain Damage and Mental Retardation: A Psychological Evaluation*. 2nd edition. Springfield: Charles C Thomas.

LOWREY, G.H. 1973. *Growth and Development of Children*. 6th edition. Chicago: Year Book Medical Publishers.

McKUSICK, V.A. 1975. *Mendelian Inheritance in Man*. 4th edition. Baltimore: Johns Hopkins University Press.

MENOLASCINO, F.J. and EGGER, M.L. 1978. *Medical Dimensions of Mental Retardation*. Lincoln: University of Nebraska Press.

MILUNSKY, A. (Ed.) 1975. *The Prevention of Genetic Disease and Mental Retardation*. Philadelphia: W.B. Saunders Co.

PENROSE, L.S. 1972. *The Biology of Mental Defect*. 4th edition. London: Sidgwick & Jackson.

SMITH, D.W. 1976. *Recognizable Patterns of Human Malformation*. 2nd edition. Philadelphia: W.B. Saunders Co.

STOELINGA, G.B.A. and VAN DER WERFF TEN BOSCH, J.J. (Eds.) 1971. *Normal and Abnormal Development of Brain and Behaviour*. Leiden: Leiden University Press.

THOMPSON, J.S. and THOMPSON, M.W. 1973. *Genetics in Medicine*. 2nd edition. Philadelphia: W.B. Saunders Co.

WARKANY, J. 1971. *Congenital Malformations*. Chicago: Year Book Medical Publishers.

24

COUNSELING PARENTS OF MENTALLY RETARDED INFANTS

Fred D. Strider, Ph.D.

Associate Professor of Medical Psychology,
Department of Psychiatry
University of Nebraska Medical Center;
Chief, Psychology Services
Chief of Staff,
Nebraska Psychiatric Institute,
Omaha, Nebraska

and

Frank J. Menolascino, M.D.

Professor of Psychiatry and Pediatrics,
University of Nebraska Medical Center,
Omaha, Nebraska

Attempts to precisely delineate the professional counseling relationship between a professional and the parents of a retarded infant are complicated. When a infant is born with obvious retardation, the "problem" has been literally thrust upon the parents; the parents, as well as the professionals involved, must explore their individual and mutual responses to the family crisis in attempting to understand the situation and help the retarded infant. Counseling in such instances ranges from an informal relationship between a parent and a professional to a structured professional helping relationship which focuses on helping the parents to grow, to accept themselves more fully, and to meaningfully care for someone apart from themselves. In this latter professional relationship, the professional counselor can provide a variety of helping services, ranging from straightforward advice and instruction to assistance in actualizing one's parenting skills in all dimensions (6).

This spectrum of the counseling services reflects the recent changes in the practice of professionals working with retarded infants and their parents. In the recent past, professionals who worked with the mentally retarded viewed their role quite narrowly; emphasis was placed upon diagnostic procedures with a literal penchant for identifying or cataloging the limitations of the retarded infant. Subsequent parental counseling involved the presentation of diagnostic information in an atmosphere of pessimism and futility, with precious little attention to the social, familial, and remedial needs of the infant. Professionals assumed that if the psychological functioning of the retarded infant could be improved through medical intervention, improvements in the parent-child relationship would automatically follow (5).

As Solomons and Menolascino (8) have noted, this role of the professional counselor has changed, since parents are now viewed as central agents in the successful treatment and management of the retarded infant. As professionals have come to more clearly understand parents of retarded infants, they have become more attuned to the parents' personal and special information needs. Parents of retarded infants are like parents everywhere, reflecting all of the strengths, weaknesses, emotions and characteristics of the human condition. They may show special qualities because of the challenges and demands placed upon them by having a family member with special needs. Their parenting challenges differ not so much in the nature of the care required, as in the timing and sequencing necessary to meet special crises over a prolonged period of time.

It is our view that the successful professional counseling relationship with parents of a retarded infant includes: crisis intervention, instructional/management functions, psychotherapy, and humanistic self-actualization functions. Combining these functions provides both opportunity and challenge for the professional. We shall examine these functions in more detail and attempt to provide the professional counselor with a framework for conceptualizing the various stages of the counseling relationship. The professional can then flexibly modify the goals and procedures of each stage of counseling to meet the presenting needs of parents and their retarded infants.

FOUNDATIONS OF THE COUNSELING RELATIONSHIP

The diagnosis of mental retardation is made on the basis of two aspects of functioning: 1) intelligence as measured by standard psychological tests;

and 2) adaptive behavior as indexed by the individual's ability to function independently and meet the cultural demands of personal and social responsibility. Other dimensions of mental retardation with respect to the diagnosis of specific syndromes and types are discussed in Menolascino and Egger (4) and will not be included in this chapter. The foundation of a successful counseling relationship is a thorough and accurate developmental evaluation by qualified professional representatives from the fields of social work, education, psychology, and developmental medicine. This evaluation forms the basis for selection of treatment and management recommendations. When coupled with a sensitive and realistic approach to parental and family problems and resources, the evaluation forms a basis for clarification and delineation of counseling goals and for the selection of specific treatment procedures for attaining these goals.

In the past, the diagnosis and definitions of mental retardation have stressed essentially negative characteristics in retarded persons, e.g., social incompetence, incurable developmental arrest, intellectual inadequacy, etc. Since the counseling relationship of the professional with the parents of a retarded child is most often initiated after (or structured by), a diagnostic evaluation of the child, this relationship has often been predicated on the negative attitudes and implications of the deficits observed and the descriptive terminology of mental retardation. Diagnostic descriptions which are outlined in negative terms almost invariably affect the understanding and expectations of the parents. The initial diagnostic information presented is all too often tragic and nihilistic, so that the counseling relationship may begin in a doomsday atmosphere which squelches parental hope. Concomitantly, the development of realistic and effective programs of care, education and training for their retarded infant is also beclouded. These negative diagnostic conceptualizations tend to activate self-fulfilling prophecies which may deny the retarded child access to educational and social experiences and effectively prevent the child from learning and developing—thus confirming the gloomy prognosis. Instead, we suggest that the modern operational definition of the symptom of mental retardation be transmitted to the parents, with sufficient attention to the potentials of the infant for learning, growth, and development (3).

The effectiveness of a professional counselor depends upon: (a) positive attitudes of the clinician towards the phenomena of mental retardation; (b) thorough knowledge of the medical syndromes which manifest mental retardation as a symptom; (c) the ability to describe and explicate diagnostic and prognostic information in a manner which not only facilitates intellectual comprehension but also addresses the emotional aspect of parental reactions effectively and appropriately; and (d) an understanding of the dynamics of the individual family and its interaction. Without these four factors, the counselor has little basis for sharing information or facilitating its interpretation (2).

The counselor's first encounter with the parents of a retarded infant is apt to be at a time of crisis when parents are reacting to the initial knowledge that their child is handicapped. We believe that a short-term crisis orientation approach, which includes both diagnostic and treatment guidelines, is most appropriate at this time. The importance of the initial interpretation interview with the parents of a retarded infant can hardly be underestimated—either in the degree to which it provides a basis for effective treatment and long-term management or in the counseling challenges it presents. The counselor must present and interpret diagnostic information which may precipitate crisis reactions in each of the parents; simultaneously, he or she must also assist the parents in effectively managing these feelings and work with them to develop and participate in realistic planning for medical services for their infant (8).

To provide the counselor with a fuller understanding of these challenges, we shall first review the general paradigm of emotional reaction to "novelty shock"—a useful model for considering the reaction of individuals to this initial crisis. We shall then consider the issues crucial to the programming of a successful management-intervention approach and review stages of management, planning, and common developmental stages which frequently precipitate crisis points for the family of a retarded infant.

A CONCEPTUAL FRAMEWORK

Menolascino (3) has described three stages of parental acceptance of the diagnosis of mental retardation in their infant. Each of these stages involves major personality repercussions in the parents. Invariably, the diagnosis of mental retardation precipitates immediate and dramatic parental emotional responses. Shock and denial are clearly in evidence, as well as common physical and psychological responses to overwhelming acute stress. These responses may be mild (when the parents have anticipated the diagnosis), or they may be severe, with associated guilt, grief, religious ruminations, and dissociative states. The use of the psychological defense mechanisms of denial and displacement is common. When guilt feelings are not successfully resolved, more pathological coping mechanisms may be adopted, including depressive, paranoid, or obsessional syndromes.

The defense mechanism of reaction formation may later appear in an effort to deny and repress unconscious wishes to be free of the child and its difficulties; this stage is characterized by overreaction and overcompensation. Further, at this stage the counselor encounters excessive protection of the child, as well as endless expressions of concern about, and aggressive demands for services and attention. Diagnostic shopping may be replaced by therapeutic shopping, a process which reflects a shift on the parents' part from the actual denial of developmental problems to grasping at diagnostic alternatives (usually vague) which usually embody more positive treatment potentials. At this point the parents may insist upon totally inappropriate diagnostic and treatment services for their infant.

When these general stages of parental reaction are successfully recognized and resolved, the parents emerge with meaningful and realistic knowledge of the child's problems and acceptance of these problems. Such resolution of the crisis aspect of the initial diagnostic information paves the way for cooperation in treatment and educational programs and for parental acceptance of differential management.

In our view, there are three major sources of the crises with which the counselor must deal: 1) *novelty shock*, the precipitation of disruptive, disorganizing and acutely painful emotional reactions when parental expectancies are precipitously shattered; 2) *reality stresses*, which inevitably occur in the demands and obligations involved in caring for a retarded person; and 3) *personal value conflicts* in one or both of the parents, related to social and cultural attitudes toward defect or deviance.

The Novelty Shock Crisis

The novelty shock crisis is precipitated whenever an individual suddenly becomes aware that one's expectations about the world, self, and others differ substantially from reality. Although the process occurs in the context of "good" and "bad" value judgments, the counselor is most apt to encounter novelty shock when the implications of the occurrence are viewed as tragic. Most commonly, novelty shock is precipitated when parents realize their child is abnormal and will be unable to fulfill their expectations of a normal child.

Birth is an especially stressful time for any parents. When novelty shock is added to this already stressful time, it may produce severe psychological symptoms of regression, bewilderment, confusion, disorganization and dissociation. Novelty shock may be precipitated by the general disruptive quality of the birth of an atypical child and by the way the event is interpreted by the parents and attending medical personnel.

The counselor generally finds that the novelty shock phenomenon, although intense and at times dramatic in the precipitation of disorganized behavior and emotions, is generally easily identified. The parents—whose personality defenses have been literally shattered—are open to direct therapeutic intervention at this time. Management of this crisis reaction involves: 1) gentle, undramatic presentation and interpretation of the known diagnostic facts within the context of a counseling relationship characterized by maximum emotional support; 2) interpretation and explanation which stress aspects of the current situation that are both realistic and positive, such as clear discussions of expected child development, available services and resources; and 3) involvement of the parents in the activity and functions of the local Association for Retarded Citizens.

The nature of novelty shock is such that parents tend to intensify their inward directed attentions; they may appear to be preoccupied, narcissistic, obsessed by a narrow spectrum of interests and activities, selfish, and, from time-to-time, steeped in self-pity. It is the task of the counselor to provide appropriate support and reassurance and to broaden each parent's concerns to include the spouse, other family members, and the new infant. One counseling approach is to emphasize future assessment of the child's progress, so as to move the parents from novelty shock to attention and concern for realistic problems and their appropriate solution(s).

The Reality Stress Crisis

Child-rearing is a demanding, challenging task even when the child is intelligent and physically healthy and the parents are capable and secure emotionally, socially and economically. It is extremely difficult for parents of average means and circumstances to rear a retarded child without provision of resources and services from outside agencies and professional persons. When the parents apply for services, signs of stress and suggestive psychopathology are almost invariably present. Their reactions may be only a normal reaction to *realistic* situational stress. It is important for the counselor to be adept at recognizing and appreciating the burden associated with rearing a retarded child, and not to mistake situational reactions and stress responses for structured psychopathology. Failure to do so results in the creation of erroneous stereotypes about the parents of retarded children and in the adoption of counseling strategies which focus erroneously on psychotherapeutic treatment—rather than on educational or concrete service delivery approaches to effectively resolve the stressing situations. The counselor must actively help the parents obtain needed services, while stressing that the parent will also benefit from joining parent advocacy groups, and work with other professionals to assure thorough follow-up services. Parents focusing on reality stresses are best served by actual developmental programs (i.e., visiting nurse program, prosthetic equipment brought to the home, special babysitting services, etc.), since these services can directly and successfully resolve the realistic difficulties facing the family. The provision of these *direct* services will concretely answer the parents' direct request for direct help.

Value Conflicts

It is only in the recent past that clinicians have begun to acknowledge the effects of attitudes and social and cultural values, not only upon the behavior of their patients, but on the counseling process itself. Parents and counselors tend to have perceptions and interpretations of mental retardation which have been learned both consciously and unconsciously in their past experience. Mental retardation is perceived as a deviancy which is negatively valued, even abhorred. Historically, retarded persons have been viewed as menaces to society or as subhuman entities; responses to them have ranged from ridicule to pity (9). Almost all parents of retarded children are, at one time or another, bound to encounter instances in which their response to the child represents conflict between the values they hold about their child as a member of their family and the negative values placed upon retarded persons by our culture and society. Subjective value conflicts frequently serve as unconscious motivational forces. They are most commonly manifested in rejection; in extreme forms, institutionalization and subsequent denial of the existence of the child are examples of behavior associated with value conflicts.

Value conflicts can be seen in parental responses of existential pain and ambivalence in acceptance of known facts about their infant's condition. Unless these unconscious values and attitudes are brought to consciousness, examined, and processed in the context of the parents' existential beliefs, these conflicts may persist unrecognized for years to the detriment of the child and the parents' relationships to him. Psychotherapeutic approaches to such conflicts focus upon the meaning of life and its ultimate values (1). Religious or pastoral counseling is an alternative and, in many instances, more realistic approach to parents whose behavior and emotional functioning suggest these value conflicts. Group therapy approaches which focus on self-worth considerations and socialization, church groups (especially those who provide congregational support), and exposure of parents to other parents who have achieved successful conflict resolution to this family issue—as in the Pilot Parent movement (4)—have been found to be helpful counseling approaches.

Counseling in this value crisis is successful when the child is conceptualized as having a positive position in the parental value system and the parents are able to invest in and have sincere concern for their infant. In some instances, the parent is able to verbalize specific value changes and to describe the resolution of the existential dilemma presented by his or her retarded infant.

Chronic perpetuation of value conflict can be seen in manifestations of chronic sorrow, with a pervading sense of emptiness and lack of fulfillment on the part of the parent. Emotional disorders, especially depression, may be prolonged. Psychological attitudes of ambivalence are frequently manifested in inconsistent management and treatment of the child. Inappropriate institutionalization and shopping for invalid diagnoses (or cures) may also reflect unresolved existential conflicts on the part of one or both of the parents.

A SUGGESTED COUNSELING APPROACH

We would suggest the following management strategy for meeting the counseling needs of parents of retarded infants. Immediately upon referral, the counselor should assess the parental response to the diagnosis of mental retardation in their child for signs of the *novelty shock crisis.* Counseling strategies must focus initially upon supportive measures for ventilation, clarification, and containment of the initial emotional aspects of the novelty shock crisis. Interpretation of the medical and diagnostic information about the child should be realistic, should be presented in ways which insure parental comprehension and understanding, and should focus upon positive developmental expectations. Immediate supportive counseling which serves to dispel unrealistic fears and to realign expectations can be of great assistance in decreasing novelty shock. The parents should be referred to parent advocacy groups for the retarded and to such groups as the Pilot Parents. At this point in the counseling process, the needs of the parent and child are well served by active participation of the parents in the initial planning and utilization of needed services. Successful resolution of the novelty shock stage is characterized by parental acceptance of current reality facts, an appropriate realization of future developmental expectations, and both short- and long-term developmental plans for their infant.

For parents who are experiencing a *reality crisis,* the counselor begins his treatment of the family with a thorough assessment of the realistic situational demands upon the family. Any concerns about suspected psychopathology (in either parent) should not be addressed until after measures have been taken to reduce the realistic stresses upon the parents. The counselor is most helpful at this point if he quickly provides entry to services or resources which have the potential to directly relieve situational demands. To the extent that these services are successful, the psychological reactions of the parents to the stressful situation will subside and an improvement in parental functioning will be noted. The counselor is able to gauge improvement at this juncture in apparent decreases in requests for support from the parents, their effective utilization of resources, and, on occasion, their participation in the creation of needed resources and services.

When parents are no longer in novelty shock, and when reality demands and burdens have been realistically assessed and relieved, it is then appropriate to assess the possible presence of primary psychopathology reactions. Although these parental problems in personal adjustments may have been aggravated by the presence of a new retarded family member, often they had their origin(s) in an earlier stage of the individual's life. Recognizable psychiatric syndromes of personality dysfunction may interfere with personal adjustment and adaptive behavior, as well as with interpersonal relationships—including the relationship with the retarded infant. These primary pathological reactions are best managed through conventional psychiatric and psychological diagnostic and treatment methods.

EMERGING INNOVATIONS

We would be remiss if we did not note some innovations in counseling of parents with retarded infants. The Pilot Parents movement, early childhood education programs for retarded infants, new parent-professional liaisons with the personnel of community-based systems of service for the retarded—all hold great promise for the retarded. Further, these changes strengthen the counselor's ability to aid these parents.

The Pilot Parents movement is an organization of parents who, having successfully adjusted to their retarded infant/child, now make themselves available as successful models to new parents. Carefully trained and well organized cadres of such parents make initial (and early!) contact with new parents in the newborn nursery, in their homes, etc. Because of their experiences, these Pilot Parents are very effective parent-to-parent intervenors—especially in instances of novelty shock crisis. Beyond this early crucial time, these Pilot Parents often form lasting relationships and provide a form of communal acceptance of both the new parents and their retarded infant.

Although early childhood educational programs for retarded infants and young children are not new, programmatic changes are increasingly being made which more actively involve the parents. Indeed, some of the programs demand an objective, individualized educational prescription which must be both explained to the parent and agreed to by them (with their signature). These programs actively utilize the parents as educational programmers in their own homes after the school day. This particular innovation brings the parents into the treatment partnership, while simultaneously training them to be more knowledgeable about their child's problems.

Lastly, the personnel of community-based programs have shown an active interest in the needs and wishes of parents of their charges. Since these programs are often in the parents' neighborhood, there are splendid opportunities for the ongoing sharing of information, feelings, and developmental expectations.

Each of these relatively recent innovations involves more individuals who can share, explore, and effectively help parents of infants who have the symptom of mental retardation.

SUMMARY

We have discussed adaptations of the conventional counseling relationship for helping parents of mentally retarded infants. In contrast to earlier counseling approaches which focused efforts narrowly upon the limitations of the retarded infant, current approaches stress counseling endeavors which bolster parental functioning to enable them to fulfill their essential role in maximizing the intellectual, social, and psychological development of their retarded infant. The foundation of such a relationship rests upon a complete, accurate, and thorough evaluation, which not only produces assessment of limitations, but contributes significantly to planning realistic programs of care and training for the infant. The stages of parental reaction to the birth of a retarded child were surveyed, with recommendations for resolving them through attention to novelty shock, reality stress crises, and value conflicts. We have suggested a paradigm for counseling the parents of the retarded infant which incorporates these considerations. Finally, we have briefly discussed some emerging innovations in the care of retarded infants which can directly enrich the armamentarium of skills of the parents and infants who come for help and, indirectly, of the counselor.

REFERENCES

1. FRANKL, V. 1970. *Man's Search for Meaning: An Introduction to Logotherapy*. New York: Simon and Schuster.
2. MATHENY, A.P. and VERNICK, J. 1969. Parents of the mentally retarded child: Emotionally overwhelmed or informationally deprived? *Pediatrics*, 74:953-959.
3. MENOLASCINO, F.J. 1977. *Challenges in Mental Retardation: Progressive Ideology and Services*. New York: Human Sciences Press, p. 14.
4. MENOLASCINO, F.J. and EGGER, M.L. 1978. *Medical Dimensions of Mental Retardation*. Lincoln, Nebr.: University of Nebraska Press.
5. MURPHY, T. 1976. Parent counselling and exceptionality: From creative insecurity toward increased humanness. In: E.J. Webster, (Ed.), *Professional Approaches with Parents of Handicapped Children*. Springfield, Ill.: Charles C Thomas.
6. OLSHANSKY, S. 1970. Chronic sorrow: A response to having a mentally defective child. In: L.N. Robert, (Ed.), *Counselling Parents of the Mentally Retarded*. Springfield, Ill.: Charles C Thomas, pp. 49-54.
7. PORTER, F. 1977. *The Pilot Parent Program: A Design for Developing a Program for Parents of Handicapped Children*. Edited by R. Coleman. Omaha, Nebraska: Greater Omaha Association for Retarded Citizens.
8. SOLOMONS, G and MENOLASCINO, F.J. 1968 Medical counseling of the parents of the retarded: The importance of a right start. *Clinical Pediatrics*, 7, 11.
9. WOLFENSBERGER, W. 1976. The origin and nature of our institutional models. In: R.G. Kugel, and W. Wolfensberger, (Eds.) *Changing Patterns in Residential Services for the Mentally Retarded*. Washington, D.C.: Government Printing Office.

25

GENETIC COUNSELING
AND THE YOUNG CHILD

CHARLES I. SCOTT, JR., M.D.

and

CHARLEEN M. MOORE, PH.D.

Department of Pediatrics,
The University of Texas Health Science Center at Houston, Texas

INTRODUCTION

Our understanding of genetic disease has expanded enormously in the past 20 years. We now recognize hereditary diseases more confidently and comprehend their genesis and mechanisms of transmission more fully. Hereditary diseases may involve single genes, multiple genes or entire chromosomes.

Man has approximately 100,000 genes which are distributed among 46 chromosomes. It is the purpose of clinical genetics to determine which gene or chromosomal aberration is associated with a given disorder, i.e., to recognize phenotypic associations with a specific gene or chromosome. Virtually any trait is the result of the combined action of genetic and environmental factors. No gene acts in a vacuum.

Hereditary disease does not confine its effects to the affected person, but has effects both on the parents, brothers, and sisters individually and on the family as a unit. For example, muscular dystrophy of Duchenne is a hereditary X-linked single gene disorder affecting males who die in the sec-

This work was supported in part by funds from Grant No. G.M. 19513 from the National Institutes of Health.

ond decade of life before reproducing. The parents' risk of having other affected sons can be high. Obviously, this information can have far-reaching consequences for the parents and their clinically normal daughters, who may be carriers of this trait. Without proper genetic counseling, such a couple might refrain from having further children, or the strain and uncertainty might lead to marital disturbance or divorce. If other affected sons are born, parental anguish and guilt can be overwhelming. Brothers and sisters of the affected boy may lead very unhappy lives if they are not provided the genetic facts concerning the risks of this disorder occurring in their offspring.

The term *congenital* refers to the fact that a particular disease or somatic abnormality is recognized at birth. Such conditions may be the result of environmental factors, as in the rubella syndrome, or they may be genetic, as illustrated by albinism. Genetic diseases may be congenital or may have a later age of onset, such as in Huntington's Chorea where the degenerative changes are not usually manifested until the fourth or subsequent decades of life. Certain disorders are *familial*, i.e., they tend to occur in certain families more frequently. The etiology can be environmental, as with pinworm infestations, or it can be associated with genetic factors and have significant recurrence risks, as in club foot deformities or cleft lip and/or palate. The term *hereditary* is generally used in referring to those disorders which are related to traits determined largely by genes or chromosomes.

MENDELIAN DISORDERS

These disorders are caused by mutant genes and follow the laws which Mendel discovered in 1866. If the gene is expressed when it exists in single dose, it is said to be *dominant*; if it must be present in double dose to show an effect, it is said to be *recessive*; if the gene is on one of the 22 pairs of non-sex chromosomes, it is said to be *autosomal*; if it is on the X-chromosome, it is referred to as *X-linked*.

Currently over 3000 single gene disorders are recognized in man (27). This is to say nothing of the large number of chromosome abnormalities now identified (5,11,47). The individual Mendelian disorders are generally quite rare in occurrence (i.e., 1 in 10,000 to 1 in 1,000,000), although in certain groups or populations some of these conditions can achieve frequencies as high as 1 in 100 to 1 in 10,000—e.g., Tay-Sachs disease in Ashkenazic Jews and sickle cell anemia in blacks. The ethnicity of those seeking counseling can, therefore, be very helpful in establishing a specific diagnosis in many genetic disorders.

Clinically similar diseases may show different patterns of inheritance—*genetic heterogeneity*. Nowhere in medicine is clinical heterogeneity better demonstrated than in the genetics of dwarfism(34,40). Over 80 types of intrinsic bone dysplasias are now delineated, of which achondroplasia is the most common. It is also the most overworked diagnostic label in the chondrodystrophies, since at least six other specific entities are routinely misdiagnosed as achondroplastic dwarfism. With close clinical, radiological, biochemical and pedigree analysis, each of these disorders can be distinguished, so that accurate genetic counseling can be given. Another area of clinical heterogeneity is that of mental retardation, in which a large number of specific hereditary disorders can be delineated(20,35,38).

Autosomal dominant traits are notoriously variable in their clinical presentation. One affected person might manifest the full syndrome with effects on multiple organ systems, while another affected person in the same kindred will often express only one feature of the syndrome. Failure to recognize this characteristic of genetic disease can result in erroneous counseling. *Penetrance* refers to whether the trait is expressed at all. When some individuals who have the appropriate *genotype* (specific genetic constitution under study) fail to express it, the trait is said to exhibit *reduced penetrance*. Clinically, this can be the basis for a *skipped generation*. Each gene has only one primary effect, in that it directs synthesis of a specific polypeptide chain; however, many varied consequences can occur from a single mutant gene—*pleiotropic effects*. For instance, in the Marfan syndrome a single autosomal dominant gene is responsible for widespread effects on the skeleton, eye and cardiovascular systems.

Many autosomal dominant traits are the result of *new point mutations*. In such instances entirely normal parents have a child affected by an autosomal dominant trait such as Apert's syndrome or achondroplastic dwarfism. These parents have virtually no risk of having another child with this specific disorder, since the occurrence of the very rare mutation was by chance only and is extremely unlikely to recur. The affected child has an autosomal dominant trait and, therefore, has a 50 percent chance of transmitting the trait to any offspring he might one day produce. An ever growing number of new autosomal dominant mutations are associated with a *paternal age effect*, i.e. there is an increased paternal age (37 years and older) at the time of conception of the affected person(21). Non-paternity must always be kept in mind whenever the family history does not support a hereditary background for the disorders, since the rate of non-paternity is a great deal higher than the rate of spontaneous new mutations.

Autosomal recessive traits are often associated with a high degree of *con-*

sanguinity of the parents, i.e., relationship by descent from a common ancestor—cousin marriages. Although it is commonly held that there is not much variability of clinical findings in autosomal recessive and X-linked traits, such variability does occur. For instance, Hunter's syndrome is an X-linked disorder of mucopolysaccharide metabolism which is manifested by severe skeletal changes, dwarfism, claw-hands, cardiovascular effects and hepatomegaly. It is now apparent that, within the same sibship, mental retardation can be variable, ranging from profoundly retarded to borderline normal intelligence(46).

Generally, one counsels parents of a child with an autosomal recessive trait that they have a one chance in four (or 25 percent) risk of having another affected child who will be homozygous for this particular gene. It is quite obvious that there is also a 75 percent chance that the child will not be affected. By stating the probabilities one way or the other, quite different connotations are presented to the family.

A trait transmitted as an X-linked recessive is expressed by all males who carry the gene, since males have only one X chromosome. Females have two X chromosomes and when one of them carries the mutant X-linked gene she is said to be a carrier. Half of her sons will receive the X chromosome bearing the trait and will be affected. Half of the carrier's daughters will be carriers just like their mother. Half of her sons and daughters will not be affected—they do not receive the mutant gene and have no risk of transmitting the X-linked trait to their offspring. The affected male will have all carrier daughters; his sons receive the father's Y chromosome and therefore cannot transmit the trait.

One of the more recently recognized X-linked disorders is Menkes syndrome(10). This condition is characterized by mental retardation, developmental delay, sparce, slow-growing hair which breaks easily leaving only scalp stubble, twisted hair (pili torti), and death by three years of age. The disorder is due to an inborn metabolic error involving copper. Only males are affected. Since these children have a tendency to develop chip or avulsion fractures at sites of muscle attachment to the large bones, it is not uncommon that the correct diagnosis is not recognized and the child's parents are charged with child abuse(1). The psychological effects of dealing with a child suffering from Menkes syndrome are great and if they are compounded by charges of child abuse, the parent may need psychiatric help.

Among women who are carriers of X-linked disorders such as Menkes syndrome, classical hemophilia, or Duchenne muscular dystrophy, feelings of guilt, depression or anxiety are common because the mothers have been identified as carrying the mutant gene. It is very helpful to advise carrier women of X-linked conditions that were it not for their mate's Y chromosome the child would not have been born a male and thereby affected. Thus, the father has an equal involvement in the genetics of the situation. Without medical advice, many relatives of the carrier and the affected child, both male and female, often incorrectly presume they are at an increased risk to transmit such traits. For example, the brother of a boy with hemophilia may be greatly relieved to learn that he cannot transmit the disorder to his offspring.

MULTIFACTORIAL DISORDERS—POLYGENIC INHERITANCE

These conditions are not associated with discrete defects of genes or chromosomes; rather they are attributed to the interaction of two or more genes of small effect which in themselves are not deleterious—the disorders are said to be *polygenic*. Since the genes are contributed by both parents and are thought to interact with a variety of environmental agents, these disorders can be considered *multifactorial* in etiology. This mechanism is thought to be involved in the five most common congenital malformations: cleft lip and palate, congenital heart disease, congenital dislocation of the hips, club feet and spina bifida cystica/anencephaly (neural tube defects). There is ample evidence that the use of birth control pills at the time of conception and/or during early embryogenesis is associated with a higher risk of congenital heart disease(18,29) and other birth defects. Most of the environmental agents which act as teratogenic agents in man have not been identified with certainty(19). In this category of genetic disease there is an increased incidence of multifactorial conditions in relatives of those who are affected, although these polygenic conditions do not follow the rules of transmission which apply to Mendelian conditions. Some of man's most common illnesses are in this category of genetic disease: diabetes mellitus, gout, hypertension, and schizophrenia. Precise genetic analysis is difficult because of the problems in evaluating the many obvious environmental variables. In general the recurrence risk for these disorders is in the range of 4 to 15 percent.

CHROMOSOMAL DISORDERS

Chromosomal abnormalities in man were first recognized in 1959 when Lejeune described an extra chromosome associated with Down's syndrome(22). This occurred three years after the diploid number in man was accurately determined to be 46 by Tjio and Levan(42). There soon followed

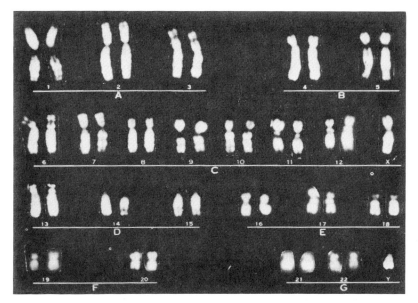

FIGURE 1. Q-banded karyotype of a normal 46,XY male chromosome pattern. Each of the 22 pairs of autosomes and the X and Y sex chromosomes has a unique pattern of bright and dull fluorescent regions allowing specific identification of each chromosome or region.

a burst of cytogenetic activity with identification of the chromosomal abnormalities associated with the classic syndromes of Turner(15), and Klinefelter(14), and identification of the extra chromosome in Patau's(32) and Edwards'(13) syndromes. Specific chromosomal aberrations associated with certain forms of cancer were also described, e.g., the association of the Philadelphia chromosome and chronic myelogenous leukemia(30).

Initially, the 46 chromosomes could be divided into seven groups, A through G, according to size and shape. This grouping of the chromosomes into a standard arrangement called a *karyotype* was established by the Chicago conference in 1966(9). Extra or missing chromosomes were described as to the group they most closely resembled, but within groups little or no distinction could be made between chromosomes. Because of the lack of definition of each pair of homologues, in the late 1960s a plateau had been reached in human cytogenetics and little new knowledge was added to this field.

The first breakthrough with new techniques was developed by Caspersson and his colleagues in 1970(8). Using the fluorescent dye, quinacrine, distinctive banding patterns were found for each of the autosomes (22 pairs) and the sex chromosomes (two X's in females and one X and one Y in males)—*Q-banding* (Figure 1). New descriptions of abnormalities, as well as many other new banding techniques, were quickly forthcoming. At a conference held in Paris in 1971(31), the nomenclature used in the descriptions of normal and abnormal karyotypes delineated with banding techniques was established.

Chromosomal abnormalities have now been reported involving virtually every segment of each of the 23 pairs of chromosomes. The segment or entire chromosome may be present in triplicate (*trisomic*, e.g., Down's syndrome —trisomy 21) or singly (*monosomic*, e.g., Turner's syndrome —monosomy X). In general, monosomy is much more severe in its effects than trisomy. Many of these abnormalities are not compatible with life, but are found only in aborted fetuses. The larger the segment or whole chromosome that is *aneuploid* (i.e., trisomic or monosomic), the more likely that it will be incompatible with life unless balanced by a second group of cells which are normal in chromosomal constitution (*mosaicism*). In extremely rare cases, a whole chromosome or segment thereof may be represented more than three times in the karyotype. This is generally described for the sex chromosomes.

Chromosomal abnormalities occur on the order of one out of every 200 live births(45). However, in certain select populations chromosomal abnormalities may be found in much higher frequency. Chromosomal abnormalities are found in about 2-3 percent of infertile men; 4-6 percent of stillbirths and early neonatal deaths; 10-15 percent of children with multiple malformations and mental retardation; 40-60 percent of spontaneous abortuses; and 80-85 percent of patients with chronic myelogenous leukemia.

Chromosomal abnormalities involve hundreds to thousands of genes and thus generally affect many organ systems. Similar features may be common to many different chromosomal aberrations; e.g., mental retardation is almost always found when any autosomal segment is trisomic or monosomic. Therefore, children with multiple congenital anomalies associated with mental retardation should be considered as prime candidates for chromosomal analysis.

Abnormalities involving the sex chromosomes are usually less severe in producing physical handicaps or mental retardation. Here again monosomy (45,X) is more severe in its effects than trisomy (47,XXX; 47,XXY; 47,XYY). Girls with Turner's syndrome (45,X) are short in stature, have webbed necks, and may have skeletal abnormalities, congenital heart defects and kidney malformations. However, triple X females (47,XXX) generally have no physical abnormalities, although some may have menstrual irregularities and relative or absolute infertility. Mental problems occurring as a result of sex chromosome monosomy or trisomy may involve specific learning disabilities (e.g., space-form blindness in Turner's syndrome) or behavior or psychiatric disorders (e.g., schizophrenia in the triple X syndrome). When chromosome numbers of 48, 49 or higher are reached (e.g., 48,XXYY or 49,XXXXX) mental retardation is virtually always a finding and skeletal abnormalities are more frequent.

The most common chromosomal abnormality found at birth (one per 600 live births) is Down's syndrome (trisomy 21)(39). The physical features are numerous and can involve many of the major organ systems. Mental retardation is a constant finding. The term mongolism was given to this syndrome because of the association of upward slanting palpebral fissures and prominent epicanthic folds. This term is no longer preferred, as the terms Down's syndrome and trisomy 21 are replacing the older terminology. Many features of the syndrome disappear or change with increasing age, so that older children may not have the same appearance as newborns, e.g., the epicanthic folds may regress and not be as prominent in late childhood. This has led to misdiagnosis or lack of recognition of the syndrome in older children who were not identified in the neonatal period.

Three different chromosomal alterations may result in Down's syndrome. Prognosis and counseling are dependent upon the type of chromosomal abnormality present and differ considerably for the various types. Thus, for accurate counseling, chromosomal studies must be initiated in all cases. Ninety-five percent of all individuals with Down's syndrome have primary trisomy 21 (47,XX or XY,+21). There are three number 21 chromosomes, rather than two, resulting in a total of 47 chromosomes. The presence of the extra number 21 is usually the result of misdivision of the 21's (nondisjunction) during formation of one of the gametes and is therefore a sporadic occurrence. This type of Down's syndrome has been related to maternal age. The older a woman, the greater her chances of nondisjunction during the formation of the egg and a resultant aneuploidy in the offspring. Age does not seem to be a factor in frequency of paternal nondisjunction. However, recent studies have shown that in one-fourth of the cases, the nondisjunctional event which results in Down's syndrome occurs on the paternal side, regardless of the ages of the parents(25). This percentage is significantly higher than originally estimated. Once primary trisomy 21 has occurred, the risk to the next offspring for a chromosomal abnormality—not necessarily trisomy 21, but any chromosomal aneuploidy—is about 4-6 percent(14). Parental studies of the origin of the nondisjunctional event may be important if the parents of a child with Down's syndrome have remarried and wish to know which parent is at increased risk for aneuploidy in future offspring(25).

About 2-½ percent of all patients with Down's syndrome have a translocation chromosomal rearrangement whereby the extra 21 is not free but has become attached to another chromosome—*translocation*. In most cases one chromosome 21 is attached to another G group chromosome or one of the D group chromosomes, although theoretically it may become attached to any of the chromosomes in the karyotype. Because the extra 21 is attached to another chromosome, children with this form of Down's syndrome have a total of 46 chromosomes but still have the equivalent of three number 21's. This is the familial form of Down's syndrome. In most instances one of the parents is found to have the same translocation chromosome, but is missing an unattached number 21 and is therefore "balanced" with no extra or missing material; the chromosomes, however, are in a rearranged state. Children with the translocation form of Down's syndrome have the same physical features as those with the primary form. Clinical examination will not distinguish between the two; only chromosomal analysis will allow this identification. Counseling is quite different for the two forms. Since one parent may also carry the translocation, there is a high risk for having other offspring with a chromosomal abnormality. For female carriers of translocations involving the 21, the recurrence risk for Down's syndrome is about 15-20 percent; for male carriers, the risk is about 1-5 percent(12). A trisomy for the other chromosome involved in the translocation is also possible and in many cases this trisomy may be incompatible with life. Thus, individuals carrying translocations are also at higher risk for spontaneous abortions.

The third form of Down's syndrome (found in 2-½ percent of affected individuals) is *mosaicism*—the presence of two or more cell lines with different chromosomal constitutions. Usually there is one cell line which is trisomic for the number 21 (47,XX or XY,+21) and one cell line with a normal constitution (46,XX or XY). The event resulting in mosaicism usually occurs after fertilization, during the early divisions of the embryo. The timing of this event may result in many cells having a normal constitution, or in many with the extra 21. Since it is a post-zygotic event, the parents should be counseled that they have no significantly increased risk for aneuploidy in future offspring. If many cells have the extra 21, the expression of the syndrome may be severe. If few cells have the extra 21, the features may be quite mild and the individual may function intellectually at a much higher level than expected. This form of Down's syndrome may be the most difficult to recognize clinically but carries a much better prognosis for the patient.

One of the newest syndromes which has been delineated through the use of the banding techniques is trisomy 8 (47,XX or XY,+8)(33). This syndrome involves mild mental retardation, skeletal malformations, eye disorders and unusual dermal patterns. Because of the large amount of chromatin material which is extra, the individuals who survive into childhood are usually mosaic, having a normal cell line to compensate for the trisomic cell line. The clinical features are variable, from mild to severe, and generally depend upon the proportion of cells with the extra number 8. In some cases, only a few tissues will have the extra 8, so that chromosomal studies may need to be done on skin as well as blood in order to identify the abnormal cell line.

Deletions (partial or complete monosomies of chromosomes) are also described for certain autosomes. These generally result in very severe disorders with multiple anomalies, severe mental retardation and, in many cases, failure to thrive. The classic conditions due to deletions are the Cri du Chat(23) and Wolf(44) syndromes. Each has a constellation of abnormalities including severe mental retardation. They are the result of small missing portions of chromosomes number 5 and 4, respectively. Some of the deletions (partial monosomies) are known to be associated with a risk of developing specific tumors, e.g., a missing portion of the number 13 is known to be associated with retinoblastoma(24). Such a deletion should alert the physician to screen these individuals regularly for such tumors.

In many partial monosomies or trisomies, a translocation is involved and is carried by one of the parents. Pedigree analysis may help in the differential diagnosis. When translocations are present in a family, there may be a history of children with multiple anomalies and mild to severe mental retardation, children who did not survive the newborn period or were stillborn, numerous spontaneous abortions with no apparent gynecological explanation, or infertility problems. Siblings of a translocation carrier may also wish to be tested since the origin of the translocation may go back several generations.

FETO-MATERNAL INTERACTIONS

Genetic differences between the fetus and mother can under certain circumstances produce abnormalities in the fetus. Most well understood is the situation of an Rh-negative pregnant mother and the Rh-positive fetus. Each genotype independently is not deleterious, but when they are present together Rh incompatibility results. Another example is that of maternal phenylketonuria. This autosomal recessive trait, if untreated, is associated with metabolic byproducts which are toxic to the developing fetus, resulting in mental retardation, behavior disorders and/or congenital heart disease(41). Although the fetus is a carrier, and as such would be normal clinically, because of the maternal milieu with derangements of phenylalanine metabolism, the fetus sustains severe impairment of brain development.

BURDEN OF GENETIC DISEASE

No one measurement can adequately reflect the total impact of genetic diseases on individuals, families and society. Morbidity estimates by the World Health Organization(43) indicate that 4 percent of live-born infants in the U.S. die each year from genetic or partly genetic disorders. Surveys show that one-third or more of admissions to a pediatric hospital are for genetic diseases. Fifty thousand or more mentally retarded individuals living in public institutions have conditions wholly or partly genetic in origin. One in every 1000 infants born is deaf; in at least 50 percent of these the deafness is caused by hereditary disease. Some 47 percent of 4,800 cases of blindness in children in a 1970 survey were attributed to genetic causes(17). How can one determine the burden of genetic disease on a personal level? The effects include grief, anxiety, despair, and unfulfilled dreams and ambitions. Life-styles and family relationships may be seriously altered or disrupted by genetic diseases.

PREVENTION AND GENETIC COUNSELING

Genetic counseling usually begins with someone wanting to know whether a disorder is heritable and if it will recur in close relatives of the patient with the condition. The need for counseling often arises retrospectively after the appearance of a genetic problem. Individuals with inherited diseases and parents of children with these conditions must face problems relating to procreation and biological fitness. Although at present we cannot favorably change actual genetic endowment, much can be done to aid individuals in living with their disease.

Typically, parents of a child with a particular genetic disorder consult the genetic counselor seeking information about the risk to any future children they might have, and the risk to their future grandchildren from either the affected or their unaffected children. Engaged couples or newlyweds may be concerned about a specific disease known to be in one of the families. Social agencies at times are concerned about the presence of a hereditary condition in a child being placed for adoption.

The birth of a child with a serious congenital deformity, mental deficiency, or serious inborn error of metabolism is a terrible shock for the parents. Frequently this shock is intensified because there was no prior indication of what was to come. It is worse still if the experience is repeated. Many difficult decisions are involved: whether to marry, whether to have another child, whether to adopt a child instead of risking another pregnancy. The demand from parents for information on genetic risks is growing as they increasingly plan, and so feel responsible for, the birth of each child and as they become more and more knowledgeable about the field of medical genetics. Parents have every right to be told what the risks are, insofar as they are currently understood, and to have these statistical figures put into proper perspective regarding the possible severity and prognosis of the condition, as well as the random risk for any couple.

To be effective, a genetic counselor must have a sound understanding of genetic principles, a broad fund of scientific knowledge, access to very specialized literature, and a good deal of tact, sympathy and common sense. The counselor must be able to effectively communicate. Certain procedural and laboratory methods are heavily relied upon: obtaining a detailed family history, cytogenetic analysis, biochemical studies of body tissues and fluids, and cell culture, including studies of amniotic fluid for prenatal diagnosis.

The initial interview requires an hour or more. This time is well invested since it nurtures a relationship between the counselor and the family. More accurate and detailed family histories and data pertinent to the disease are obtained when both parents are present. A joint interview also gives the counselor insight into domestic interactions. Information given one parent is often misinterpreted to the spouse, creating additional problems.

Assessment of genetic risk and probabiliy depends on an *accurate, quite specific diagnosis—the cornerstone of genetic counseling.* Thus, the first requirement in the counseling process is the establishment of a diagnosis or validation of one previously made. Confirmatory tests and consultations with appropriate specialists may be necessary. Attention to details on physical examination is essential, especially in recognition of syndromes and other patterns of malformation(4,16,20,39).

Once a diagnosis is determined and found to be genetic, the precise mode of inheritance must be determined. Specific risk figures can be calculated based on the family pedigree. For conditions which are multifactorial in origin, empirical risk figures can be used. Such figures are usually available from large surveys in which the frequency with which relatives of individuals with specific defects are themselves affected are determined. Empirical risk figures also exist for cytogenetic abnormalities. Theoretically, the frequency of transmission of chromosomal translocations from parent to child can be calculated. However, on clinical grounds the observed data do not agree with the a priori estimates—the observed cases are considerably less than would be theoretically expected.

It is important that those counseled know what the recurrence risk means in their situation. Risks are usually presented in terms of a probability. When presented in cold, hard figures the concept may be very difficult to comprehend. The task of making the concept clear is aided by charts, illustrations, karyotypes or diagrams. Time must be spent helping the family adjust emotionally to the information. The common feeling of guilt that parents may harbor should be ameliorated and eased with knowledge and understanding. It is useful to compare the risk figure quoted with the random risk. True random risks apply when there is an environmental etiology that is unlikely to recur in a later pregnancy—for example, maternal rubella. Near-random risks of recurrence in later sibs also apply when the patient's condition is genetically determined but is the result of a fresh chromosomal or gene mutation. Genetic counseling can allay anxiety rather than give the counselee additional worry. Patients with an autosomal recessively inherited condition such as galactosemia or Wilson's disease will have children who are clinically normal—provided they marry unrelated persons who are not carriers of the specific gene.

Once the family understands the meaning of probability, prognosis of the disorder must be explained. The usual behavior of the disorder and its natural history are explained, as well as the range of severity, complications to be expected, goals to be attained, social consequences, and availability of therapy. Although most genetic diseases are not amenable to specific treatment, a sizable and growing number are responsive to therapy(41). Most of the latter are disorders of metabolism which are inherited as autosomal recessive traits, e.g., congenital adrenogenital syndrome and glycogen storage disease.

Next in the counseling process an informed decision must be made. Much depends on the nature of the condition—the burden perceived by the affected person and the family. Counseling will depend to some extent on prognosis: Early death is quite different from long years of invalidism. Relatively minor disabilities and those that are readily treatable are again different. The counselor should not impose his view of the appropriate decision. He should assist the family in reaching a decision based on as much factual information as can be obtained. Options regarding future children should be identified and explained: sterilization, artificial insemination, adoption, and conception with amniocentesis or prenatal diagnosis.

INTRAUTERINE—PRENATAL DIAGNOSIS

Amniocentesis transabdominally during the second trimester of pregnancy had increasingly been employed in the prenatal diagnosis of a host of genetic diseases. Amniotic taps for genetic reasons are done at the 14th-16th week of pregnancy following an ultrasound examination to determine the position of the placenta and fetus. The amniotic fluid may be assayed directly for the level of alpha-fetoprotein; other biochemical assays and chromosomal analysis must use cultured amniotic cells. Three-to-five weeks in culture are required to accumulate sufficient cells for these determinations. Timing of the tap is crucial in order to act if termination of the pregnancy is elected. Amniocentesis during the midtrimester is very safe, with a risk of less than one percent(37). In rare instances, complications have included infections, spontaneous abortion, or injury to the fetus.

Open neural tube defects (meningomyeloceles and anencephaly) result in the leakage of alpha-fetoprotein (AFP) into the amniotic fluid. A high AFP value may indicate defects in the closure of the neural tube. About 90 percent of neural tube defects have open meninges and thus are detectable by this assay(6). Since the assay is reliable and inexpensive, and since the incidence of neural tube defects is sufficiently high in the general population(36), most amniocenteses performed for other indications employ this test as well.

The cultured cells may be analyzed for many defects, both biochemical and chromosomal, but only for specific indications. Every pregnancy cannot be monitored for every known genetic defect. It is important to realize that amniocentesis can never insure the birth of a "normal" baby, but can only exclude specific defects for which the family is at risk.

Prenatal diagnosis is used to detect well over 60 specific metabolic diseases and all of the chromosomal disorders(7). Sex determination is used in the case of X-linked conditions where specific biochemical markers are not known. Amniocentesis is indicated in the following cases: advanced maternal age (35-37 or older); a previous child born with a chromosomal abnormality; individuals who carry a chromosomal translocation; parents who are carriers for metabolic disorders which can be identified in cultured cells from the amniotic fluid; and a family history of neural tube defects (28).

New tools, such as fetoscopy, are being developed to visualize the fetus and to take blood and skin samples directly. Many of the hemoglobinopathies are now being identified prenatally by fetal blood samples obtained from the placenta(2). An increasing number of dwarfing conditions are being identified by fetoscopy, real-time ultrasound and the judicious use of x-rays(26).

At the present time, there is treatment for only a limited group of genetic disorders. One of the few treatments available is the use of vitamin B^{12} therapy for the fetus affected with methylmalonic aciduria(3). When an affected fetus is detected, often the only alternative one can offer the parents is termination of the pregnancy.

Amniocentesis has been of outstanding benefit to parents at high risk of having a child with a chromosomal or metabolic disorder. Before the test was available, many parents would not have considered having offspring because of the high recurrence risk. Amniocentesis, followed by medically induced abortion, allows these parents the option of selecting children unaffected for specific genetic disorders.

SCREENING SELECTED GROUPS

Screening for genetic disease may be retrospective or prospective. Once an affected individual (e.g., a patient with galactosemia) has been identified, a certain population, the immediate family and many of the close relatives, may then retrospectively be determined to be at risk for this disorder. Depending on the genetic basis, determination of carrier status may be desirable.

Prospective screening may involve a newborn population (e.g., PKU screening), a defined group with a population (e.g., Tay-Sachs screening in Ashkenazic Jews), or prenatal screening (e.g., alpha-fetoprotein levels in the British Isles). Several criteria must be met for a successful screening program: 1) There must be a high incidence of the disorder in a defined population; 2) a simple, accurate, inexpensive test must be available; 3) treatment or intervention must be available; and 4) there must be no overlap in differentiating between the affected individual and those that are carriers.

Selected screening tests are increasingly required by law in the newborn population because of the availability of treatment for many of the metabolic genetic diseases. Many governments have instituted mandatory screening for PKU (i.e., the Gutherie test), galactosemia, hypothyroidism and other inborn errors of metabolism. When such an error is suspected in an older child, a battery of simple, rapid, inexpensive, and nonspecific screening tests can be performed on blood or urine which, if positive, is followed by specific tests to identify the exact defect.

Certain ethnic groups in the population are known to have a high incidence of different disorders. One in 10 Blacks carries the gene for sickle cell disease, one in 20 Caucasians carries the gene for cystic fibrosis and one in 30 Ashkenazic Jews carries the gene for Tay-Sachs disease. Carriers for sickle cell and Tay-Sachs disease can be identified. However, a reliable test for carriers of cystic fibrosis has not yet been developed. Among the British population, neural tube defects occur in one-tenth of all pregnancies. Prenatal screening is provided through determination of alpha-fetoprotein levels in maternal serum and in amniotic fluid.

As screening tests become more common and are made mandatory, certain legal and moral issues arise concerning: privacy; the right not-to-know; insurance coverage of affected individuals or carriers; who shall reproduce; and the stigma which may be associated with carrier status. The rights of individuals have been strongly debated not only as to whether to give birth to an affected fetus, but how aggressive to be in treatment once the affected child is born. There is considerable controversy over offering or requiring prenatal diagnosis for chromosomal abnormalities for all women over 35. As prenatal screening becomes more accepted, those individuals who give birth to children with certain abnormalities may be increasingly ostracized when the parents do not choose to have the test performed or to abort the affected fetus. As screening programs develop and technology expands the knowledge about genetic makeup, there will be a need to identify the impact of this screening not only on the affected individual and his family but also on society and the species. Guidelines must be established before technology gives us power and knowledge without wisdom and understanding.

CONCLUSION

Wholly or partly genetically determined conditions are increasingly prominent as public-health problems, in part because of the success of environmental-health services in reducing the incidence of environmentally determined disease. The diagnostic armamentarium of clinical genetics has increased greatly in recent years through newly developed chromosomal and biochemical methods, and through better clinical delineation of genetic and congenital disorders. An accurate diagnosis is of the utmost importance to sound genetic counseling. New techniques for the detection of heterozygous carriers for genes responsible for autosomal recessive and X-linked recessive diseases offer new hope for preventing such diseases through counseling. Detection of chromosomal aberrations and selected inborn errors of metabolism early in pregnancy in cells obtained by amniocentesis offers the prospect of reducing the frequency of such anomalies at birth. Today it is possible to treat genetic diseases of metabolism by dietary restrictions and modification or administration of required substances. In other instances, transplantation of vital organs has shown great promise. Genetic counseling has emerged as a new discipline with a variety of means to detect, diagnose, prevent, and treat hitherto enigmatic genetic disease.

REFERENCES

1. ADAMS, P.C., STRAND, R.D., BRESNAN, M.J., and LUCKY, A.W. 1974. Kinky Hair Syndrome. Serial study of radiological findings with emphasis on the similarity to the Battered Child Syndrome. *Radiology*, 112, 401.

2. ALTER, B.P., MODELL, C.B., FAIRWEATHER, D., HOBBINS, J.C., MAHONEY, M.J., FRIGOLETTO, F.D., SHERMAN, A.S., and NATHAN, D.G. 1976. Prenatal diagnosis of hemoglobinopathies. *New Eng. J. Med.*, 295, 1437.

3. AMPOLA, M.G., MAHONEY, M.J., NAKAMURA, E. and TANAKA, K. 1975. Prenatal therapy of a patient with vitamin B12 responsive methylmalonic acidemia. *New Eng. J. Med.*, 293, 313.

4. BERGSMA, D.B. 1973. *Birth Defects Atlas and Compendium.* Baltimore: Williams and Wilkins Co.

5. BORGAONKAR, D.S.1977. *Chromosomal Variation in Man: A Catalog of Chromosomal Variants and Anomalies.* 2nd Edition. New York: Alan R. Liss, Inc.

6. BROCK, D.J.H. and GOSDEN, C. 1977. Are second-trimester amniotic fluids being properly examined? *Lancet*, 1, 1168.

7. BURTON, B.K., GERBIE, A.B., and NADLER, H.L. 1974. Present status of intrauterine diagnosis of genetic defects. *Am. J. Ob. Gyn.*, 118, 718.

8. CASPERSSON, T., ZECH, L., JOHANSSON, C. and MODEST, E.J. 1970. Identification of human chromosomes by DNA-binding fluorescing agents. *Chromosoma*, 30, 215.

9. *Chicago Conference 1966: Standardization in Human Cytogenetics.* 1966. Birth Defects: Original Article Series, II, 2. New York: The National Foundation.

10. DANKS, D.M. CAMPBELL, M.B., STEVENS, B.J., MAYNE, V. and CARTWRIGHT, E. 1972. Menkes Hair Syndrome. An inherited defect in copper absorption with widespread defects. *Pediatrics*, 50, 188.

11. DEGROUCHY, J. and TURLEAU, C. 1977. *Clinical Atlas of Human Chromosomes.* New York: Wiley.

12. DUTRILLAUX, B. and LEJEUNE, J. 1969. Etude de la descendance des porteurs d'une translocation t(21qDq). *Ann. Genet.*, 12, 77.

13. EDWARDS, J.H., HARNDEN, D.G., CAMERON, A.H., CROSSE, V.M., and WOLFF, O.H. 1960. A new trisomic syndrome. *Lancet*, 1, 787.

14. FORD, C.E., JONES, K.W., MILLER, O.J., MITTWOCH, U., PENROSE, L.S., RIDLER, M.A.C., and SHAPIRO, A. 1959. The chromosomes in a patient showing both mongolism and the Klinefelter syndrome. *Lancet*, 1, 709.

15. FORD, C.E., JONES, K.W., POLANI, P.E., DEALMEIDA, J.C., and BRIGGS, J.H. 1959. A sex-chromosome anomaly in a case of gonadal dysgenesis (Turner's syndrome). *Lancet*, 1, 711.

16. GORLIN, R.G., PINDBORG, J.J., and COHEN, M.M., JR. 1976. *Syndromes of the Head and Neck.* Second Edition. New York: McGraw-Hill Book Co.

17. HATFIELD, E.M. 1972. Blindness in Infants and Children. *Sight Saving Review*, 42, 69.

18. HEINONEN, O.P., SLONE, D., MONSON, R.R., HOOK, E.B. and SHAPIRO, S. 1977. Cardiovascular birth defects and antenatal exposure to female sex hormones. *New Eng. J. Med.*, 296, 67.

19. HEINONEN, O.P. SLOAN, D., and SHAPIRO, S. 1977. *Birth Defects and Drugs in Pregnancy.* Littleton, Mass: Publishing Sciences Group, Inc.

20. HOLMES, L.B., MOSER, H.W., HALLDORSSON, C.S., MACK, C., PANT, S.S. and MATZILEV-
ICH, B. 1972. *Mental Retardation: An Atlas Of Diseases With Associated Physical
Abnormalities.* New York: Macmillan.

21. JONES, K.L., SMITH, D.W., HARVEY, M.A., HALL, B.D., and QUAN, L. 1975. Older paternal
age and fresh gene mutation. *J. Pediat.*, 86, 84.

22. LEJEUNE, J. 1959. Le mongolisme. Premier exemple d'aberration autosomique humaine.
Ann. Genet., 1, 41.

23. LEJEUNE, J., LAFOURCADE, J., BERGER, R., VIALATTE, J., BOESWILLWALD, M., SERINGE, P.,
and TURPIN, R. 1963. Trois cas de deletion partielle du bras court d'un chromosome
5. *C. R. Hebd. Seances Acad. Sci.*, 257, 3098.

24. LELE, K.P., PENROSE, L.S., and STALLARD, H.B. 1963. Chromosome deletion in a case of
retinoblastoma. *Ann. Hum. Genet.*, 27, 171.

25. MAGENIS, R.E., OVERTON, K.M., CHAMBERLIN, J., BRADY, T., and LOVRIEN, E. 1977.
Parental origin of the extra chromosome in Down's syndrome. *Hum. Genet.*, 37, 7.

26. MAHONEY, M.J., and HOBBINS, J.C. 1977. Prenatal diagnosis of chondroectodermal dys-
plasia (Ellis-van Creveld syndrome) with fetoscopy and ultrasound. *New Eng. J. Med.*,
297, 258.

27. MCKUSICK, V.A. 1978. *Mendelian Inheritance In Man. Catalogs Of Autosomal Dominant,
Autosomal Recessive, And X-linked Phenotypes.* Fifth Edition. Baltimore: The John
Hopkins Press.

28. MILUNSKY, A. 1973. *The Prenatal Diagnosis of Hereditary Disorders.* Springfield, Ill:
Charles C Thomas.

29. NORA, J.J. 1971. Etiologic factors in congenital heart disease. *Pediatric Clin. North Am.*,
18, 1059.

30. NOWELL, P.C., and HUNGERFORD, D.A. 1960. Chromosome studies on normal and leukemic
human leukocytes. *J. Natl. Cancer Inst.*, 25, 85.

31. *Paris Conference 1971: Standardization in Human Cytogenetics.* 1972. Birth Defects:
Original Article Series, VIII, 7. New York: The National Foundation.

32. PATAU, K.A., SMITH, D.W., THERMAN, E.M., INBORN, S.L., and WAGNER, H.P. 1960.
Multiple congenital anomalies caused by an extra autosome. *Lancet*, 1, 790.

33. PFEIFFER, R.A. 1977. Trisomy 8. In: J.J. Yunis (Ed.), *New Chromosomal Syndromes.*
New York: Academic Press.

34. SCOTT, C.I., JR. 1972. The Genetics of Short Stature. *Progress in Medical Genetics*, VII,
243.

35. SCOTT, C.I., JR. and THOMAS, G.H. 1973. Genetic Disorders Associated with Mental Retardation. Clinical Aspects. *Ped. Clinics Nor. Am.*, 20, 121.

36. SHULMAN, K. 1974. Anencephaly. In: D. Bergsma (Ed.), *Birth Defects: Atlas and Compendium.* Baltimore: Williams & Williams Co.

37. SIMPSON, N.E., DALLAIRE, L., MILLER, J.R., SIMINOVICH, L., HAMERTON, J.L., MILLER,
J., MCKEEN, C. 1976. Prenatal diagnosis of genetic disease in Canada: Report of a
collaborative study. *Canad. Med. Assoc. J.*, 115, 739.

38. SLATER, E. and COWIE, V. 1971. *The Genetics of Mental Disorders.* New York: Oxford
University Press.

39. SMITH, D.W. 1976. *Recognizable Patterns of Human Malformation.* Second Edition. Philadelphia: W.B. Saunders.

40. SPRANGER, J.W., LANGER, L.O., JR., and WIEDEMANN, H.R. 1974. *Bone Dysplasias. An
Atlas Of Constitutional Disorders Of Skeletal Development.* Philadelphia: W.B. Saunders.

41. STANBURY, J.B., WYNGAARDEN, L.B., and FREDERICKSON, (Eds.). 1978. *The Metabolic
Basis of Inherited Disease.* Fourth Edition. New York: Blakiston Division, McGraw-
Hill.

42. TJIO, J.H., and LEVAN, A. 1956. The chromosome number of man. *Hereditas*, 42, 1.

43. WHO 1969. Genetic counseling, third report of the expert committee on human genetics.
Technical Report Series, 416.

44. WOLF, U. and REINWEIN, H. 1967. Klinische und Cytogenetische Differentialdiagnose de Defizienzen au den Kurzen Armer der B-Chromosomen. *Z. Kinderheilkd*, 98, 235.
45. WRIGHT, S.W., CRANDALL, B.F., and BOYER, L. 1972. *Perspective in Cytogenetics*. Springfield: Charles C Thomas.
46. YATZIN, S., ERICKSON, R.P. and EPSTEIN, C.L. 1977. Mild and severe Hunter Syndrome (MPS II) within the same sibship. *Clinical Genetics*, 11,319.
47. YUNIS, J.J. 1977. *New Chromosomal Syndromes*. New York: Academic Press.

26

GROUP DAYCARE AND
MENTAL HEALTH

J. F. Saucier, M.D., Ph.D.

Associate Professor,
Department of Psychiatry,
University of Montreal, Canada
and
Raquel Betsalel-Presser, Ph.D.,

Associate Professor,
Faculty of Education,
University of Montreal, Canada

During the last three decades, important economic, social and cultural changes in most industrialized countries have contributed to the emergence of a new "institution," the day-care center for groups of children under the age of six.

This paper will be concerned only with *regular* group day-care for children under the age of three; that is, centers which receive infants and toddlers from 9 a.m. to 4 or 5 p.m., five days a week, for a duration of nine or ten months a year.

INTRODUCTION

At least in most Western countries, four major factors seem to be mainly responsible for this innovation in child-rearing practices. First, we have the ever-increasing proportion of women of child-bearing age participating in the labor force, many of these women going back to work at an earlier time following delivery of the infant. Second, we have the steady decline of the social support system of the nuclear family, a decline that is so advanced in some urban regions that this support system cannot provide help, even in emergencies, let alone ensure the regular supervision of an infant when his mother is busy at work. Third, we have the movement of women's liberation that has been favoring the day-care of children as a way to free the mothers from exclusive preoccupation with their children. And fourth, we have an educationally oriented movement which is promoting the day-care institution with the rationale that the inclusion of an infant in a group setting might improve his psychological development and his social adaptation.*

Whatever the justification for a day-care center might be, the day-care movement has met with some resistance. Whether it is supported by private or public funds, this institution is costly, and most governments are slow to finance it. Besides, even in families that can afford day-care, a large number of mothers, employed or not, are reluctant to entrust their infants to other adults for long periods of time at such an early age. The traditional concept of the mother's role as the main and only educator of her young children makes the acceptance of a group care experience still rather difficult. Fein and Clarke-Stewart(17) report a study of Low and Spindler(32) where they note:

> A surprisingly large percentage of children under six years of age are cared for by relatives, including their own mothers. Family ties are preserved for 53 percent of the children of full-time working mothers, and this proportion increases to 80 percent for the children of part-time working mothers (p. 39).

Furthermore, these statistics find stronger support when one reviews the values in our Western societies, where legislation for adequate developmental and educational centers for young children is rather poor, as compared to the provisions for instructional and special programs geared to compensate whatever loss in development could have been prevented at an earlier age.

Researchers are also cautious in promoting day-care centers as a universal "solution," on the ground that this experience could disrupt the mother-infant relationship, and so hinder the basic development of attachment in the child. In a very recent publication, Williams(47) compared the main basic and applied research on child development and supplemental care,

---

*See chapter 9 in Vol. 3 of this series, *Modern Perspectives in International Child Psychiatry.*

raising some of the unanswered questions on this matter. The following pages will deal with some of these studies.

This paper will cover the following: 1) a review of the main shortcomings of research done on the relationship between regular group day-care and the psychological development of the child; 2) an outline of some relevant research findings; 3) an outline of what remains to be done in this field of research, with some light on a few promising hypotheses; 4) discussion of the practical management of separation; and 5) discussion of some problems of public policy, focusing on the relevance of new approaches in the day-care field.

SHORTCOMINGS OF RESEARCH

Because of financial and structural limitations, research on group day-care has been replete with shortcomings. Among the most important are the following:

1) Most of the solid data now available on day-care come from demonstration "model" centers operated on university campuses (Children's Center, Syracuse, N.Y.; Demonstration Center, Greenboro, N.C.; Frank Porter Graham Child Development Center, Chapel Hill, N.C.; Yale Study Center, New Haven, Ct., etc.). These experimental centers can afford a high ratio of adults per infants, that is, a minimum of one adult for four or five children. In spite of the great need for further research, we are, at this point, particularly concerned with the application of these data to ordinary day-care programs, since they are operating under totally different ideological and practical conditions.

2) A most frequent weakness encountered in the research design is the absence of the pre-test measurement of the developmental level of the children not exposed to day-care (the "control group"). Most often, children exposed to day-care are measured on different scales after a period of time, and then children not exposed to day-care are matched for sex, age and social class. It is then impossible to know whether the children of day-care were similar or not to the others when they started being exposed to that institution, and this impossibility precludes any valid post-test. For instance, Lézine(30) reported that some of the children who manifested greater difficulties on adapting to the center were already exposed to stress in their family context.

3) In order to compare the intensity of attachment of the infants to their mothers among subjects exposed and not exposed to day-care, many authors use Mary Ainsworth's(5) "strange situation" as a way of measuring this

primary aspect of psychological development. The problem is that this measure was never normalized, i.e., we still do not know which behaviors are normal and which ones are pathological. As a result, some studies easily conclude that this certain group of children cries more when the mother leaves the room, without being able to assess whether such a reaction, at that particular age, is an "expected" one or a "non-expected" one. Furthermore, often this instrument is still used with children up to the age of three, while the data available recognize its decreasing validity after the age of 21 months(18).

4) The number of longitudinal studies on the behavior of day-care and home-reared children is still limited(12,20,25,37,41).

These are some of the numerous shortcomings encountered in the available data. One should be wary of making sweeping generalizations, and the interpretation of the findings ought to be treated with considerable caution. Caldwell(12) and Williams(47) present detailed analyses on this topic.

OUTLINE OF SOME RELEVANT RESEARCH FINDINGS

The quality and quantity of data are sufficiently good only concerning the particular group of day-care centers that have the high ratio of one adult for four or five children. Recent studies give solid, although still preliminary, evidence of the impact of this type of group day-care on the psychological development of the child.

Age of Entry in Day-care

From another research perspective, we have been concerned with the problem of the minimal age for admission to the day-care program. This question has a direct bearing on the considerable work on attachment and on the effects of the day-care experience, but it has not received sufficient attention. At issue here is whether the infant should be admitted to the center before his primary attachment has been achieved (i.e., during the first six months), or whether the child should only be exposed to multiple mothering after his primary attachment has been clearly established.

The literature is particularly scarce on this matter, and the implications must be carefully considered from sociological as well as psychological perspectives.

At this point, we will empirically state that *if* the child is to attend a day-care center, he (or she) should be admitted during the first six months of life. This statement is based on two assumptions: 1) that the mother is unable (for economical, cultural, emotional or physical reasons) to offer a stimulating and nurturing contact at home during the day, and thus has no choice but to send her child to a center; 2) that the chosen day-care center can be relied upon to provide a stable, loving adult who will carefully adapt the program to the child's needs and interests. However, our preferred choice remains the home environment where the child is in close interaction with one adult.

The next few pages will attempt to explain our position, and will conclude with some recommendations.

Sociological Considerations

In a previous study, Betsalel-Presser(6) examined the infant programs in the U.S., France, the Soviet Union and the Israeli kibbutz, and found considerable variability in the criteria for establishing the minimal age of admission. These criteria vary either along the stages of biological growth, motor development and emotional maturity of the child, or along the norms of a country's social policy.

In some countries, such as France, Chile, the Soviet Union, and some states in the U.S., the minimal age for admission to the day-care center coincides with the end of maternity leave. The infant can be sent to day-care somewhere between the first six weeks and the third month, depending on the specific local legislations. The present social reality shows that if the child is not admitted following the end of the maternity leave, the family must find a temporary solution, until the infant reaches the minimal age for admission to the program. This "solution" usually implies that the mother will stay home without earning an income, or that a babysitter will be hired, with no guarantee that he or she will ensure a stable and stimulating contact during the months prior to admission to the center. Whatever the choice, we believe that it is preferable for the infant to experience a stable and unchanging setting than to be exposed to different people and arrangements during the first months of life. Once attachment becomes manifest, it is not advisable to subject the child to an abrupt shift in his emotional ties to people and places. This issue is further elaborated on in our next section on psychological implications.

A second important aspect to underline here is the implicit age criteria adopted in the U.S. and Canada, as shown in the study of Stevenson and Fitzgerald(45). Indeed, this survey on standards for day-care indicates that only 27 states and five provinces issue licenses to day-care centers for infants. It is quite evident that the rest of the states and provinces fix their minimal age somewhere after the age of two. As this same study also demonstrated, the definition of "infant" varied across 33 states and provinces.

Finally, we would like to express our skepticism on the coherence and practicality of most license policies and governmental measures in providing the necessary help or incentive for the creation of adequate facilities. For instance, Quebec is among the five provinces who license centers for infants aged three weeks, but the proportion of centers who really admit these babies is very low, with virtually no technical assistance to ensure an adequate program.

Therefore, we must strongly impress upon governments that the quality of experience during the first years is the key to a healthy development. Day-care centers admitting babies and mothers who choose to stay at home with their youngsters ought to be able to do so on a stimulating, stable and continuous basis, since these conditions are essential to adequate attachment and proper development.

Psychological Considerations

The above sociological considerations reflect the existence of two psychological schools of thought. The first one places the admittance age between three weeks and six months (6,7,12,13,15,26,30,37,39,41). The second one suggests that admittance take place after the age of three (9,11). This latter principle is implicitly supported by the limited number of states and provinces who have legislated on this matter. Williams' (47) comparative review of basic and applied research in infant development discusses this issue in depth.

Both these views find their roots in the psychoanalytical studies of the mother-child relationship, and in the developmental psychology work on the cognitive and emotional evolution during the first six months of life. Some essential factors, such as the effects of early institutionalization, the mother-child attachment, sensorimotor stimulation, and multiple mothering, must be considered individually in an attempt to delineate the complexity of the problem.

The effects of early institutionalization

The long-standing fears of negative effects of early separation on the child's intellectual, motor, and emotional development have been recently proven wrong by sufficient data where day-care children exposed to a warm, loving, stable and consistent staff, on a high child-adult ratio, showed no difference in their cognitive or social development from the totally home-reared children (12,20,25).

The Mother-child attachment

Although the literature on mother-child attachment is now considerable, very little consideration is given to the specific issue of the effects of mother-child separation before or after the attachment is achieved. The data gathered are sometimes contradictory. Roughly speaking, three main tendencies can be observed. The first tendency favors separation before the critical age of six months; the second disapproves of separation before six months of age; and the third seems to give more importance to the environmental conditions than to the age itself. However, all three schools of thought support the principle that an early separation must be avoided unless major reasons impose it.

The researchers likely to be identified with the first trend (6,10,14,40,41,44,48,51) assume that a mother-child separation before the age of six months would be less harmful for the emotional stability of the child than a separation produced after the establishment of attachment. This argument rests on the fact that during the first three months, the child does not seem to differentiate the care given by his mother from that of other people. Hence, the care can be split without necessarily affecting the mother-child relationship.

The researchers associated with the second tendency (1-5,9,12,13,29,33,37) believe that the child who has had enough time to "attach" to his mother, receiving all the necessary care and stimulation almost exclusively from her, would be in a better position to develop emotional ties to other people than the child whose relationship has been divided at an earlier stage.

As for the researchers of the third group (20,43,48-52), their main preoccupation is with the importance of the perceptual motor stimulation during the first months of life. Thus, the origins and stages of attachment are of relatively secondary interest to them when compared to the environmental changes that the child must confront when he is separated from home.

Clearly, much research remains to be done before answers can be provided to such complex questions. In the meantime, we maintain our support of the option of placing the child in group care as soon as the maternity leave is over, whenever home-rearing is not available.

Multiple mothering

In a review of the literature concerning infant-rearing practices in the kibbutz, Betsalel-Presser (6) reports that the mother and the "metapelet" share responsibility for the baby's care and that the quality of the affective bonds created among the adults is projected upon the infant. In most cases, the child does not seem to be affected by this double mothering, even if his mother has been the main provider of care during the first six months.

The same phenomenon is observed on the Russian "yasli-sad," where infants are cared for by different people from the first month of life. This multiple care does not appear to interfere with the intensity of the mother-child relationship (15).

While the Israeli and Soviet experiences can hardly be used as models in our occidental society, which is politically, culturally and demographically different, we must consider the accumulated data (12,13,19,20,25,37,42) as convincing evidence that, if the mother substitute is loving and stimulating, the child's emotional stability is not affected by double or even multiple mothering. These studies have not found any significant differences between infants reared at home or at day-care centers.

On closing this section on minimal age of admission, some *practical considerations* are pertinent:

> 1) The accessibility of day-care centers should be extended to very young infants because of the urgent social reality. However, the ideal situation remains legislation offering mothers the option of a substantial family allowance for staying at home, at least during the first two years of life of their children, or the possibility of going back to their previous activities, secure in the knowledge that their child is in an adequate day-care center.
>
> 2) Whatever the choice, there is a great need for educating the public on the positive as well as the negative effects of a day-care experience, under the conditions which prevail today.
>
> 3) Parents should be made aware, before registration, of the possible reactions of their child to this new experience.

Peer Relationships

Exposure to day-care does not seem to give a *permanent* advantage in the specific field of peer relationships. As in some previous studies, Kagan, Kearsley and Zelazo (25) found that day-care children, at the age of 20 months, were significantly less apprehensive with an unfamiliar peer. However, when the same two groups of children were retested nine months later, this advantage of the day-care children had vanished, because spontaneous maturation had permitted the home-care children to catch up.

This finding is also important because it does away with the often heard claim that day-care experience gives definite superiority in social relationships. Moreover, this finding warns us against research studies that claim permanent differences based on measures taken at a single period of life.

Social Class

As far as social class is concerned, when a high adult-child ratio is kept stable, there is no significant difference in the impact of day-care between middle-class and working-class white children.

In summary, in group day-care with a high ratio of caretakers, children are not likely to be harmed by exposure to this institution, nor are they likely to have their social development significantly enhanced by it. One can thus see how influential the home environment is on early development of the child.

AREAS FOR SUBSEQUENT RESEARCH

Since we only have solid evidence for the small and non-representative group of day-care centers with a high ratio of caretakers, much ground remains to be covered by future research. Here are a few directions for exploration that could be fruitful:

1) It is important to find out, for each age group of children, what is the threshold in adult to child ratio where exposure to day-care can become harmful. Is it one adult for ten children among the infants of less than one year of age? Is it one adult for 15 children for toddlers between one and two years of age?

2) Very few studies have been done regarding the importance of staff selection, their psychological, educational and social characteristics, the variety of competencies among the staff, and the specific roles.

3) What are the main variables which help a young child to adapt easily to day-care environment? Some hypotheses can be advanced, but they need to be verified. Which child would adapt more easily:

(a) a child who has had the opportunity to develop more than one attachment;
(b) a child who has had the opportunity to develop an attachment to another child (sibling, friend);
(c) a child who has a high imaginative capacity (hypothesis suggested by Mireille Steinberg, M.A. in psychology)?

4) Also relevant is the development of better ways to improve continuity of care between parents and day-care personnel, either by requiring parental presence at certain periods, especially during the first week or two of exposure, or by a system of intensive feedback between parents and personnel, to monitor at home and in the center the adaptation of the child to the new situation, etc.

5) Equally important is a systematic exploration in group formation. The usual routine of a day-care center includes a summer break, after which some of the children come back to the center, to which is added a group of newcomers. One often notices problems of adaptation in these circumstances.

A preliminary study done by McGrew (34) has revealed that one efficient method of group formation is, when the day-care center reopens, to first have only the children of the previous year for a few days, in order to let them readapt to each other. Then the newcomers are introduced *one by one* during a period of five days for each, thus allowing the group to fully incorporate this newcomer; the process is then repeated every five days until all newcomers are assimilated into the group. This is a slower method than the instantaneous one, but the quality of adaptation of each new child, as well as of each "oldtimer," seems to be much higher.

MANAGEMENT OF SEPARATION

The routine in any day-care center implies the daily separation of the young child from his parents. Contrary to the expectations of many parents, problems emerging from the daily separation are not settled quickly and completely after one or two weeks of regular attendance at the center, even with the presence of the mother for the first few days.

Importance of Parents' Awareness of Separation Anxiety

Parents are not usually aware of what daily separation means to the young child. Even in the best conditions, with a high ratio of staff and individualized care, separation remains a potential problem. The adaptation of the young child does not follow a simple and ascending linear curve; rather, separation anxiety is a very complex and fluctuating phenomenon, with periods of easy adaptation followed abruptly by periods of crisis. As the psychology of the child becomes more complex with increasing age, daily separations take on new meanings. For example, most authors believe that during the first year of life, separation means fear of loss and abandonment, a fear that can be alleviated by the care of a warm person. But during the second year, and sometimes during the third year, many separation situations may be interpreted by the toddler as punishment given by the parents for misbehaving the previous day. This gradual inclusion of internalized aggression and guilt feelings makes separation anxiety more complex and much more difficult to manage, both at the center and at home.

The day-care staff need the training and the time to make parents aware of the complexity and subtlety of separation anxiety. In order to enable parents to fully understand the situation, they should be informally taught the basics of the concepts of attachment and separation, concepts which are essential to the understanding of the young child. The staff should also be aware that the resistance parents will demonstrate in the acceptance of these notions is not only due to idiosyncratic or neurotic tendencies, but also to strong cultural factors.

Our Western culture has indeed been preoccupied, if not obsessed for centuries, by the requirement of early autonomy in the young child. Normal and usual attachment behavior during the first three years of life seems to upset many parents who become afraid that their children will remain "dependent" on them for the rest of their lives—hence their preoccupation with suppressing any "spoiling" gesture in the interaction with their children. Some parents even go further than not spoiling; they take steps, sometimes before the end of the first year, to "train" their children in autonomy. Sending children to the day-care center is often part of this "autonomy training."

Day-care personnel have to be very patient when they meet strong parental resistance to separation anxiety. It seems that the best way to handle it is for one member of the staff to establish a personal relationship with the parents and gradually, when the occasion arises, to point out, explain and suggest ways of alleviating the emotional reaction of the child to separation. With time, tact, and repeated exposure to such situations, parents will become aware of the basic attachment needs of their child, and they will be more likely to adequately cope with them.

The discussion above points to the need to better educate day-care personnel in the affective development of the young child, with particular emphasis on the dimensions of attachment and separation. Unfortunately, in many training centers, most of the teaching on the development of the child is limited to *cognitive* stages of development, as if the affective aspect did not matter much. The curriculum of these schools urgently needs to be revised in order to achieve a better balance between all facets of a healthy development.

Time Spent in the Day-care Center

It appears that the stress of separation increases with the amount of time spent every day at the center; young children who attend four hours a day seem to manage better than the ones who are there for the whole day. Indeed, Provence and associates (37), after thorough observation, are convinced that the children who regularly attend a day-care center for half-days are the ones who profit most from it. For those who spend the whole day at the center, special measures should be taken in the afternoon to alleviate their increasing stress.

Fundamental Principle in the Management of Separation

The basic idea is to *integrate* the family and day-care environments as much as possible, in order to maximize the *sharing of information* about the child, and in order for the child to feel *continuity* between the two environments. Provence and associates (37), who made the most systematic efforts in this area, talk about the *creation of bridges* between family and day-care. Not only should day-care personnel inform the parents of problems encountered by the child during the day, but reciprocally, parents should inform the staff of problems experienced by the child at home. It sometimes happens that a child succeeds in bravely adapting to the day-care experience, but this may be accomplished at the cost of some disturbance in eating, sleeping or other activities at home. Thus, it is imperative that both parents and staff share a global picture of the child's behavior.

Recommendations

The following is not an exhaustive list of measures to be taken, nor is it intended to be followed rigidly. We present these suggestions as examples of ways to alleviate the child's separation anxiety. Let us remember that each child is unique, and that one measure might function very well for one child, but not at all for another.

We subscribe to the following:

> —that parents *and child* visit the day-care center at least once before entry, in order to get acquainted with the personnel, the curriculum and the physical surroundings;
> —that parents be assigned to a specific stable member of the staff who will be more often in charge of the child, and who will thus gather all information from both parents and staff about that particular child. The assignment of only one person greatly eases communication and enhances the likelihood of establishing a significant relationship with the parents;
> —that the child be witness to the interactions between his parents and his assigned member of the staff, since children become more easily attached to persons who have a positive relationship to at least one of their parents;
> —that, during the one or two weeks following the entry of the child, parents see to it that one of them spends most of the day with the child

at the center. If this is not possible, another member of the family (grandmother, aunt, older sibling) can replace them. If that is also not possible, one parent spends half an hour at the beginning of the day. In the case of the child who must spend the whole day at the center, the parent should go back for one hour at lunch time. All this is done *even if* the child does not show manifest signs of distress;

—that parents who bring the child to the center arrange to spend some time for relaxed interaction with the staff, rather than rushing in and out. The daily separation is best handled when parents take time to get the child settled comfortably at the center. It is at this time that the assigned member of the staff can be informed of particular events that occurred at home the previous evening or night;

—that parents bring with the child objects that connect home to the center, either toys that he likes, or something like a blanket on which he depends;

—that parents also bring to the center objects that belong to each of them, which will be a symbolic replacement of them during their absence. Photos of parents are especially appropriate. These photos could be deposited in the child's locker, and should be accessible to him whenever he feels like looking at them to reassure himself;

—that children be permitted by staff to express their feeings of loss and separation after the departure of the parents, or when they feel lonesome;

—that for children who stay the whole day at the center, special means be used to alleviate the long separation. For example, parents should be encouraged to come for a short mid-day visit. If this is not possible, the telephone can be used: According to Provence, this is most meaningful for children over two and a half, but children as young as 18 months can also profit from hearing their parents' voice. Not only could parents phone the child, but, in special situations, staff should help the child to phone his parents;

—that staff encourage the child to take part in make-believe activities in which separation from loved ones is a direct or indirect item of the play. This gives the child the opportunity to gradually *master* his separation anxiety and feel more at ease when being away from home.

These are just a few examples of ways to better integrate home life to the day-care experience. Parents and staff will no doubt be able to find other ingenious ways to achieve this highly desirable goal, in a manner adapted to each particular child.

SOME POLICY ISSUES

Most governments have been reluctant, at the beginning, to support day-care centers, either by helping private organizations or by creating a public system of day-care. But the pressure on Western governments is now so strong that they have been obliged to increase steadily the funding of these institutions.

Three main issues seem to be the most salient in the field of public policy. They are

(a) the quality of the staff;
(b) the optimal number of children in a group experience;
(c) the administrative framework of public day-care centers.

The Quality of the Staff

It is usually rather difficult to talk of quality of staff without considering simultaneously the number and the variety of adults in a day-care center. But let us particularly focus on the need for improving the adult understanding of the children's world, their needs, and the best way to enhance their interactions.

There is an urgent need to create and promote regular training sessions, workshops and field experiences for people working in day-care centers, and these should be available at different specialized or semi-specialized levels. Both universities and colleges have an important role to play as coordinators of the day-care staff, as well as being responsible for pertinent research studies in the field. Very few studies deal directly with the effects of the staff training and their attitudes and actions on children (36). Since this crucial variable can only be assured by long-term studies, most governments have ignored the data and neglected the following facts:

1) Whatever kind or type of continued experience the child has (routine or play), it has an effect on his personality and, thus, carries an educational component that must always be carefully respected.

2) the *younger* the child, the more competent the adult must be, since communication with infants is more subtle and requires a greater understanding of their needs, desires and thoughts. At the present time, the usual practice is the reverse, directing the better trained staff to the older groups.

3) Day-care staff are underpaid, and the working conditions are far from being equivalent to those of the school board personnel. This becomes a complex, vicious circle, since well trained personnel seldom accept such a low salary, and without competent staff, the quality of the program is necessarily affected. Low paid personnel have low working motivations and are low on stimulating the children. A poor program discourages the parents from entrusting their youngsters to the center, and this institution can hardly find its needed place in society.

The Optimal Number of Children in a Group Experience

Much discussion centers on whether or not there is such a thing as "the" optimal place for young children, and which place this should be.

Briefly, in terms of day-care centers, two models are now competing in the minds of most policymakers: The first one, that can be called the "bureaucratic service" model, has for its main objective an ideal of efficient centralization and minimal cost in big centers, allowing 100 children or more. The second model, called by its authors, Christopher Heinicke et al. (23) the "extended family" model, puts much emphasis on maximum continuity between family and day-care personnel, and allows between 30 and 60 children in each center.

Although the second model appears to be the best one to most of us, we still need hard evidence to prove its superiority and to convince the policymakers that cost-benefit analysis, in terms of material organization, should not be the first factor in the field of day-care. Lourie (31) has already emphasized this topic in an earlier publication.

However, the day-care issue has also been analyzed in terms of whether it should continue in the form of group care, or under other forms such as parent-child centers (24,46), family day-care (17,27,35), or under parent education programs (21,22,28).

Some of these programs seem quite compatible and we would only support the principle that alternative solutions must be looked for, experimented with and evaluated in order to help families choose the solution most suitable for them.

The Administrative Framework of Public Day-care Centers

Should day-care fall under the responsibility of a ministry of education, or under a ministry of health and welfare? In many Western countries, because of the significant decrease in the birth rate, a lot of primary school facilities are not completely utilized, and there is now an increasing pressure to put the nursery schools, as well as the day-care centers, in the school system.*

We are strongly opposed to such solutions, since, on one hand, once in the school system, the program of day-care would be under an enormous pressure to evolve towards an instructional model. It would also have a bad influence on the children exposed to day-care, because of premature insistence on systematic learning, conformity and discipline. Rather, nursery

---

*See chapter 27 in this volume.

schools and, still more, day-care centers should be inspired by a rationale of stimulation, play and creative imagination.*

On the other hand, if day-care falls under a ministry of health and welfare, we fear too much accent would be put on custodial care, with a low quality educational experience.

We feel that an independent and autonomous "consortium" of several concerned ministries, such as education, health and welfare, labor, immigration and justice, would be ideal, and at least worthwhile to try out. Each of these ministries has an important role to play in representing a specific policy, incorporated in a more flexible and open structure, which would allow the harmonious coexistence of alternative child care services.

REFERENCES

1. AINSWORTH, M.D. 1967. Patterns of infantile attachment to mother. In: Y. Brackbill and G.G. Thompson (Eds.), *Behavior in Infancy and Early Childhood*. New York: The Free Press.
2. AINSWORTH, M.D. 1969. Object relations, dependency and attachment: A theoretical review of the infant-mother relationship. *Child Development, 40,* 969.
3. AINSWORTH, M.D. 1973. The Development of Infant-Mother Attachment. In: B. Caldwell and H.N. Ricciuti (Eds.), *Review of Child Development Research*, III. Chicago: University of Chicago.
4. AINSWORTH, M.D. and WITTIG, G. 1969. Attachment and exploratory behavior of one-year olds in a strange situation. In: B.M. Foss (Ed.), *Determinants of Infant Behavior*, I. London: Methuen.
5. AINSWORTH, M.D. and BELL, S. 1970. Attachment, exploration and separation illustrated by the behavior of one-year olds in a strange situation. *Child Development, 41,* 49.
6. BETSALEL-PRESSER, R. 1974. Centre de jour éducatif: implications psychopédagogiques d'un programme destiné aux enfants de moins de deux ans. Ph.D. dissertation, Université de Montréal, Dept. of Psychology.
7. BETTELHEIM, B. 1965. *Children in Collectives: Child Rearing Aims and Practices in the Kibbutz.* Springfield, Ill.: Charles C Thomas.
8. BETTELHEIM, B. 1969. *The Children of the Dream.* New York: Macmillan.
9. BLEHAR, M.C. 1974. Anxious attachment and defensive reactions associated with daycare. *Child Development, 40,* 683.
10. BOWLBY, J. 1951. *Maternal Care and Mental Health.* Geneva: World Health Organization, Monography series No.2.
11. BOWLBY, J. 1969. *Attachment and Loss: I. Attachment.* London: Hogarth Press.
12. CALDWELL, B.M. 1977. Child Development and Social Policy. In: M. Scott and S. Grimnett (Eds.), *Current Issues in Child Development.* Washington: Nat. Assoc. for the Educ. of Young Children.
13. CALDWELL, B. M., WRIGHT, C. M., HONIG, A. S. and TANNENBAUM, J. 1970. Infant daycare and attachment. *Amer. J. Orthopsychiat., 40,* 397.
14. CASLER, L. 1961. Maternal deprivation: a critical review of literature. *Monographs of the Society for Research in Child Development, 26,* Series No.8, 1.
15. CHAUNCEY, H. 1969. *Soviet Preschool Education: Vol. I. Program of Instruction.* Educational testing service. New York: Holt, Rinehart & Winston.

*See chapter 28 in this volume.

16. DOYLE, A. B. 1975. Infant development in daycare. *Developmental Psychology, 11,* 5, 655.
17. FEIN, G. and CLARKE-STEWART, A. 1973. *Day Care in Context.* New York: Wiley.
18. FELDMAN, S. S. and INGHAM, M. E. 1975. Attachment behavior: A validation study in two age groups. *Child Development, 46,* 319.
19. FOWLER, W. 1972. A developmental learning approach to group care in a group setting. *Merrill-Palmer Quarterly, 18,* 145.
20. FOWLER, W. and KHAN, N. 1976. *The Comparative Effects of Group and Home Day Care on Early Development.* Ontario Institute for Studies in Education.
21. GORDON, I. 1967. *A Parent Education Approach to Provision of Early Stimulation for the Culturally Disadvantaged.* Final report, Eric Clearinghouse for early childhood education, Urbane: University of Illinois.
22. GORDON, I. 1969. Stimulation via parent education. *Children, 16,* 58.
23. HEINICKE, C.M. et al. 1973. The organization of daycare: Considerations relating to the mental health of child and family. *Amer. J. Orthopsychiat., 43,* 8.
24. HUNT, V. J. 1970. Parent and child centers: Their basis in the behavioral and educational sciences. Paper presented at the American Association of Orthopsychiatry, San Francisco, Cal.
25. KAGAN, J., KEARSLEY, R. B. and ZELAZO, P. R. 1976. The effects of infant daycare on psychological development. Paper presented at the A.A.A.S. Meeting, Boston, Mass.
26. KEISTER, M. E. 1970. *"The Good Life" for Infants and Toddlers.* Washington: National Association for the Education of Young Children.
27. KEYSERLING, M. D. 1972. *Windows on Day Care.* New York: National Council of Jewish Women.
28. LALLY, J. R. 1973. The family development research program. Progress report, Syracuse, New York.
29. LEWIS, M. and BAN, P. 1971. Stability of attachment behavior: A transformational analysis. Paper presented at the National Meeting of the Society of Research in Child Development, Minneapolis.
30. LÉZINE, IRÈNE 1972. L'influence du milieu chez le jeune enfant. In: F. Duyckaertz et al. (Eds.), *Milieu et Développement.* Paris: Psychologie d'aujourd'hui, P.U.F.
31. LOURIE, N. V. 1972. Maximizing legislation opportunities for early child development and daycare program. *Journal of American Academy of Child Psychiatry, 11,* 314.
32. LOW, S. and SPINDLER, P. G. 1968. *Child Care Arrangements of Working Mothers in the United States.* U.S. Department of Health, Education and Welfare, Children's Bureau Publication No. 461.
33. MACCOBY, E. and FELDMAN, S. F. 1972. Mother attachment and stranger reactions. *Monographs of the Society for Research in Child Development, 37,* No. 1.
34. McGREW, W. C. 1974. Interpersonal Spacing of Preschool Children. In: K. Conneley and J. Bruner (Eds.), *The Growth of Competence.* London: Academic Press.
35. PRESCOTT, E. 1978. Is daycare as good as a good home? *Young Children, 33,* 2, 13.
36. PRESCOTT, E., JONES, E. and KRITCHEWSKY, S. 1972. *Day Care as a Child Rearing Environment,* Vol. II. Washington: National Association for the Education of Young Children.
37. PROVENCE, S., NAYLOR, A. and PATTERSON, J. 1977. *The Challenge of Day Care.* New Haven: Yale University Press.
38. RABIN, A. I. 1959. Attitudes of kibbutz children to family and parents. *Amer. J. Orthopsychiat., 29,* 172.
39. RICCIUTI, H. N. and PORESKY, R. 1973. Development of attachment to caregivers in an infant nursery during the first year of life. Preliminary report presented to the Society for Research in Child Development, Philadelphia.
40. ROBINSON, H. B. 1967. A Proposed Daycare Experiment and its Physical Plant. In H. Witmer (Ed.), *On Rearing Infants and Young Children in Institutions.* U.S. Depart-

ment of Health, Education and Welfare, Children's Bureau Research Report No. 1, Social and Rehabilitation Service.

41. ROBINSON, H. B. and ROBINSON, N. B. 1971. Longitudinal development of very young children in a comprehensive daycare program: the first two years. *Child Development*, *42*, 1673.

42. ROMAINE, M. and TEETS, S. 1972. A comparison of attachment behavior observed in daycare and home reared infants. Report presented at the Southwestern Conference on Research in Child Development, Section Infancy, Williamsburg, Va.

43. SCHAFFER, H. R. 1963. Some issues for research in the study of attachment behavior. In: B.M. Foss (Ed.), *Determinants of Infant Behavior*, II. London: Methuen.

44. SCHAFFER, H. R. and CALLENDER, W. N. 1959. Psychological effects of hospitalization in infancy. *Pediatrics*, *24*, 528.

45. STEVENSON, M. and FITZGERALD, H. E. 1972. Standards for infant daycare in the United States and Canada. *Child Care Quarterly*, *1*, 2, 89.

46. WEBER, E. 1970. *Early Childhood Education: Perspective on Change*. Ohio: Charles A. Jones.

47. WILLIAMS, T. M. 1977. Infant development and supplemental care: A comparative review of basic and applied research. *Human Development*, *20*, 1.

48. YARROW, L. J. 1964. Separation from parents during early childhood. In: M.L. Hoffman and L. W. Hoffman (Eds.), *Review of Child Development Research*, I. New York: Russell Sage Foundation.

49. YARROW, L. J. 1965. Mesures et définitions des effets du milieu pendant la toute première enfance. In: *Les Soins aux Enfants dans les Crèches*. Cahiers de Santé publique, No. 24, Genève: O.M.S.

50. YARROW, L. J. 1967. The development of focused relationship. In: J. Hellmuth (Ed.), *Exceptional Infant, I. The Normal Infant*. New York: Bruner-Mazel.

51. YARROW, L. J. and GOODWIN, M. S. 1965. Some conceptual issues in the study of mother-infant interaction. *Amer. J. Orthopsychiat.*, *35*, 473.

52. YARROW, L. J., RUBENSTEIN, J. and PEDERSON, F. 1975. *Infant and Environment, Early Cognitive and Motivational Development*. Washington: Hemisphere Publ. Corp.

27

THE NURSERY SCHOOL
AND THE DISTURBED CHILD

STUART FINE, M.B., F.R.C.P.(C)

Assistant Professor and Head,
Division of Child Psychiatry,
Department of Psychiatry,
University of British Columbia,
Vancouver, Canada

and

P. SUSAN STEPHENSON, M.B., F.R.C.P.(C)

Associate Professor,
Department of Psychiatry,
University of British Columbia,
Vancouver, Canada

INTRODUCTION

Nursery schools provide a rich site for the study of emotional, cognitive, physical, and language development of the preschool child. The social development of these children in a small group can also be studied intensively, over a period of time, in a nursery school.

The nursery school, either intended for "normal" children or organized with a special group of children in mind, plays a very important role in prevention, early detection, and treatment of emotional disturbance and

The authors acknowledge the cooperation of the Children's Hospital Diagnostic Centre, Vancouver, B.C. for allowing them to take photographs included in this chapter, and the parents of the children for giving them permissin to use these photographs.

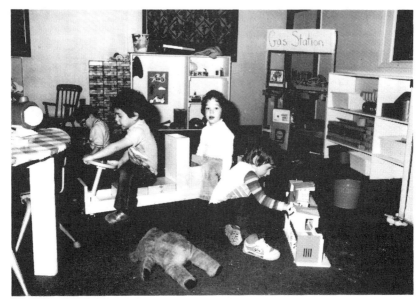

FIGURE 1. Nursery schools provide an opportunity for children to exercise their cognitive, physical, language, and social skills.

developmental delay. It is also a suitable supervised venue for introducing a disturbed or physically disabled child to peers.

This peer interaction may be very important for these children. Disturbed and physically disabled children are often isolated from peers. Health care professionals may advise this isolation, or parents may elect to isolate their child because they fear what other adults and children may say or do to the child. There is evidence that exposing maladapted and physically disabled children to "normal" peers may be salutory to them, as well as to the normal peers. With adequate planning and structure in the nursery school, some maladaptive behaviour may be eliminated (8,16,20). The nursery school is, however, no magic answer to all behavior problems and developmental delay in preschool children. It is only one part of a range of services.

The nursery school can become a rallying point for parents of normal and disturbed children, and these parents may then learn how wide is the variety of skills and behaviours in preschool children.

The nursery school, especially if disturbed and physically disabled children are included, is an excellent site for teaching students and doing research. The students may be in the medical, social science, or educational spheres. Many students and, for that matter, even experienced professionals have remarked with surprise how fine the dividing line is between normal and maladaptive behaviour in the preschooler. It would be helpful for high school students to work in a nursery school so that they have some idea of the range of behaviours that preschoolers show. They would then know what to expect when they become parents.

CULTURAL AND SOCIETAL FACTORS

The role of the nursery school in prevention and treatment of emotional disorder has to be looked at in the context of the basic philosophies of the society in question and the attitudes of that society towards children. This enables one to be wary of the narrow but still prevalent view that more and more services are the answer to children's problems (49).

Nursery schools in different countries have widely ranging objectives, ranging, from transmission of cultural values to preparation for an educational setting. The availability of nursery schools, the status of the staff and the importance attached to their work, and the general view of child care as an individual, family or community responsibility are some factors which affect the usefulness of the nursery school and its acceptance as a community resource.

Children are a national priority in some countries, less so in others. Many writers have emphasized the wealth of the U.S.A., and its apparent disregard for millions of children. Pasamanick (36) emphasized the futility of "years-long piddling commission after commission on the needs of children," Kempe (28) asks "whether one of our cherished democratic freedoms is the right to maim our own children," while Meier (33) stresses that sensational stories of violence and neglect must be used to focus the public's attention on children, "a resource on which we spend less than 10 percent of our G.N.P., yet which represents 40 percent of our population and 100 percent of our future." Viano (51) states that as many as 1,000,000 U.S. children are malnourished or actually starved to the point where both physical and mental growth is stunted. The plight of poor Canadian children has been similarly documented (44,54). Writing about the future of services to Canadian children, Ricks (41) stresses that society must place a priority on the well-being of all children and their families.

The broader societal context must be kept in mind so that we can critically examine whether a child's disturbance is symptomatic, for instance, of his own individual problem, his mother's pathology, or his family's dysfunction, or whether it is related to much wider social pressures and cultural malaise.

Descriptions of nursery schools and their philosophies in a variety of cultures may serve to emphasize these points. Many visitors to the nursery schools of Russia, China and the kibbutz have remarked on the apparent lack of behaviour problems. Sidel(45), accenting the multiplicity of approaches in Western pluralistic societies, asks whether children in these three locations are benefitting from basic agreements as to beliefs and purpose, and ". . .instead of getting multiple messages, the child gets basically one, even if from different people."

Goals of Soviet upbringing, according to Bronfenbrenner(4), include a focus on maternal and child health and nutrition, heavy use of modelling and group forces to achieve desired behaviours, and assignment of responsibilities for achieving the goals of the classroom, school and community. In nursery schools collective play is emphasized with special complex toys designed to be operated by several children. Children are assigned many responsibilities such as gardening, caring for animals, cleaning up, serving at table. Bronfenbrenner feels that the Soviet child gains a more stable and gratifying sense of himself via learning, early in life, the skills and rewards of service to his own community.

Chinese nursery schools have a similar emphasis on preparing the child to serve his community. Preschool children gain experience of manual labour and production by such activities as testing flashlight bulbs and folding cartons. Kessen(29) highlights the "ideological saturation" of the school programme. It is presumed that all activities must foster the child's moral, intellectual, and physical development and work towards the ultimate goal of a classless society. Spiro(47) lays emphasis on similar socialist ideals in kibbutz nursery school, pointing out that the absence of social classes leaves no room for invidious comparisons. He describes less structure and more aggression in kibbutz nursery schools, and stresses the marked identification with the group which is a crucial part of socialization.

In presenting some practical details about nursery schools and disturbed children, we will have to limit ourselves to describing our own experience in North America and to related literature.

THE NURSERY SCHOOL FOR NORMAL CHILDREN

Philosophies about the most effective way of educating preschoolers vary. Some people doubt whether preschoolers should be sent to a school. A study 30 years ago showed that preschool children exposed to nine months in a nursery school showed greater independence, initiative, social adaptability, and interest in the environment than peers who had not had a nursery school experience(24). A more recent study, however, suggests that a nursery school experience may make children more ready to complain and to contradict the teacher(38).

Some nursery schools are very highly structured with an emphasis on cognitive development, and others stress the importance of the social and emotional growth of the child. The latter tend to emphasize creative play, the need to relate to peers, sharing, and cooperation.

Jones(26) suggests that children who do not interact with peers in the preschool years may have difficulty in understanding certain nonverbal cues from other adults in later life. Exposing a young rhesus monkey, which has suffered maternal deprivation, to a small group of slightly younger monkeys may overcome the effects of maternal deprivation(23). If this is true in humans, the importance of the peer group experience, as in a nursery school, is confirmed.

ROLE WITH THE DISTURBED CHILD

Prevention and Early Identification

Early identification of behavioural, physical, or learning difficulties can take place in the nursery school and the appropriate intervention may be initiated. There are, however, difficulties in predicting behavioural, physical, and learning disabilities. Some children who are identified as having developmental delays in preschool years are found, at a later age, to have no difficulties(10). Although there is a core group which continues to have difficulties, in the preschool years, this core group is hard to distinguish from those who "catch up."

Predictors of later behaviour disorders are certain temperamental characteristics. Graham et al.(19) found that low fastidiousness, low habit regularity, and poor malleability were important predictors of later behaviour disorders.

Parents and professionals need to recognize that each child has a different temperamental constellation. This constellation is established at birth. Nine different temperamental traits have been described by Thomas and Chess(50), including the child's activity level; regularity of sleeping, eating, defecating, and urinating; threshold and intensity of response to stimuli; adaptability to new situations, quality of mood; approach or withdrawal responses; distractibility and perseverence. Certain constellations lead to "difficult" or "easy" children or children who are slow to warm up to new situations. If there is "a poor fit" in parental expectations and the child's temperament, conflict occurs.

Parenting a "difficult" child is much more challenging, anxiety-provoking, and more likely to erode parents' self-esteem than bringing up an "easy child." Thomas and Chess(50) highlight the still prevalent traditional assumption, based on psychoanalytic theory, that a parent's attitude towards a child is solely determined by the adult's personality patterns, defences, and conflicts. They point out that it is all too easy for parents and a "difficult" child to get caught up in a vicious cycle of increasingly negative interactions, and for a professional to assume that the parents' pathological attitude and behaviour are the cause of the problem.

If parents are told about these different temperamental variables and understand how their expectations may be at variance with the child's temperament, some behaviour problems, as well as much parental guilt, may be averted. This instruction may be given by the preschool teacher. Some children who are particularly distractible may be given practice at tasks that interest them, so that their attention spans lengthen. Some children may need some time to absorb and consider instructions and follow them. With these children, an immediate response is not likely; however, if a little more time is allowed, they may be able to involve themselves constructively.

The nursery school teachers should help mothers and children separate from one another. This is a task of development at this age and can sometimes cause difficulties. By intervening, if separation anxiety is a problem, and providing the necessary support for both mother and child, a preventive role for the nursery school teacher is further established.

Parent education programmes help parents to understand how children develop emotionally, physically, and socially. Understanding the child's temperament, cognitive style, and above all, how they, as parents, can have mutually enjoyable encounters with their children, can prevent emotional disturbance.

Intervention: Introducing Disturbed Children into this Setting

Some parents and professionals may have magical expectations of the nursery school, while others tend to believe that the child will "grow out" of his problem. Both these attitudes need to be explored and, if possible, modified.

The assessment of the disturbed child and his family should determine which, of a variety of therapeutic approaches, would be most appropriate. When placement of the child in a nursery school is considered, the needs of the child and the composition, philosophy, and general orientation of available nursery schools must be balanced. The child may benefit most from an integrated nursery school (disturbed and normal children); a ther-

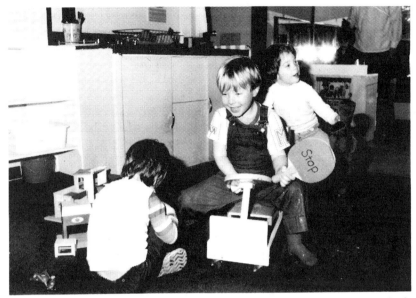

FIGURE 2. Specific tasks can be given to a child recently introduced to a nursery school so that he does have a specific role.

apeutic nursery school (usually only disturbed children); or a nursery school in the community. Some community nursery schools have easy access to psychologists, social workers, or child psychiatrists. These professionals consult about behavioural controls, cognitive skills, and emotional development.

Professionals working with preschool children should get to know the nursery schools in the community. Some disturbed children may do better in a structured programme(22), some in a programme with special approaches(34,37), and some in a free programme where creative play and socialization with peers are stressed(12,16,25).

When a referral to a particular nursery school is planned, a conference, which includes staff from that school, is useful. An initial plan of action about how to work with the child and his family may be decided on. On entering the nursery school, a child must be closely observed by the nursery school teachers as they decide how best to help him. Individual work may be embarked upon first so that the child makes a relationship with an adult other than his usual caretaker. This adult may then accompany him to the small group activities or the larger group. Initially, the disturbed child may spend very little time with the larger group. Sometimes, only after several months is he ready to spend longer times each day with this larger group(12,16,25).

Goals for these children need to be planned, and periodic reassessments or discussions with the referring agency should take place. The modelling of "good" socially acceptable behaviour by the majority of the children and the effect of peer group pressure (for example, on the child who hits his peers and has sufficient peers to retaliate) help to modify overactive and overaggressive behaviours. Teachers need to support the children who are showing acceptable behaviour and they need to reinforce any behaviours that are acceptable in the disturbed child.

Some Difficulties in Integrating Disturbed Children

1) Possessiveness of one preschool teacher

The amount of time each week that a disturbed preschool child should spend in a nursery school varies according to the disturbance, nursery school philosophy, and staffing arrangements. If a disturbed child works individually for some time with a nursery school teacher, we have found that the teacher is often very reluctant to integrate the child. She may be concerned that all the work done in individual sessions will be undone, or she may feel that no one else can manage to help the child as well as she. The nursery school director or consulting professionals may need to be very persuasive about this integration.

2) Fear of contamination

When disturbed children are introduced into a nursery school setting, parents and teachers often fear that the normal children will acquire their disturbed behaviours. There are no reports that this has occurred. However, groups of preschool children do respond to some examples of behaviour. For instance, they behave more aggressively after they have seen television programmes or films with much violence. It is important for the teachers to make clear what behaviour is socially acceptable and to counteract noxious television programmes!

3) Determining the ratio of disturbed to normal children

Different proportions of normal and maladapted children have been recommended. Gesell(17) described integrating maladapted children with normals. He composed his groups so that half were well-adjusted, outgoing children, and half were children who had problems causing them to be referred for assessment and treatment.

In another programme(11,12), a maximum of four maladapted and/or physically disabled children were introduced to a group of 11 normal children. In this setting there were two teachers and an aide for 15 children, and often there were students from other disciplines to offer a helping hand. This particular programme was set up as a model programme on a university hospital campus. It was hoped that other nursery school teachers would be prepared to accept "maladapted children" in their schools after they had seen how these exceptional children improved and how the normal children may have gained from this exposure by learning tolerance and compassion. No conclusion about the best proportion of normal to disturbed preschoolers has been drawn.

4) Relationship of nursery school to overall programme

In another programme, Project Enlightenment in Raleigh, North Carolina, there is a demonstration nursery school where disturbed children were mixed with normals, but the nursery school is one very small element in the total range of services. One other service of this project is consultation to 100 private nursery schools and kindergartens in the city of Raleigh(18).

5) Specials needs for the disturbed child

Guralnick(22) described a programme for handicapped and nonhandicapped children, stressing the need for systematically designed interactions. Rutter and Mittler(43) have pointed out that simply exposing a child with language delay to a peer group will not necessarily help that child with language. However, with planned interaction, the child may be helped.

6) The nature of the "normal" peer group

The level of skills of the "normal" peer group is important, as is defining goals and working towards them. Karnes et al.(27) have compared a structured nursery school programme with three others: a traditional nursery school programme with middle-class children; a traditional nursery school programme with a mix of middle class and disadvantaged children; and a Montessori programme. Children in the structured programme acquired several skills best. Those children in the traditional nursery school with a mix of middle-class and disadvantaged children acquired skills more slowly, while those in the other two programmes were the slowest. The groups of children were well matched for other variables. The argument for defined goals is further developed by Pines(37). She describes remarkable gains cognitively and socially in some experimental nursery schools.

Not all preschool children who are maladapted, disabled, or disadvantaged(46) will benefit from even the best organized nursery school. Each "normal" peer group is also going to differ as to how it can handle a new arrival; for example, for the inhibited child with small stature, a preschool group of children of younger age may be more supportive.

Some programmes make use of a small number of aggressive, acting-out children to modify the behaviour of autistic children(8,14). Another introduces psychotic children into a group of "normal" children from one-parent families(25).

7) Placement after the nursery school experience

It is often difficult to obtain an appropriate placement for the disturbed child after he has been placed in a therapeutic nursery school. The teachers in community schools may be reluctant to accept him, even with advice from his nursery school teachers. If they do accept him they seldom invite his previous nursery school teachers to give advice about how best to control his behaviour and interest him in tasks.

SPECIAL NURSERY SCHOOLS

In some centres special nursery schools for disturbed and/or retarded children have been developed(9,16,25). Many of these therapeutic nursery schools are attached to hospital facilities or closely associated with university departments.

There are different admission criteria and intake procedures for each of these nursery schools. Many insist on doing their own thorough assessment of the whole family initially, although Coleman et al.(9) suggest that one should be very gentle in enlisting family participation. A contract is worked out with the parents as to how often they will be seen. Often the parents are seen as a couple, as well as in couple groups. Work with the parents usually includes providing them with information about their child's diagnosis and prognosis and attempting to explain to them how their methods of discipline and communication of information and feelings may affect his progress. Emphasis is placed on how parents and their preschool child can have a mutually enjoyable time together. Often parents observe their children in the special preschool and may eventually work with their own or other

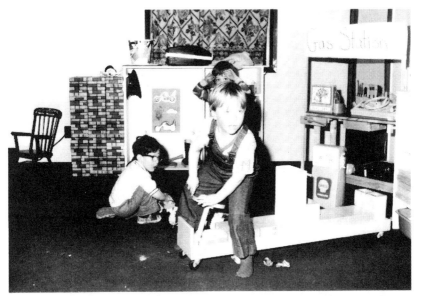

FIGURE 3. Various parts of a nursery school can be assigned specific functions. Children can learn to practice real life skills. This picture was taken in a nursery school for children with communication disorders, i.e., developmental dysphasia, deafness, or autism.

children in the school. As traditional and "parent-blaming" approaches dissolve, there is growing emphasis on the importance of parents as primary therapists for their own children. This change is seen clearly in recent approaches to autistic children(13).

The child may require psychotherapy, cognitive stimulation in language, motor, and sensory areas, and the experience in a peer group where there is a very high pupil/teacher ratio. Some children may benefit from medicines, such as the phenothiazines or antidepressants, which can be monitored in the nursery school.

THE CHILDREN

Prevalence of Disorder

Bateman(2) has estimated that 5 percent to 15 percent of the school population have serious difficulty in reading, 2 percent to 10 percent have speech problems, and 20 percent to 30 percent have less than adequate

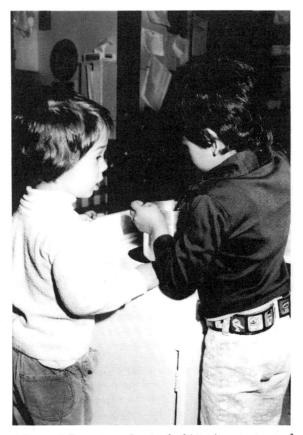

FIGURE 4. Preparing and eating food is an important part of
the program for preschool groups. Certain social skills can be
learned at snack time.

motor development. He suggests that many of these disorders could have
been helped if discovered earlier.

Robinson and Robinson(42) have suggested that there are three factors
involved in not referring children for help when they are under the age of
five. Firstly, young children are rarely exposed to adult observation outside
the family. Secondly, observations are often brief and sporadic in those
situations to which most children are brought for routine professional care
and therefore do not uncover many signs of emotional or developmental
maladjustment. Thirdly, even in those children identified as having prob-

lems, the professionals' attitude is often incorrectly that "the child will grow out of it."

Problems of Classification

Kolvin et al.(31) and Kolvin(30) have pointed out the difficulty in identifying disturbance in preschool children. Frommer et al.(15) differentiate depressed, anxious, or aggressive preschool children. Even if there is good agreement as to whether the child is disturbed or not, there might be disagreement about the particular diagnostic category. Coleman et al.(9) have found four major referral problem categories in preschoolers: management problems (e.g., conduct disorders), neurotic disorders (e.g., separation difficulties, eating and sleeping difficulties), development delay (including language delay and general backwardness), and social stress (e.g., lack of language stimulation, neglect, and abuse).

The development of aberrant attitudes seems to be established by the age of three or four years(32). This applies to establishing racial stereotypes and gender identity(21). Changing these attitudes and behaviours, even at this age, may be difficult.

The Disadvantaged Child

A multidimensional approach to the problems of disadvantaged preschool children and their families is vital. Headstart programmes in the United States, which started with a focus on the individual child, have given way to a diversity of programmes which include home tutoring and parent training(52).

Both Coleman et al.(9) in London, and Stephenson(48) in Vancouver stress that treatment along traditional lines, whether psychoanalytic or behavioural, is rarely appropriate to, or sufficient for, disadvantaged children. The child's problem is a result of a host of factors, including parental isolation, cramped accommodation and lack of play space, parental unemployment, financial problems, alcohol, drugs, minority group status, single parenthood, poor marital situations, and parents' personality problems. Both programmes stress meeting the emotional needs of the adults as well as the child, helping the child and family in a wide range of areas, and making the programme acceptable, readily available, and nonthreatening to the parents. Picking the children up daily from their families and taking them to "school" serve this purpose and seem far more appropriate than expecting a depressed, isolated family to bring one of their children, via public transport, for sessions at a psychiatric clinic.

Although many such programmes show results, at least initially, we have to realize that early intervention cannot function as an "inoculation." Ongoing programmes are needed(53) and, furthermore, as stressed by Chilman(7), "It seems inescapable that basic income maintenance for poor people must undergird any programme that seeks to deal effectively with poverty and disadvantaged parents and children."

THE FAMILIES

Frommer(14) has found 15 percent of the fathers of disturbed preschoolers have psychiatric illness, and 50 percent of their mothers have a depressive illness.

In other studies of mothers of preschool children, investigators have found that 30 percent of mothers of three-year-olds may have been significantly depressed over a 12-month period(35,40) and of those children with behaviour problems there was a significant association with strained marital relationships between parents, and with social stresses(39). Most of these mothers did not seek help, and those who did went to their general practitioner. He would often respond by giving tranquilizers, sedatives, or other medication, but no emotional support to help them cope with raising their preschoolers was provided(35). Bernard(3) has described the many problems and pitfalls of motherhood in modern industrialized society.

If marital strife and poor housing do indeed contribute to behaviour disorders, then emotional support to the caretakers, by using as many community resources as possible, is necessary. Although personnel from most therapeutic nursery schools and some community nursery schools provide some counselling and training for mothers, only some will do home visits and reach out to those caretakers who find it difficult to keep office appointments.

THE TEACHERS

Teacher training for nursery school varies in content and the length of the course. Although lectures on child development are usually included, the teachers are often surprised at the maladaptive behaviour of "normal" children and the occasional normal behaviour of disturbed children. Observation of children over a period of months is essential in order to do adequate assessments and to appreciate these fluctuations in behaviour. Medical students, as well as pediatric and psychiatric registrars, know even less about the ranges of behaviour of preschoolers than the teachers.

Some nursery school teachers are interested in having contact with the parents of the child, and there has been a proliferation of literature about "parent education." These parent education programmes are effective if carefully planned and executed(1). Consultants should encourage teachers to do as much work with parents as possible.

It is unfortunate that many nursery school teachers see themselves as inferior in training to teachers in elementary schools and high schools. They are paid much less than teachers in the higher grades and their status is lower. These teachers are expected to call upon and use other professionals. It is not surprising that Chazan and Jackson(6) have found preschool teachers to be reluctant to use consultation, and "they would on the whole prefer to cope with children's behaviour problems by means of internal resources, including aides and extra teachers, rather than by enlisting outside help." If their status is low, they are hardly likely to enlist other professionals to help.

CONSULTATION

Despite the nursery school teachers' hesitation, consultation from a visiting mental health professional can help them understand the needs of child and family and identify appropriate intervention strategies.

Case Example

Four-year-old Johnny, with hyperactive, aggressive and disruptive behaviour, was of great concern to his parents and teachers. Methylphenidate prescribed by the family doctor merely made him more irritable and whiney, and a variety of commonsense measures did not work. An interview with Johnny and his parents was illuminating. Johnny, a very active and rambunctious child with a short attention span, was the adopted and only child of two quiet perfectionists who strove to contain and control Johnny's behaviour at home.

In this case Johnny's behaviour did not settle down until parents and school agreed on similar management techniques which emphasized both structure and the need to let Johnny "blow off steam" periodically.

INDIRECT CONSULTATION

The mental health professional meets with the staff on an individual or group basis and attempts to understand management problems without a formal assessment of child and parents, although the consultant may have observed the child in the nursery school. The consultant attempts to both understand the problem being presented and tune in to why this particular situation is of concern. Does the report suggest lack of experience, gaps in knowledge, deficiencies in understanding, or problems with objectivity? The first three factors indicate a need for inservice training; coping with the fourth is more complicated. When the consultant gets a sense that the consultee's own emotions and personal experiences are causing loss of objectivity, it is important that this be sorted out in a way that is not threatening to the working relationship and does not cause the consultee to feel labelled as neurotic or put in a patient role. Some nursery school staffs have group meetings where personal feelings come up for discussion. Caplan(5) describes indirect methods for working on the consultee's "thematic interference," such as "examining the evidence" for a particular set towards a child.

Case Example

A nursery school supervisor insisted, repeatedly and anxiously, that the potential for Jane had been missed and that she should not be sent to a resource for retarded children. Together with the supervisor, the consultant did a careful reevaluation of all the information pertinent to the child's development. As Jane's limitations became really clear, the supervisor's anxiety subsided, and she stopped opposing the child's move. Several months later, in a staff meeting, the supervisor connected her feelings about Jane with those about a sister, painfully shy and nervous, who had been wrongfully dismissed as a retarded child.

CONCLUSION

While national priorities and political ideologies in various societies affect the availability of nursery schools, their scope, status, and philosophy, a few basic principles may apply to all cultures. Nursery schools allow for socialization of young children, shaping of behaviour, interaction with peers, and the introduction to skills which prepare them for school. Potential problems can be identified within nursery schools and appropriate intervention planned.

The nursery school for "normal" children is a resource for a few specially chosen disturbed children who will use the other children as models. At the present time, in many areas, there are obstacles which stand in the way of the most constructive use of the nursery school. These include lack of communication between professionals, general lack of knowledge about early childhood development, the low status of the nursery school teacher and resulting defensiveness about using other professionals as consultants, lack of communication or competitiveness between parents and teachers and among teachers themselves, failure to perceive the nursery school as part of a network of services to young children in a community, and problems with administration and funding.

Special nursery schools are sometimes necessary for groups of children with special needs: autistic, blind, deaf, mentally retarded, and severely psychiatrically disabled children. There is a growing trend towards parent involvement, working collaboratively with parents and viewing them as primary therapists for their children.

Nursery schools are important training settings for a variety of students, so that university and medical school settings might, with advantage, establish their own child study centres which would include nursery schools. There would then be freer access for students from different disciplines and possibilities for continued learning and research.

Liaison with community nursery schools and with the school authorities for the higher grades of education is essential to allow some continuity of care after the disturbed child leaves the nursery school setting. A good working relationship with these other institutions can be facilitated only by frequent meetings with their personnel and the establishment of mutual trust and respect.

The community nursery schools should not work in isolation. Nursery schools should be part of the programmes for prevention and treatment of disorders in the preschooler. Therapeutic nursery schools should be part of an outpatient, inpatient, and community consultation programme.

The overall planning for preschoolers should be done at a regional and also at a national level. Also, the nursery school intervention needs to be followed by adequate programmes for the children in their later years. Finally, the most difficult task of evaluation of nursery school programmes requires funding, as well as professional interest and attention.

REFERENCES

1. AUERBACH, A. 1968. *Parents Learn Through Discussion*. New York: Wiley.
2. BATEMAN, B. 1966. Learning disorders. *Review of Educ.*, 36, 93.
3. BERNARD, J. 1974. *The Future of Motherhood*. New York: Penguin Books.
4. BRONFENBRENNER, U. 1970. *Two Worlds of Childhood: U.S. and U.S.S.R.* New York: Russell Sage Foundation.

5. CAPLAN, G. 1970. *The Theory and Practice of Mental Health Consultation.* New York: Basic Books.
6. CHAZAN, M. and JACKSON, S. 1971. Behaviour problems in the infant school. *J. Child. Psychol. Psychiat., 12,* 191.
7. CHILMAN, C.S. 1973. Programs for disadvantaged parents, some major trends and related research. In: B. Caldwell and H.N. Ricciuti (Eds.), *Rev. Child Develop. Res., 3.* New York: Russell Sage.
8. COFFEY, H. and WIENER, L. 1967. *Group Treatment of Autistic Children.* Englewood Cliffs, N.J.: Prentice Hall, Inc.
9. COLEMAN, J., BURTENSHAW, W., POND, D., and ROTHWELL, B. 1977. Psychological problems of preschool children in an inner urban area. *Brit. J. Psychiat., 131,* 623.
10. DE HIRSCH, K., JANSKY, J.J., LANGFORD, W.S. 1966. *Predicting Reading Failure.* New York: Harper & Row.
11. FINE, S. 1974. A high proportion of maladjusted preschool children in a group of normal preschoolers. *Can. Ment. Health, 22,* 3.
12. FINE, S. 1973. The assessment and treatment of the preschool child with maladaptive behaviour in a hospital nursery school. *Clin. Ped., 12,* 240.
13. FREEMAN, B.J. and RITVO, E.R. 1976. Parents as paraprofessionals. In: E.R. Ritvo (Ed.), *Autism: Diagnosis, Current Research and Management.* New York: Spectrum Publications.
14. FROMMER, E.A. 1967. A day hospital for disturbed children under five. *Lancet, 1,* 377.
15. FROMMER, E.A., MENDELSON, W.B., and REID, M.A. 1972. Differential diagnosis of psychiatric disturbance in preschool children. *Brit. J. Psychiat., 121,* 71.
16. FURMAN, R. and KATAN, A. 1969. *The Therapeutic Nursery School.* New York: International Universities Press.
17. GESELL, A.L. 1930. *The Guidance of Mental Health in Infant and Child.* New York: Macmillan.
18. GLASSCOATE, R. and FISHMAN, M.E. 1974. *Mental Health Programs for Preschool Children. A Field Study Joint Information Service.* Washington: American Psychiatric Association and the National Association for Mental Health.
19. GRAHAM, P., RUTTER, M., and GEORGE, S. 1973. Temperamental characteristics as predictors of behaviour disorders in children. *Am. J. Orthopsychiat., 43,* 328.
20. GRANTHAM, E. 1971. Handicapped children in preschool groups. *Brit. Med. J., 4,* 346.
21. GREEN, R. 1974. *Sexual Identity Conflict in Children and Adolescents.* New York: Basic Books.
22. GURALNICK, M. 1976. The value of integrating handicapped and nonhandicapped preschool children. *Am. J. Orthopsychiat., 46,* 236.
23. HARLOW, H.F. and SUOMI, S. 1971. Social recovery by isolation-reared monkeys. *Proc. Nat. Acad. Sci, U.S.A., 68,* 1534.
24. HATTWICK, B.W. 1936. The influence of nursery school attendance upon the behavior and personality of the preschool child. *J. Exptl. Educ., 5,* 180.
25. HAVELKOVA, M. 1968. Follow-up study of 71 children diagnosed as psychotic in the preschool age. *Am. J. Orthopsychiat., 38,* 846.
26. JONES, B. 1966. An ecological study of some aspects of social behavior of children in nursery schools. In: D. Morris (Ed.), *Primate Ethology.* Chicago: Aldine.
27. KARNES, M., TESKA, J., and HODGINS, S.A. 1970. Effects of four programs of classroom intervention on the intellectual and language development of 4-year-old disadvantaged children. *Am. J. Orthopsychiat., 40,* 58.
28. KEMPRE, C.H. 1976. Approaches to preventing child abuse: The health visitor's concept. *Am. J. Dis. Child, 130,* 941.
29. KESSEN, W. (Ed.) 1975. *Childhood in China.* New Haven and London: Yale University Press.
30. KOLVIN, I. 1971. Studies in the childhood psychoses. I. Diagnostic criteria and classification. *Brit. J. Psychiat., 118,* 381.

31. KOLVIN, E., WOLFF, S., BARBER, L.M., TWEDDLE, E.G., GARSIDE, R., SCOTT, D.McI, and CHAMBERS, S. 1975. Dimensions of behaviour in infant school children. *Brit. J. Psychiat.*, *126*, 114.

32. KONOPKA, G. 1973. Formation of values in the developing person. *Am. J. Orthopsychiat.*, *43*, 86.

33. MEIER, J.H. 1976. In: R.E. Helfer, C.H. Kempe, and W.F. Mondale, (Eds.), *Child Abuse and Neglect: The Family and the Community*. Cambridge, Mass.: Ballinger.

34. MONTESSORI, M. 1964. *The Montessori Method*. New York: Schocken Books.

35. MOSS, P. and PLEWIS, I. 1977. Mental distress in mothers of preschool children in Inner London. *Psychol. Med.*, *7*, 641.

36. PASAMANICK, B. 1971. A child is being beaten. *Am. J. Orthopsychiat.*, *41*, 540.

37. PINES, M. 1966. *Revolution in Learning*. New York: Harper & Row.

38. RAPH, J., THOMAS, A., CHESS, S., and BIRCH, H. 1968. The influence of nursery school on social interactions. *Am. J. Orthopsychiat.*, *38*, 144.

39. RICHMAN, N. 1977. Behaviour problems in preschool children. Family and social factors. *Brit. J. Psychiat.*, *131*, 523.

40. RICHMAN, N. 1976. Depression in mothers of preschool children. *J. Child Psychol. Psychiat.*, *17*, 75.

41. RICKS, F. 1977. Evaluation. In: J. Shamsie, (Ed.), *Experience and Experiment*. Toronto: Leonard Crainford.

42. ROBINSON, H. and ROBINSON, N. (Eds.) 1973. In: Task Force I Studies of Infancy Through Adolescence. Mental Health: From Infancy Through Adolescence. *Reports of Task Forces I, II, and III and the Committees on Education and Religion by the Joint Commission on Mental Health of Children*. New York: Harper & Row.

43. RUTTER, M. and MITTLER, P. 1972. Environmental influences on language development. In: M. Rutter and J.A. Martin (Eds.), *The Child with Delayed Speech. Clinics in Developmental Medicine Monographs*, *43*, 64.

44. RYAN, T.J. (Ed.) 1972. *Poverty and the Child*. Toronto: McGraw-Hill Ryerson.

45. SIDEL, R. 1973. *Women and Child Care in China: A Firsthand Report*. Baltimore, Md: Penguin Books.

46. SILVERMAN, M.A. and WOLFSON, E. 1970. The use of small educational-therapeutic groups in a program for disadvantaged preschoolers. *Psychosocial Process*, *1*, 47.

47. SPIRO, M.E. 1965. *Children of the Kibbutz*. New York: Schocken Books.

48. STEPHENSON, P.S. 1976. Project toddler. *Can. Ment. Health*, *24*, 20.

49. SUSSMAN, A. and COHEN, S.J. 1975. *Reporting Child Abuse and Neglect: Guidelines for Legislation*. Cambridge, Mass.: Ballinger.

50. THOMAS, A. and CHESS, S. 1977. *Temperament and Development*. New York: Brunner/Mazel.

51. VIANO, E.C. 1977. From the editor: Special issue: Child abuse and neglect. *Victimology*, *2*, 175.

52. WILKINSON, J.E. and MURPHY, H.F. 1976. Differential methods of enhancing growth in urban preschool children. *Child Care, Health and Development*, February, 2.

53. WILLIAMS, T.M. 1977. Infant development and supplemental care: A comparative review of basic and applied research. *Human Develop.*, *20*, 1.

54. *Poverty in Canada: A Report of the Special Senate Committee* 1971. Ottawa: Information Canada.

28

PRESCHOOL PLAYGROUPS

ELIZABETH GRANTHAM, M.B.,B.S.(LONDON)

*Part-time Children's Physician, Child Development
Unit, Peterborough District General Hospital, England*

and

JANE GRUBB, M.B. Ch.B. (Edin)

*Part-time Clinical Medical Officer, Avon Health
Authority and Research Associate (Child Health)
University of Bristol, England*

INTRODUCTION

In many countries the importance of play in promoting children's development is now acknowledged and studied(52); arrangements for spontaneous and structured play for children, as a group or individually, are often an integral part of professionally organised systems of preschool education and day-care.

In the Organisation for Economic Cooperation and Development countries the demand for early childhood education increased rapidly from 1960 to 1970 and further rapid growth is foreseen(31). However, internationally, information about community playgroups is scanty. There are several reasons for this. Statistics for all preprimary provisions are confused by the difference in age at which schooling becomes compulsory; the terminology is inconsistent both within and between countries; the whole non-statutory sector is usually termed "private" with no distinction between profit- and

The authors would like to express their thanks to the many playgroups they have known, from whom they have learned so much. They also acknowledge the help of Mr. J. Eatough, A.R.P.A., Medical Photographer, Bristol Royal Hospital for Sick Children.

non-profit-making organisers and with no definition of the extent of parental responsibility.

However, some published material is now available which brings into focus the varied approaches to early child care and education, and outlines current practice in more than 20 countries (32,33,34). To summarise these would be misleading, but it is relevant to pick out two items. The U.S. and Yugoslavia are reported as exceptional (among the countries described) in the degree to which parental control and staffing of publicly sponsored child care programmes have developed. Secondly, a forum sponsored by the Centre for Educational Research and Innovation has been established among a few member countries (W. Germany, Netherlands, Australia, Sweden, U.S.) to discuss experimental preschool projects which include some element of parental involvement.

We surmise that in countries where, for one reason or another, there is a high level of state provision and often full-day-care for preschool children, for instance U.S.S.R., China and some European countries, there has been little scope for parents to initiate and organise provision themselves.

Conversely, in other countries where state provision has been low, but the benefits of early education have been perceived, parents have been instrumental in setting up schemes. In the U.S. the Parent Cooperative Preschool Movement started 50 years ago, later spreading to Canada. Largely middle-class at first, preschool programmes have incorporated and extended some of the principles of this organisation in disadvantaged communities. In New Zealand in the 1930s, the Play Centres involved parents more directly in realising their potential and responsibility as educators of their own children. Their system of parent-controlled preschool schemes spread to Australia, where, however, there is a strong lobby for state-sponsored, professionally-run kindergartens. In both countries the playgroup movement has put considerable effort into reaching ethnic minorities, notably the Maori and the Aborigine.

The New Zealand Play Centres built up an effective system of supervision and advice, publishing useful booklets which were of practical value in Britain when the playgroup movement began there. To some extent the U.S. Cooperative ideas, through visiting lecturers and an international journal, also had an influence in Britain.

By the mid '60s the British playgroup influence had begun to spread across the channel. In the Netherlands playgroups have multiplied rapidly since 1970. The Werkgemeenschap Kinderen Nederland (WKN) is an advisory and supportive foundation which also encourages cooperation between playgroups and nearby day centres(7). In Brussels playgroups are proliferating.

Since Britain entered the European Economic Community (EEC) there has been more interchange of ideas. Playgroup representatives, and tutors of playgroup training courses can now participate in seminars and discussions with their counterparts from other member states.

Parents familiar with playgroups in their own country have often initiated similar groups if they go to work abroad; for instance, in Iran a number of playgroups are well established in Tehran, and in Zahedan (near the Pakistan border) they are just beginning. Though these groups may be multiracial, they are in no sense indigenous. A letter from Iran(43) describes these playgroups in Tehran and comments: "The growth of playgroups will only come with the infiltration of more European and Western ideas. Here the woman is still regarded as one whose duties lie entirely within the home."

Developments in Rhodesia are of particular interest: Over the past five years, with help from the National Playgroups Association, preschool education training courses have been given in African communities. "The courses' aim was to alert mothers and grandmothers to what could be done with their own children at home and to demonstrate the value of community playgroups." There is "the nucleus of a really impressive movement that is slowly gathering momentum"(44). In tribal villages, as well as in urban areas, the imported playgroup concept is showing its relevance in very different settings.

An important factor in Rhodesia was undoubtedly the support given by the Playgroups Association and the past experience of the tutors. It would be more difficult to establish such courses in countries where children's actual survival is still a pressing problem, where all education, especially for girls, is scarce, and resources for play are negligible. However, it is possible that the influence of play schemes run in conjunction with emergency relief, or in refugee camps, or with health and nutrition programmes could make a significant impact by breaking into a cycle of play deprivation(27).

DEFINITION

In 1976, for the first time, the Concise Oxford Dictionary defined the word playgroup—"group of young children who play together regularly under supervision," thus giving recognition to what had become common English usage over the last 25 years, for one category of nursery provision. There are several different kinds of playgroup(56) and here we are mainly concerned with those which in Britain are often called *community playgroups* and are for preschool children of about three-to-five years old. These groups are likely to be *voluntary*, i.e., non-statutory, *non-profit-making*, and organised by a committee which includes *parent representatives* or sometimes by a less formal group of all or some of the parents. Expenses are met by parental contributions which may be supplemented by public or charitable funding. A supervisor, i.e., playleader, is in charge of the session (two-three hours several times a week) with assistant(s) and/or additional help from a roster of parents. Once certain conditions(30) laid down by the local government authority have been satisfied, each playgroup is largely autonomous, with its own character, and may also show considerable changes over time as different parents bring their own experiences to it. Nevertheless, while the playgroup movement in Britain has retained this dynamic variety, it has taken on a corporate identity, not only as a new type of preschool provision, but also as a voluntary enterprise, making a distinctive contribution to a long tradition in national life.

DEVELOPMENT OF PLAYGROUPS IN BRITAIN

Since the first "nursery playgroup" for 25 deprived children in London was set up in 1945 by the Save the Children Fund (SCF), the growth of playgroups has accelerated to almost 15,000 groups in 1976 in England(14) and Wales(57), providing places for about one in four of all children in the three- and four-year-old age groups. A substantial increase has also taken place in Scotland and Northern Ireland.* A small proportion are run as business concerns, but the great majority are non-profit-making and are connected with voluntary and charitable bodies, particularly the Preschool Playgroups Association (PPA), which has 10,000 member groups(39).

In this chapter we consider briefly some reasons for this phenomenon and, in more detail, the aims and functioning of playgroups. We also give our view of their significance for young children.

In Britain, in 1961, a group campaigning for more nursery schools to be established by the Government brought together parents who discovered that some of them had already independently found ways to start their own nursery playgroups. These "self-help" parents set up the PPA, which was quickly recognised as a source of advice and support. At first these groups sprang up mainly in relatively affluent areas where parents realised the value of early socialisation and learning through play, but at the same time there was a steady growth of groups set up by local authorities and by charities in disadvantaged areas, so that the idea spread widely. Further impetus to the movement came in the late 1960s from programmes of urban aid and community development in which the Government funded many

---

*In Scotland, playgroup information can be obtained from S.PPA, 7 Royal Terrace, Glasgow, 63 7NT. In Northern Ireland it can be obtained from NI.PPA, 6 Lower Crescent, Belfast BT 7 INR.

preschool projects. The first results of research monitoring these programmes suggested that the self-help or community playgroup could have
a distinctive role in early childhood education, chiefly because of the way
in which it could engage the active interest of parents(23). Consideration of
the apparent cost-effectiveness of playgroups has encouraged serious debate
about how voluntary playgroups might retain an identity within an expanding system of statutory preschool provision(15).

In disadvantaged areas organisations tended to set up playgroups with
trained staff to work with the children and to "give the mothers a break."
The Liverpool Priority scheme was a notable exception. This scheme grew
from Government-sponsored action research projects undertaken 1969-71,
which recognised the "interlock of parent and child in educational produc-
tivity." It aimed to create a more confident and informed awareness in
mothers of their own influence on their young children both at home and
in group settings(29). More agencies now see their workers as enablers,
helping parents to formulate their own solutions to neighbourhood needs
for young children. Parents may decide that a playgroup is their first objective, or they may have other priorities such as welfare rights, women's
liberation, adult education classes, or bulk-buy schemes to purchase food
cooperatively. To enable them to attend they may organise ad hoc care
arrangements, which they later develop into a playgroup.

Probably all playgroup organisations would now agree with the substance
of this statement, made in 1974:

> Preschool Playgroups Association (PPA) exists to help parents to un-
> derstand and provide for the needs of their children. It aims to pro-
> mote community situations in which parents can with growing enjoyment
> and confidence make the best uses of their own knowledge and re-
> sources in the development of their children and themselves(42).

THE AIMS AND FUNCTIONING OF PLAYGROUPS

Thus the aims of playgroups concern parents, children and the community
in which they operate. These aims are interdependent but are considered
separately below.

Parents and Parent Involvement

The self-help playgroups were influenced at first by the New Zealand Play
Centres, which emphasised the benefit to the children of the parents' participation in play organisation(24). In Britain, "it was only later the parents

realised how much *they* were benefiting themselves, and the principle of parent involvement was born''(9,p.107).

However, it is still difficult to determine just how and how much parents are involved. PPA figures suggest that, overall, 82 percent of member playgroups have some parents helping at sessions regularly, but on average this help is given by only 27 percent of the total number of parents(39). Three playgroup characteristics seem to favour involvement: medium size; rural area; and the management being by a parent committee. A scale devised(13) to rate parent involvement in decision-making in preschool programmes could perhaps be developed further to help define what involvement actually implies.

Some of the factors in families and in playgroups which may hinder parent involvement in the playgroup, or use of a playgroup at all, are brought out in studies by Shinman(50), and by Ferri and Niblett(20). Shinman emphasises how crucial is the mother's own psychological situation, and Ferri and Niblett how the playgroup must be able to offer resources which the mother sees as relevant.

A paper from the U.S. by Datta(12) sets out the issues related to the trend towards parent involvement and urges further study of about 12 topics, including what parents actually want and need; what are the real costs of parent involvement; and whether special programmes to involve parents are justified.

Two recent British studies throw some light on what parents say they want. Bradley and Kucharski(4), in a Liverpool survey, found that parents wanted more information on the types of preschool provision, and also on what teachers would expect children to know at school entry. Bone(3), in a survey to find the extent of need for day-care, found that most mothers preferred a break from their child and, of those who did spend time in the group or school, only about half liked doing so. However, twice as many mothers felt *welcome* to participate in a playgroup, as against other provisions. Forty-six percent of the mothers whose children were not yet using day-care said they would like to be involved if their child were to become a user. This implies initial willingness to be involved but some disappointment with it when it occurred.

A study by Watt(56) explored attitudes towards involvement and towards professionalism in relation to possible integration of voluntary and statutory preschool facilities. She suggests that the particular model of parent involvement used is of less importance than the nature of the relationships within which it takes place. Shinman(50) makes the same point.

A recent report on the future of voluntary organisations in Britain(58) points out the need to keep under review the effectiveness of services which they provide, and suggests that client satisfaction may be a useful indicator. When there is client participation, the degree of satisfaction can more easily be assessed and PPA is cited as a good example of a mutual aid organisation demonstrating the principle of participation. PPA evidence quoted in the report referred to the young mother suddenly finding that she had a role to play herself, which increased her confidence in handling her child and in relating to other adults. We see this as a valuable antidote to the feeling of inferiority which a woman often experiences when she is "just a mother"—a job devalued by present-day society. We note too, that Zigler, in discussing the American headstart concept, emphasised how parents' belief in their competence to influence their environment is an important variable related to subsequent school performance.(60)

One index of the effectiveness of the playgroup movement in encouraging participation is the steady increase in demand by playgroup mothers, irrespective of social and educational background, for opportunities to learn more about the play needs of their children and about how to meet them(40).

Parents and Training

Nurturing involvement of parents (father *and* mother) and increasing adults' sensitivity to children's needs have become important objectives in the training courses which PPA has developed. Closely linked with observation and assignments in the playgroups themselves, the flexible system of training helps mothers and playgroup staff to share in learning processes which parallel those of the children. It is as much a matter of discovering human relationships as of learning to "manage" a finger-painting session and we feel it to be one of the most significant features of the playgroup movement.

A new development has been the collaboration of PPA with the Open University (TV and radio) on a course in child development designed to interest mothers at home with their young children. If students wish (8,000 have applied for the first two course presentations), they can be linked up in local groups to discuss the programmes with a coordinator.

The Children and the Playgroup

All playgroups must comply with conditions set by the local authority. These concern mainly premises and staff:child ratios (usually 1:8 or 1:10). There are considerable variations among authorities. A study in progress of most preschool institutions in Britain is analysing all their main features.

Until that is completed PPA is the main source of information for England and Wales.

An average PPA group meets in a rented hall for four sessions (of two-and-a-half hours) weekly. The supervisor is likely to have attended a play-group course and may have an assistant as well as mother helpers. The group offers 24 places but has 37 children on the register so not all can attend every session. Thirty-one percent of groups receive some grant aid (1978 figures). In 38 percent, secondary school girls and boys visit or help; 16 percent also run a mother and toddler group (1978 figures)(39).

Social Aspects

Analysis of 5,800 PPA groups in 1975 showed the following distribution: rural areas, 38 percent; urban, "better off," 10 percent; urban, mixed, 40 percent; urban, "poor," 12 percent(39). A clearer picture will emerge from the national study mentioned above which will compare uptake by different social and ethnic groups, and the extent of support and advice systems.

Activities in a Playgroup Session

In general, equipment and materials are similar to those found in a nurs-ery school, but are often limited by the shared premises or cost. Access to outdoor play space is often restricted. By exploiting what *is* available, a session usually offers an enjoyable blend of active and quiet play, painting, dough, sand and water, dressing up and "home corner" play, as well as stories, music and, increasingly, time to talk with the children. We feel it is the sustained interest, the ability to observe, and the resourcefulness of the adults that help the play of individual children and of the group to grow into rich and appropriate learning opportunities in which formal teaching is unnecessary. Perceptive guidelines on this have been written by Crowe(10).

Effects on the Children's Development

There has so far been little research to assess how far *playgroups*, as distinct from other forms of nursery facilities, succeed in meeting children's needs. The individuality of playgroups and their vulnerability to changes in local demand complicate attempts to measure effectiveness. The child's re-sponse to his experiences in the play session is influenced by his parents' feelings about the playgroup and the impact it has on his family. Shinman's study(50) has shown that, in spite of difficulties associated with interview techniques, the parents' feelings can be elucidated, though more research

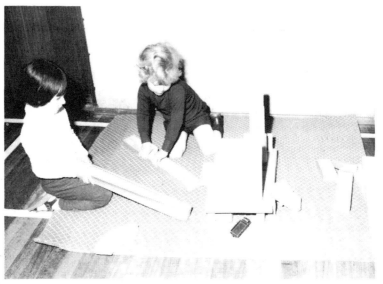

FIGURE 1. Large wooden blocks in playgroup offer learning opportunities in many ways.

is still needed. Parents' feelings may also be related to their use of preventive health services for their children. One study has shown that a substantial proportion of children identified as non-attenders at traditional Child Health Clinics do make use of private day-care and playgroups rather than statutory preschool groups(17). Experiments to integrate health surveillance effectively with these non-statutory groups are long overdue. Positive attitudes towards their child's full development can be among the objectives of parent education, but in Europe generally there is a serious lack of research to compare different approaches(51).

Turner's study of playgroups for deprived children in Belfast, Northern Ireland, is of particular importance(55). It is the first major research project to examine in detail the usual programme of a playgroup session and to evaluate its effectiveness. She compared the development of children attending four-to-five sessions a week over a six-month period with that of children not attending any type of preschool provision. Of particular interest is the use of a new measure of children's competence in social skills, the first experimental version of the Turner Pre-School Social Progress Scale (TPSPS). Her scrutiny of the playgroup setting and activities elicited several factors likely to influence the effects on the children. An unusually practical

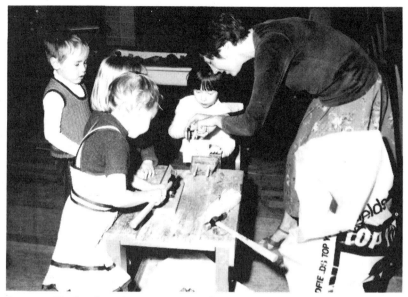

FIGURE 2. Woodwork in playgroup (not only for boys) always needs an adult on hand.

outcome of the project is the concise and clear summary of the main findings which the author has written for the Northern Ireland PPA(55A).

We summarise very briefly some of the findings discussed in Turner's evaluative study of Belfast playgroups and refer to some other studies. In certain circumstances it appears that playgroups can provide a setting which favourably influences children's development in cognitive, socioemotional, general reasoning, verbal and gross motor aspects. Some success may relate more to warmth, consistency and responsiveness in the attitudes of the staff(53,55) and to positive parental attitudes(55) than to buildings and equipment. (See Figures 1 and 2.) However, premises lacking adequate storage and outdoor play space may make a full range of play difficult to achieve(35). Outdoor space seems particularly valued by children from working-class backgrounds and there may be scope for staff to take more advantage of this in structuring play for aspects of learning(54).

In Belfast, which we suggest may be a special case in this respect because of civil unrest, gains in children's development seem to be related to the regularity of attendance and to the number of sessions children attend(55). Meeting the same children on consecutive days enables more progression of play to take place(35). There is some evidence, however, that some mothers prefer their children not to attend every day and that afternoon sessions are not favoured(3,56). Many playgroups have to ration places because of the demand so that many more premises and more funding would be required to enable those who wished for more frequent sessions to have them. As school numbers drop in the next few years, more classrooms could, in theory, be used for playgroups, but, as discussed by Turner(55), some parents find schools unapproachable, and would be less comfortable in participating.

Teachers' attitudes towards parent involvement are relevant here; some may not be prepared as yet for all that is implied by parent management of a playgroup(56). A further aspect of some importance is the teacher's view, at school entry, of the effects of playgroup attendance. One study(47) found that, while most teachers considered the effects beneficial, some teachers in working-class areas had reservations about the way local playgroups tended to preserve cultural modes of behaviour and communication in the children. This links with a view expressed by Poulton and James(38) suggesting that if the gains from home-orientated early education are to be maintained once "proper" school begins, then schools may need to find ways to move towards the community, on the community's terms.

Playgroups, the Community and Statutory Authorities

We have shown playgroups' concern for the children and parents and it is no surprise that increasingly this concern extends beyond the playgroup itself. This has been facilitated by PPA, which now has a comprehensive local and regional support system, usually available not only to members but to all playgroups. Mother and toddler groups, play schemes among ethnic minorities, in hostels for homeless families or for battered wives, and with child minders are examples of situations where insight derived from playgroups is being used. This has often required approaching statutory authorities for financial help. Some authorities have generously encouraged this kind of voluntary response to unmet needs, but others have been unwelcoming and have planned services without any consultation.

These contrasting attitudes highlight a longstanding lack of coherent policy for under-fives(59), partly due to fragmented administrative systems. Education authorities are responsible for state nursery schools and classes, social service departments for all playgroups and day nurseries, and health authorities for medical care in state groups. Some steps towards cooperation have been taken recently(16) and it is now acknowledged that voluntary bodies have a permanent contribution to make to services for under-fives and should be involved in planning them. This acknowledgement was undoubtedly hastened by a discussion paper from a new body set up in 1976(28). This—the Voluntary Organisations Liaison Council for Under-Fives (VOL-CUF)—will try to define common aims and objectives among all those concerned with under-fives. VOLCUF is sufficiently representative for its views to be given some weight by statutory authorities. This will have implications for playgroups in relation to local authorities' plans for preschool education, and also in exploring more deeply how the idea of parent involvement can be fostered within a national strategy for under-fives and their families.

Some families and their children have special problems of handicap or disturbance and we now consider some aspects of playgroup provision for them.

PLAYGROUPS AND HANDICAPPED CHILDREN

Psychiatric Aspects

Some child guidance clinics and hospitals have run small day centres for children with various difficulties where the activities are planned on a nursery school model and the parents are expected to participate(1). In an article on disobedience and violent behavior in school-age children, Bentovim(2) suggests, as others do(8), that preschool settings which help parents and offer appropriate models of behaviour for children are greatly needed. Recent work has shown what a high proportion of junior school children are at risk of maladjustment and educational difficulty(26). We have found that community playgroups can diversify to complement professionally run centres.

Special Playgroups for Handicapped Children

The continued shortage of nursery education, especially for handicapped children, resulted in a number of experimental playgroups being established to cater for children with needs thought to be too specialised for the "ordinary" group of 20 to 30 active three and four year olds.

The first of several for the physically handicapped was started by a social worker for children with spina bifida and/or hydrocephalus(25). Others were started for mentally handicapped children. Both varieties met real needs in children and parents, and the experience gained in the search for suitable equipment and activities was invaluable. The Spastics Society made a further contribution by correlating and disseminating some of this experience in multidisciplinary training sessions.

Special groups were set up too for disadvantaged and deprived children—some by social services departments and some by other organisations such as the National Society for Prevention of Cruelty to Children (NSPCC). The NSPCC monitored ten therapeutic playgroups and a preliminary report(48) suggested that the scheme was successful in identifying families and children from backgrounds of substantial material deprivation, financial hardship, and, in many cases, considerable emotional disturbance. It provided an ongoing service for the children for a considerable time and showed that there was a clear tendency for an increase in language development and sociability in play and an improvement in peer relationships.

Without denying the pioneer value of the groups set up for particular handicapping conditions, some practical difficulties became apparent; for example, funds donated to an organisation dealing with one handicap could not necessarily be used to benefit a child with a different disability. Children might have to be brought long distances so it was not always practicable to involve the parents, or to include siblings who might themselves be at risk of developmental or emotional problems.

Opportunity Playgroups

It was in response to a request by the mother of a mongol child, who wanted somewhere where she could take both her handicapped child and the normal twin to play, that an "Opportunity Playgroup" was started in 1966(19), and over the next few years many more opened. These groups, which are usually voluntary, and run by a committee representing parents, professionals, and community, aim to help handicapped children from birth onwards and to have about half the places for non-handicapped under-fives. Most also help the mothers by providing a place where they can meet together, perhaps with a social worker. The adult:child ratio is usually 1:2 or:3 or even 1:1. Such groups often offer a useful halfway house to an ordinary playgroup for children with any type of handicap, including those recovering from severe illness, accident, or hospitalisation. (See Figure 3.)

PPA has a subcommittee with special responsibility for handicapped children in playgroups, which, working closely with a National Adviser, is in touch with more than 80 opportunity groups. PPA also produces publications to help special groups and the ordinary groups where handicapped children attend(45).

Children in Hospital

In 1963, the Save the Children Fund (SCF) appointed a trained play leader to a children's ward. Since then play programmes of various kinds

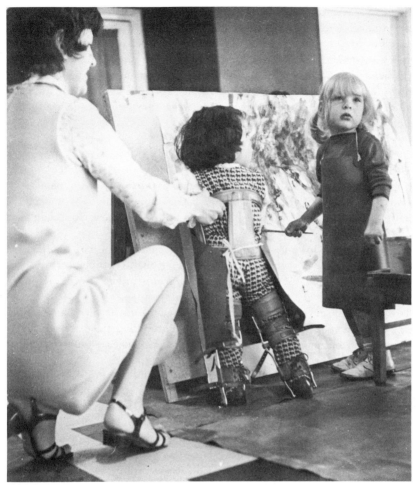

FIGURE 3. Opportunity playgroup provides freedom to explore paint for a 2½year-old with a high spinal bifida lesion and a 3-year-old with cerebral palsy.

have been started in wards, outpatient departments, or waiting areas; additional helpers are often recruited from among playgroup-experienced people. The National Association for the Welfare of Children in Hospital (NAWCH), SCF and PPA set up a Play in Hospital Liaison Committee (PHLC) in 1971, whose aim is the provision of play for all children in hospital. This sharing of experience has had useful repercussions, not least of which is encouraging community playgroups to help parents to understand the needs of their own child when ill or hospitalised. A well-knit family can often prepare its child and help him very positively through traumatic experiences(37). A further result has been that in some areas the playgroup organisation has made contact with a mental subnormality hospital, initiating play opportunities for patients of any age and, through the numerous volunteers, opened up relationships between the patients and the outside community(41).

Ordinary Playgroups and Handicapped Children

We referred earlier to the possibility of an opportunity group being a step towards an ordinary playgroup. It has been estimated by PPA that in 1977 about 3,000 of the half million children attending ordinary playgroups were handicapped.

A survey done by one of us(21) gave information on 114 handicapped children attending playgroups in the Peterborough (Cambridgeshire, England) area. In 1966 there were three playgroups open serving about 145 children, and one of these children was handicapped. By 1974 there were 42 groups open serving over 1,600 children, of whom 40 were handicapped. Over 75 percent of the handicapped children attending playgroups benefited from this arrangement and were accepted by their peer group. (See Figure 4.)

Children with hearing problems went to a special nursery school unit run by the education authority, but apart from that most types of handicap were represented in the playgroups. The commonest handicap (shown by 35 percent of the children) was a communication problem, usually delay or difficulty with speech; many of these children, as well as those with physical, visual or intellectual problems, also showed symptoms of emotional disturbance. Jenny, for example, a child with partial vision, also had a difficult mother/child relationship. Playgroup was the only place where Jenny would allow someone to brush her hair and put in her eye-drops. About 20 percent of the handicapped children were placed in the playgroup because of developmental delay or behaviour problems associated with poor social conditions and/or marital disharmony.

In 1975 and 1976 further information was obtained on another 38 children recognised as having special needs but not classified by the playgroups as being handicapped. Most of these children were known to the Social Services Department and the majority came from the New Town area of Peterborough. Eighty percent of these children had social and behaviour problems

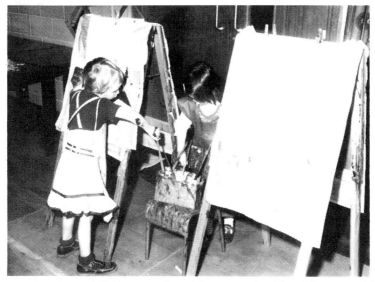

FIGURE 4. Handicapped child in an ordinary playgroup—the girl on left, now aged 4, has had successful surgery for congenital heart disease since she joined the playgroup.

and 25 percent had communication problems. Only two of these 38 children had difficulty in being accepted by their peer group. One had communication problems and one, whose mother could not cope with her, was rather aggressive.

Peterson et al.(36) have noted, in an Illinois study of mixed handicapped and normal children attending preschool classes, that the children are influenced by and more likely to model their behaviour on a non-handicapped child rather than on a handicapped one. Our own observations confirm this, provided that only about 10 percent of the children have special problems. We also have found, like Guralnick(22), that non-handicapped peers can improve the social quality of a handicapped child's play.

The Value of the Ordinary Playgroup to the Child

A playgroup can offer any child opportunities for play which may not be possible at home. He has the chance to gain courage and master skills with large equipment, to explore the messy materials and to learn to manipulate various "educational" playthings. He can begin to choose and make decisions himself. There is time for him to repeat his experimenting as long as he needs to. No one will say, "Stop making a mess," or "Get out of my way." The playgroup adults are interested in his activities and encourage him to talk about them and ask questions. They can prevent undue frustration and, when appropriate, structure play to extend his experience. He learns to interact with adults outside his family, who at the same time welcome his mother and are careful to ensure her approbation, or at least tolerance, of his play.

Such interactions help not only language development and understanding of local social norms, but also the development of personal identity. Meeting in the same group several times a week, the children get to know one another and the range of their social play increases. Four-year-olds often play out quite complicated situations. Along with the usual domestic play in the "home corner," the children may play out experiences they have had in common and which have disturbed or stimulated them. For example, a frightening television programme will often be played out by a group of children. On one occasion the children saw a nearby house catch fire. For weeks afterwards they played fires and evacuated their "house." This helped them to come to terms with this alarming incident. Hospital experiences—the ambulance, injections, IVs and so on—are often played out with other children or with dolls and "soft" toys. This type of play can be very helpful for handicapped children who may often have to attend or stay in hospital.

An individual child can play out his own anxieties within the secure framework of the playgroup. Jealousy of a new baby was resolved by one small boy who allowed himself to be mothered by a group of girls in a game involving mothers and babies. Another child with the same problem viciously cut up dough babies made for him by the understanding supervisor.

Angry or even violent encounters which a child may have watched, or to which he has been subjected, may also find some outlet through play materials or in socio-dramatic play. A change in a child's play or behaviour is likely to alert an observant supervisor to the possibility of previously unrecognised stress in the family.

Advisory Help Needed by the Playgroup Taking Handicapped Children

As suggested above, it may be in a playgroup that a suspicion of some abnormality in child or family may first arise. The playgroup supervisor then needs to know where she can turn for help without delay. When there is good liaison with a Health Visitor, this can be the person to advise and support the supervisor, and to act as a link between parent, general practitioner and specialists. Professionals who refer a child to a playgroup, as many do, need to be aware of some of the difficulties which may arise, and should be prepared to discuss particular problems with the playgroup supervisor. It is also appreciated if they inquire about progress at intervals and offer the playgroup constructive comments. Whenever possible, a referral should be made in consultation with a Playgroup Adviser (who is usually based in the Social Services Department of the local authority) or a local organiser who knows the playgroup circumstances at the time and can discuss with the supervisor whether the group can cope with the problem presented by this particular child.

Even when referrals are restricted so that only one in ten of the children present at one play session are handicapped, there may well be other children going through "normal" developmental problems who require extra attention. If an "ordinary" playgroup has more than 10 percent of problem children to cope with, it can cease to be an "ordinary" playgroup and become a "special" playgroup needing more support and extra adults present. If the arrangement breaks down through insufficient preparation, it is extremely distressing for both the playgroup and the parents and child who may have been referred.

While most types of handicapped children (using the widest definition of handicap(61)) can usually be successfully accommodated in a playgroup, there are some who may present more problems than the playgroup can handle. Hyperkinetic, very aggressive, and autistic children and, in some cases, severely emotionally disturbed children need special care with placement, as well as follow-up support. Brenda Crowe's warning(9) about clinically diagnosed maladjusted children should be noted:

> No such child should be placed in a playgroup unless someone knowledgeable (preferably from the Child Guidance Clinic) has visited the playgroup to ascertain that the group is well established, happy and stable; that the playgroup leader is gifted in handling difficult children; and does not even consider them to be difficult; and that the parents involved are mature enough to accept the child with tolerance and affection, whilst taking the same attitude towards his behaviour as that of the playgroup leader (p. 47).

Less severe emotional problems or behavioural difficulties, such as feeding fads, wetting, or tics, can be helped when tension in the mother/child relationship is relieved by the attitudes in the playgroup. Soiling is a difficult problem for a playgroup to accept, often because of practical hygienic considerations in premises with few amenities, and used by other people.

Some playgroup supervisors have found that mothers deprived of loving early relationships themselves have great difficult in accepting warm care for their own children from other adults. These mothers need "mothering" like the children, which can be extremely demanding. In these situations playgroup staff themselves need support.

The value of an experienced playgroup adviser who can be readily available is described by Ferri and Niblett(20). They point out that many advisers have a heavy work load and cannot visit groups often. Confirmation of this comes from preliminary findings in a survey(6) which indicate that a third of preschool institutions had not been visited by a health visitor in the previous 12 months, and only a quarter of the groups had an arrangement for routine visiting by advisers. While voluntary PPA organisers do visit groups and give as much support as they can, anyone referring a child with a problem should try to ensure that sympathetic and knowledgeable follow-up will be available.

MEETING THE MOTHERS' NEEDS IN THE PLAYGROUP

In the Peterborough study it was found that about 75 percent of the mothers of handicapped children seemed to benefit from their child's placement in a playgroup. About 50 percent of the mothers of handicapped children became involved in playgroup activities. These mothers were helped in much the same way as all mothers of playgroup children are helped. The majority of mothers of under-fives are at home with their children; they want to enjoy their children and do their best for them. Playgroups, by enabling them to understand more about their children and how their needs can be met, have strengthened mothers' confidence in themselves; there is then a boomerang effect which further helps the children.

Mothers have the chance to go somewhere outside the home, meet other mothers and share the everyday problems of living with active preschool children. (See Figure 5.) Often they feel isolated when they are far from relatives and husbands are out at work all day. In the playgroup they are reassured about particular anxieties—other children suck their thumbs and wet their beds; other mothers on occasion scream at their children and feel they can't stand the sight of them.

Mothers with young children are very liable to develop depression(5,46). Sometimes they reach the stage where their own need to survive as a person is their top priority. Then their concern with their child is of lesser importance and they may not avail themselves of playgroup provision(60). It may be possible for some of these very vulnerable mothers to be helped to take advantage of playgroup support and provision for their child if they find a genuine welcome—always—in the playgroup. Other mothers who *do* become

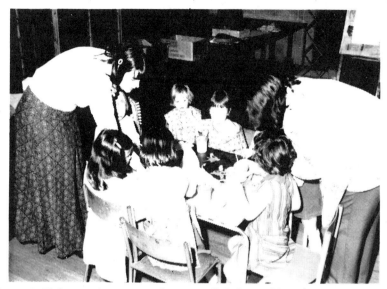

FIGURE 5. Mothers in playgroup—making a giraffe before a visit to the zoo.

actively involved with their playgroup may find openings for personal growth. Many have discovered to their surprise that they can cope with being a committee member or officer. They may find that working in the group on a rotating basis gives them confidence to consider assisting regularly and later becoming a supervisor. PPA's training and development structure may often provide an opportunity for a mother to develop as a person in her own right, in a sphere which she finds absorbing, and which is not necessarily dependent on formal educational qualifications. Some mothers may, when their children are older, go with enhanced confidence to train for work in the community or in teaching, taking with them concepts and understanding discovered in the playgroup.

The Mother Who Has a Handicapped Child

The mother of a handicapped child has the same needs as other mothers, but she may also have additional needs, just as her child has needs in addition to those of all children. She may be going through a sequence of reactions after having realised that her child is in some way different.

If she is still in the stage of shock, grief and mourning, any group may be too big a step for her. Her greatest need is a sympathetic listener. At this stage she may not want to meet other "normal" children and their mothers, nor may she want to meet other "abnormal" children and their mothers, yet have come to terms with her own child's particular problem. We know of one mother who was introduced to an Opportunity Group by a well-intentioned friend, but the sight of other handicapped children so upset her that she went home and wept for a week. However, many months later she went to an ordinary playgroup and found it a great success for her child and herself.

After this initial reaction, she may pass into a stage of isolation. Not only will she feel that because her child is different, she is different and wants to withdraw, but she also has to contend with the changed attitudes towards her from familiar friends and neighbours. Many people are apprehensive or frightened by any abnormality, and do not know how to make contact with the mother. This changing attitude can cause these mothers added distress. During the stage of isolation she may still find it difficult to face going to a big playgroup. With the help of friendly neighbours or an understanding health visitor, she can meet a few other mothers, perhaps at coffee mornings or in a small mother and toddler club. She can then progress on to a playgroup with them(45). In many cases some assessment of a child's problems is made well before three years old—the age when he would normally start at a playgroup. By the time he is three years old, his mother may have had the chance to begin to come to terms with his difficulties, but she may also become overanxious and overconcerned with this child, so that the whole family is handicap-orientated. Involvement in a playgroup can help her to put her problems into perspective. She can begin to balance the needs of the handicapped child with the needs of the rest of the family, including her own needs.

With children who have Down's syndrome this stage of wanting to "do something" and meet others is often reached about the end of the first year(11), and at this point a mother and toddler club or a special group can be helpful. Having somewhere specific to go outside the home is of value.

If she can meet other mothers as an ordinary mother, not as someone different, and if she can be involved in playgroup activities, the mother's confidence in herself is given a boost. She may still need additional opportunities to meet other parents with handicapped children, which may be possible through a toy library or local club.

When her child has settled in the playgroup (and PPA policy is for mother to remain as long as the child needs her), she will be free for a couple of hours to go shopping, or get her hair done, or just have time to herself.

Separation between mother and child is not always easy, particularly when there is an unusual mother/child relationship. If the child has a problem, he may give mother more than the usual number of cues indicating that he needs protection and care. The dependent phase of childhood may be prolonged unduly. Because of this the mother may be more wrapped up in her child, for a longer period, than she would be with a normal child. This may isolate her from the rest of her family, even from her husband, and she may come to feel that this child has become her only reason for existence.

In the playgroup, the separation of mother and child can take place gradually, so neither loses confidence.

Having separated herself from her child, even if it is only to the other end of the room, the mother can stand back and look at her child, perhaps seeing him in a different light. She can see him in relation to his peers, see how his behaviour differs or is the same, see how he copes with the same problems that the other children are coping with. Sometimes this experience brings about an understanding of the reality of the child's situation better than any conversations with the doctor. It can also bring hope and an understanding that the child is capable of more than she thought. She can see how other people handle his problems. However, the playgroup has to be sensitive to her feelings and not undermine her confidence in her own ability to be a mother.

There are also mothers who have experienced quite normally rewarding relationships with their other children, but with one this has not happened. Sometimes the playgroup can help this mother/child pair(49) by making a kind interpretation of each to the other, and by trying to ensure that the separation and the reunion at either end of the session are achieved in a context of happy anticipation(9).

CONCLUSION

We have shown how "playgroups offer the possibility of bringing together mothers and children in order that they should *both* have support and stimulation"(18) and thus have a *preventive* role for the family in its normal developmental disturbances and a *therapeutic* role when there is a handicapped child or when relationships are impaired. There is a *community* role also when a playgroup is a focus for the involvement of fathers, grandparents, teenagers and others in various related activities. From the *educational* aspect, there are learning opportunities for children and for parents, both in the play session and in the way they can take ideas back into the home. Playgroup training courses offer new challenges to tutors. Students of medicine and other disciplines can gain insight into needs of parents and children by practical experience in a playgroup during their training.

The keystone of the playgroup movement is the participation by parents.

For some of them this may at times be minimal, but when conditions are favourable parents have the option to modify and control the setting they have chosen for their child in their light of what they observe, learn and decide together as a group. We recognise that this kind of parent participation requires adequate and skilled support from professionals; nevertheless, it has possibilities for growth and change in attitudes, as well as for greater enjoyment of child-rearing. We believe this principle to be crucial to the healthy development of children during their most formative years. It is this feature, peculiar to the voluntary playgroup component of British preschool facilities, which we see as most significant.

REFERENCES

1. BENTOVIM, A., and LANSDOWN, R. 1973. Day hospitals and centres for disturbed children in the London area. *Brit. Med. J.*, 2, 536.
2. BENTOVIM, A. 1976. Disobedient and violent behaviour in children: family pathology and family treatment. Part 1, *Brit. Med. J.*, 1, 947; Part 2, *Brit. Med. J.*, 1, 1004.
3. BONE, M. 1977. *Pre-school Children and the Need for Day Care*. HMSO.
4. BRADLEY, M. and KUCHARSKI, R. 1977. *They Never Asked Us Before . . .* Voluntary Pre-school Groups Aid/Research Project. Liverpool Institute of Higher Education.
5. BROWN, G., and BHROLCHAIN M. 1975. Social class and psychiatric disturbance among women in an urban population. *Sociology*, 9, 225.
6. BUTLER, N.R., OSBORN, A.F., DOWLING S.F.O., and HOWLETT, B.C. (In preparation). Child Health and Education (CHES). National nursery/playgroup survey University of Bristol.
7. CHAZAN, M. (Ed.) 1978. *International Research in Early Childhood Education*. Slough: NFER (for SSRC).
8. COLEMAN, J., BURTENSHAW, W., POND, D. and ROTHWELL, B. 1977. Psychological problems of pre-school children in inner urban areas. *Br. J. Psychiat.*, 131, 623.
9. CROWE, B. 1973. *The Playgroup Movement*. London: Allen and Unwin.
10. CROWE, B. 1974. *Playgroup Activities*. London: PPA, Alford House, Aveline St., SE11 5 DJ.
11. CUNNINGHAM C., and SLOPER P. 1977. Down's Syndrome infants. A positive approach to parent and professional collaboration. *Health Visitor*, 50: 2, 32.
12. DATTA, L. 1975. Parent involvement in the United States. In: *Developments in Early Childhood Education*. Paris: Organisation for Economic Cooperation and Development (OECD).
13. DEITCHMAN, R., NEWMAN, I., and WAISH, K. 1977. Dimensions of parental involvement in pre-school programmes. *Child Care Health and Development*, 3: 3, 213.
14. DEPARTMENT OF HEALTH AND SOCIAL SECURITY. 1976. Children's day care facilities at 31st March 1976. England: DHSS Statistics and Research, 6. Obtainable from DHSS Store, Scholefield Mill, Brunswick St., Nelson, Lancs. B89 OHU.
15. DEPARTMENT OF HEALTH AND SOCIAL SECURITY, DEPARTMENT OF EDUCATION AND SCIENCE. Low cost day provision for under-fives. Papers from Sunningdale Conference. Obtainable from DHSS Store, Scholefield Mill, Brunswick St., Nelson, Lancs. B89 OHU.
16. DEPARTMENT OF HEALTH AND SOCIAL SECURITY, DEPARTMENT OF EDUCATION AND SCIENCE. Co-ordination of services for children under 5 Ref. DHSS LASSL (78) 1. DES S 47/24/013. Obtainable from DHSS Store, Scholefield Mill, Brunswick St., Nelson, Lancs. B89 OHU.

17. DOWLING, S. 1977. The inter-relationship of children's use of Child Health Clinics and day care facilities in the pre-school years. Paper given at a seminar *0-5: A Changing Population*. London: VOLCUF. 11, South Hill Park, NW.3.
18. DYKINS, M.E. 1976. Profile: The Pre-school Playgroups Association—Playgroups in the Community. *Child Care Health and Development*, 2, 125.
19. FAULKNER, R. 1971. Opportunity classes—Study of voluntary integrated nursery classes for handicapped and normal children. *Community Medicine*, No. 32, 95, vol. 120, No. 16, p. 213.
20. FERRI, E., with NIBLETT, R. 1977. Disadvantaged families and playgroups. *National Children's Bureau report*. Slough:NFER.
21. GRANTHAM, E. A study to determine the feasibility of admitting handicapped children to their local playgroup. (in preparation.)
22. GURALNICK, M. 1976. The value of integrating handicapped and non-handicapped pre-school children. *Amer. J. Orthopsychiatr.*, 42(2).
23. HALSEY, A.H. (Ed.) 1972. *EPA Problems and Policies*. Vol. 1 of Educational Priority D.E.S. London: HMSO.
24. HILL, C., SOMERSET, G., and GREY, A. 1965. *Living and Learning with Children—New Zealand Play Centre Federation*. Wellington, N.Z.: Price Milburn.
25. HODGES, D. 1972. Handicapped adventure. *Social Work Today*, 13, 10, p. 7.
26. KOLVIN, I., GARSIDE, R.F., NICOL, A., LEITCH, I. and MACMILLAN, A. 1977. Screening school children for high risk of emotional and educational disorder. *Br. J. of Psychiatr.*, 131, p. 192.
27. JOLLY, H. 1969. Play is work. *Lancet*,2, 484.
28. LOCAL AUTHORITY ASSOCIATIONS STUDY 1977. *Under Fives* (Appendix 3). Association of County Councils, 66a Eaton Square, London, SW1W 9BH.
29. MIDWINTER, E. 1978. Pre-school priorities. *Where*, No. 135 p. 45.
30. NURSERIES AND CHILDMINDERS ACT 1948 (Section 60). Amended 1968. London: HMSO.
31. ORGANISATION OF ECONOMIC COOPERATION & DEVELOPMENT Report 1974. *The Educational Situation in O.E.C.D. Countries*. Paris: OECD.
32. ORGANISATION OF ECONOMIC COOPERATION & DEVELOPMENT Report 1977. *Early Childhood Care and Education. Objectives and Issues*. Paris: OECD.
33. OFFICE OF CHILD DEVELOPMENT USA 1976. *Child Care Programs in Nine Countries*. Washington: U.S. Department of Health, Education and Welfare.
34. ORGANISATION MONDIALE POUR L'EDUCATION PRE-SCOLAIRE OMEP. Report to World Council 1978. *Survey of Child Care Practices*. Obtainable from Caulfield Institute of Technology, Caulfield East 3145. Australia.
35. PARRY, M. and ARCHER, H. 1974. *Pre-school Education Schools Council Research Studies*. New York: Macmillan.
36. PETERSON, C., PETERSON, J., and SCRIVEN, G. 1977. Peer imitation by non-handicapped and handicapped pre-schoolers. *Exceptional Children*, January, 223.
37. PETRILLO, M., and SANGER, S. 1972. *Emotional Care of Hospitalised Children. An Environmental Approach*. Philadelphia: J.P. Lippincott.
38. POULTON, G.A. and JAMES, T. 1975. *Pre-school Learning in the Community*. London and Boston: Routledge and Kegan Paul.
39. PRE-SCHOOL PLAYGROUPS ASSOCIATION (PPA) 1975, 1976 and 1977. *Facts and Figures*. Obtainable from PPA, Alford House, Aveline St., London SE11 5DJ.
40. PRE-SCHOOL PLAYGROUPS ASSOCIATION (PPA) 1975. *Guidelines for a Foundation Course*, p 3. Obtainable from PPA, Alford House, Aveline St., London SE11 5DJ.
41. PRE-SCHOOL PLAYGROUPS ASSOCIATION (PPA) 1977. *Contact October 1977 (Subnormality Hospital)*, p. 20. Obtainable from PPA, Alford House, Aveline St., London SE11 5DJ.
42. PRE-SCHOOL PLAYGROUPS ASSOCIATION (PPA) 1974. *Contact Heading since June 1974*. Obtainable from PPA, Alford House, Aveline St., London SE11 5DJ.
43. PPA CONTACT Sept. 1977, p. 8. Obtainable from PPA, Alford House, Aveline St., London SE11 5DJ.

44. PPA CONTACT Jan. 1978, p. 8-11. Obtainable from PPA, Alford House, Aveline St., London SE11 5DJ.

45. PRE-SCHOOL PLAYGROUPS ASSOCIATION (PPA). Three pamphlets concerned with handicap: i. Notes for Opportunity Groups; ii. The handicapped child and his mother; iii. Guidelines for playgroups with a handicapped child. Obtainable from PPA, Alford House, Aveline St., London SE11 5DJ.

46. RICHMAN, N. 1977. Behaviour problems in pre-school children. *Br. J. Psychiatr.*, 131, 523.

47. ROGERS, S., WHEELER, T., and MCLAUGHLIN, S. 1977. Playgroups—Their effects on the language and socialisation of children. *Child Care Health and Development*, 3, 3, 175.

48. ROSE, N. 1973. *Ten Therapeutic Playgroups. A Preliminary Study of the Children Attending and their Families.* NSPCC, London.

49. SCHAFFER, R. 1977. *Mothering.* London: Fontana—Open Books.

50. SHINMAN, S. 1975. *Parental Response to Pre-school Provision.* Brunel University, Dept. of Educ. (mimeo).

51. STUKAT, K-G. 1976. *Current Trends in European Pre-school Research.* Council of Europe. European Trend Reports on Educational Research. Slough: NFER. National Foundation for Education Research.

52. TIZARD, B., and HARVEY D. (Eds.) 1977. Biology of play. *Clinics in Developmental Medicine*, No. 62. Spastics International Medical Publications. London: Heinemann.

53. TIZARD, B., PHILPS, J., and PLEWIS, I. 1976. Staff behaviour in pre-school centres. *J. Child Psychol. Psychiatr.*, 17, 21.

54. TIZARD, B., PHILPS, J., and PLEWIS, I. 1976. Play in pre-school centres. II. *J. Child Psychol. and Psychiatr.*, 17, 265.

55. TURNER, I. 1977. *Pre-school Playgroups—Research and Evaluation Project Report.* Queen's University of Belfast, Dept. of Psychology. (Mimeo).

55A. TURNER, I. 1977. *Pre-school Experience and Psychological Development.* Northern Ireland Pre-school Playgroups Association.

56. WATT, J. 1977. *Co-operation in Pre-school Education.* London:SSRC.

57. WELSH OFFICE 1977. *Activities of Social Service Departments.* Cardiff:Economic Services Division.

58. WOLFENDEN COMMITTEE Report 1978. *The Future of Voluntary Organisations.* London: Croom Helm.

59. YUDKIN, S. 1967. *0-5 A Report on the Care of Pre-School Children.* London: Allen and Unwin.

60. ZIGLER, E. 1976. Head Start: Not a program but an evolving concept. In: J.D. Andrew (Ed.), *Early Childhood Education. It's an Art? It's a Science?* Washington: The National Association for the Education of Young Children.

61. SHERIDAN, M. 1973. *Children's Developmental Progress.* Slough: NFER, p. 14.

29

FOSTER CARE

Richard Galdston, M.D.

Assistant Clinical Professor of Psychiatry,
Harvard Medical School;
Senior Consultant in Psychiatry,
Children's Hospital Medical Center, Boston, Mass.

INTRODUCTION

Foster care has been defined as "child welfare service which provides substitute family care for a planned period for a child when his own family cannot care for him for a temporary or extended period and when adoption is neither desirable nor possible"(4, p. 2). The need for such care of young children arises out of the failure of the child's biological parents to provide adequate parenting for their issue. The causes of such failure are varied, complex, and difficult to evaluate in epidemiological terms. Death, divorce, mental and/or physical illness, poverty and abandonment are among the causes cited. Once placed in the care of those other than its parents, there is little likelihood that a child will be reclaimed. It has been estimated that fewer than 17 percent of children placed ever return to their own homes (4, p. 75). A child who has been placed in foster care as a temporary measure will likely remain indefinitely in a state of limbo as far as his family context is concerned.

The choice, implementation, and supervision of foster placement involve a network of public and private agencies that defies standardization because of its complexity and variation among the states. A certain number of placements are de facto, within an extended family structure, without official sanction or supervision. It has been estimated that, in the U.S. in 1972, there were 315,000 children in foster placement at a public cost of

585

$450,000,000 (7). The numbers and costs have probably increased greatly since the time of this report.

The legal implementation of foster care requires the courts to make an evaluation and to render a judgment, followed by placement in a foster home under the supervision of an agency, either public or private. The role of public welfare agencies in making and supervising such placements involves economic, administrative, and psychological services. Most public welfare agencies are ill-equipped to assume such burdens and they are severely taxed by the demands of the responsibility. The administrative burden is considerable, and the requirements for specialized skills often exceed the training and support available to the personnel upon whose shoulders responsibility falls. The rigors of expediency and the hazards of fiscal constraint often dictate the policies, or lack thereof, that govern the placement of these children.

Oliphant, in a study of federal funding for foster care concludes, "The Aid to Families of Dependent Children (A.F.D.C.) foster care program has been a matter of little concern or attention, at either the federal or state level, and has not been subject to examination, study or comparison with other methods for funding and development of foster care or child welfare services. A continuing disregard may well allow its vices to flourish, its potential virtues to go unrealized, and its real value for the long run to remain obscure" (5, p. 38).

The following observations and comments are based upon clinical experience gained from psychiatric consultation to the In-Patient Services of the Children's Hospital Medical Center in Boston, Massachusetts, from 1960-1972, and from work as the Principal Investigator of the Parents' Center Project for the Study in Prevention of Child Abuse. The effects of foster care upon children and adults who came under psychiatric study are presented in summary form with no attempt to determine their prevalence or incidence. The consequence of foster placement is subject to infinite variation in accordance with the many factors that contribute to human experience. The effects of foster placement cannot be isolated from all of the other forces that impinge upon the development of individual character. One can only hope to form a general impression of the impact of the experience as it appears to present among the children and adults who have been party to such arrangements for the upbringing of children.

STRESSES UPON THE CHILDREN IN FOSTER CARE PLACEMENT

Stresses stem initially from the conditional basis of foster placement, which is, by definition, understood to be a temporary affair. The terms of foster placement render impermanent the relationship of child to foster home, subject to change without the consent of the child. Such an arrangement strikes at the heart of the child's needs for constancy. The consensus of research into the requirements for optimal growth among children point clearly to the child's need for a set of object relationships that affords a predictable and constant matrix (1). The attachments to adult figures that afford the child a basis for the development of healthy psychic structures depend upon the enduring presence of persons with whom to identify. When these attachments are interrupted, the child soon learns to restrict the quality and extent of his attachments in order to protect himself from the ravages of repeated loss. This foreshortening of attachment results in constriction in the formation of an identification with the adult world. It leaves the child with a deficient superego and with a conscience which has been blighted by the needs to provide for self-protection in the absence of adequate parental protection. Children who have to learn to take care of themselves too soon do so at the expense of their relationship to others. They learn to become "street-wise," developing precocious competence at manipulating their immediate surroundings. They fail to develop a historical sense of self. Robbed of a feeling for the continuity of their past, they fail to form a sense of a personal future.

Therapeutic interviews with parents who had suffered repeated foster placements during their own childhood reveal a foreshortening in their expectancy of life. They view their lives as of the present, bracketed between repression of their past and an absence of future ambitions. Their lives take on a two-dimensional quality, limited to place and person in the here and now. The dimension of personal past, so essential to the formation of identity, is deficient for these adults. They rely upon their present for a sense of their being. They are here today and gone tomorrow. Such parents are ill-equipped to provide their own children with a sustaining experience of parenting. One adult said of his childhood, "When I look back, it's not me that I see going all the way back. . .I'm just waiting. . .waiting for something. . .waiting for my life to begin. . .I just spit it out and leave it behind. . .and go on."

STRESSES UPON FOSTER PARENTS

The same sense of conditional commitment has its effect upon parents who take in a child for foster care. The relationship lacks the definition of biological reproduction; further, it does not contain the deliberate commitment of adoption. The personal motivations for foster care are subject to revision and interruption by the state, the biological parents or the foster parents themselves. It is a relationship made with the fingers crossed, with the reservations of ambivalence written into the contract.

For some parents, foster care is an economic endeavor, for others it is made to promote some idea, and for others it is an act of love. Whatever their motivations, the foster parents are also constrained by the threat of possible loss. For some, this imposes a certain form of anxiety, a need to prove themselves as "good parents" worthy of their charge. Such anxiety can exert an intimidating effect, leading them into attitudes and practices towards the foster child that are fraught with the threat of possible failure and inadequacy.

Some foster parents charge the child with a need to prove the validity of an idea, a principle of child-rearing which takes on a moral imperative. If the child fails to corroborate the idea, the parents become deeply disappointed and reject the child out of their disillusionment. On the surface, the ideas may have an intellectual, social, or psychological appeal, but if the child fails to live up to them, it is the child who is sacrificed.

In many instances, the child is taken into foster care to replace a lost figure—a parent, another child, a spouse, or someone else. The foster child is burdened with a replacement value that precludes his own identity; to the extent that he falls short of that value, the foster parent will be further disappointed.

The vicissitudes of foster care are many and complex. Under optimal circumstances professional consultation in support of the foster relationship could go far to ameliorate the stresses upon the home. Unfortunately, such help is seldom forthcoming. Studies show that Massachusetts loses 29 percent of its public casework personnel each year. With such a turnover, the likelihood of continuity of supervisory consultation to foster parents is slight (6).

STRESSES UPON BIOLOGICAL PARENTS

A mother who gives birth and then places her child will suffer a loss that she must grieve. The grieving process requires time, supportive relationships, and a certain amount of intrapsychic work (2). Mothers who place their children in foster care seldom have the opportunity for adequate grieving. Gruber's study of parents who placed children revealed that 82 percent of those interviewed said that they had seen a social worker six times or less before placement. He reports that 30 percent of the sample interviewed felt that placing their child in foster care was unnecessary, and 23.3 percent said that they thought placement could have been avoided with quicker or more extended family counselling. Seventy-five percent declared that they would never consider foster care for their children again, even if faced with a situation which made it appear necessary (4). These comments lend objective substance to the clinical observation that, although foster placement removes the child physically from its parents, the psychic attachment remains.

The persistence of psychic attachment to an absent child can function as a force powerful in its influence upon subsequent parental behavior. Some mothers seek relief from the pain resulting from their loss through repression of the experience. Other women try to replace their lost child by conceiving again, or through taking on another woman's child, or by busying themselves in child-care activities of a surrogate sort. Whatever course of action they may pursue, it seldom affords them relief from the pangs of an unmourned loss.

The traumatic effects of foster placement upon biological parents are difficult to evaluate systematically because the parents seldom seek psychiatric consultation. Some inkling of the range of hazards can be obtained from the comments of a group of women studied in the Parents' Center Project for the Study in Prevention of Child Abuse (3). These women, overwhelmed by psychic and physical adversity, were at high risk for the physical and mental abuse of their young children, yet almost all had refused to consider foster placement. In group and individual meetings, they observed, "I could never give her up. . .I might never get her back, and then she would always be out there somewhere looking for me." Another woman said of her son whom she had violently assaulted on several occasions, "If I gave him up, he wouldn't know who I was. He might even grow up and marry his own sister without knowing who she was!"

These, and similar comments, reflect a deep, pervasive recognition of relationship as the basis of identity. The sense of *belonging to*, the proprietary dimension of parenthood, affords a mutual base for identity, for both parent and child. The adult, especially the woman, is as much defined by being the *mother of*, as the child is by being the *son* or *daughter of*. The mother who relinquishes her child to foster care gives up a piece of her own identity that goes with the child. The loss is of herself. The ramifications of such loss can be far-reaching and delayed in recognition. Sometimes they can be detected among women in mental hospitals whose earlier losses of their children can be recognized in the deluded and hallucinatory restorations of their missing memories.

The alternatives to foster placement—adoption, or more prolonged counselling in support of the biological parents in their reproductive relationship—appear to offer a better solution in many instances. Adoptive parents agree to commit themselves to their new child without reservation of time, a circumstance essential for optimal growth and development. When properly presented by professionally trained personnel, counselling can allow for a clinical trial that is helpful in distinguishing those parents who have the potential to rise to the occasion of their parenthood from those who are unlikely to attain it with a promptness sufficient to meet the needs of their child. Many decisions for foster placement are made impulsively under duress of adversity from within and without. Many of the agencies responsible for implementing foster care lack the personnel or the philosophy to support a clinical trial of parenthood sufficient to make an informed and deliberately considered decision about the necessity for foster placement.

DISCUSSION

The foster home care system was pioneered in the Commonwealth of Massachusetts during the latter half of the nineteenth century. It was developed to be an alternative to public orphanages or private servitude as a solution to the plight of homeless children. The alternative probably had substantial merit during an era when a largely agricultural society afforded the likelihood that another helping hand would be an addition welcomed within a rural family. This advantage has been eliminated with the rapid industrialization of the country. The implementation of laws preventing child labor have further reduced the economic desirability of having an extra child in the home.

Other socioeconomic changes have reduced the potential of the foster home care system as a solution to the problem of the homeless child. Urbanization, with all of its physical constraints upon living space, has resulted in crowding that precludes the comfortable addition of another child in many homes. Changes in marital patterns, the rise in divorce, and decline in birth rates reduce the resilience of the family as an institution capable of absorbing the addition of another parent's child in an equitable fashion. In the U.S., it can no longer be said that any family is better than none. In many instances, it can be demonstrated that no home would be better than the foster placement in which these children find themselves.

Public declarations that children be considered as a natural resource often prove to be hollow words when it comes to the spending of government monies. Within the adversarial bodies that decide the allocation of public funds, the welfare of children seldom receives a responsive audience. Their needs are often championed by parties more endowed with political aspiration than with professional expertise. This results in the creation of bureaucracies marked by a potential for patronage and self-aggrandizement, rather than a capability for effective, professional service to children.

In the shell-game of shifting public responsibility, there is a popular notion that the community should take care of its own. This idea results in the assignment of responsibility for the disbursal of federal funds for the care of homeless children to state and local administrators. The practice is predicated upon a fantasy of a local community which seldom exists in reality. Foster children tend to come from outside of the community in which they live; they are born to parents at the lower socioeconomic fringes of society. They come under the care of agencies limited by insufficient staffing with underpaid and inadequately trained personnel whose tenure on their jobs is brief.

The foster child can be described as one who lacks a community, who has fallen between the cracks of the social structure. The foster child needs the services of a body of professionals whose training has been specialized to supplement the deficits that result from having been deprived of a community in which to grow up. Provision of these services requires an order of training sufficiently professional to support a life's career devoted to the work. It cannot be accomplished by the present administrative apparatus, burdened with a political superstructure that isolates those whose decisions determine policy from the clinical realities of their charges.

A possible improvement lies in the creation of a corps of career public servants trained in a profession devoted to the care of children, even as governments maintain career public servants to husband other natural resources, parks, forests, waters, and minerals. Such a body of professionals could offer unwanted children representation by an informed advocacy capable of responding to their needs with actions based upon experience and knowledge.

REFERENCES

1. BOWLBY, J. 1969. *Attachment and Loss. Vol. 1 Attachment*, New York: Basic Books, Inc.
2. FREUD, S. 1949. Mourning and melacholia. In: *Collected Papers, Vol. 4*, London: Hogarth Press.
3. GALDSTON, R. 1975. Preventing the abuse of little children. *Am. J. Orthopsychiatry*, 45(3), pp. 372-381.
4. GRUBER, A.R. 1973. *Foster Home Care in Massachusetts*. Commonwealth of Massachusetts, Governor's Commission on Adoption and Foster Care.
5. OLIPHANT, W. 1974. *A.F.D.C. Foster Care: Problems and Recommendations*. Child Welfare League of America.

6. Social and Rehabilitation Service, 1968. National Center of Social Statistics Public Welfare Personnel; Annual Statistical Data. Washington, D.C.: Department of Health, Education, and Welfare, Table 6.

7. WERNER, R.M.1976. Public Financing of Voluntary Agency, Foster Care Child Welfare League.

30

HIRED MOTHERING
THROUGH THE AGES

M. Livia Osborn

Clinical Research Officer,
The Institute of Family Psychiatry,
The Ipswich Hospital,
Ipswich, England

INTRODUCTION

There are many forms of mothering and, indeed, many forms of parenting. There is care of children by the natural mother; there is adoption of children by relatives or strangers; there is fostering, and group or community upbringing. There is good mothering and bad mothering; adequate care, and deprivation. The quality of care varies from excellent to appalling, from enlightened to primitive, and this variation applies to all forms of mothering. Most of these forms have been explored in depth and the studies they have inspired have produced a vast literature.

There is, however, one form of mothering which has remained shadowy, rarely identified and seldom referred to. This is the auxiliary mothering provided by women who are hired to take care of infants and children other than their own. The care they provide is seldom that of a substitute mother, nor do they wholly replace for long the physical and emotional care usually provided by natural parents. They are usually hired by the mother or the head of the family to help with the care of children in a stipulated way, which may be agreed verbally and informally or be detailed by a formal written contract backed by legislation. Thus we have the wet-nurse, the children's nurse, the nanny, the oriental amah, the ayah—a term introduced into India by the Portuguese—and the baby-sitter or au pair girl of more recent and egalitarian times.

The term "*nanny*" to denote a children's nurse is not found in the English language until the end of the 18th century and its etymology is not clear. Many dictionaries of the English language do not list this term. Webster's dictionary suggests that it is a short version of Anne, or that it derives from nanny goat and thus is linked to the wet-nurse's function. Other dictionaries, including the Oxford English Dictionary, state that it is a word used in young children's language only, hence it means a children's nurse. *To nanny* has come to mean to be overprotective.

However, if the terminology is varied and at times of uncertain etymology, the practice is old, stretching into antiquity. Indeed, archaeological findings have shown that infant feeding bottles, which made the infant independent from the mother, were used in prehistoric times (25). Specimens have been found in graves of infants of the bronze and iron ages. They demonstrate that prehistoric families were at pains to preserve the life of young children by providing alternatives when breast-feeding was unavailable.

In the space of a chapter it is impossible to give a description of all the geographical variances of hired mothering in time and place; hence, a few examples have been selected to demonstrate the universality of this practice from antiquity to the 20th century. The 19th and the 20th centuries are well covered by available literature; thus they will not be discussed in detail here.

ANCIENT HISTORY

Mesopotamia and Egypt

When in c.2100 B.C. Hammurabi unified the Mesopotamian peoples, he collected the laws of the various regions and organized them into one body, the Code of Hammurabi, which he ordered to be engraved upon a stone shaft and preserved in Babylon, in the temple of the god Marduk. This, the oldest preserved code of the ancient law, depicts several aspects of the way of life of the Babylonians and shows that they had the welfare of their children very much to heart (39). In the Code we find a description of the legal contracts that were drawn up to detail the obligations of a nurse to the child entrusted to her. Sumerian nurses, who often took care of infants for periods of two or three years, were sometimes able to buy their charges. This was possible if, at the end of the period stipulated in the contract, the parents were unable to pay the price agreed for her services (22). Moreover, if parents entrusted a nurse with their child and he died while in her care, she was not allowed to undertake further nursing without first divulging this

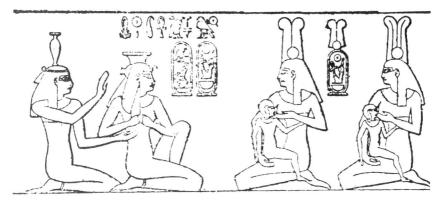

FIGURE 1. Egyptian nurses—Bas-relief, c.1300 B.C.

death to prospective employers. The penalty for concealment was the extirpation of the breasts (7).

In Mesopotamia, as in many other early cultures, nurses were believed to be particularly vulnerable to harm from demons and other supernatural forces, which could cause their milk to dry up, or the babies to be snatched from their arms. Amulets, prayers and incantations were used to protect them and prevent Labartu (or Lamashtu), a malevolent demon particularly vicious to children, from doing his worst (40).

Again, in ancient Egypt, although maternal nursing was more or less general, the women of the harem were allowed to entrust their children to hired nurses or to slaves (See Figure 1). The position of royal nurse was much sought after, especially if it involved suckling the "infant god." The royal nurse was an important personage, invited to all the official ceremonies and to the coronation of the king (7). Her importance is demonstrated by the fact that at the height of Egyptian civilization, we find a figure of great power in the political intrigues of the court—she is Tey, the nurse of Nefertiti (c.1372-1350 B.C.) (12).

The term of "nurse" was also applied to the prince's tutor, in charge of his cultural nourishment, and many sages were proud to add to their titles that of "royal nurse."

Sparta and Athens

Plutarch suggests that Spartan women who were liberated from domestic tasks and, according to Cicero (8), were often unwilling to bear children,

employed nurses to look after their infants and that these were usually
helots (serfs) or slaves (37).

In democratic Athens, in the 4th century B.C., citizen-women (that is
those women who had full membership of the state) were expected to practice
a great deal of self-help, but wealthy women still employed wet-nurses, often
from good families, who had been driven by the war conditions to seek a
remunerative employment. The mother of Euxitheus, the speaker of De-
mosthenes in book LVII, was among those and in her poverty she was reduced to sell ribbons and to work as a wet-nurse. (26).

Greek nurses were considered, more often than not, to be ignorant, negligent and indiscreet. Moreover, they had the reputation of being gluttons
who would consume food intended for the children. Their stupidity was
proverbial, and Aristophanes made fun of them in his comedies, while Plato
has a telling, if metaphorical, phrase in *The Republic*," she (the nurse) lets
you go on snivelling, and does not wipe your nose when you need it. . . ."
Hence, prosperous Greek families preferred to employ Spartan nurses, who,
as already mentioned, were readily available and demanded small remu-
neration. They took the infant to their own abode and rarely remained in
the household of the family (7).

Plato's *Republic* detailed what should be the ideal method of child care
and envisaged a system with a strangely modern approach to job equality
for the sexes:

> Then the children as they are born will be taken in charge by the
> officers appointed for the purpose, whether these are men or women
> or both. . . The children of good parents, . . .they will put into the
> rearing pen, handing them over to nurses who will live apart in a
> particular portion of the city (36).

Good nurses, however, were highly thought of by the Greeks; if slaves,
they were often freed and statues were erected to honour them after their
death. A common theme in Greek sculpture from the 6th century B.C. until
Roman times is the tomb of a young girl with an older woman in attendance.
A delicate terracotta figurine of the 4th century B.C. shows an old woman
nursing a baby (Figure 2).

Indirectly, we owe the slender Corinthian column to the loving gesture of
a nurse. Vitruvius records that the invention of the capital of the Corinthian
column was due to Callimachus, a Greek sculptor of the 5th century B.C.,
who was inspired by the sight of a basket placed over the grave of a girl by
her nurse. The nurse had covered it with a tile to protect its contents—goblets
which had delighted the child when living—and placed it accidentally over

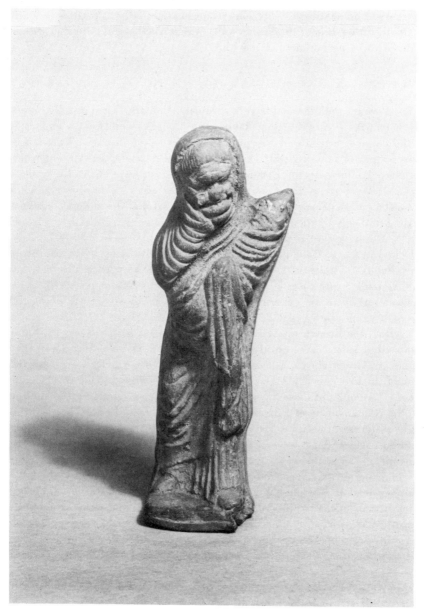

FIGURE 2. Nurse and child—Attic terracotta, 4th century B.C. (Reproduced by courtesy of the Trustees of the British Museum.)

the roots of an acanthus. The roots, thus compressed, put forth leaves and shoots by either side of the basket and these formed elegant curving volutes destined to be perpetuated in marble.

Rome

The Romans took family life very seriously. Roman women usually breast-fed their infants until a higher standard of living, brought by the expansion of the empire, introduced the practice of hiring wet-nurses. Women who were prepared to sell their services in this way would gather under the *Columna Lactaria* in the Forum (11). In the later part of the Republic, it was a sign of poverty in a family if the mother was seen to nurse the child herself. Cato's wife was the exception: He insisted that she undertake breast-feeding not only of their infants, but also of some of the children of their slaves, believing that both would benefit by it (7).

Octavius, Nero, Caligula and Tiberius were brought up by hired nurses. The cruelty of Caligula and the drunkenness of Nero were attributed to habits instilled into them by their nurses, as it was a Roman belief that the character of the nurse was communicated to the child, who acquired through the milk virtues or vices (42).

Tacitus, the Roman historian, just before the fall of the Roman Empire, commented with regret on the fact that Roman matrons entrusted their infants to Greek slaves. These slaves were not necessarily wet-nurses, as around the first century A.D. the Romans were manufacturing glass feeding vessels. Examples of these have been found during excavation at Colchester, an old Roman town in England (18). Other infants' feeding bottles were made of terracotta with a leather covered nipple—a most insanitary com-bination, which must have been a contributing factor to the high infant mortality, even in the upper classes. Thus we find that of Marcus Aurelius' 12 children, only five reached adulthood (2).

Breast-feeding was often prolonged. For instance, according to Hieroni-mous Mercurialis, Platinus, the Roman Neoplatonic philosopher of the third century A.D., was still being breast-fed at the age of eight years and would run away from his lessons and demand that his nurse feed him.

A number of medical authors concerned themselves with matters of child care (41). Celsus, in *De Medicina* (c.A.D.50), advises that the nurse of a suckling child should take walks, be sent to the baths, feed on light foods and, should the child be feverish, she—not the child—should drink water in abundance.

Soranus's(A.D.98-117) work περι γυναικειων (on diseases of women) contains a very comprehensive account of the care of infants in sickness and in health. Among other subjects, Soranus deals with the choice of a wet-nurse, with the correct way of swaddling a baby and with the manner in which he should be handled during the crawling stage to assist him towards learning to walk without straining his developing limbs. He too stresses that diseases in suckling infants should be treated by prescribing remedies for the nurse.

Less than half a century after the death of Soranus, Galen (c.A.D.130-A.D.200) of Pergamus, called to Rome by the Emperor Marcus Aurelius, became so authoritative that he influenced medical practice at least until the 16th century. In his writing he covers the care of the healthy infant and young child. He has advice for the nurse on how to use swaddling clothes and on how to quieten crying babies by placing the teat in their mouths and by moderate movement and singing. Experienced nurses—he says—know how to soothe a fretting child by rocking him in their arms and singing lullabies.

Oribasius (A.D.325-403), a Roman physician renown for his charm and modesty, wrote, among other works, a homely treatise dedicated to his friend Eunapius. In this work the first chapter deals with the feeding of infants and contains advice not found in previous writers. He wrote that the nurse, in addition to the suckling duties, should be given a certain amount of physical work, especially of a kind that would bring into play movements of the chest and shoulders, as grinding, weaving and walking would, as this exercise promotes a good flow of milk. A nurse, he advised, should be a healthy woman, aged between 25 and 35 years, recently delivered, prefer-ably, of a male child. He also advised about her diet and that she should "abstain from venery."

For centuries to come Western physicians based their advice on the works of these Roman authors.

THE MIDDLE AGES

Contemporary Opinions

In the Middle Ages there were no theories on child development, but nevertheless childhood was regarded as a special period when the vulnera-bility and fragility of the infant demanded particular care (24). Medical writers, however, were mostly silent on the subject of day-to-day child care. Rhazes (A.D.850-932), the famous Arabian physician, wrote an entire trea-tise on the diseases of children. This was the first large work completely dedicated to paediatrics, but it contained no advice on the care and nurturing of normal, healthy children. Likewise Avicenna (A.D.980-1037) and Averroes (1126-1198), other Arabian physicians of great fame, made only incidental references to the care of healthy infants.

Leech books of between the tenth and twelfth century also seldom refer to infants and only occasionally make suggestions about suckling difficulties in the nurse or the infants, or mention herbal treatments for childhood disorders.

The exception was Bartholomew the Englishman, a Franciscan friar better known by his Latin name of Bartholomeus Anglicus, who flourished between 1220 and 1250. His work, *De Proprietatibus Rerum*, a kind of handbook for his parishioners, was so constructed as to give easily located answers; it proved so popular that, even before the invention of the printing press, it was widely copied and translated into five modern languages. In this book he wrote specifically on the child's nurse and her duties (19):

> . . .A nurse rejoices with a boy when it rejoices and weeps with him when he weeps, just like a mother. She picks him up when he falls, gives the little one milk when he cries, kisses him as he lies, holds him tight and gathers him up when he sprawls, washes and cleans the little one when he makes a mess of himself, feeds him with a finger when he pushes, teaches the boy to talk and babbles at him in his ignorance, and almost breaks his tongue to teach him to talk more easily. She gives him medicine when proper and nurses him through sickness. She takes him and lifts him up when he howls, now in her hands, now on her shoulders and now on her knees. She chews up his food first and by chewing it makes it ready for the toothless boy so that he can swallow better, and thus she eases his hunger. When the boy is asleep she soothes him with whistlings and lullabies. She binds up his limbs with splints and rags while they are young and corrects them so that the little one does not contract any ugly bandiness. She cherishes the little one's flesh with bath and ointments.

Francesco Barberini, an Italian poet, friend of Dante, in a valuable source book of 13th century manners, also listed the qualities required in a nurse (7)—he included the usual good points outlined by previous writers, and added that she should not be haughty, irascible, melancolic, mad, or too lazy; most of all, however, she must not be a redhead!

The nursing supersititions of past centuries continued. Breast milk was still believed to have almost magic qualities; it could transmit to the baby not only the physical characteristics of the nurse, but also something of her psychological makeup. Numerous voices raised against young children being cared for by hired mother substitutes stridently stressed this point. Thus, the behaviour of that saintly but formidable woman, the Countess Yde de Boulogne, was much admired and cited as an example of good mothering. She was determined that her children would inherit no other qualities than her own and on finding that her baby son Eustace had been suckled by a nurse because he had "wailed sore and howled," trembling with rage, "her face as black as coal with the wrath that seethed within," she shook him violently and "he delayed not to give up the milk." She then suckled him herself until, satiated, he fell asleep. The guilty nurse is reported to have "stood more benumbed than worm in winter-time" (20).

Position in the Family

Examples of hired nurses in the Middle Ages are to be found in numerous lives of saints and in royal or aristocratic biographies (29). Their presence is undisputed, but their image remains somewhat elusive, as they are seldom described. A few individuals, however, must have experienced beneficial relationships with their nurses, if we accept that they projected them in their writings. For instance, a long poem entitled *The Rape of Proserpine*, written by Claudian towards the end of the 4th century, presents the nurse in a favourable light as one who loved the child "like a mother" and was "companion, guardian and almost mother."

The link between the wet-nurse and the child was often very strong and universally recognised. In Ottoman Turkey, for instance, she was thought of as the nurseling's "milk mother." Her own children were regarded as its brothers and sisters and their relationship as being in the prohibited degree for purposes of marriage. Child and parents treated her with respect, no matter how humble she was, and she remained one of the family not only during the breast-feeding period, but also subsequently (28).

Even when the nurse was a slave, she was sometimes given consideration. Thus, Leoba, the Anglo-Saxon abbess of Tauberbischofsheim, was nursed by a slave, who was rewarded with liberty by the family after her prediction that her charge would become eminent in the church became true (33). Eastern girls of 11 or 12 were often bought by Italian merchants to be used as little nurses, but they seldom became integrated in the family and were required to wear distinguishing clothes marked with black (32).

The importance of the nurse in the medieval castle is also demonstrated by the fact that members of her own family became known by the term indicating her occupation. *Norris*, a surname still shared by many, is derived from "nourrice," the French term for nurse (31).

Conditions of Employment

It is difficult to assess the amount nurses were paid for their services. Among the Normans it was the practice to send children to be fostered and educated in families of other chiefs, thus establishing close relationships. These children received free board and lodging and, in theory, also small wages. As soon as they were old enough, the girls were often employed as child minders and their wages were little more than pocket money and gifts of clothes (13). It was a system very similar to that of the present-day au pair girls.

In France, a royal decree dated 1350 fixed the fees for nurses and for the "recommandaresses," women who recommended them to families with new-born children. The same decree clearly stated their duties (7).

Legal documents of the period at times shed some light on the kind of compensation a good nurse may have looked forward to. For instance, wills of some aristocratic families in 13th century Italy contain bequests to nurses, who were referred to with the affectionate name of "mamma," an appellative usually reserved for the natural mother. Jewelry and items of personal clothing were often left to nurses (21). The will of Ralph de Nevill, Earl of Westmoreland, who died in 1424, is another example; it contains the following lines: "I give and bequeath to every gentlewoman of other degree, then being occupied in the nurture of my children 40s" (38). Again, a York chaplain in 1432, left his maid a book of fables (38), suggesting that this book was of particular significance to her and that perhaps she had read it to him in his childhood.

Not all presents, however, came to the wet-nurse after the death of her employer; gifts were often given to her to sweeten her disposition and her milk. She certainly had reasons enough to feel aggrieved now and again; medicine prescribed for the baby was administered to her, as Bartholomaeus Anglicus had written ". . .if the chylde be syke, medicines shall be gyven to the nouryce, and not to the chylde." Her diet was closely controlled, again, as the same author had decreed ". . .she shall be ruled according to good diet" (9). Nor could she be sexually active, as this was forbidden her until the child was weaned. For hours on end she was expected to rock the cradle, so that fumes from the child's hot and moist humors would mount to his brain and produce sleep (15). Even her dress was sombre as, according to the household accounts of Philip-Augustus of France for the years 1202-1203, the nurses were dressed in dark-coloured gowns made of a woollen stuff called brunette (27). Moreover, at least in England, she could not freely choose her employers, as a law of Henry III, passed in 1235, forbade Christian nurses to serve Jews (23).

Contemporary Practice and Opinions

The importance of the nurse, especially the wet-nurse, is no less evident in this period than in previous centuries, as there was still almost no alternative to breast-feeding and feeding bottles had remained a crude affair, mostly made from cow's horns.

Moreover, it was the custom to put children to nurse despite the disapproval voiced by learned men, who would have had every child nursed by his own mother, but in practice disregarded what they preached. Rousseau, for instance, did not hesitate to consign his five children to the foundling hospital. The wet-nurse was usually a country woman who took the baby to her cottage, although in some instances she would move into the home of her employers. Many country women abandoned their infants in search of employment as nurses. Instances have been recorded of the nursing being shared by mother and nurse, or by several nurses (30). In Normandy, by the 18th century, even children of small craftsmen were nursed by hired women (3). As late as 1780, it was estimated that, in Paris, of 21,000 children born in a year, 17,000 were sent to country wet-nurses, 2,000 or 3,000 were placed in nursery homes, 700 were breast-fed by a nurse at home and only 700 were nursed by their mothers (11). Mothers in Colonial America were equally dependent on nurses and, again, the practice was condemned. For instance, *The New York Mercury*, on May 6th, 1754, printed an article on the "Inconvenience of Hired Nurses."

The new learning of the Renaissance was beginning to question many of the health practices which had been blindly followed for centuries because they originated in the writings of the great Greek and Arabian physicians. Galen's authority, however, still remained supreme and physicians, parents and nurses were afraid to reject too readily those remedies for which they had no substitutes.

Printed books on paediatrics began to appear towards the end of the 15th century. The first of them, by Paolo Bagellardo, was printed in Padua in 1472 and contained the usual advice on the choice of a wet-nurse. He suggested that the newborn infant should be fed by a nurse, unless he was a pauper, in which case the feeding would have to be undertaken by his own mother—a good pointer to the practice of the time, even if some of his contemporaries disagreed.

The management and feeding of infants were dealt with at length in a book principally dedicated to midwifery—this was the *Rosengarten* of Eucharius Roesslin (c.1512), which was translated into many European lan-

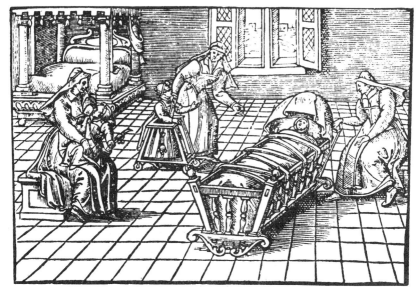

FIGURE 3. Nurses and children—Engraving on wood, 1570. Note strapping on the cradle to prevent the baby falling out during vigorous rocking.

guages. It was the first book of its kind to be translated into English. With the title *The byrth of mankynde* it was printed in London in 1540 and dedicated by the translator, Richard Jones, to Henry VIII's fifth wife, Catherine Howard. She was never to use it, as she remained childless and her short marriage ended when she lost her head on the scaffold.

The first English book wholly dedicated to the care of children was written by Thomas Phaire in 1545. The author, said by Fuller in his *Worthies of England* to have been born in Wales (while others make him a native of Norwich), was not only a physician, but also a lawyer, a poet and a translator of classic Latin works. He translated the *Aeneid* into English verse and dedicated it to Queen Mary. As a champion of the English language, he wrote *The Boke of Chyldren* in the vernacular, so that it could "be read by as many as would." In this work he writes in detail on children's diseases and gives advice on the management of minor disorders, as, for instance, those due to teething and to disturbed sleep. He suggested a number of herbal remedies for epilepsy (peony root, violets, lind flowers, rosemary, thistle and chicory), alongside charms and amulets made of coral, sapphire or emerald. On the choice of a nurse, he wrote that she should be "not of ill complexion and worse manners: but suche as shalbe sobre, honeste and chaste, well fourmed, amyable and chearefull, so that she may accustome the infant vnto mirth, no dronkarde, vicious nor sluttysshe, for suche corrupteth the nature of the chylde" (34).

Another book written in the vernacular with the aim of instructing nurses rather than physicians was a work by Simon de Vallambert. It was the first such book written in French and was published at Poictiers in 1565 with the title *De la maniere de nourrir et governer les enfants des leur naissance.* Like Phaire, although following the ancient writers, this author sounds a new note of common sense and attacks many unhygienic practices still prevalent among the nurses of his time.

In Spain, Lobero de Avila was also writing in his own language with the same aim in mind; his book, published in 1551, was an indication that the Spaniards, too, were becoming more concerned about the education of mothers and nurses in child care.

Precepts for the nurse are also to be found in the writings of Omnibonus Ferrarius, whose treatise on children, this time in Latin, was published in Verona in 1577. He deals not only with the physical side of child care, but also with what we would now call emotional aspects. Ferrarius insists that a young child must not be subjected to stress, fear or sadness as "many through depression have become ill." And again, "Let the nurse always cheer the child with a bright and loving countenance when the child comes to her." This is followed by an injunction not to utter "blasphemies, curses or abuse or wicked and unchaste language" in the presence of an infant. Ferrarius wrote also a series of aphorisms in which he stresses that the feeding of infants by the mother is always to be preferred to that of a wetnurse, unless this is impossible because of illness, inability or—and this is very revealing—bad character. Infants, he says, grow to love the woman who nurture them more than their natural mother and they will "savour of the nature of the person by whom they are suckled" (41). This belief was taken very seriously and was debated at Oxford in 1605 (41).

Johannes Ceckius of Bologne compiled a work on the disease of children in 1604; it was more or less a summary of the views of ancient physicians, but gives us another glimpse of what he and his contemporaries thought of nurses when, in a chapter on burns, he states that, because of the carelessness of nurses, children often tumble into the fire or come into contact with boiling water (41).

Jacques Guillemeau, physician to four Kings of France, in his book on the nursing of children, *De la nourriture et gouvernement des Enfants* (1609), exhorted mothers to nurse their children themselves and obviously had a very poor opinion of hired wet-nurses. He thought that the "great inconveniences" that they may cause are infinite, but, to be brief, he mentioned just four: They may substitute the baby; the baby's affection for the mother would diminish; the baby could inherit bad conditions and inclinations from the nurse; and, finally, the nurse may pass on to the child some imperfection of her own body (41). However, if one must have a nurse, Guillemeau decreed that she must have an agreeable face, with clear eyes, well-made nose, red mouth and white teeth; her neck must be round and strong and her chest deep. Moreover—and most important—the nurse was required to have firm and resilient breasts; she must "shun all disquietness of mind," have the ability to sing in a pleasing voice and be not over interested in food, drink, her own husband or, for that matter, the husband of her employer. This said, he reserved his admiration for Blanche of Castile, mother of King Louis IX of France, who nursed her child with no help from wet-nurses and was very angry when she found that a lady of the Court had suckled him; she promptly put her finger down his throat and made him vomit (41). Her behaviour is reminiscent of that of Yde de Boulogne, already mentioned.

François Mauriceau, a distinguished French surgeon and accoucheur, writing in 1668, had this to say regarding the choice of a nurse:

> As the Nurse is, so will the Child be, by means of the nourishment which it draweth from her, and in sucking her it will draw in both the vices of her Body and Mind. She ought to have a sweet voice to please and rejoyce the Child, and likewise it ought to have a clear and free pronunciation that he may not learn an ill accent from her as usually red-hair'd have. The milk must be of a sweet and pleasant smell which is a testimony of a good temperament, as may be seen in red-haired Women whose Milk hath a soure stinking and bad scent.

His aversion to redheads is reminiscent of Francesco Barberini, the 13th century Italian poet, mentioned earlier.

Dr. William Cadogan in his *Essay on the Nursing and Management of Children from their Birth to Three Years of Age*, published in 1748, repeated the recommendations of his predecessors, but added that the nurse should keep the child awake and amused during the day, not lull it to sleep to save trouble "to the great detriment of Children's Health, Spirits and Understanding." Moreover, she should bring them up to be ambidextrous (16)!

William Buchan (1766-1805), a man of the church, thought that hired nurses "were mainly destitute of all reason, knowledge and principle: in short of almost everything except mercenary prospects" (42).

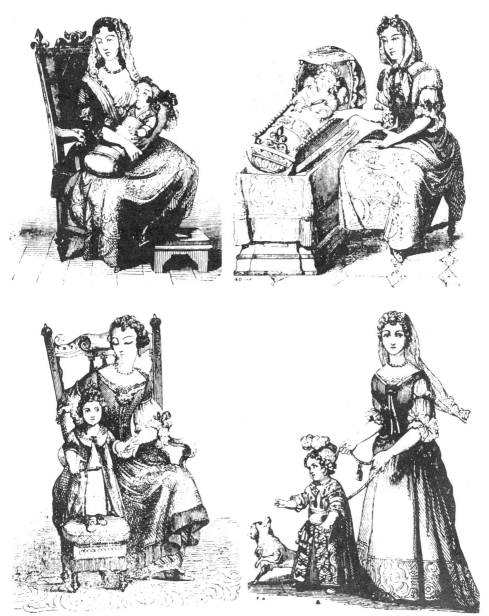

FIGURE 4. Wet-nurse and three dry-nurses of the Duc de Bourgogne (1687-1712).

The stress put on the danger of inheriting personality traits with the milk went so far as to suggest that if the milk was too hot for a boy or too cold for a girl, the boy would be effeminate and the girl mannish (30).

The unfortunate child fed on animal milk was at an even greater risk. Thomas Muffett (1553-1604) quoted the case of ". . .Aegyrthus, who being fed in a Shepheard's Cottage only with goat's milk, waxed thereupon so goatish and lecherous, that he defiled not only Agamemnon's bed, but also neighed (in a manner) at every man's wife" (42).

The same author reinforced his argument with the case of old Dr. Caius, at Cambridge, who was "so peevish and so full of frets" when he "suckt one woman froward of conditions—and so quiet and well when he suckt another of a contrary disposition" (42).

Yet, despite all this, a collection of tales entitled *Tales and quicke answeres, very merry and pleasant to rede*, first published in 1532, contains a passage which implies that nurture was more important than heredity transmitted through the milk ". . .nourysshynge, good bryngynge up, and exercyse ben more apte to leade folke to humainte and the doynge of honest thynges than Nature her selfe." Hence, Hugh Rhodes, in his *Book of Nurture* (1577) found it necessary to advise to ". . .take good heede of anye newe servauntes that you take into your house, and howe yee put them in authorytye among your children" (17). And Robert Burton mused that "if a man escape a bad nurse, he may be undone by evill bringing up" (4).

The opinion of the nurseling, however, is well expressed by the 17th century French moralist Coustel, who describes a nurseling's return home as an adult. He has gifts for his nurse and criticism for his mother, whom he addresses as follows:

> I show more affection and gratitude to the one to whome I owe the most. When the time for your lying-in came you rid yourself of me as of a burden that was inconvenient. . .while instead my nurse continually caressed me, nourished me for two years with her own milk and by her care and trouble brought me to the vigorous manhood in which you see me at present (10).

Didactic Poems

It is unlikely that the ordinary mother or the illiterate hired nurse knew about the precepts contained in learned treatises or even about the advice offered in books written in the vernacular. Simple folk learned the good rules of house management and child care in a more homely way—from rhymes, often no more than doggerel verses, which were easy to memorise with their direct appeal to the imagination and their musical cadences.

These didactic poems were to be found in many countries and continued to be popular for a long time. For instance, Germany had the *Verschung des Leibs* (care of the body) written by Heinrich von Louffenburg in 1429; Italy had *La Balia* (the nurse) by Luigi Tansillo, written in 1552. Tansillo advocated mothers' breast-feeding their own children and warned against unscrupulous nurses' substituting their own baby for the one entrusted to them by careless parents. France is represented by Scévole de Ste Marthe's *Paedotrophia* (1629)—the work of a concerned father rather than a physician. The part referring to the nurse starts:

Chuse one of middle age, nor old nor young,
Nor plump nor slim her make, but firm and strong,
Upon her cheek, let health refulgent glow
In vivid colours, that good-humour show.
(Translated by H.W. Tytler in 1797.)

A poem on education, partially translated from Erasmus by Edward Hake in 1574, describes how a nurse teaches a child to say his first words and how she carefully feeds him (5).

"Dad dad" for father first they give,
and "bead" they teach for bread:
And when they teach him drink to ask
then "din" to him is said.
And prettily they lisp their words
whereto it prates again,
And thus at length as proof doth teach
the baby speaketh plain.

. . .

. . . their child they never feed
With all that comes to hand, but they
observe with careful heed
Both what to give and how to give:
what quantity to use:
And eke to feed it leisurely:
for if they should infuse
And pour it in with reckless hands
they know they either should
Their baby choke, or at the least
his clothes would be foul'd.

The Preservation of Health, written in 1744 by John Armstrong, is a later example of didactic poems.

Conditions of Service and Legislation

Wet-nursing was a highly organized occupation in this period and the good rate of pay made it a popular choice for many poor girls. It was not unknown for young, often unmarried, women to contrive to become pregnant and destroy the infant before seeking employment. In England, doctors and accoucheurs kept a "nurse book" for the benefit of their prosperous patients.

In France, as we have seen, nurses had organized themselves from the 12th century. Later, Louis XIII had granted patent letters to their agents, limiting their number and confirming a kind of monopoly. By 1715, in Paris, there were four municipal employment bureaux where nurses registered. These were later augmented by private bureaux.

Legislation was enacted in 1762 which forbade nurses to leave their own infants before they were nine months old. From this date they were also subjected to medical inspection and forbidden to sleep with the baby in the same bed; the provision of cradles was made compulsory to prevent overlaying (42). The same law fixed a scale of pay for nurses and, until 1792, employers were threatened with prison if they failed to honour their part of the bargain. Each year, Parisian prisons held between 500 to 600 such defaulters and special charitable organizations were founded to help them pay their debts to the nurses (7).

No other country had such careful legal provisions to regulate the employment of nurses. In England, nurses employed by foundling hospitals were subjected to more controls than nurses in private families. The former were not allowed to nurse a third child if two had died while in their care (35).

Superstitions

This was an age of superstitions and the newborn infant was surrounded by many credulous notions. The midwife was often believed to be a witch (14) and hired nurses fared little better. If a child did not thrive, they were accused of bewitching him. The unbaptized baby could be lost to the Devil, fairies lurked round every cradle and the evil eye was blamed for many childhood disorders.

Amulets against poison and jealousy continued to hang from children's necks as they had done in antiquity. Thus, the children of the rich cut their teeth on precious emeralds or coral hanging on gold chains, and the children of the poor bit equally vigorously, and perhaps less painfully, on roots of violets, bramble or liquorice. Starsmare, a 17th century English physician, advised: "If the child is bewitcht a Saphir or Carbuncle hung about the Childs Neck is conceived good" (41).

The time of weaning was particularly wrapped in superstition. For instance, it was considered unwise for the nurse to wean an infant when the moon was waxing. Moreover, she was to be careful to place the cradle in such a place that the beams of the moon may not reach the infant.

Nurses seem to have been specially superstitious and full of folkloristic beliefs. John Aubrey, in his *Miscellanies* (1696) recalls his nurse telling him about changelings and how fairies would steal a human baby from the cradle and replace him with one of their ailing or deformed offspring. Other tales were equally frightening and it is no wonder that most physicians of the time discussed "sleep terror and terrible dreams," and prescribed tranquillisers in the form of oil of violets, white opium, or juice of mandragora (41).

Nurses in Literature

The figure of the nurse is no stranger in the literature of this period. Since there are many references to her, it is impossible to quote them all. Two examples are selected here, both from the Elizabethan period. The first author, Shakespeare, needs no introduction. The second, Peter Erondell, is less well known. He was born in Normandy, but towards the end of the 16th century he came to England where he earned his living by teaching French. In 1605 he wrote a conversation manual entitled *The French Garden*. In this work he gives vivid descriptions of ordinary daily life events of his time (6).

Shakespeare. In the plays of Shakespeare the imagery of the nurse is used in many situations. In *Anthony and Cleopatra* the Queen compares the asp at her breast to a baby who suckles the nurse asleep. In *Much Ado About Nothing* we find "If you hear a child cry in the night you must call the nurse and bid her still it. . .if the nurse be asleep. . .let the child wake her with crying." "The baby beats the nurse" in *Measure for Measure*, and "a testy baby will scratch the nurse" in *Two Gentlemen of Verona*. In *Pericles* there is Lychorida, nurse to Marina.

But it is in *Romeo and Juliet* that we have the best example in that "good sweet nurse," to whom Lady Capulet had entrusted her baby daughter, Juliet, some 14 years before the action of the play. The nurse, now a widow 40 years old, is depicted as a bawdy, garrulous and vindictive woman, but also full of affection, warmth and energy despite her "aking bones" and breathlessness. Her position in the noble household of the Capulets is indicated by the manner in which she is allowed to speak to the lady of the house and to her adolescent charge. She reminisces how she nursed Juliet alongside her own child Susan, how she weaned her by putting wormwood on the nipple, and how her husband once picked up Juliet when, learning to walk, she fell on her face. The good man lifted up the toddler and made jokes to stop her crying. The nurse remained in the household as Juliet grew up and to her she was loyal to the point of conspiring to bring about her secret and fateful marriage to Romeo. So in *Romeo and Juliet* we have a vignette of a practice of infant care in England at the time of Shakespeare. The nurse was part of the family; the baby was brought up with the family of the nurse. In Juliet's case, the nurse was a secure and happy young woman with a husband, who "was a merry man."

Peter Erondell. In *The French Garden*, we have a vigorous sketch of the nursery. The nurse's duties can be surmised from the mother's comments. The lady of the house, having settled the older children with their French tutor, sweeps into the nursery. She has hardly heard the answer to her "good morrow, Nurse" when she starts on the poor woman, who has been unwise enough to say that the infant was "somewhat wayward the last night." She bids the nurse to undo the swaddling and bath the baby in her presence. "How now, how does the child?. . . Unswaddle him, undo his swaddling bands. . .wash him, before me. Wash his ears. . .hath he not a pimple upon his nose?. . . His gums be sore, show me his tongue. . . His thumb and little finger are flea-bitten. . .is there any fleas in your chamber?. . . Forget not to make clean his toes, the great toe and all. Now swaddle him again. . . Give him his coat of changeable taffeta and his satin sleeves. . . Where is his bib? Where is his little petticoat? Let him have his gathered apron with strings, and hang a muckinder to it; you need not yet to give him his coral with the small golden chain, for I believe it is better to let him sleep until the afternoon. . . Give him some suckle. God send thee good rest, my little Boykin." A maid (not the nurse) is ordered to fetch the cradle and make it ready and finally, having told the nurse to "rocke him till he sleepe" and "have a care of him," the lady leaves and peace descends on the nursery (5).

The Nurse in Art

The nurses of the statuary of antiquity have already been mentioned. Euricleia washing Ulysses appears on ancient vases. Egyptian friezes, too, often represented nurses, usually together with royal infants. Family life, however, did not become a popular subject in western art until the 16th century and this trend continued until the 19th century (1), although the nurse is represented in some earlier works. Here are just a few examples from the Renaissance to the 18th century.

A line engraving by the German Master ES, c.1440, shows the Madonna watching the Child being bathed. This is not a nativity scene. The Madonna looks on from a high seat, quite relaxed, holding an open book, while an angelic nurse kneels on the floor by a wooden tub, in which the child sits with all the appearance of enjoying the experience.

François Clouet executed a painting (c.1550) said to represent Diane de Poitiers, mistress of Henry II, showing a lady in her bath and immediately behind her a nurse of strong features and generous proportions suckling a child.

Both Botticelli's (c.1440-1510) and Mantegna's (c.1431-1506) pictures of Judith with the head of Holofernes show an old woman, a nurse in the tradition of Julliet's nurse, that is to say still with the grown-up child.

Fragonard (1732-1806) depicted a visit to the nurse—a country cottage, an elegant couple looking at a child in a cradle and the nurse sitting by it. The child's face is firmly turned towards the nurse. The same theme, very fashionable in the 18th century, was taken up by Etienne Aubry (1745-1781), while Jean-Baptiste Greuze (1725-1805) shows a young mother being deprived of her child, who is handed over to a wet-nurse—"The Painful Loss" is the title of this picture.

Again, Pietro Longhi (1702-1785), who took as his subjects many studies of intimate social life, painted "The Nurse," a young woman taking charge of a baby with the elegant but sad mother patting his head.

However, Franz Hals' "Nurse and Child," painted in 1620, is a much happier image: Both nurse and child looking contented, relaxed and very prosperous.

But the final apotheosis of the nurse must be the large canvas by Jean Dumont (1700-1781), depicting Madame Mercier, nurse to Louis XV. There she sits in majesty holding a large portrait of her royal charge surrounded by no less than ten bewigged members of her own family, plus a small dog.

THE NINETEENTH AND TWENTIETH CENTURIES

As was explained in the introduction, this period is so well covered by available literature that it is not covered in detail here.

Child care underwent radical changes in the 19th century. The practice of wet-nursing shifted from prosperous families to families of manual workers of little means. This may have been due to four factors: contemporary opinion, fashion, necessity, and availability of alternatives. The nanny, rather than the nurse, was now more common than in the past.

With few exceptions, official opinion about whom should breast-feed, nurse and bring up young children has not changed throughout the ages. The mother was, and still is, the first choice. Many authors wrote stressing this preference; the difference from the past was in the fact that now their books were, at least in part, veritable child-care manuals in the future tradition of Spock and were more likely to be read and heeded by a greater number of mothers than previously.

At the beginning of the present century, social conditions and taxation started to erode in to upper-class opulence. Families became smaller; the number of servants decreased. The new trend was towards a do-it-yourself attitude, dictated more by the economic situation than by fashion. The role of the nanny, especially towards the mid-century, was to enable the mother to continue her career or her job. In small households, the nanny may live as one of the family and qualities of kindness, common sense, good-humour, firmness, understanding, sympathy and adaptability are regarded as more important than the qualifications offered by specialized college training.

CONCLUSION

Our culture has conditioned us to regard the mother as the sole person fit to nurse and bring up young children. But the qualities needed to give a child a happy, secure and rewarding environment are not necessarily found in every woman who becomes a mother. Other women, even those who perhaps have never experienced a biological maternity, may have those qualities. When they offer their mothering for sale, they are hired and paid a wage. When they leave, they are forgotten. But they deserve more, in terms of gratitude, for the priceless gift of love.

The Daily Telegraph for the 23rd March, 1975, published a picture of an important man in full evening dress, affectionately embracing a lady equally formally dressed—it was a photograph of President Giscard d'Estaing welcoming his former nanny Mathilde Zervas to an official dinner at the Elysée Palace. He had not forgotten.

REFERENCES

1. ARIES, P. 1973. Centuries of Childhood. Harmondsworth: Penguin Books.
2. BIRLEY, A. 1964. Life in Roman Britain. London: Batsford.
3. BOURDIN, P.M. 1968. La plaine d'Alençon. In: M. Bouvet and P.M. Bourdin (Eds.), A Travers la Normandie des XVIIe et XVIIIe Siécles. Caen.

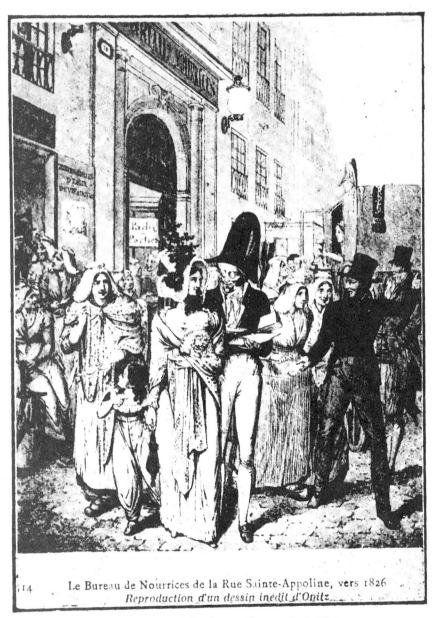

Le Bureau de Nourrices de la Rue Sainte-Appoline, vers 1826
Reproduction d'un dessin inédit d'Opitz

199 FIGURE 5. Nurses' Employment Bureau, Paris 1826.

4. BURTON, R. 1628. *The Anatomy of Melancholy.* Reprinted 1968. London: Dent.
5. BYRNE, M. ST. CLARE, 1949. *The Elizabethan Home, Discovered in Two Dialogues.* London: Methuen.
6. BYRNÈ, M. ST. CLARE, 1961. *Elizabethan Life in Town and Country.* London: Methuen.
7. CABANES, A. 1920. *Usages et Coutumes Disparus.* Paris: Albin Michel.
8. CICERO, 1945. *Tusculan Disputations.* London: Heinemann.
9. COULTON, C.G. 1956. *Social Life in Britain.* Cambridge: Cambridge University Press.
10. COUSTEL, P. 1687. *Les Règles de l'Education des Enfants.* Paris.
11. DE MAUSE, L. (Ed.), 1976. *The History of Childhood.* London: Souvenir Press.
12. DESROCHES-NOBLECOURT, C. 1965. *Tutankhamen.* Harmondsworth: Penguin Books.
13. DUGGAN, A. 1962. *Growing Up in the 13th Century.* London: Faber & Faber.
14. FORBES, T.R. 1966. *The Midwife and the Witch.* New Haven and London: Yale University Press.
15. GIES, J. and GIES, F. 1969. *Life in a Medieval City.* London: Barker.
16. GORDON, J.E. 1972. Nurses and nursing in Britain. *Midwife and Health Visitor, 8,* 25.
17. HARRISON, M. and ROYSTON, O.M. 1963. *How They Lived 1485-1700.* Oxford: Blackwell.
18. HASKELL, A. and LEWIS, M. 1971. *Infantilia.* London: Dobson.
19. HASSALL, W.O. 1962. *How They Lived 55B.C.-1485.* Oxford: Blackwell.
20. HIPPEAU, C. (Ed.), 1874-77. *Chanson du Chevalier du Cygne et de Godefroid de Bouillon.* Paris. (quoted by de Mause, reference No. 11).
21. HUGHES, D. 1975. Domestic ideals and social behavior. In: C.E. Rosenberg (Ed.), *The Family in History.* Philadelphia: University of Pennsylvania Press.
22. JASTROW, M., JR., 1915. *The Civilization of Babylonia and Assyria.* Philadelphia and London: Lippincott.
23. KING-HALL, M. 1958. *The Story of the Nursery.* London: Routledge & Kegan Paul.
24. KROLL, J. 1977. The concept of childhood in the middle ages. *J. Hist. Behav. Sci., 13,* 384.
25. LACAILLE, A.D. 1950. Infant feeding-bottles in prehistoric times. *Proc. Roy. Soc. Med., 63,* 565.
26. LACEY, W.K. 1968. *The Family in Classical Greece.* London: Thames & Hudson.
27. LACROIX, P. 1963. *France in the Middle Ages.* New York: F. Ungar.
28. LEWIS, R. 1971. *Everyday Life in Ottoman Turkey.* London: Batsford.
29. MCLAUGHLIN, M.M. 1976. Survivors and surrogates: Children and parents from the ninth to the thirteenth centuries. In: L. de Mause (Ed.), *The History of Childhood.* London: Souvenir Press.
30. MARVICK, E. WIRTH, 1976. Nature versus Nurture: Patterns and trends in 17th century french child-rearing. In: L. de Mause (Ed.), *The History of Childhood.* London: Souvenir Press.
31. MATTHEWS, C.M. 1966. *English Surnames.* London: Weidenfeld & Nicholson.
32. ORIGO, I. 1955. The Domestic Enemy: The Eastern Slaves in Tuscany in the 14th and 15th Centuries. *Speculum, 30,* 321.
33. PAGE, R.I. 1970. *Life in Anglo-Saxon England.* London: Batsford.
34. PHAIRE, T. 1553. *The Boke of Chyldren.* Reprinted 1965. London: Livingstone.
35. PINCHBECK, I. and HEWITT, M. 1969. *Children in English Society.* London: Routledge & Kegan Paul.
36. PLATO, 1937. *The Republic,* Vol. V. Translated by P. Shorey. London: Heinemann.
37. PLUTARCH, 1914. *Lycurgus.* London: Heinemann.
38. POWER, E. 1975. *Medieval Women.* Cambridge: Cambridge University Press.
39. RADBILL, S.X. 1973. Mesopotamian pediatrics. *Episteme, 7,* 283.
40. SIGERIST, H.E. 1951. *History of Medicine.* Vol. 1. Oxford: Oxford University Press.
41. STILL, G.F. 1931. *The History of Paediatrics.* Oxford: Oxford University Press.
42. WICKES, I.G. 1953. A history of infant feeding. *Arch. Dis. Childh., 28,* 151, 232, 332, 416.

The author wishes to thank Mr. P. Dove of the Medical Illustration Department, The Ipswich Hospital, for his help with the illustrations.

NAME INDEX

SUBJECT INDEX

Ability
  tests of, 78–82
Abortion
  mother's feelings, 395–396
Adolescence
  motherhood in, 185, 232
Adoption, 589–590
  disinhibited children, 187
  mourning by mother, 399–400
Adrenocorticotropic hormone release, 151–153
Affect
  maternal deprivation and, 143–144, 156
Amniocentesis, 482–485, 517, 518
  indications, 517
  timing, 517
Anaclitic depression, 328, 445
Animal studies
  bonding, 243
  fathering, 215–216, 243
  imprinting, 284–291
  mothering, 177–178
Anorexia nervosa
  psychological factors and, 147
Anthropology
  child development, 298–305
  fathering, 216
Anxiety
  in children, 438
  depression and, 438
  separation and, 443–444
Apert's syndrome, 486
Arginiosuccinic aciduria, 485
Arousal
  through play, 134–135
Asthma
  effect on family, 274
Attachment (see also Bonding and Imprinting)
  age of separation, 529
  conditioning and, 292
  culture and, 305–308
  development of, 292–293, 443
  father-infant, 224–225
  loss and, 443–444
  multiple, 307
  need for, 587
Attention
  direction of, 26–27, 34
  at preconceptual stage, 34–35, 39–40
Authoritarian homes, 14

Autistic children
  development deviations, 464–466
  diagnosis, 355, 453, 468–469
  explorative behavior, 116
  male-female ratio, 356
  onset, 469
  parents' educational level, 356
  play, 116
  prevalence, 355–357
  prognosis, 368
  symptoms, 453
Autonomy
  development of, 5, 7–9

Basal metabolic rate
  maternal deprivation and, 154–155
Battered child syndrome
  accidents and, 384
  adolescent parents, 232
  age prevalence, 411
  causative factors, 416–421
  childhood of parents, 178
  clinical manifestations, 410–415
  corporal punishment, 418, 423–424
  custody disputes, 422–423
  definition, 409–410
  diagnosis, 410–411, 431
  epidemiology, 415–421
  failure to thrive, 414–415
  father and, 229–230, 232
  follow-up studies, 415
  high-risk infants, 230–231
  historical background, 406–408
  hospitalization, 430
  illegitimacy and, 419
  intervention programs, 230
  legal aspects, 410, 416, 418, 421–426
  mothering of parents, 429
  parental psychopathology, 229–230, 419–420, 427
  practical management, 430–431
  prevalence, 385, 409, 415–416
  psychotherapy of child, 427–428
  psychotherapy of parents, 427
  radiographic examination, 414
  Society for the Prevention of Cruelty to Children, 425
  treatment, 426–431
Bedwetting (see Enuresis)

638